T0228907

Gynecologic Pathology: Practical Issues and Updates

Editor

BROOKE E. HOWITT

SURGICAL PATHOLOGY CLINICS

www.surgpath.theclinics.com

Consulting Editor
JASON L. HORNICK

June 2019 • Volume 12 • Number 2

ELSEVIER

1600 John F. Kennedy Boulevard • Suite 1800 • Philadelphia, Pennsylvania, 19103-2899

http://www.theclinics.com

SURGICAL PATHOLOGY CLINICS Volume 12, Number 2
June 2019 ISSN 1875-9181, ISBN-13: 978-0-323-68117-9

Editor: Stacy Eastman
Developmental Editor: Donald Mumford

© **2019 Elsevier Inc. All rights reserved.**

This periodical and the individual contributions contained in it are protected under copyright by Elsevier, and the following terms and conditions apply to their use:

Photocopying

Single photocopies of single articles may be made for personal use as allowed by national copyright laws. Permission of the Publisher and payment of a fee is required for all other photocopying, including multiple or systematic copying, copying for advertising or promotional purposes, resale, and all forms of document delivery. Special rates are available for educational institutions that wish to make photocopies for non-profit educational classroom use. For information on how to seek permission visit www.elsevier.com/permissions or call: (+44) 1865 843830 (UK)/(+1) 215 239 3804 (USA).

Derivative Works

Subscribers may reproduce tables of contents or prepare lists of articles including abstracts for internal circulation within their institutions. Permission of the Publisher is required for resale or distribution outside the institution. Permission of the Publisher is required for all other derivative works, including compilations and translations (please consult www.elsevier.com/permissions).

Electronic Storage or Usage

Permission of the Publisher is required to store or use electronically any material contained in this periodical, including any article or part of an article (please consult www.elsevier.com/permissions). Except as outlined above, no part of this publication may be reproduced, stored in a retrieval system or transmitted in any form or by any means, electronic, mechanical, photocopying, recording or otherwise, without prior written permission of the Publisher.

Notice

No responsibility is assumed by the Publisher for any injury and/or damage to persons or property as a matter of products liability, negligence or otherwise, or from any use or operation of any methods, products, instructions or ideas contained in the material herein. Because of rapid advances in the medical sciences, in particular, independent verification of diagnoses and drug dosages should be made.

Although all advertising material is expected to conform to ethical (medical) standards, inclusion in this publication does not constitute a guarantee or endorsement of the quality or value of such product or of the claims made of it by its manufacturer.

Surgical Pathology Clinics (ISSN 1875-9181) is published quarterly by Elsevier Inc., 360 Park Avenue South, New York, NY 10010. Months of issue are March, June, September, and December. Business and Editorial Office: Elsevier Inc., 1600 John F. Kennedy Blvd., Ste. 1800, Philadelphia, PA 19103-2899. Accounting and Circulation Offices: Elsevier Inc., 3251 Riverport Lane, Maryland Heights, MO 63043. Periodicals postage paid at New York, NY and at additional mailing offices. Subscription prices are $213.00 per year (US individuals), $279.00 per year (US institutions), $100.00 per year (US students/residents), $272.00 per year (Canadian individuals), $318.00 per year (Canadian Institutions), $263.00 per year (foreign individuals), $318.00 per year (foreign institutions), and $120.00 per year (international & Canadian students/residents). Foreign air speed delivery is included in all *Clinics*' subscription prices. All prices are subject to change without notice. **POSTMASTER:** Send address changes to *Surgical Pathology Clinics*, Elsevier, 3251 Riverport Lane, Maryland Heights, MO 63043. **Customer Service: 1-800-654-2452 (US). From outside the United States, call 1-314-447-8871. Fax: 1-314-447-8029. E-mail: JournalsCustomerServiceusa@elsevier.com (for print support) and JournalsOnlineSupport-usa@elsevier.com (for online support).**

Reprints. For copies of 100 or more, of articles in this publication, please contact the Commercial Reprints Department, Elsevier Inc., 360 Park Avenue South, New York, NY 10010-1710. Tel. 212-633-3874; Fax: 212-633-3820; E-mail: reprints@elsevier.com.

Surgical Pathology Clinics of North America is covered in *MEDLINE/PubMed (Index Medicus)*.

Contributors

CONSULTING EDITOR

JASON L. HORNICK, MD, PhD
Director of Surgical Pathology and
Immunohistochemistry, Brigham and
Women's Hospital, Professor of Pathology,
Harvard Medical School, Boston,
Massachusetts, USA

EDITOR

BROOKE E. HOWITT, MD
Assistant Professor, Department
of Pathology, Stanford University
School of Medicine, Stanford, California,
USA

AUTHORS

JOSEPH W. CARLSON, MD, PhD
Senior Consultant Pathologist,
Associate Professor, Department of
Oncology–Pathology, Department of Clinical
Pathology and Cytology, Karolinska Institutet,
Karolinska University Hospital, Stockholm,
Sweden

LAURA CASEY, FRCPath
Department of Pathology, Queen's Hospital,
Romford, United Kingdom

KELLY A. DEVEREAUX, MD, PhD
Resident, Department of Pathology, Stanford
University School of Medicine, Stanford,
California, USA

ELIZABETH D. EUSCHER, MD
Professor, Department of Pathology,
The University of Texas MD Anderson
Cancer Center, Houston, Texas, USA,
USA

OLUWOLE FADARE, MD
Department of Pathology, Anatomic Pathology
Division, University of California San Diego
Health, La Jolla, California, USA

ANN K. FOLKINS, MD
Assistant Professor, Department of Pathology,
Stanford University School of Medicine,
Stanford, California, USA

KRISZTINA Z. HANLEY, MD
Associate Professor, Department of Pathology,
Emory University Hospital, Atlanta, Georgia,
USA

BROOKE E. HOWITT, MD
Assistant Professor, Department of Pathology,
Stanford University School of Medicine,
Stanford, California, USA

DAVID L. KOLIN, MD, PhD
Associate Pathologist, Division of Women's
and Perinatal Pathology, Department of
Pathology, Brigham and Women's Hospital,
Instructor in Pathology, Harvard Medical
School, Boston, Massachusetts, USA

TERI A. LONGACRE, MD
Richard L. Kempson Endowed Professor of
Surgical Pathology, Department of Pathology,
Stanford University School of Medicine,
Stanford, California, USA

WESLEY DANIEL MALLINGER, DO
Resident of Anatomic and Clinical Pathology,
Department of Pathology, University of
Arkansas for Medical Sciences, Little Rock,
Arkansas, USA

ANNE M. MILLS, MD
Assistant Professor, Department of Pathology,
University of Virginia, Charlottesville, Virginia,
USA

MARINA B. MOSUNJAC, MD
Associate Professor, Department of Pathology,
Grady Memorial Hospital, Atlanta, Georgia,
USA

DENIS NASTIC, MD
Consultant Pathologist, Department of
Oncology–Pathology, Department of Clinical
Pathology and Cytology, Karolinska Institutet,
Karolinska University Hospital, Stockholm,
Sweden

MARISA R. NUCCI, MD
Vice Chair, Division of Women's and Perinatal
Pathology, Department of Pathology, Brigham
and Women's Hospital, Professor of
Pathology, Harvard Medical School, Boston,
Massachusetts, USA

KAY J. PARK, MD
Associate Attending Pathologist, Department
of Pathology, Memorial Sloan Kettering
Cancer Center, New York, New York,
USA

VINITA PARKASH, MD
Departments of Pathology and Obstetrics and
Gynecology, Yale School of Medicine, New
Haven, Connecticut, USA

CARLOS PARRA-HERRAN, MD
Department of Laboratory Medicine,
Sunnybrook Health Sciences Centre,
University of Toronto, Toronto, Ontario,
Canada

CHARLES MATTHEW QUICK, MD
Associate Professor, Department of Pathology,
University of Arkansas for Medical Sciences,
Little Rock, Arkansas, USA

J. KENNETH SCHOOLMEESTER, MD
Assistant Professor, Department of Laboratory
Medicine and Pathology, Mayo Clinic,
Rochester, Minnesota, USA

ELISHEVA D. SHANES, MD
Gynecologic Pathology Fellow, Department of
Pathology, University of Virginia,
Charlottesville, Virginia, USA

NAVEENA SINGH, MD, FRCPath
Department of Cellular Pathology, Barts Health
NHS Trust, The Royal London Hospital,
London, United Kingdom

**GULISA TURASHVILI, MD, PhD, FRCPC,
FCAP**
Assistant Professor, Department of Pathology
and Laboratory Medicine, Mount Sinai
Hospital, University of Toronto, Toronto,
Ontario, Canada

JACLYN C. WATKINS, MD, MS
Assistant Professor, Department of Pathology,
Microbiology and Immunology, Vanderbilt
University Medical Center, Nashville,
Tennessee, USA

ERIC J. YANG, MD, PhD
Clinical Assistant Professor, Department of
Pathology, Stanford University School of
Medicine, Stanford, California, USA

Contents

Preface: Practical Issues and Updates in Gynecologic Pathology   xi

Brooke E. Howitt

Human Papillomavirus–Independent Squamous Lesions of the Vulva   249

Jaclyn C. Watkins

The pathogenesis of vulvar squamous neoplasia has 2 pathways: human papillomavirus (HPV)-dependent and HPV-independent. The HPV-dependent pathway in the vulva follows the same progression as HPV-dependent lesions elsewhere in the gynecologic tract—HPV infection results in high-grade squamous intraepithelial lesion with subsequent progression to basaloid squamous cell carcinoma. The HPV-independent pathway is more complex, with a variety of precursor lesions and molecular alterations. Although the most recognized form of HPV-independent vulvar lesion is differentiated vulvar intraepithelial neoplasia, recent explorations have elucidated new precursors. This review provides an update on HPV-independent risk factors and precursor lesions for squamous cell carcinoma of the vulva.

Human Papilloma Virus–Associated Squamous Neoplasia of the Lower Anogenital Tract   263

Eric J. Yang

HPV-associated squamous neoplasias of the lower anogenital tract are biologically and morphologically equivalent; a unified, two-tiered nomenclature system is recommended to reflect this. Low-grade squamous intraepithelial lesion represents the morphologic manifestation of transient HPV infection with high rate of regression. High-grade squamous intraepithelial lesion (HSIL) represents the morphologic manifestation of persistent high-risk HPV infection and viral integration with a significant rate of progression to invasive carcinoma. Despite these shared attributes, SILs encounter unique diagnostic challenges by anatomic site. This article discusses the LAST project recommendations, challenges associated with their application, and site specific diagnostic challenges in their relevant clinical context.

Cervical Glandular Neoplasia: Classification and Staging   281

Gulisa Turashvili and Kay J. Park

Endocervical adenocarcinomas (EAs) account for 25% of all primary cervical carcinomas. Approximately 90% of EAs are driven by high-risk human papillomavirus (HPV) infection, the most common of which is the so-called usual type endocervical adenocarcinomas. Non-HPV-driven subtypes harbor distinct clinicopathologic features and prognosis and have been increasingly recognized in recent years, which has led to efforts to improve classification of EA based on clinically relevant and reproducible criteria. This review discusses a recently proposed classification system, the International Endocervical Adenocarcinoma Criteria and Classification, which uniquely integrates morphology, cause/pathogenesis, and biological behavior of HPV and non-HPV-driven subtypes of EA.

Benign and Premalignant Lesions of the Endometrium   315

Wesley Daniel Mallinger and Charles Matthew Quick

> In this review, we highlight the benign and premalignant lesions of the endometrium that the pathologist may encounter in daily practice. We begin by detailing our current understanding of excess estrogen in the progression of endometrial neoplasia. We outline the currently accepted terminology to be used when evaluating proliferative endometrial lesions, while highlighting their key features. Attention is then turned to the molecular underpinnings of neoplastic progression and how this can be exploited with immunohistochemical stains when appropriate. Finally, we discuss types of metaplasia and their associations, including so-called papillary proliferations of the endometrium.

Endometrial Carcinoma: Grossing, Frozen Section Evaluation, Staging, and Sentinel Lymph Node Evaluation   329

Vinita Parkash and Oluwole Fadare

> This article gives an overview of the pathologic assessment of resection specimens removed for uterine carcinoma. Areas of controversy and recent developments in pathologic staging are addressed. This includes assessment of myometrial invasion in the setting of adenomyosis, fallopian tube involvement, and vascular invasion. An overview of the role and evaluation of sentinel node assessments in the staging of endometrial carcinoma is provided.

High-Grade Endometrial Carcinomas: Classification with Molecular Insights   343

Joseph W. Carlson and Denis Nastic

> This article provides an overview of the current diagnosis of endometrial carcinoma subtypes and provides updates, including the most recent molecular findings from The Cancer Genome Atlas and others. Interpretation of relevant immunohistochemistry and critical diagnostic differential diagnosis with pitfalls are discussed.

Uterine Mesenchymal Tumors: Update on Classification, Staging, and Molecular Features   363

Carlos Parra-Herran and Brooke E. Howitt

> The spectrum of mesenchymal neoplasia in the uterus has expanded in recent years. First, the identification of prevalent, recurrent molecular alterations has led to a more biologically and clinically congruent classification of endometrial stromal tumors. Likewise, the diagnostic criteria of several rare and miscellaneous tumor types have been refined in recent case series (Perivascular Epithelioid Cell tumor, inflammatory myofibroblastic tumor). Pure mesenchymal tumors are still broadly classified based on morphology according to the tumor cell phenotype. Smooth muscle tumors predominate in frequency, followed by tumors of endometrial stromal derivation; the latter are covered in depth in this article with an emphasis on defining molecular alterations and their morphologic and clinical correlates. The remaining entities comprise a miscellaneous group in which cell derivation does not have a normal counterpart in the uterus (eg, rhabdomyosarcoma) or is obscure (eg, undifferentiated uterine sarcoma). This article discusses their clinical relevance, recent insights into their molecular biology, and the most important differential diagnoses. Regarding the latter, immunohistochemistry and (increasingly) molecular diagnostics play a role in the diagnostic workup. We conclude with a few considerations on intraoperative consultation and macroscopic examination, as well as pathologic staging and grading of uterine sarcomas as per the most recent American Joint Cancer Commission and the Fédération Internationale de Gynécologie et d'Obstétrique staging systems.

Smooth Muscle Tumors of the Female Genital Tract 397

Kelly A. Devereaux and J. Kenneth Schoolmeester

Smooth muscle tumors are the most common mesenchymal tumors of the female genital tract. However, awareness of tumor variants and unconventional growth patterns is critical for appropriate classification and patient management. For example, recognition of fumarate hydratase–deficient leiomyomas allows pathologists to alert providers to the potential for hereditary leiomyomatosis and renal cell carcinoma. Furthermore, myxoid and epithelioid smooth muscle tumors have different thresholds for malignancy than spindled tumors and should be classified by criteria specific to these variants. This article provides an overview of smooth muscle tumors of each major organ of the gynecologic tract and discusses diagnostic challenges.

Fallopian Tube Neoplasia and Mimics 457

David L. Kolin and Marisa R. Nucci

This review discusses select fallopian tube entities and their associated mimics. It first focuses on adenomatoid tumors, the most common benign tumor of the fallopian tube. High-grade serous carcinoma and its precursor, serous tubal intraepithelial carcinoma, are then addressed. Finally, attention is turned to endometrioid proliferations of the fallopian tube. A diagnostic approach is provided for these lesions, with an emphasis on differential diagnoses and situations in which a benign lesion may appear malignant, and vice-versa.

Low-grade Serous Neoplasia of the Female Genital Tract 481

Ann K. Folkins and Teri A. Longacre

Low-grade serous neoplasia of the gynecologic tract includes benign (serous cystadenomas), borderline, and malignant lesions (low-grade serous carcinoma). Classification of these lesions relies on rigorous attention to several pathologic features that determine the prognosis and the need for adjuvant therapy. Risk stratification of serous borderline tumor behavior based on histologic findings and criteria for low-grade serous carcinoma are the primary focus of this article, including the redesignation of invasive implants of serous borderline tumor as low-grade serous carcinoma based on the similar survival rates. The molecular underpinnings of these tumors are also discussed, including their potential for prognostication.

Ovarian High-Grade Serous Carcinoma: Assessing Pathology for Site of Origin, Staging and Post-neoadjuvant Chemotherapy Changes 515

Laura Casey and Naveena Singh

High-grade serous (HGSC) stands apart from the other ovarian cancer histotypes in being the most frequent, in occurring as part of a genetic predisposition in a significant proportion of cases, and in having the poorest clinical outcomes. Although the pathologic diagnosis of HGSC is now made with high accuracy, there remain areas of disagreement regarding viewpoints on tissue site of origin and designation of primary site, with impact on staging in low-stage cases, as well as difficulties in reproducible and clinically relevant reporting of HGSC in specimens taken after neoadjuvant chemotherapy. These areas are discussed in the current article.

Pathology of Endometrioid and Clear Cell Carcinoma of the Ovary 529

Oluwole Fadare and Vinita Parkash

This review is an appraisal of the current state of knowledge of 2 enigmatic histotypes of ovarian carcinoma: endometrioid and clear cell carcinoma. Both show an association endometriosis and the hereditary nonpolyposis colorectal cancer (Lynch) syndrome, and both typically present at an early stage. Pathologic and immunohistochemical features that distinguish these tumors from high-grade serous carcinomas, each other, and other potential mimics are discussed, as are staging, grading, and molecular pathogenesis.

Mucinous Ovarian Tumors   565

Anne M. Mills and Elisheva D. Shanes

Ovarian mucinous tumors range from benign cystadenomas to borderline tumors to frankly malignant adenocarcinomas, and may display either intestinal-type morphology or, less frequently, endocervical-type differentiation. The latter category has been the subject of recent controversy owing to its morphologic overlap with so-called "seromucinous" ovarian tumors, a group that shares more molecular features with endometrioid tumors than it does with either serous or mucinous ovarian neoplasias. Endocervical-type differentiation in ovarian mucinous tumors may also represent an endocervical metastasis. Distinction of primary ovarian mucinous tumors from gastrointestinal metastases can be difficult, as the morphology of intestinal-type ovarian mucinous primaries sometimes differs only subtly if at all from gastrointestinal metastases.

Practical Review of Ovarian Sex Cord–Stromal Tumors   587

Krisztina Z. Hanley and Marina B. Mosunjac

Ovarian sex cordestromal tumors are uncommon tumors and clinically differ from epithelial tumors. They occur across a wide age range and patients often present with hormone-related symptoms. Most are associated with an indolent clinical course. Sex cordestromal tumors are classified into 3 main categories: pure stromal tumors, pure sex cord tumors, and mixed sex cordestromal tumors. The rarity, overlapping histomorphology and immunoprofile of various sex cordestromal tumors often contributes to diagnostic difficulties. This article describes the various types of ovarian sex cordestromal tumors and includes practical approaches to differential diagnoses and updates in classification.

Germ Cell Tumors of the Female Genital Tract   621

Elizabeth D. Euscher

Ovarian germ cell tumors are a histologically diverse group of neoplasms with a common origin in the primitive germ cell. The vast majority are represented by mature cystic teratoma. In the minority are malignant germ cell tumors including immature teratoma, dysgerminoma, yolk sac tumor, embryonal cell carcinoma, and choriocarcinoma. This article reviews the histologic and immunohistochemical features of the most common ovarian germ cell tumors. The differential diagnoses for each are discussed.

SURGICAL PATHOLOGY CLINICS

FORTHCOMING ISSUES

September 2019
Hematopathology
Mina Luqing Xu, *Editor*

December 2019
Endocrine Pathology
Justine A. Barletta, *Editor*

March 2020
Pulmonary Pathology
Kirk Jones, *Editor*

RECENT ISSUES

March 2019
Soft Tissue Pathology
Elizabeth G. Demicco, *Editor*

December 2018
Genitourinary Pathology
Sean R. Williamson, *Editor*

September 2018
Cytopathology
Vickie Y. Jo, *Editor*

SERIES OF RELATED INTEREST

Clinics in Laboratory Medicine

THE CLINICS ARE AVAILABLE ONLINE!
Access your subscription at:
www.theclinics.com

Preface
Practical Issues and Updates in Gynecologic Pathology

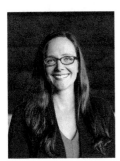

Brooke E. Howitt, MD
Editor

I am pleased to serve as the editor for this issue of *Surgical Pathology Clinics*, focusing on selected practical issues and updates in gynecologic pathology. Gynecologic specimens account for a significant volume of general surgical pathology case load and encompass a wide variety of entities frequently encountered in cervical and endometrial biopsies and resections as well as rarely encountered tumors such as uterine sarcomas and germ cell tumors. It is an exciting time to be a gynecologic pathologist as we continue to expand our understanding of molecular underpinnings of gynecologic tumors and preinvasive lesions. However, it can be difficult to stay up-to-date when new tumor subtypes are continually emerging and new classification systems are established. While this issue certainly cannot comprehensively address all updates in gynecologic pathology, we collectively touch on a number of relevant issues for the practicing pathologist.

First, there are some recently proposed changes in classification systems in gynecologic pathology that deserve critical review and attention. For example, histotyping in endocervical adenocarcinoma may undergo significant changes to more accurately reflect tumor biology and specifically the association with human papillomavirus (HPV). In addition, we now appreciate that in HPV-associated endocervical adenocarcinoma, the morphologic pattern of invasion is prognostic. For tubo-ovarian high-grade serous

carcinoma (HGSC), the diagnosis may not often be challenging, but there is the age-old question of site of origin (fallopian tube vs ovary). The fallopian tube has, over the last 10 to 15 years, garnered much attention and has indeed shifted from a forgotten organ to one of critical importance with regard to the pathogenesis of (so-called) ovarian HGSC. Because we now tend to examine more, if not all, of the fallopian tube, we are also looking more closely. This has allowed us to detect less obvious preinvasive lesions, including atypias and lesions for which we have no name, or we give many names, but importantly do not precisely know the clinical significance of such lesions. In addition, frequent use of neoadjuvant chemotherapy in HGSC has led to a reproducible and clinically relevant scoring of response to chemotherapy, the "chemotherapy response score." In the field of uterine mesenchymal tumors, there has been, in recent years, description of a number of new entities with specific molecular findings, most notably in high-grade endometrial stromal sarcomas and smooth muscle tumors.

Other topics covered in this issue include frequently encountered epithelial neoplasias, including vulvar and cervical squamous lesions, premalignant lesions of the endometrium, classification of high-grade endometrial carcinomas, and both clear cell and endometrioid ovarian carcinomas. The Lower Anogenital Squamous

Surgical Pathology 12 (2019) xi–xii
https://doi.org/10.1016/j.path.2019.03.001
1875-9181/19/© 2019 Published by Elsevier Inc.

Terminology Standardization Project for HPV-associated lesions has resulted in unifying terminology across all anatomic sites and also addresses the use of p16 immunohistochemistry. One review herein is dedicated entirely to intraoperative evaluation and challenging staging issues in endometrial carcinoma and addresses how we can recognize and measure depth of invasion from sites of involvement by adenomyosis. Based on experience from consultation practices, some areas of gynecologic pathology continue to be troublesome despite few changes in diagnosis and classification; these include low-grade serous neoplasia, specifically drawing the line between noninvasive implants and low-grade serous carcinoma and classification of ovarian mucinous tumors, sex-cord stromal tumors, and germ cell tumors (the latter being even more difficult to recognize and diagnose outside the ovary).

I would like to thank all of the authors for their wonderful contributions to this issue of *Surgical Pathology Clinics*. It has been a pleasure to work with and learn from each and every one of you. Many of the authors in this issue are pathologists whose guidance, mentorship, and friendship have been invaluable to my professional development and career as a gynecologic pathologist, whether across a hallway or across the country (and beyond!).

Brooke E. Howitt, MD
Department of Pathology
Stanford University School of Medicine
300 Pasteur Drive H2128E
Stanford, CA 94305-5324, USA

E-mail address:
bhowitt@stanford.edu

Human Papillomavirus–Independent Squamous Lesions of the Vulva

Jaclyn C. Watkins, MD, MS

KEYWORDS

- Verrucous carcinoma • Differentiated vulvar intraepithelial neoplasia
- Vulvar acanthosis with altered differentiation • Vulvar dermatoses
- Differentiated exophytic vulvar intraepithelial lesion

Key points

- Vulvar squamous cell carcinoma pathogenesis is divided broadly into human papillomavirus (HPV)-dependent and HPV-independent pathways.
- The HPV-independent pathway is growing increasingly complex in the molecular era.
- Precursor lesions in this pathway may be *TP53*-mutated (eg, differentiated vulvar intraepithelial neoplasia) or *TP53*–wild type.
- The *TP53*–wild-type pathway includes newly introduced entities, such as vulvar acanthosis with altered differentiation and differentiated exophytic vulvar intraepithelial lesion, as well as more well-established lesions, such as verrucous carcinoma.

ABSTRACT

The pathogenesis of vulvar squamous neoplasia has 2 pathways: human papillomavirus (HPV)-dependent and HPV-independent. The HPV-dependent pathway in the vulva follows the same progression as HPV-dependent lesions elsewhere in the gynecologic tract—HPV infection results in high-grade squamous intraepithelial lesion with subsequent progression to basaloid squamous cell carcinoma. The HPV-independent pathway is more complex, with a variety of precursor lesions and molecular alterations. Although the most recognized form of HPV-independent vulvar lesion is differentiated vulvar intraepithelial neoplasia, recent explorations have elucidated new precursors. This review provides an update on HPV-independent risk factors and precursor lesions for squamous cell carcinoma of the vulva.

RISK FACTORS FOR HUMAN PAPILLOMAVIRUS–INDEPENDENT VULVAR SQUAMOUS CELL CARCINOMA

LICHEN SIMPLEX CHRONICUS

Introduction

Lichen simplex chronicus (LSC) arises in the setting of repeated physical trauma, often secondary to an underlying pruritic lesion (eg, eczematous processes, stasis dermatitis, vulvar intraepithelial neoplasias [VINs], and infections). It is most often observed in the fourth through sixth decades of life.

Microscopic Features

LSC demonstrates hyperkeratosis, psoriasiform epidermal hyperplasia (eg, elongated rete ridges), hypergranulosis, vertical papillary dermal fibrosis,

Disclosure Statement: Nothing to disclose.
Department of Pathology, Microbiology and Immunology, Vanderbilt University Medical Center, MCN C-3306A, 1161 21st Avenue South, Nashville, TN 37232-2582, USA
E-mail address: Jaclyn.c.watkins@vumc.org

Surgical Pathology 12 (2019) 249–261
https://doi.org/10.1016/j.path.2019.01.001
1875-9181/19/© 2019 Elsevier Inc. All rights reserved.

and sparse chronic inflammation (typically peri-vascular) (**Fig. 1**A). Given that the lesion arises secondary to trauma, pigment incontinence also may occur.

Differential Diagnosis

LSC lacks basal atypia and abnormal keratinocyte maturation, 2 key features necessary for a diagnosis of differentiated VIN (DVIN), the most clinically important differential diagnostic consideration.

Diagnosis

Diagnosis of LSC is largely morphologic. In cases where DVIN enters the differential, however, p53 staining may be used. Although LSC may demonstrate some mild basal layer up-regulation of p53 secondary to inflammation,[1] the overall p53 pattern in LSC is still wild type (heterogenous) and confined to the basal layer[2–4] (see **Fig. 1**B).

Prognosis

LSC is a risk factor for squamous cell carcinoma (SCC), but it is not considered a direct precursor lesion. So-called verruciform LSC, a variant of LSC with a verrucoid growth pattern, has been associated with an increased risk of progression to SCC or verruciform carcinoma (VC).[5] However, the operational usage of verruciform LSC is still in question, with some fraction of such lesions likely representing newer entities (such as differentiated exophytic vulvar intraepithelial lesions [DE-VILs]/verruciform acanthosis with altered differentiation [discussed later]). Although typical LSC does not need to be excised, verruciform LSC should be conservatively excised. Patients with LSC should be monitored for new or changing lesions.

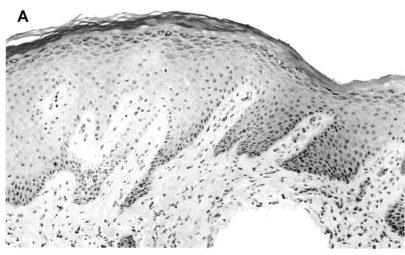

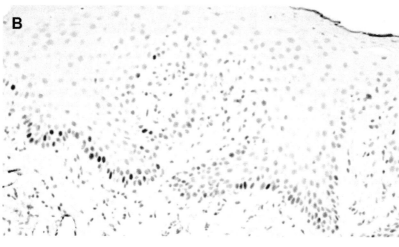

Fig. 1. LSC (*A*) demonstrates hyperkeratosis, hypergranulosis, vertical papillary dermal fibrosis, and psoriasiform epidermal hyperplasia (H&E, original magnification). Such lesions are p53 wild-type in the basal layers (*B*).

> ### Key Features
> #### LICHEN SIMPLEX CHRONICUS
>
> - Hyperkeratosis
> - Psoriasiform epidermal hyperplasia (eg, elongated rete ridges)
> - Hypergranulosis
> - Vertical papillary dermal fibrosis
> - Sparse chronic inflammation (typically perivascular)

LICHEN SCLEROSUS

Introduction

Lichen sclerosus (LS) presents as pruritic to painful "porcelain white" plaques in women typically over 40 years old. From a molecular standpoint, LS is not believed to harbor mutations and, therefore, is considered a risk factor rather than a true precursor for *TP53*-mutated SCC. Documentation of the same *TP53* mutations in invasive SCC and adjacent LS,[1,6] however, provides some evidence that LS may provide a background in which *TP53*-mutated clones may arise.[7]

Microscopic Features

LS displays variable histologic features depending on lesion age. Early LS may present with subtle findings, including psoriasiform epidermal hyperplasia, basal vacuolization, mild papillary dermal fibrosis, and a superficial lichenoid lymphocytic infiltrate. Established lesions (**Fig. 2**) generally present as more readily recognizable LS, with quintessential dermal homogenization/hyalinization, hyperkeratosis, loss of dermal vasculature, deeper lymphocytic infiltrates, epidermal atrophy, rete effacement, and dermal edema.

Differential Diagnosis

Early LS may raise the possibility of spongiotic dermatoses, including LSC. Lichen planus also enters the differential and should be considered when basal colloid bodies, hypergranulosis, and prominent acanthosis (instead of atrophy) is present.

Diagnosis

Diagnosis is largely based on histomorphology. Elastic stains may be of use in more challenging cases—decreased elastic fibers are seen in the areas of homogenization. Although p53 and p16 are generally not used for the diagnosis, p53 may show mild basal layer overexpression due to inflammatory upregulation, but the overall staining pattern is wild-type.[1–4,6,8]

Prognosis

Because 5% of LS cases progress to VIN or invasive SCC, regular clinical follow-up is recommended.[9]

> ### Key Features
> #### LICHEN SCLEROSUS
>
> - Early LS—psoriasiform epidermal hyperplasia, basal vacuolization, mild papillary dermal fibrosis, and a superficial lichenoid lymphocytic infiltrate
> - Established LS—dermal homogenization/hyalinization, hyperkeratosis, loss of dermal vasculature, deeper lymphocytic infiltrates, atrophy, rete effacement, and dermal edema

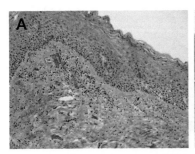
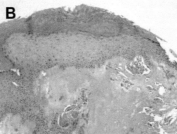
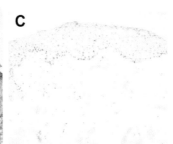

Fig. 2. The inflammatory stage of LS has a lichenoid infiltrate of chronic inflammatory cells, and subtle papillary dermal fibrosis (H&E, original magnification) (*A*). Established LS (H&E, original magnification) (*B*) demonstrates characteristic dermal homogenization/hyalinization, hyperkeratosis, loss of dermal vasculature, deep lymphocytic infiltrates, epidermal atrophy/rete effacement, and dermal edema. Although p53 may be mildly upregulated in the basal layer, the overall pattern (*C*) is wild type. If a p53 appears mutant in the basal 2 to 3 cell layers, DVIN arising in a background of LS should be considered.

⚠️ **Differential Diagnosis**

Lichen Sclerosus versus	Helpful Distinguishing Features
• Lichen planus	• Basal colloid bodies
	• Hypergranulosis
	• Prominent acanthosis

DIFFERENTIATED VULVAR INTRAEPITHELIAL NEOPLASIA: AN HPV-INDEPENDENT, TP53-DEPENDENT PRECURSOR LESION

Introduction

DVIN, a precursor to vulvar SCC, harbors mutations in TP53[4] and is associated with background dermatoses (eg, LSC and LS).[10–12] DVIN only accounts for 10% of VIN; however, this may be due to under-recognition.[13,14] It is most commonly diagnosed in the setting of coexisting SCC.[13]

Molecularly speaking, DVIN is defined by TP53 mutations (most commonly exons 5–9).[3,4] These mutations are considered pathogenic because subsequent SCCs share the same TP53 mutational profile as the precursor DVIN.[3]

Microscopic Features

DVIN demonstrates 2 key histologic features: abnormal keratinocyte maturation and basal atypia[2,4,13,15–17] (Figs. 3 and 4). Abnormal keratinocyte maturation occurs in the form of premature keratinization (eg, hypereosinophilic keratinocytes in layers beneath the stratum granulosum and squamous eddies/keratin pearls). Cytologic atypia in DVIN is confined to the basal-most 2 to 3 cell layers and is defined by hyperchromasia, nuclear enlargement,

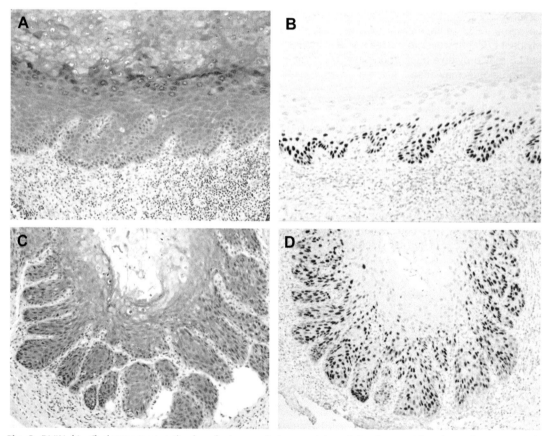

Fig. 3. DVIN (*A*, *C*) demonstrates the key features of abnormal keratinization and basal atypia. Less-specific features include parakeratosis, rete ridge elongation/anastomosis, acanthosis, and spongiosis (H&E, original magnification). P53 staining tends to be overexpressed in the basal 2 to 3 cell layers (mutant phenotype [*B*, *D*]) or may be entirely negative (null mutant phenotype). (*Courtesy of* Dr Christopher Crum, Brigham and Women's Hospital/Harvard Medical School, Boston, MA.)

Fig. 4. A third example of DVIN (*A*) with mutant p53 expression (*B*). Note the prominent basal atypia and premature keratinization at higher power (*C*) (H&E, original magnification). (*Courtesy of* Dr Christopher Crum, Brigham and Women's Hospital/Harvard Medical School, Boston, MA.)

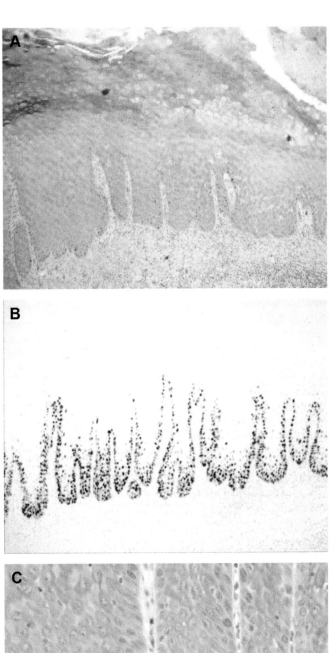

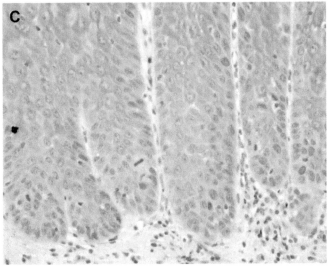

and prominent nucleoli (see **Fig. 4**C). Mitoses also may be seen. Other less-specific DVIN features include parakeratosis, rete ridge elongation/anastomosis, acanthosis, and spongiosis, with prominent intracellular bridges. Inflammation is not a typical feature of DVIN; however, a superimposed dermatosis may confound the picture and introduce inflammation.

Differential Diagnosis

The differential diagnosis for DVIN includes usual-type VIN with superimposed LSC, LS, and pseudoepitheliomatous hyperplasia.

The first differential diagnostic consideration, usual type (human papillomavirus [HPV]–associated) or classic VIN (CVIN) with superimposed LSC, can be particularly challenging because there may be near-perfect morphologic overlap with DVIN. In this setting, immunohistochemistry proves invaluable as CVIN with superimposed LSC demonstrates p16 block positivity in the lower epithelium. Additionally, p53 demonstrates unique staining in CVIN with superimposed LSC-p53 staining is entirely negative in the basal layer with wild-type expression noted in the parabasal/midepithelial layers. In contrast, p53 typically demonstrates mutant expression in the basal layers of DVIN.[18]

In cases of LS or pseudoepitheliomatous hyperplasia, the absence of significant basal atypia should distinguish between DVIN and these 2 benign entities. In ambiguous cases, however, p53 staining can be used.

Diagnosis

Although the presence of characteristic morphologic findings is sufficient to render a diagnosis of DVIN, immunohistochemical evidence suggestive of an underlying *TP53* mutation can be useful in distinguishing DVIN from its mimics. In particular, mutant p53 staining (overexpression or null expression) in the atypical basal layers supports the diagnosis (see **Figs.** 3B, D and 4B).[4,13,19] In the author's practice, such cases are routinely stained for p53, requiring a mutant phenotype to render the diagnosis. DVIN is p16 negative, reflecting its HPV-negative status.[13,16]

Prognosis

When identified as an independent precursor, DVIN is believed to have a higher rate of progression to SCC than HPV-related VIN, with some literature suggesting that 30% to 90% of lesions progress.[14,20–23]

Key Features
DIFFERENTIATED VULVAR INTRAEPITHELIAL NEOPLASIA

- Abnormal keratinocyte maturation (premature keratinization)
- Basal atypia in first 2 to 3 cell layers
- Parakeratosis, rete ridge elongation/anastomosis, acanthosis, spongiosis

 Differential Diagnosis

Differentiated Vulvar Intraepithelial Neoplasia vs	Helpful Distinguishing Features
• Usual VIN with superimposed LSC	• Block p16 positivity in lower epithelium
	• p53 demonstrates negativity in basal layer with wild-type expression in parabasal to midepithelium
• LS	• Absence of significant basal atypia
	• Typically wild-type p53 in basal layer
• Pseudoepitheliomatous hyperplasia	• Absence of significant basal atypia
	• Wild-type p53 in basal layer

HUMAN PAPILLOMAVIRUS–INDEPENDENT, TP53-INDEPENDENT SQUAMOUS LESIONS

VERRUCOUS CARCINOMA

Introduction

VC, a subtype of HPV-negative vulvar SCC, affects women in their seventh and eighth decades. Although there is no established precursor for VC, both vulvar acanthosis with altered differentiation (VAAD)[5] and DE-VIL,[6] discussed later, have a putative relationship with the development of VC.

Microscopic Features

VC is an extremely well-differentiated form of SCC. The tumor shows minimal cytologic atypia, superficial epithelial pallor, and parakeratosis. It is characterized by blunt invasion with bulbous rete ridges and a smooth epithelial-stromal interface (**Fig. 5**). The pattern of invasion is best appreciated at low power (**Fig. 6**), using uninvolved background epithelium as a comparison. Importantly, if any degree of infiltrative invasion is present, the tumor should be designated SCC or SCC arising in a background of VC.

Differential Diagnosis

Both verruciform LSC and giant condyloma, 2 exophytic entities with verruciform architecture,

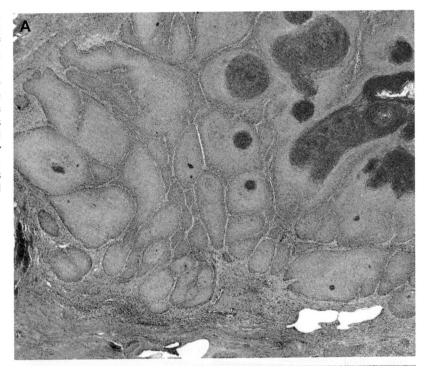

Fig. 5. Verrucous carcinoma (*A*) is characterized by a blunt pattern of invasion (*B*). Bulbous rete ridges and a smooth epithelial-stromal interface as well as an absence of invasion by single cells or small angulated nests are typical (H&E, original magnification). (*Courtesy of* Dr Christopher Crum, Brigham and Women's Hospital/Harvard Medical School, Boston, MA.)

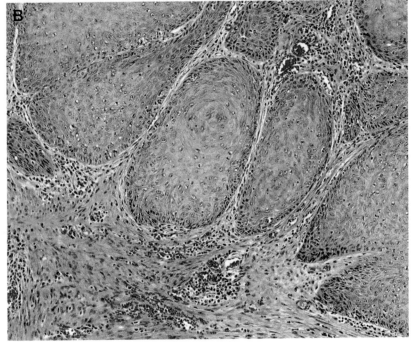

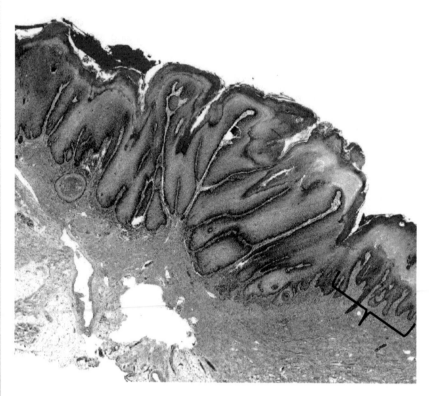

Fig. *6.* The invasive pattern of verrucous carcinoma is most readily identified at low power. Here, an early verrucous carcinoma is arising in association with a putative precursor, VAAD (*bracketed region*). Note the blunt pattern of invasion in the verrucous carcinoma that is absent in the VAAD (H&E, original magnification). (*Courtesy of* Dr Christopher Crum, Brigham and Women's Hospital/Harvard Medical School, Boston, MA.)

may enter the differential diagnosis for VC. However, both entities lack blunt invasion. Additionally, giant condylomas generally demonstrate HPV-related viral cytopathic change (ie, koilocytosis) and often are associated with low risk HPV infection.

Diagnosis

Diagnosis of VC is largely based on morphology and the exclusion of an infiltrative invasive component (eg, invasion by single cells or small clusters of cells). Immunohistochemistry demonstrates wild-type/heterogenous p53 staining,[24] reflecting VC's *TP53*-independent status. Although the relationship between VC and HPV infection has been debated,[25–31] p16 staining generally is negative.[24]

Prognosis

Without evidence of invasion, VC is clinically indolent with essentially no risk of lymph node or distant metastasis.[32]

Key Features
VERRUCOUS CARCINOMA

- Blunt invasion with bulbous rete ridges
- Smooth epithelial-stromal interface
- Minimal cytologic atypia
- Superficial epithelial pallor
- Parakeratosis

  Differential Diagnosis

Verrucous Carcinoma vs	Helpful Distinguishing Features
• Giant condyloma	• Koilocytosis
	• Exophytic without blunt invasion
• VAAD/DEVIL	• Absence of blunt invasion

Pitfall
IN THE DIAGNOSIS OF
VERRUCOUS CARCINOMA

! If any degree of infiltrative invasion is present, the tumor should be designated typical SCC or SCC arising in a background of VC

VULVAR ACANTHOSIS WITH ALTERED DIFFERENTIATION

Introduction

VAAD, a putative precursor of VC,[5] is an HPV-independent, *TP53*–wild-type lesion that recently was shown to harbor frequent mutations in *HRAS* (71.4%) and *NOTCH1* (28.6%).[7] The lesion was first described in a case series of VC, in which 7 of 9 VCs demonstrated a noninvasive adjacent squamous proliferation that failed to meet criteria for DVIN or other established precursors.[5]

Microscopic Features

VAAD displays morphologic overlap with VC, namely epithelial pallor and a lack of cytologic atypia (**Fig. 7**). It lacks, however, downward expansile growth (ie, blunt invasion) (see **Figs. 6** and **7A**). The lesion also displays acanthosis, plaque-like parakeratosis, loss of the granular cell layer, and variable verruciform architecture (see **Fig. 7**). Koilocytes are absent, reflecting the lesion's HPV-independent nature.

Differential Diagnosis

The main differential for VAAD is VC, the latter of which is distinguished from VAAD by the presence of blunt invasion. Verruciform LSC can appear quite similar; however, verruciform LSC generally lacks plaque-like parakeratosis and epithelial pallor.[5] The absence of cytologic atypia helps distinguish VAAD from DVIN.

Fig. 7. VAAD (*A*) shares some features with verrucous carcinoma, including an absence of basal atypia (*B*) and the presence of epithelial pallor (*C*). The lesion, however, lacks downward expansile growth (ie, blunt invasion) (*A*). Other features include acanthosis, plaque-like parakeratosis, loss of the granular cell layer, and variable verruciform architecture (H&E, original magnification).

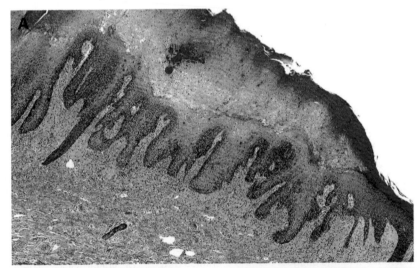
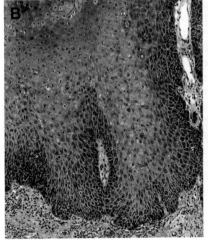
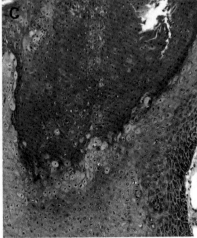

Diagnosis

p53 IHC is typically wild type/heterogenous and p16 staining is negative, reflecting the lesion's *TP53* and HPV-independent nature.

Prognosis

Given the presence of pathogenic mutations and the association with VC, conservative excision is recommended for these lesions.

Key Features
VULVAR ACANTHOSIS WITH ALTERED DIFFERENTIATION

- Epithelial pallor
- Absence of cytologic atypia
- Acanthosis
- Plaque-like parakeratosis
- Loss of the granular cell layer
- Variable verruciform architecture

DIFFERENTIATED EXOPHYTIC VULVAR INTRAEPITHELIAL LESION

Introduction

DE-VIL[6] was initially derived from a group of "atypical verruciform lesions" that failed to meet criteria for VIN (differentiated or usual type) and displayed histologic overlap with VAAD and/or VC. They are HPV-negative and *TP53*-independent lesions that are putative precursor lesions to a subset of well-differentiated vulvar SCC.

Although a vast majority of VAAD lesions fall under the umbrella of DE-VIL morphologically, some molecular findings suggest that the 2 entities may be unique. Namely, VAAD has been associated with a high percentage of *HRAS* (71.4%) and *NOTCH1* (28.6%) mutations.[7] In contrast, DE-VILs are largely defined by activating *PIK3CA* mutations, which are found in 73% of lesions, and *HRAS* mutations were identified in only 7%.[6] Further studies are required to aid in the distinction, if any, between these lesions. For diagnostic purposes at the moment, the author prefers the term DE-VIL over VAAD when the criteria for DE-VIL are met.

Microscopic Features

DE-VIL lesions are defined by the following microscopic features: (1) an exophytic growth pattern, (2) prominent verruciform or acanthotic architecture, (3) absence of HPV-related histology (eg, koilocytosis or full-thickness atypia), and (4) absence of basal atypia sufficient for a diagnosis of DVIN (**Fig. 8**). Thus, DE-VIL is an umbrella term for any verruciform lesion with altered differentiation and bland nuclear features at the lesion-stromal interface.

Differential Diagnosis

DVIN enters the differential for DE-VIL; however, DE-VIL lacks basal atypia and mutations in *TP53*, as evidenced by typically wild-type p53 staining (see **Fig. 8C**). Additionally, DVIN is not often exophytic, particularly when occurring in the absence of associated SCC.

Diagnosis

DE-VIL shows variable p53 positivity in the basal cell layers, leading to overlap between DE-VIL and verruciform DVIN. From a molecular standpoint, however, DE-VIL lacks *TP53* mutations, suggesting that the increased expression seen with IHC is likely inflammatory or reactive in nature.

Prognosis

PIK3CA mutations have been demonstrated in only 8% of HPV-independent vulvar SCC.[7,33] Furthermore, most keratinizing SCCs harbor *TP53* mutations[6]; therefore, classifying DE-VIL as a direct precursor for SCC, rather than a risk factor for SCC, is not entirely possible with the current data available. Nevertheless, the presence of known carcinogenic mutations in DE-VIL justifies their neoplastic, rather than hyperplastic, role in the development of vulvar SCC. Therefore, complete excision, when feasible, and monitoring for regrowth/progression is recommended in all cases of DE-VIL.

Key Features
DIFFERENTIATED EXOPHYTIC VULVAR INTRAEPITHELIAL LESION

- Prominent verruciform or acanthotic architecture
- Exophytic growth
- Absence of HPV histology (eg, koilocytosis)
- Lack of significant basal cytologic atypia

Fig. 8. DE-VIL (*A*), a putative precursor of keratinizing vulvar SCC, demonstrates prominent verruciform or acanthotic architecture, exophytic growth, an absence of HPV-type changes, and an absence of significant basal cytologic atypia (*B*) (H&E, original magnification). P53 staining (*C*) is generally wild type, reflecting an absence of *TP53* mutations in these lesions.

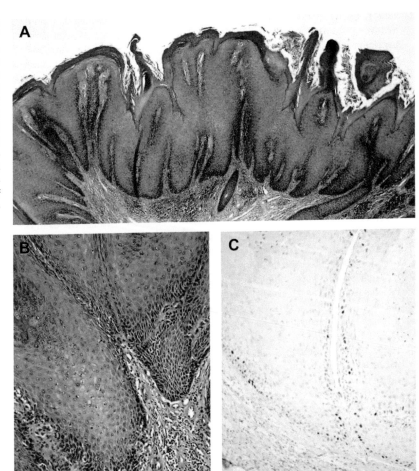

SUMMARY

In the molecular era, the landscape of HPV-independent vulvar neoplasia is increasingly complex. Of particular note is recent work suggesting a third pathway to vulvar SCC that is both HPV-independent and *TP53*–wild type. The putative precursors in this pathway, VAAD and DE-VIL, demonstrate considerable morphologic overlap and require additional study to further delineate if they are independent processes. Nevertheless, the molecular exploration of these lesions is particularly valuable, because it may provide new therapeutic targets for what, until now, has been a disease with major morbidity and mortality.

REFERENCES

1. Rolfe KJ, MacLean a B, Crow JC, et al. TP53 mutations in vulval lichen sclerosus adjacent to squamous cell carcinoma of the vulva. Br J Cancer 2003;89(12):2249–53.

2. Liegl B, Regauer S. p53 immunostaining in lichen sclerosus is related to ischaemic stress and is not a marker of differentiated vulvar intraepithelial neoplasia (d-VIN). Histopathology 2006;48(3):268–74.

3. Pinto AP, Miron A, Yassin Y, et al. Differentiated vulvar intraepithelial neoplasia contains Tp53 mutations and is genetically linked to vulvar squamous cell carcinoma. Mod Pathol 2010;23(3):404–12.

4. Yang B, Hart WR. Vulvar intraepithelial neoplasia of the simplex (differentiated) type: a clinicopathologic study including analysis of HPV and p53 expression. Am J Surg Pathol 2000;24(3):429–41.

5. Nascimento AF, Granter SR, Cviko A, et al. Vulvar acanthosis with altered differentiation: a precursor to verrucous carcinoma? Am J Surg Pathol 2004; 28(5):638–43. Available at: http://www.ncbi.nlm.nih.gov/pubmed/15105653.

6. Vanin K, Scurry J, Thorne H, et al. Overexpression of wild-type p53 in lichen sclerosus adjacent to human papillomavirus-negative vulvar cancer. J Invest Dermatol 2002;119(5):1027–33.

7. Yap JKW, Fox R, Leonard S, et al. Adjacent Lichen Sclerosis predicts local recurrence and second field tumour in women with vulvar squamous cell carcinoma. Gynecol Oncol 2016;142(3):420–6.

8. Chiesa-Vottero A, Dvoretsky PM, Hart WR. Histopathologic study of thin vulvar squamous cell carcinomas and associated cutaneous lesions: a correlative study of 48 tumors in 44 patients with analysis of adjacent vulvar intraepithelial neoplasia types and lichen sclerosus. Am J Surg Pathol 2006;30(3):310–8.

9. Carlson JA, Ambros R, Malfetano J, et al. Vulvar lichen sclerosus and squamous cell carcinoma: a cohort, case control, and investigational study with historical perspective; implications for chronic inflammation and sclerosis in the development of neoplasia. Hum Pathol 1998;29(9):932–48. Available at: http://www.sciencedirect.com/science/article/pii/S0046817798901988.

10. Hantschmann P, Sterzer S, Jeschke U, et al. P53 expression in vulvar carcinoma, vulvar intraepithelial neoplasia, squamous cell hyperplasia and lichen sclerosus. Anticancer Res 2005;25(3A):1739–45. Available at: http://www.ncbi.nlm.nih.gov/pubmed/16033093.

11. Micheletti L, Preti M, Radici G, et al. Vulvar lichen sclerosus and neoplastic transformation: a retrospective study of 976 cases. J Low Genit Tract Dis 2016;20(2):180–3.

12. Rolfe KJ, Eva LJ, MacLean AB, et al. Cell cycle proteins as molecular markers of malignant change in vulvar lichen sclerosus. Int J Gynecol Cancer 2001;11(2):113–8. Available at: http://www.ncbi.nlm.nih.gov/pubmed/11328409.

13. Mulvany NJ, Allen DG. Differentiated intraepithelial neoplasia of the vulva. Int J Gynecol Pathol 2008;27(1):125–35.

14. van de Nieuwenhof HP, Bulten J, Hollema H, et al. Differentiated vulvar intraepithelial neoplasia is often found in lesions, previously diagnosed as lichen sclerosus, which have progressed to vulvar squamous cell carcinoma. Mod Pathol 2011;24(2):297–305.

15. van den Einden LC, de Hullu JA, Massuger LF, et al. Interobserver variability and the effect of education in the histopathological diagnosis of differentiated vulvar intraepithelial neoplasia. Mod Pathol 2013;26(6):874–80.

16. Reyes MC, Cooper K. An update on vulvar intraepithelial neoplasia: terminology and a practical approach to diagnosis. J Clin Pathol 2014;67(4):290–4.

17. Hart WR. Vulvar intraepithelial neoplasia: historical aspects and current status. Int J Gynecol Pathol 2001;20(1):16–30.

18. Watkins JC, Yang E, Crum CP, et al. Classic vulvar intraepithelial neoplasia with superimposed lichen simplex chronicus: a unique variant mimicking differentiated vulvar intraepithelial neoplasia. Int J Gynecol Pathol 2018. https://doi.org/10.1097/PGP.0000000000000509.

19. Singh N, Leen SL, Han G, et al. Expanding the morphologic spectrum of differentiated VIN (dVIN) through detailed mapping of cases with p53 loss. Am J Surg Pathol 2015;39(1):52–60.

20. van de Nieuwenhof HP, Massuger LFAG, van der Avoort IAM, et al. Vulvar squamous cell carcinoma development after diagnosis of VIN increases with age. Eur J Cancer 2009;45(5):851–6.

21. Eva LJ, Ganesan R, Chan KK, et al. Differentiated-type vulval intraepithelial neoplasia has a high-risk association with vulval squamous cell carcinoma. Int J Gynecol Cancer 2009;19(4):741–4.

22. Eva LJ, Ganesan R, Chan KK, et al. Vulval squamous cell carcinoma occurring on a background of differentiated vulval intraepithelial neoplasia is more likely to recur: a review of 154 cases. J Reprod Med 2008;53(6):397–401.

23. McAlpine JN, Kim SY, Akbari A, et al. HPV-independent differentiated vulvar intraepithelial neoplasia (dVIN) is associated with an aggressive clinical course. Int J Gynecol Pathol 2017;36(6):507–16.

24. Santos M, Montagut C, Mellado B, et al. Immunohistochemical staining for p16 and p53 in premalignant and malignant epithelial lesions of the vulva. Int J Gynecol Pathol 2004;23(3):206–14. Available at: http://www.ncbi.nlm.nih.gov/pubmed/15213596.

25. Crowther ME, Shepherd JH, Fisher C. Verrucous carcinoma of the vulva containing human papillomavirus-11. Case report. Br J Obstet Gynaecol 1988;95(4):414–8. Available at: http://www.ncbi.nlm.nih.gov/pubmed/2838068.

26. Della Torre G, Donghi R, Longoni A, et al. HPV DNA in intraepithelial neoplasia and carcinoma of the vulva and penis. Diagn Mol Pathol 1992;1(1):25–30. Available at: http://www.ncbi.nlm.nih.gov/pubmed/1342951.

27. Kondi-Paphitis A, Deligeorgi-Politi H, Liapis A, et al. Human papilloma virus in verrucus carcinoma of the vulva: an immunopathological study of three cases. Eur J Gynaecol Oncol 1998;19(3):319–20. http://www.ncbi.nlm.nih.gov/pubmed/9641242.

28. Gualco M, Bonin S, Foglia G, et al. Morphologic and biologic studies on ten cases of verrucous carcinoma of the vulva supporting the theory of a discrete clinico-pathologic entity. Int J Gynecol Cancer 2003;13(3):317–24.

29. Gupta J, Pilotti S, Shah KV, et al. Human papillomavirus-associated early vulvar neoplasia investigated by in situ hybridization. Am J Surg Pathol 1987;11(6):430–4. Available at: http://www.ncbi.nlm.nih.gov/pubmed/3035953.

30. Milde-Langosch K, Becker G, Löning T. Human papillomavirus and c-myc/c-erbB2 in uterine and vulvar lesions. Virchows Arch A Pathol Anat Histopathol 1991;419(6):479–85. Available at: http://www.ncbi.nlm.nih.gov/pubmed/1661047.

31. Liu G, Li Q, Shang X, et al. Verrucous carcinoma of the vulva: a 20 year retrospective study and literature review. J Low Genit Tract Dis 2016;20(1):114–8.

32. Japaze H, Van Dinh T, Woodruff JD. Verrucous carcinoma of the vulva: study of 24 cases. Obstet Gynecol 1982;60(4):462–6. Available at: http://www.ncbi.nlm.nih.gov/pubmed/7121933.

33. Trietsch MD, Spaans VM, ter Haar NT, et al. CDKN2A(p16) and HRAS are frequently mutated in vulvar squamous cell carcinoma. Gynecol Oncol 2014;135(1):149–55.

Human Papilloma Virus–Associated Squamous Neoplasia of the Lower Anogenital Tract

Eric J. Yang, MD, PhD

KEYWORDS

- Human papillomavirus (HPV) • Low-grade squamous intraepithelial lesion (LSIL)
- High-grade squamous intraepithelial lesion (HSIL) • Dysplasia • Squamous cell carcinoma
- Lower anogenital tract

Key points

- HPV-related squamous intraepithelial lesions of the lower anogenital tract are morphologically and biologically equivalent.
- A unified, two-tiered nomenclature that represents current understanding of HPV biology and is clinically relevant is recommended:
  ○ Low-grade squamous intraepithelial lesion (LSIL).
  ○ High-grade squamous intraepithelial lesion (HSIL).
- p16 immunohistochemical stain is an extensively studied surrogate biomarker of high risk HPV infection that is recommended as a diagnostic adjunct in specific circumstances.
- The term "superficially invasive squamous cell carcinoma" is recommended for the group of minimally invasive carcinoma that may be amenable to conservative management.
- Squamous intraepithelial lesions of the vulva can be divided into HPV and non-HPV related etiologies.

ABSTRACT

HPV-associated squamous neoplasias of the lower anogenital tract are biologically and morphologically equivalent; a unified, two-tiered nomenclature system is recommended to reflect this. Low-grade squamous intraepithelial lesion represents the morphologic manifestation of transient HPV infection with high rate of regression. High-grade squamous intraepithelial lesion (HSIL) represents the morphologic manifestation of persistent high-risk HPV infection and viral integration with a significant rate of progression to invasive carcinoma. Despite these shared attributes, SILs encounter unique diagnostic challenges by anatomic site. This article discusses the LAST project recommendations, challenges associated with their application, and site specific diagnostic challenges in their relevant clinical context.

Disclosure Statement: No relevant financial relationships to disclose.
Department of Pathology, Stanford University School of Medicine, 300 Pasteur Drive H2128B, Stanford, CA 94305-5324, USA
E-mail address: ericyang@stanford.edu

Surgical Pathology 12 (2019) 263–279
https://doi.org/10.1016/j.path.2019.02.001
1875-9181/19/© 2019 Elsevier Inc. All rights reserved.

OVERVIEW

Human papillomavirus (HPV) infection is the necessary cause of a disproportionately large subset of carcinomas in the lower anogenital tract. Virtually all cervical squamous cell carcinomas are considered attributable to HPV infection, whereas 90% of anal carcinomas and 40% of vulvar, vaginal, and penile carcinomas are HPV-attributable.[1] Despite the common causes and morphologic similarities of HPV-related squamous neoplasia of the lower anogenital tract, the classification systems used by pathologists, gynecologists, and dermatologists lacked uniformity until recently. With the goal to establish a biologically and clinically relevant histopathologic nomenclature system, the Lower Anogenital Squamous Terminology (LAST) project, cosponsored by the College of American Pathologists and the American Society for Colposcopy and Cervical Pathology made the following recommendations[2]:

1. A unified, 2-tiered nomenclature for all noninvasive HPV-associated squamous neoplasia of the lower anogenital tract, further qualified with the appropriate intraepithelial neoplasia (-IN) designation by site
2. The criteria for use and interpretation of the p16 immunohistochemical stain
3. Adopting the category of superficially invasive squamous cell carcinoma (SISCCA) as a group of minimally invasive carcinomas that may be amenable to conservative treatment, with accompanying site-specific size criteria.

The practical applications, pearls, and pitfalls of these recommendations are discussed primarily in the cervix section, with the understanding that the overall principles are applicable to all sites in the lower anogenital tract. However, each site within the lower anogenital tract possesses a unique microanatomy that raises distinct differential diagnoses, diagnostic challenges, and management considerations; these site-specific aspects are further discussed in the corresponding anatomically subdivided sections. Although cytology is not the focus of this review, the subject is briefly discussed in the context of clinical management and the author's approach to cytology–histology correlation for quality assurance purposes.

CERVIX

HPV infection is a necessary but not sufficient cause of virtually all squamous neoplasia of the cervix. The interaction of HPV with squamous epithelium can be conceptualized and simplified into 2 major pathways:

1. Transient infection
   - Biology: maturing squamous epithelium supports virion production
   - Histopathology: low-grade squamous intraepithelial lesion (LSIL; cervical intraepithelial neoplasia 1)
   - Clinical relevance: high rate of regression
2. Persistent infection
   - Biology: viral genome integration and expression of oncogenes E6 and E7 that promote accumulation of DNA damage and cell cycle progression through dysregulation of p53 and retinoblastoma protein (Rb) pathways
   - Histopathology: high-grade squamous intraepithelial lesion (HSIL; CIN2-3)
   - Clinical relevance: high rate of progression to cancer.

Therefore, the current understanding of HPV biology, its morphologic manifestations, and associated clinical implications support a 2-tiered nomenclature. The recommended nomenclature (LSIL and HSIL) parallels those of the Bethesda system,[3] which was created to standardize reporting terms and criteria for gynecologic and anal cytology.

LOW-GRADE SQUAMOUS INTRAEPITHELIAL LESION

GROSS FEATURES

The cervix is most commonly visualized by colposcopy to direct biopsies to the most grossly abnormal-appearing areas.[4] The transformation zone is a critical landmark to visualize because most cervical precancers and cancers arise within this area from a distinct population of squamocolumnar junctional (SCJ) cells of embryonic derivation.[5,6] The overall principle of colposcopy is that the illuminated cervical mucosa appears whiter with increasing nuclear-to-cytoplasmic (N/C) ratio and epithelial thickness due to increased intensity of reflected white light and decreased red color of the transilluminated blood vessels. The application of acetic acid (3%–5%) elicits a transitory swelling of cells with intensity and duration of epithelial whitening (acetowhite changes) proportional to the increasing N/C ratio and other abnormalities of the cells. The important features of colposcopic abnormality include epithelial color (ie, acetowhite changes), vascular pattern, surface topography, and margin characteristics. LSIL usually appears faintly acetowhite (slightly translucent), which can be difficult to distinguish from changes seen in immature metaplasia. Clearly demarcated irregular (geographic) margins and vessel prominence may help distinguish LSIL from metaplasia.

MICROSCOPIC FEATURES

Cytology

Lesional cells demonstrate nuclear enlargement (>3 times normal intermediate nuclei), anisonucleosis, nuclear contour irregularity, coarse hyperchromasia, abundant dense cytoplasm (low N/C ratios), binucleation or multinucleation, and koilocytosis (crisp perinuclear cavitation with a dense, darkly stained peripheral rim of cytoplasm). Atypical squamous cells that do not meet these diagnostic criteria are designated atypical squamous cells of undetermined significance (ASC-US).

Histology

The maturing squamous epithelium demonstrates acanthosis and cytologic atypia most conspicuously at the superficial layers (Fig. 1A). Disarray of nuclear distribution is perceivable from low power. On higher power, the nuclei demonstrate anisonucleosis, hyperchromasia, coarse chromatin, occasional binucleation or multinucleation, and koilocytosis, which are features similar to those seen on cytology. These cytopathic changes are most prominently seen in the superficial epithelial layers of lesions involving maturing squamous epithelium and are more subtle in areas of immature squamous metaplasia (see later discussion in the differential diagnosis sections of cervical LSIL and HSIL). The basal layer may exhibit a subtle expansion (limited to the lower one-third of the epithelial thickness) but the cells are usually evenly aligned and demonstrate minimal cytologic atypia. Mitotic activity is typically confined to the base. The lesions may be flat or exophytic (condyloma).

DIFFERENTIAL DIAGNOSIS

Versus Reactive Mimics

Glycogenation of normal maturing squamous epithelium (Fig. 1D), as well as small, indistinct perinuclear halos seen in reactive squamous epithelium, may mimic koilocytic changes. If perinuclear cytoplasmic clearing is appreciated at low power, nuclear atypia as previously defined needs to be confirmed at high-power examination for the diagnosis of LSIL; the presence of perinuclear halos in the absence of nuclear atypia is not sufficient for the diagnosis of LSIL. Although the lower end of nuclear atypia seen in LSIL may overlap with the higher end of reactive atypia, significant nuclear size variation (vs uniformly enlarged nuclei) and disarrayed nuclear distribution (vs uniform distribution) can be helpful in distinguishing low-grade dysplastic changes from reactive changes. Mild nuclear atypia in the background of severe inflammation favors reactive changes. Especially in the setting of severe inflammation and ulceration, the viral cytopathic changes of herpes simplex virus (multinucleation, chromatin margination, and nuclear molding) and cytomegalovirus (cellular enlargement, nuclear inclusions with owl's eye morphology) should be considered and excluded.

Versus High-Grade Squamous Intraepithelial Lesion

The LAST project recommends the classification of LSIL-appearing lesions with marked cytologic atypia (Fig. 1B) or atypical mitotic figures as HSIL. The literature on this topic is sparse; however, Park and colleagues[7] found that LSIL with marked cytologic atypia (5 or more cells with nuclear enlargement of at least 5 times the size of an intermediate cell nucleus or multinucleation with 5 or more nuclei) may have a higher rate of progression to HSIL. In contrast, a study by Fadare and Rodriguez[8] found no difference in progression to HSIL based on the presence of marked cytologic atypia in LSILs. Given that (1) there is no significant body of evidence establishing the progressive potential of LSIL with marked atypia, (2) the inherently subjective nature of atypia classification is expected to cause issues with reproducibility, and (3) patients with an LSIL diagnosis are initially followed with increased frequency,[9] the author recommends designating these lesions as LSIL to prevent overtreatment.

A major distinguishing factor of LSIL from HSIL is epithelial (squamous) maturation. Therefore, LSIL involving areas of immature metaplasia (Fig. 1C) may mimic HSIL due to lack of prominent squamous maturation (see later discussion in HSIL differential diagnosis).

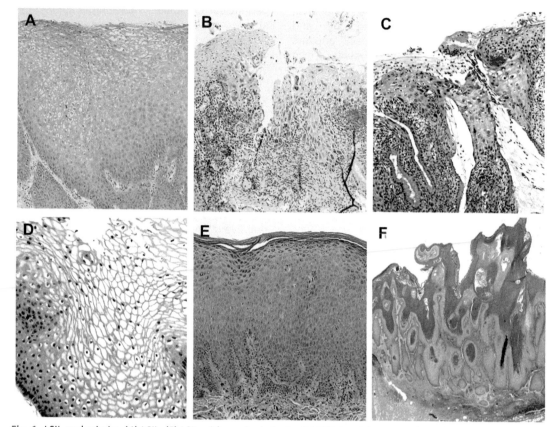

Fig. 1. LSIL and mimics. (*A*) LSIL. (*B*) LSIL with marked atypia. (*C*) LSIL involving metaplasia. (*D*) Squamous mucosa with glycogenation. (*E*) Lichen simplex chronicus (LSC). (*F*) Verrucous carcinoma.

DIAGNOSIS

The diagnosis of LSIL relies on hematoxylin-eosin (H&E) morphology. The LAST project specifically discourages the use of p16 immunohistochemical stain for the diagnosis of LSIL because it may demonstrate block-positive, patchy, or completely negative p16 expression and, in the context of a morphologic LSIL, the p16 staining pattern is not predictive of outcome. Therefore, a negative p16 result (patchy or complete absence of staining) should not serve as justification to downgrade a lesion to be negative or reactive, and a positive p16 result (strong and diffuse nuclear and cytoplasmic staining, block-positivity) should not serve as justification to upgrade a lesion to HSIL.

PROGNOSIS

Most cervical LSILs regress spontaneously (60%) with much less persistence (30%) and progression (10% to HSIL, 1% to invasive carcinoma) compared with HSIL.[10] In keeping with this favorable prognosis, an LSIL

diagnosis on cytology and/or histology are generally amenable to increased screening frequency without a diagnostic excisional procedure.

Key Features
Low-Grade Squamous
Intraepithelial Lesion

Biology

Transient HPV infection with high rate of regression

Morphology

Low-power

- Thickened mucosa

- Irregularly dispersed, enlarged hyperchromatic nuclei with cytoplasmic halos in upper layers

- Lower third without significant squamous maturation, mitotic figures usually limited to lower layer

High-power

- Enlarged nuclei with coarse chromatin, irregular nuclear contours

- Binucleation

- Sharply punched out nuclear halos (koilocytosis)

HIGH-GRADE SQUAMOUS INTRAEPITHELIAL LESION

GROSS FEATURES

On colposcopy, HSIL appears distinctly acetowhite (opaque vs the slightly translucent white color of LSIL and immature metaplasia) for a longer time. These features are largely due to the increased density of abnormal nuclei in the lesion. The margins are almost always well-defined and possibly raised. Abnormalities in the vessels may be seen due to the expansile growth of neoplastic epithelium occluding blood flow, causing vessel prominence and irregular distribution.

MICROSCOPIC FEATURES

Cytology

Lesional cells are basaloid and may be present as single cells, sheets, or syncytial crowded aggregates. The nuclei are typically hyperchromatic, coarsely chromatic, have irregular nuclear contours, demonstrate anisonucleosis, and are overall enlarged but not always to the degree of LSIL nuclei. The high N/C ratio is a defining feature of HSIL; the cytoplasm frequently appears dense and metaplastic but may also be keratinizing or delicate. Atypical squamous epithelium with some of the previous features (ie, high N/C ratio) but not sufficient for the diagnosis of HSIL are designated atypical squamous cells–cannot exclude HSIL (ASC-H).

Histology

On low power, acanthotic squamous mucosa characterized by a crowded proliferation of atypical basaloid cells lacking any significant squamous maturation is seen (**Fig. 2**A); some hyperkeratotic cytoplasmic maturation may be seen in the upper one-third layer. On higher power, the irregular, hyperchromatic, and coarsely chromatic nuclei demonstrate variable degrees of anisonucleosis. Nucleoli are generally inconspicuous. Cytoplasm is scant (high N/C ratio) with indistinct cytoplasmic borders, imparting a syncytial appearance. The nuclei are overlapping and demonstrate loss of epithelial polarity. Dyskeratotic cells and mitotic figures, including atypical forms, may be seen in all layers of the epithelium.

DIFFERENTIAL DIAGNOSIS

Atrophy and Immature Squamous Metaplasia

CIN2 is a poorly reproducible, indeterminate diagnostic category that has no biological correlate (**Fig. 2**B). The designation likely represents a mixture of morphologically equivocal reactive lesions, LSIL, and HSIL. As expected, the risk of progression of CIN2 is intermediate between CIN1 and CIN3.[10] The LAST project recommendation to retain the CIN2 designation is mainly to accommodate the current guideline to conservatively manage young, reproductive-age women with CIN2.[9] Although CIN2 has no defining criteria, the author conceptualizes the designation as a morphologically low-end HSIL, which may be practically described as a CIN3 that lacks significant cytologic atypia, with maintained epithelial polarity and a greater degree of squamous maturation in the superficial layers. This appearance may closely mimic other physiologic conditions that lack significant squamous maturation, such as atrophy and immature squamous metaplasia. Notably, true atrophic changes are seen more diffusely and should lack mitotic activity. Superimposed inflammatory or reactive changes may make these nondysplastic processes morphologically indistinguishable from CIN2 without the aid of ancillary studies. The LAST project recommends the use of p16 immunohistochemical stain when the pathologist is considering a diagnosis of CIN2 to prevent the overcalling of such benign mimics. The definition of p16 positivity is strong and diffuse nuclear and cytoplasmic staining, termed block-positivity (**Fig. 3**A). Cytoplasmic only and patchy or focal (**Fig. 3**B) staining patterns are considered negative. Diagnostic discrepancies arise most commonly in these morphologically ambiguous situations, and p16 may also be used as an adjudication tool for professional disagreement. Block-positive p16 staining should be used to confirm the morphologic impression of a CIN2 with the understanding that p16 positivity has no prognostically predictive value outside of its morphologic context; rather, the superb negative predictive value of p16 is of essence here, helping exclude benign mimics in the setting of a histologic lesion that is suspicious for high-grade dysplasia.

Key Features
CRITERIA FOR USE AND INTERPRETATION OF P16

Positive p16

Strong, diffuse nuclear and cytoplasmic staining (block-positive)

Negative p16

Absent, focal, patchy, and cytoplasmic-only staining.

Use p16

- To confirm the diagnosis of CIN2

- To exclude benign mimics such as atrophy, immature metaplasia, and so forth

- As an adjudication tool for professional disagreement

- LSIL or less biopsy diagnosis in the setting of a high-risk Papanicolaou (Pap) test result (HSIL, ASC-H, ASC-US or HPV 16+, atypical glandular cells)

Do not use p16

- Morphologically unequivocal LSIL, HSIL, negative

- LSIL versus reactive

- LSIL versus HSIL

Low-Grade Squamous Intraepithelial Lesion Involving Metaplasia

The cervix is composed of squamous, transformation zone, and endocervical mucosa. Within the transformation zone is a population of embryonically derived cells termed SCJ cells. Most HSIL and squamous cell carcinoma are now thought to arise from this unique cell population,[6,11] which explains the topographic propensity of cervical carcinoma to arise within the transformation zone. LSIL derived from these SCJ cells or involving immature squamous metaplasia may lack obvious squamous maturation and could be confused with HSIL (see **Fig. 1**C, top right area). It is emphasized here that p16 should not be used to differentiate LSIL from HSIL. LSILs in this setting may frequently demonstrate p16 block positivity and the distinction needs to be made on morphology. Although metaplastic LSIL may mimic HSIL on low-power evaluation, high-power evaluation reveals neither significant cytologic atypia nor expansion of the basal layer cells. The nuclei maintain polarity and are evenly spaced. Subtle squamous maturation is seen past the basal or parabasal layers with perceptible increase in cytoplasmic volume and eosinophilia. The superficial-most cells may demonstrate some koilocytic changes but these findings are usually more subtle given that viral cytopathic effect depends on epithelial maturation.

Squamous Intraepithelial Lesion, Indeterminate Grade

The reader may question if there is any meaningful difference between CIN2 and a squamous intraepithelial lesion (SIL) of indeterminate grade (**Fig. 2**F). In keeping with the LAST project recommendations, a CIN2 designation implies commitment to an HSIL diagnosis and its associated management. SIL, indeterminate grade, makes no such commitment and its use is only appropriate when evaluation is limited by the quality of the specimen. Some scenarios in which the author uses this designation include (1) significant erosion is appreciated in the setting of a thin, dysplastic epithelium and (2) detached, unoriented fragments of dysplastic epithelium are present. In the first scenario, although the thin dysplastic epithelium may appear to demonstrate the full-thickness atypia (suggestive of HSIL), this may represent just the basal layer of an eroded LSIL. In the second scenario, the detached and unoriented nature of the dysplastic epithelium precludes optimal evaluation of squamous maturation. The immunohistochemistry of p16 cannot resolve these issues. Rather, repeat sampling can potentially resolve these issues and a diagnostic comment suggesting consideration for rebiopsy may be appropriate.

Stratified Mucin-Producing Intraepithelial Lesion

Stratified mucin-producing intraepithelial lesion (SMILE) is characterized by overlapping morphologic features of HSIL and adenocarcinoma in situ (AIS), in which stratified dysplastic epithelial cells with mucinous cytoplasmic vacuoles are seen throughout the epithelial thickness (**Fig. 2**C). Neither definite squamous differentiation nor gland formation is seen. This is an uncommon premalignant lesion that mimics HSIL and is considered a high-grade dysplasia of stem or reserve cells with potential for multidirectional differentiation.[12,13] It may be seen in association with HSIL and AIS, as well as invasive squamous cell carcinoma, adenocarcinoma, and adenosquamous carcinoma. Given its diffuse mucin production and lack of definitive squamous differentiation by immunohistochemistry, it is currently considered a stratified variant of AIS for management purposes.

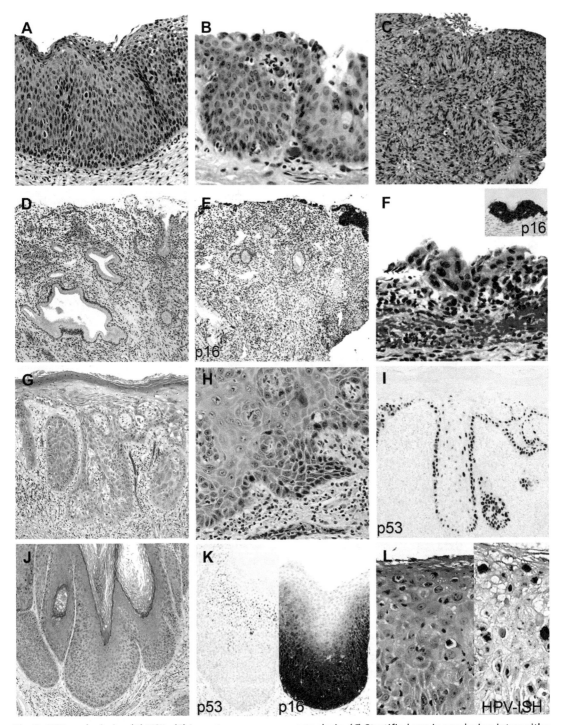

Fig. 2. HSIL and mimics. (*A*) HSIL. (*B*) Immature squamous metaplasia. (*C*) Stratified mucin-producing intraepithelial lesion. (*D, E*) HSIL that may be missed without p16. (*F*) Squamous intraepithelial lesion, indeterminate grade. (*G, H*) Differentiated vulvar intraepithelial neoplasia (dVIN). (*I*) p53 staining pattern in dVIN. (*J*) HSIL with superimposed LSC. (*K*) HSIL with superimposed LSC; p53 (*left*) and p16 (*right*). (*L*) HSIL with pagetoid spread (*left*) and HPV–in situ hybridization (*right*).

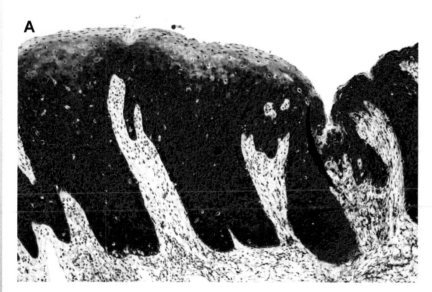

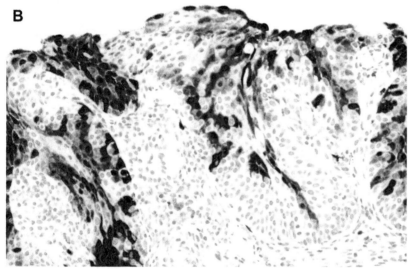

Fig. 3. p16 interpretation. (A) Diffuse nuclear and cytoplasmic p16 positivity (block-positive). (B) Patchy staining is interpreted as negative.

DIAGNOSIS

The diagnosis of HSIL relies on H&E morphology with the option of confirmation by p16 immunohistochemical stain for cases in which (1) the pathologist is considering a diagnosis of CIN2, (2) benign mimics need to be excluded, or (3) there is professional disagreement. Additionally, the use of p16 is recommended if a colposcopy was performed for a prior cytologic interpretation of HSIL, ASC-H, ASC-US positive for HPV 16, or atypical glandular cells, and if the biopsy is interpreted as LSIL or nonlesional. In this situation, p16 may pick-up an area of high-grade dysplasia missed on initial review

(Fig. 2D, E). HSIL involving areas of thin epithelium, as well as small foci of HSIL, in a background of inflammation are common scenarios in which dysplasia is missed on initial review. Of course, the area of p16 block-positivity must be rereviewed on H&E to confirm that the lesion qualifies morphologically as HSIL.

In the author's practice, if the colposcopic biopsy is interpreted as negative (based on H&E and p16), the prior high-risk Pap test is also reviewed. In some cases, the atypical cells may correlate with reactive cells seen on the biopsy specimen, in which case the correlated findings are reported in a diagnostic comment. In other cases, the atypical cells are truly worrisome for a high-grade lesion and are not represented in the colposcopic biopsy specimen. In such cases, the discrepancy is noted in the diagnostic comment and consideration for additional sampling to exclude the possibility of an unsampled lesion is suggested. Although such reviews of discordant Pap test and biopsy results are required by regulatory bodies, the timing is not specified; the author chooses to correlate (high-risk Pap test and negative biopsy) at the time of biopsy review because the results can change immediate management.

PROGNOSIS

HSIL precedes most invasive squamous cell carcinomas and, without treatment, 30% of untreated HSIL become invasive carcinoma within 30 years; however, adequate treatment reduces this risk to 0.7%, which emphasizes the overall preventable nature of cervical cancer, as well as the critical importance of screening and treatment.[14]

Key Features
HIGH-GRADE SQUAMOUS INTRAEPITHELIAL LESION

Biology
  Persistent HPV infection and viral genome integration with a high rate of progression to invasive carcinoma

Morphology
  Low-power
  • Thickened mucosa
  • Crowded proliferation of atypical basaloid cells with hyperchromatic irregular nuclei
  • Minimal squamous maturation; some keratinization may be seen in the superficial layers

  High-power
  • High nuclear to cytoplasmic ratios
  • Enlarged crowded nuclei with coarse chromatin and irregular nuclear contours
  • Dyskeratotic cells
  • Mitotic figures may be found in the all layers of the epithelium

INVASIVE SQUAMOUS CELL CARCINOMA

GROSS FEATURES

On colposcopy, invasive squamous cell carcinoma appears distinctly acetowhite; yellowish color may be seen in association with necrosis. The surface is irregular with granular texture, with erosions and frank necrosis in advanced disease. Markedly abnormal angioarchitecture is seen and may manifest as red coloration, as well as easy bleeding.

MICROSCOPIC FEATURES

Early stromal invasion is appreciated by irregular outpouching of dysplastic epithelium, frequently characterized by paradoxic maturation (abundant dense eosinophilic cytoplasm at the invasive front) and stromal response (inflammation, desmoplasia, and edema). Single dyskeratotic cells with nuclear atypia may also be seen infiltrating reactive stroma (**Fig. 4**). Large tumors may demonstrate infiltrative patterns with invasive tongues, a confluent pattern with solid growth, and a spray-bud pattern with numerous small nests.

DIFFERENTIAL DIAGNOSIS

Invasive squamous cell carcinoma may be mimicked by florid squamous metaplasia or SIL. Ectopic decidua in the setting of pregnancy may also mimic invasive nests of squamous cell carcinoma. Appropriate history and keratin immunohistochemical stain can resolve this issue.

The commonest pitfall for overcalling stromal invasion is tangential sectioning of HSIL with endocervical glandular involvement. The presence of adjacent partially involved glands, smooth or rounded contours, and maintained basal cell palisading at the periphery favor tangential sectioning with or without endocervical glandular involvement. Detached smooth-contoured nests may attach to adjacent endocervical crypts on deeper level sections.

DIAGNOSIS

Early cervical carcinomas are staged histologically, whereas larger tumors are staged clinically. Depth of invasion defines early stage tumors, which is measured from the base of the epithelium at the point of origin (squamous epithelium basement membrane or deepest point of endocervical glandular involvement) to the deepest extent of the invasive front. SISCCA corresponds to International Federation of Gynecology and Obstetrics (FIGO) stage IA1 and the American

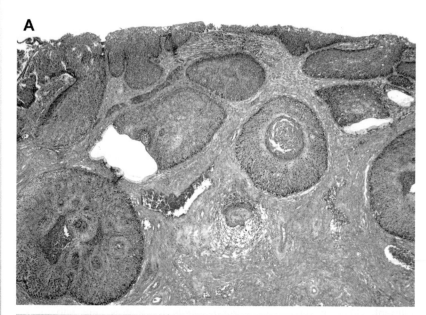

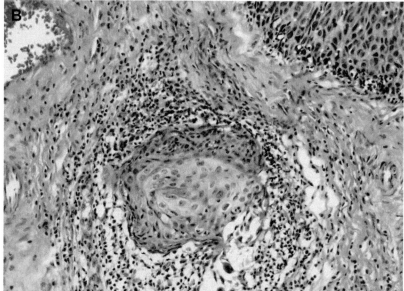

Fig. 4. (*A*) SISCCA and adjacent HSIL with expansile endocervical glandular involvement (*B*) Close-up view of invasive focus.

Joint Committee on Cancer (AJCC) tumor (T) stage 1a1, and is defined as follows by the LAST project:

- No grossly visible lesion
- Size measurement
  - Less than or equal to 3 mm in depth of invasion
  - Less than or equal to 7 mm in maximal linear extent
- Completely excised.

If the tumor is not completely visualized but otherwise meets size criteria, the tumor may be designated as at least SISCCA. If multiple foci of invasion are present, each focus is measured separately and the measurements are not added. The focality of the tumor, as well as presence of lymphovascular space invasion, should be noted, although neither changes the staging of the tumor.

PROGNOSIS

Stage is the most important prognostic factor for cervical cancer. FIGO stage IA1 tumors (SISCCA) have a negligible risk of nodal spread and may be treated conservatively by cone biopsy or LEEP if the resection margins are negative.

Key Features
SUPERFICIALLY INVASIVE SQUAMOUS CELL CARCINOMA

Cervix (AJCC T1a1, FIGO IA1)

- No grossly visible lesion
- Size measurement
  - Less than or equal to 3 mm in depth of invasion
  - Less than or equal to 7 mm in maximal extent
- Completely excised

Vagina

- No recommendations due to lack of data

Vulva (AJCC T1a, FIGO 1A)

- Tumor 2 cm or less in size
- Confined to the vulva or perineum
- Stromal invasion is 1 mm or less

Anus (AJCC T1)

- Size measurement
  - Less than or equal to 3 mm in depth of invasion
  - Less than or equal to 7 mm in maximal extent
- Completely excised

VAGINA

A unified 2-tiered nomenclature (previously described in the cervix section), qualified by the site-specific -IN designation is recommended for the classification of HPV-related squamous lesions of the vagina:

1. LSIL; VaIN 1
2. HSIL; VaIN 2–3.

HPV-related squamous lesions of the vagina are uncommon (incidence of 0.3–0.7 per 100,000[1]) and are seen most commonly in association with lesions of the cervix.

GROSS FEATURES

The vaginal mucosa is characterized by an undulating rugal pattern unlike the flat cervical mucosa. At the time of colposcopy, special attention is given to the upper third of the vagina where most lesions are identified. It is a site commonly subject to trauma (eg, intercourse, diaphragm, tampons) and inflammation or infection; the associated benign changes (abrasions, erythema, increased vascularity, bruising, petechiae, leukoplakia, thrush patches) must be distinguished from neoplastic lesions (see previous discussion described in the cervix section).[4]

MICROSCOPIC FEATURES

The vaginal mucosa is anatomically in continuation with the cervical mucosa and the nonkeratinizing squamous epithelium is microscopically indistinguishable. Likewise, the microscopic features of LSIL, HSIL, and invasive squamous cell carcinoma are identical to those of the cervix.

DIFFERENTIAL DIAGNOSIS

Although the morphologic features of HPV-related precancer and cancer of the vagina are identical to those of the cervix, the unique anatomic features of the vagina and their associated lesions raise a distinct set of differential diagnoses.

Squamous Metaplasia

There is no transformation zone in the vagina; however, glandular epithelium may be present in the form of vaginal adenosis. These benign endocervical or tuboendometrioid-type epithelium may give rise to squamous metaplasia, which could mimic HSIL. As in the cervix, immature squamous metaplasia is distinguished from HSIL by the lack of significant cytologic atypia, nuclear crowding, dyskeratosis, mitotic activity, and negative p16 staining. Although adenosis with florid metaplasia may mimic invasive squamous cell carcinoma, the lack of dysplastic cytologic features, as well as smooth epithelial contours and lack of stromal response would argue against invasive carcinoma.

Radiation Change

Postradiation atypia may be seen after treatment of cervical cancer, and is a common diagnostic challenge in the setting of surveillance Pap tests and biopsies. Although the atypia of radiation may be alarming, preserved N/C ratios (enlarged nucleus and cytoplasm), smudgy or degenerated chromatin, or metachromatic and vacuolated cytoplasm in the setting of known radiation should point the pathologist away from a diagnosis of dysplasia.

Prolapse

Acanthotic and hyperkeratotic or parakeratotic changes may be seen in the setting of prolapse and may mimic LSIL. Although superimposed reactive nuclear atypia may make the distinction challenging, significant anisonucleosis, coarse hyperchromasia, and architectural disarray are uncommonly seen in reactive processes.

Epithelial Polyps

Exophytic condylomas are classified as LSIL and are more commonly associated with low-risk HPVs (HPV 6 and 11). Fibroepithelial and tubulosquamous polyps of the vagina may architecturally mimic condylomas at low power. Fibroepithelial polyps (also commonly seen in the vulva) can be distinguished from condylomas based on the lack of bulbous rete and acanthosis. Surface glycogenation may mimic koilocytosis but the nuclei in glycogenation are typically centrally located and have smooth nuclear contours and bland or fine chromatin. Fibroepithelial stromal polyps can be recognized by the presence of stellate and multinucleated stromal cells, similar to those seen in the native vaginal stroma. Tubulosquamous polyps are thought to originate from the Skene glands, and are characterized by nests of glycogenated or nonglycogenated squamous cells, as well as small tubules lined by bland cuboidal cells. The appearance of this unique mixed epithelial polyp should be easily distinguishable from condylomas as long as one is aware of this entity.

DIAGNOSIS

The diagnosis of vaginal LSIL, HSIL, and squamous cell carcinoma largely mirror those of the cervix (see previous discussion).

PROGNOSIS

Most vaginal LSILs regress and are generally managed by observation. HSILs are more likely to progress and may be treated topically (5-fluorouracil, imiquimod), ablation (carbon dioxide laser), or surgical excision. The most important prognostic factor for vaginal squamous cell carcinoma is stage. Vaginal carcinomas are staged clinically, and there is currently no recommendation to classify a subset of these tumors as SISCCA. Given the rarity of primary vaginal squamous cell carcinoma, there is insufficient evidence to define early lesions for conservative treatment.

VULVA

Vulvar SILs are unique within the lower anogenital tract because there are at least 2 well-defined, major pathways for the development of dysplasia: HPV-dependent and HPV-independent. The HPV-dependent pathway is commonly referred to as classic or usual vulvar IN (VIN) and demonstrates biologic and morphologic characteristics in keeping with those previously described in the cervical and vaginal sections. Accordingly, a unified 2-tiered nomenclature, qualified by the site-specific -IN designation is recommended for the classification of HPV-related squamous lesions of the vulva:

1. LSIL; VIN 1
2. HSIL; VIN 2–3.

In contrast, the most well-defined non–HPV-dependent vulvar dysplasia is termed differentiated (or simplex) VIN (dVIN), and demonstrates epidemiology, biology, morphology, and clinical behavior that are distinct from the HPV-related lesions. The distinguishing features of these non–HPV-dependent lesions are discussed in the differential diagnosis section. (See Jaclyn C. Watkins's article, "HPV-Independent Squamous Lesions of the Vulva," in this issue.)

GROSS FEATURES

Plaque-like, papular, or verruciform lesions of variable color (white, pink, red, pigmented) may be present in association with itching or burning. The lesions may be barely visible or extensively involving the entire vulva. Multifocal lesions are common. Specifically, multifocal small cutaneous papules with the appearance of HSIL on histology are termed Bowenoid papulosis and represent a clinically distinct entity that has a high rate of spontaneous regression.[15] Therefore, although terminologies such as Bowen disease (a term traditionally used for cutaneous precancerous lesions) is no longer recommended, the designation of Bowenoid papulosis may warrant special consideration given its clinical significance and favorable natural history.

MICROSCOPIC FEATURES

The externally visible portion of the vulva is lined by squamous epithelium, which is nonkeratinized within the vulvar vestibule and keratinized elsewhere. Major and minor vestibular glands, paraurethral glands, and pilosebaceous units may be found within the subepithelial stromal tissue with connections to the squamous epithelium. Although surface keratinization is observed more frequently in cutaneous lesions, this does not reliably distinguish cutaneous from mucosal lesions. Warty changes (spiky surface with marked hyperkeratosis, and prominent granular layer) are more frequently seen but these features are also not specific to cutaneous lesions. Overall, the microscopic features of HPV-related vulvar squamous lesions are considered indistinguishable from those of other lower anogenital sites.

DIFFERENTIAL DIAGNOSIS

Differentiated Vulvar Intraepithelial Neoplasia

A critical differential diagnostic consideration for vulvar HSIL is dVIN. dVIN is an HPV-independent high-grade dysplastic lesion strongly linked to keratinizing squamous cell carcinoma (**Fig. 2**G–I). It predominantly occurs in postmenopausal women and is frequently seen arising in a background of chronic anogenital inflammatory skin disease such as lichen sclerosus. *TP53* mutations are often present, and the same mutation has been identified in dVIN and the adjacent invasive squamous cell carcinoma, supporting the progressive relationship between the 2 lesions.[16] dVIN is morphologically characterized by basal cell atypia (nuclear enlargement and elongation, hyperchromasia), abrupt and premature cytoplasmic maturation (marked increase in cytoplasmic volume and eosinophilia in the parabasal cells), and prominent intercellular bridges. Mitotic activity is usually limited to the basal and parabasal cells but dyskeratotic cells can be seen throughout the epithelial thickness. Low-power view demonstrates acanthosis with elongated, branching rete ridges. Immunohistochemical staining for p53 typically demonstrates abnormal staining in the form of strong continuous staining of the basal cells (with possible extension into the parabasal layers) or complete absence (consistent with null-mutation). In their most classic forms, HSIL and dVIN are not difficult to distinguish. However, basaloid forms of dVIN closely mimicking HSIL have been described.[17] Conversely, HSIL with superimposed lichen simplex chronicus (LSC) may be histologically indistinguishable from dVIN (**Fig. 2**J).[18] The use of p16 and p53 immunohistochemical stains make the distinction of HSIL and dVIN relatively straightforward, given that HSIL demonstrates p16 block positivity with negative p53 and dVIN demonstrates basal p53 positivity with negative p16. A potential pitfall here is a newly described p53 staining pattern seen in HSIL with superimposed LSC in which there is weak to moderate staining of parabasal and midepithelial cells with sparing of the basal layer (**Fig. 2**K); without careful evaluation, this may be misinterpreted as the basal layer p53 staining of dVIN.[18]

> ### Key Features
> #### DIFFERENTIATED VULVAR INTRAEPITHELIAL NEOPLASIA
>
> Biology
> - HPV-independent high-grade dysplastic squamous lesion strongly linked to keratinizing squamous cell carcinoma by association
> - Occurs in postmenopausal women and is frequently seen arising in a background of chronic anogenital inflammatory skin disease such as lichen sclerosus
> - *TP53* mutations are typically present
>
> Morphology
> Low-power
> - Elongated, branching rete ridges
> - Adjacent lichen sclerosus or invasive squamous cell carcinoma
>
> High-power
> - Nuclear atypia of the basal cell layer
>   - Hyperchromasia
>   - Enlargement or elongation
>   - Prominent nucleoli
> - Abnormal, abrupt epithelial maturation
>   - Enlarged keratinocytes with abundant markedly eosinophilic cytoplasm, enlarged nuclei, prominent nucleoli
>   - Loss of cellular cohesion
>   - Dyskeratosis, hyperkeratosis, or parakeratosis
> - Abnormal p53 expression by immunohistochemistry
>   - Strong, continuous p53 staining in the basal and parabasal layers
>   - Complete absence (null-pattern)

Reactive or Inflammatory Skin Conditions

LSC (**Fig. 1**E) is the histologic manifestation of chronic scratching and is characterized by epidermal hyperplasia with a prominent granular layer and overlying hyperkeratosis. Although acanthosis and reactive epithelial changes may be present, there is normal maturation of the keratinocytes and absence of significant, diffuse cytologic atypia. Reactive squamous epithelium tends to be spongiotic with visible nucleoli, whereas the cytoplasm of HSIL tends to be syncytial and nucleoli are not conspicuous. Block positive p16 staining may easily distinguish HSIL versus reactive changes. If reactive, special stains, such as periodic acid-Schiff stain with diastase (PAS-D) and Gomori methenamine silver stain to exclude fungal infection is recommended in this setting.

Seborrheic Keratosis

Seborrheic keratosis consists of a proliferation of basaloid epithelial cells leading to a thickened epidermis with keratin horn cysts and bland nuclear features, as well as a flattened interface with the dermis. The surface exhibits basket-weave orthokeratosis but no parakeratosis or compact hyperkeratosis. There is significant morphologic overlap with condyloma (especially those with minimal cytopathic changes) and, in fact, whether or not vulvar seborrheic keratosis represents HPV-related lesions is controversial because studies have detected HPV (mostly type 6) in a significant subset of genital seborrheic keratosis.[19,20] The distinction here may not be critical for clinical management because both lesions have low risks of progression to carcinoma, although inappropriate labeling of a lesion as associated with a sexually transmitted disease may have social implications.

Versus Well-Differentiated Verrucopapillary Neoplasms

Giant condyloma (Buschke-Lowenstein tumor) and verrucous carcinoma can be difficult to distinguish histologically from exophytic condylomas on a superficial biopsy specimen. Verrucous carcinoma and giant condyloma are considered by some to be synonymous in the anogenital region; however, the author thinks they are best classified as different entities distinguished by HPV-status. Verrucous carcinoma is not HPV-associated[21,22] and is a tumor characterized by markedly acanthotic squamous epithelium that invades underlying stromal tissue with a broad, well-defined pushing border (Fig. 1F). By definition, cytologic atypia (including viral cytopathic change) is not present in verrucous carcinoma. Clinical history is essential because verrucous carcinomas can present as what seems to be a slow-growing, large condyloma that recurs and is resistant or poorly responsive to therapy. In contrast, giant condylomas are commonly associated with low-risk HPV (HPV 6 or 11)[23] and demonstrate exophytic growth with viral cytopathic effect. Giant condylomas can be indistinguishable from typical condylomas on small biopsies without the clinical context of a large mass. Rare cases of invasive squamous cell carcinomas arising from giant condylomas have been reported.

Versus Extramammary Paget Disease

Extramammary Paget disease (EMPD) is an epidermotropic apocrine neoplasm characterized by large malignant cells scattered throughout the epidermis singly and as small nests. The neoplastic cells have enlarged nuclei, vesicular chromatin, prominent nuclei, and abundant pale cytoplasm with occasional intracytoplasmic vacuoles. Typical EMPD mimics include synchronous or metachronous colorectal or urothelial primaries with pagetoid spread. However, rare cases of HSIL with pagetoid growth pattern have been seen, in which the dysplastic squamous cells (with dense to unusually pale cytoplasm) are dispersed singly and in nests throughout the epithelial thickness (Fig. 2L). In this setting, HPV in situ hybridization (ISH) may be the most useful ancillary study because EMPD and secondary EMPD are not HPV-related neoplasms. Potential pitfalls of other more commonly used immunohistochemical stains include p16 positivity in a rare subset of EMPD and Cytokeratin 7 (CK7) positivity in some HSILs. Pagetoid spread of urothelial carcinoma can be particularly treacherous because urothelial carcinoma can be p16 and p63 positive, and HSIL can be weakly GATA3 positive.

DIAGNOSIS

The diagnoses of vulvar LSIL and HSIL rely primarily on H&E morphology and selected use of the p16 immunohistochemical stain as recommended by the LAST project. Given the host of other neoplastic mimics, vulvar HSIL may require additional studies such as p53 immunohistochemistry and HPV-ISH.

SISCCA of the vulva corresponds to AJCC T1a and FIGO 1A and is defined as

- Tumor 2 cm or less in size
- Confined to the vulva or perineum
- Stromal invasion is 1 mm or less (depth of invasion is defined as the distance from the adjacent superficial most epithelial-stromal interface of the dermal papillae to the deepest point of invasion).

SISCCA may be treated by excision alone without lymph node dissection. Similar to endocervical glandular involvement, tangential sectioning of vulvar HSIL involving pilosebaceous units may mimic superficial invasion.

PROGNOSIS

Vulvar LSIL is expected to regress in most cases and progression to HSIL is rare. Although the natural history of untreated HSIL is unclear owing to the ethical considerations of investigative trials, a significant portion is expected to progress to invasive carcinoma with transit time to invasion less than 8 years.[24] Given the potential of occult invasion, wide-local excision with negative margins (0.5–1.0 cm from visible lesion) is the preferred treatment, although ablation and topical treatments may be considered in cases without concern for invasion.[25] Of note, dVIN is thought to have a significantly higher and faster rate of progression to invasive carcinoma compared with vulvar HSIL,[26] emphasizing the importance of timely recognition of dVIN.

ANAL CANAL AND PERIANUS

Anal cancer incidence has been rapidly increasing by about 2% per year in the last several decades and its risk is alarmingly high among HIV-positive men who have sex with men, with an incidence of 131 per 100,000.[27] Most anal carcinoma is squamous cell carcinoma (85%), of which approximately 90% is attributable to HPV infection.[1,28] HPV-related anal and perianal SILs are considered biologically and morphologically equivalent to lesions arising in all other sites of the lower anogenital tract. A unified 2-tiered nomenclature (as described in the cervix section), qualified by the site-specific -IN designation is recommended for the classification of HPV-related squamous lesions of the anal canal and perianus:

1. LSIL; anal intraepithelial neoplasia 1 (AIN 1) or perianal intraepithelial neoplasia 1 (PAIN 1)
2. HSIL; AIN 2–3 or PAIN 2–3.

GROSS FEATURES

High-resolution anoscopy (HRA) may be used to visualize the anal canal for biopsies. Similar to colposcopy, acetic acid is applied to observe differential acetowhite changes and blood vessel abnormalities. The anal transitional zone (ATZ) is a region of squamous metaplasia that extends from the dentate line (old squamocolumnar junction) to the new squamocolumnar junction, which is the most important and readily identifiable landmark at the time of anoscopy because most lesions are thought to arise in this region. Additionally, the site of origin (above or below the dentate line) is clinically significant because the dentate line marks the division of vascular, lymphatic, and neural supply. Lesions arising above the dentate line spread primarily to the internal iliac nodes, whereas those arising below spread primarily to the superficial inguinal nodes.

MICROSCOPIC FEATURES

The anal canal is composed of 4 histologic zones (from proximal to distal): (1) colorectal zone, (2) ATZ, (3) squamous zone, and (4) perianal skin. Although the colorectal and squamous zone or perianal skin are defined by epithelial type (pure glandular and squamous epithelium, respectively), the ATZ is defined by its relative location to the adjacent histologic zones because the epithelial types present in this zone are variable. The ATZ is composed of a mixed population of the prototypical ATZ epithelium (multilayered columnar to cuboidal cells with an underlying squamous-type basal cell layer), squamous epithelium (immature metaplastic or glycogenated), and glandular (colorectal) epithelium. The SCJ cells appear unique to the cervix; an analogous cell population with similar topographic distribution is not present in the anal canal.[29] These subtle differences in cervical and anal epithelium may help explain the significantly lower incidence of anal cancer compared with cervical cancer despite an ostensibly similar microanatomy with squamocolumnar junctions.

LSIL, HSIL, and invasive squamous cell carcinoma arising from the ATZ, squamous zone, and perianal skin cannot be reliably distinguished but, in general, those arising from the ATZ and squamous zone tend to resemble cervical lesions, and those arising from the perianal skin tend to resemble cutaneous vulvar lesions.

DIFFERENTIAL DIAGNOSIS

The differential diagnosis of SIL arising from the ATZ and squamous zones overlap with those arising in the cervix and revolve around the diagnostic challenges associated with immature squamous metaplasia (see cervix section). The differential diagnosis of SIL arising from the perianal skin overlap with those arising in the vulva, and include fibroepithelial polyps, LSC, seborrheic keratosis, well-differentiated verrucopapillary neoplasms, and EMPD (see vulva section). Although a small subset of anal squamous cell carcinoma is HPV-independent, an in situ lesion analogous to dVIN has not yet been identified.

Reactive Anal Transitional Zone Epithelium

The ATZ epithelium is unique to the anal canal and raises diagnostic issues similar to those of immature squamous metaplasia given its stratified appearance without significant squamous epithelial maturation. A useful diagnostic tool to distinguish reactive ATZ from HSIL may be p16. LSIL arising from ATZ appear similar to metaplastic LSIL of the cervix and may be confused with

HSIL; the use of p16 is inappropriate in this setting because the distinction must be based on morphologic features.

Hemorrhoids

Hemorrhoids may mimic a condyloma (LSIL) on low power. They are common in the perianal region and are recognizable by the markedly dilated vessels that are often thrombosed. The epithelium may be acanthotic but lacks papillary projections and bulbous rete. The nuclei are typically bland, except reactive nuclear atypia can be seen in inflamed hemorrhoids.

DIAGNOSIS

The diagnosis of anal LSIL and HSIL rely primarily on H&E morphology and selected use of p16 immunohistochemistry as recommended by the LAST project. SISCCA of the anus is defined as

- Size measurement
  - Less than or equal to 3 mm in depth of invasion
  - Less than or equal to 7 mm in maximal linear extent
- Completely excised.

SISCCA of the anal canal is included in the T1 category (tumor less than or equal to 2 cm), which is not further subdivided. There is specific treatment recommendation for SISCCA of the anal canal and, given the limited outcome data available, the defining measurements are largely based on cervical data. The intention here is to collect prospective data on this early invasive category that may be amenable to conservative therapy, given the morbidity associated with surgical procedures of the anal canal.

PROGNOSIS

The natural history of anal SIL is not well-characterized. Although LSIL is generally thought to have a low rate of progression at other anogenital sites, anal LSIL may be associated with a higher rate of progression to HSIL,[30] possibly due a combination of the immunocompromised status of the susceptible population (eg, HIV-positive, transplant), as well as the technical challenges of the HRA-guided biopsies. The progression of HSIL to invasive carcinoma seems to take approximately 5 years,[31] although well-controlled prospective studies are lacking. Currently, there is no standardized screening program implemented for the prevention of anal cancer. To address this issue, a multicenter phase III clinical trial, the Anal Cancer/HSIL Outcomes Research (ANCHOR) study, is currently underway.[32]

REFERENCES

1. Parkin DM, Bray F. Chapter 2: the burden of HPV-related cancers. Vaccine 2006;24(Suppl 3). S3/11–25.
2. Darragh TM, Colgan TJ, Thomas Cox J, et al. The Lower Anogenital Squamous Terminology Standardization project for HPV-associated lesions: background and consensus recommendations from the College of American Pathologists and the American Society for Colposcopy and Cervical Pathology. Int J Gynecol Pathol 2013;32(1):76–115.
3. Wilbur DC, Nayar R. Bethesda 2014: improving on a paradigm shift. Cytopathology 2015;26(6):339–42.
4. American Society for Colposcopy and Cervical Pathology, Mayeaux EJ, Thomas Cox J. Modern colposcopy textbook and atlas. Lippincott Williams & Wilkins; 2011.
5. Marsh M. Original site of cervical carcinoma; topographical relationship of carcinoma of the cervix to the external os and to the squamocolumnar junction. Obstet Gynecol 1956;7(4):444–52.
6. Herfs M, Yamamoto Y, Laury A, et al. A discrete population of squamocolumnar junction cells implicated in the pathogenesis of cervical cancer. Proc Natl Acad Sci U S A 2012;109(26):10516–21.
7. Park K, Ellenson LH, Pirog EC. Low-grade squamous intraepithelial lesions of the cervix with marked cytological atypia-clinical follow-up and human papillomavirus genotyping. Int J Gynecol Pathol 2007;26(4):457–62.
8. Fadare O, Rodriguez R. The significance of marked nuclear atypia in grade 1 cervical intraepithelial neoplasia. Hum Pathol 2009;40(10):1487–93.
9. Saslow D, Solomon D, Lawson HW, et al. American Cancer Society, American Society for Colposcopy and Cervical Pathology, and American Society for Clinical Pathology screening guidelines for the prevention and early detection of cervical cancer. Am J Clin Pathol 2012;137(4):516–42.
10. Ostör AG. Natural history of cervical intraepithelial neoplasia: a critical review. Int J Gynecol Pathol 1993;12(2):186–92.
11. Herfs M, Vargas SO, Yamamoto Y, et al. A novel blueprint for "top down" differentiation defines the cervical squamocolumnar junction during development, reproductive life, and neoplasia. J Pathol 2013;229(3):460–8.
12. Park JJ, Sun D, Quade BJ, et al. Stratified mucin-producing intraepithelial lesions of the cervix: adenosquamous or columnar cell neoplasia? Am J Surg Pathol 2000;24(10):1414–9.
13. Boyle DP, McCluggage WG. Stratified mucin-producing intraepithelial lesion (SMILE): report of a

case series with associated pathological findings. Histopathology 2015;66(5):658–63.

14. McCredie MRE, Sharples KJ, Paul C, et al. Natural history of cervical neoplasia and risk of invasive cancer in women with cervical intraepithelial neoplasia 3: a retrospective cohort study. Lancet Oncol 2008;9(5):425–34.

15. Ackerman AB. Bowenoid papulosis. JAMA 1981; 246(7):732.

16. Pinto AP, Miron A, Yassin Y, et al. Differentiated vulvar intraepithelial neoplasia contains Tp53 mutations and is genetically linked to vulvar squamous cell carcinoma. Mod Pathol 2010;23(3):404–12.

17. Ordi J, Alejo M, Fusté V, et al. HPV-negative vulvar intraepithelial neoplasia (VIN) with basaloid histologic pattern: an unrecognized variant of simplex (differentiated) VIN. Am J Surg Pathol 2009;33(11): 1659–65.

18. Watkins JC, Yang E, Crum CP, et al. Classic vulvar intraepithelial neoplasia with superimposed lichen simplex chronicus: a unique variant mimicking differentiated vulvar intraepithelial neoplasia. Int J Gynecol Pathol 2018. https://doi.org/10.1097/PGP. 0000000000000509.

19. Tardío JC, Bancalari E, Moreno A, et al. Genital seborrheic keratoses are human papillomavirus-related lesions. A linear array genotyping test study. APMIS 2012;120(6):477–83.

20. Reutter JC, Geisinger KR, Laudadio J. Vulvar seborrheic keratosis: is there a relationship to human papillomavirus? J Low Genit Tract Dis 2014;18(2): 190–4.

21. del Pino M, Bleeker MCG, Quint WG, et al. Comprehensive analysis of human papillomavirus prevalence and the potential role of low-risk types in verrucous carcinoma. Mod Pathol 2012;25(10):1354–63.

22. Zidar N, Langner C, Odar K, et al. Anal verrucous carcinoma is not related to infection with human papillomaviruses and should be distinguished from giant condyloma (Buschke-Löwenstein tumour). Histopathology 2017;70(6):938–45.

23. Wells M, Robertson S, Lewis F, et al. Squamous carcinoma arising in a giant peri-anal condyloma associated with human papillomavirus types 6 and 11. Histopathology 1988;12(3):319–23.

24. Jones RW, Rowan DM, Stewart AW. Vulvar intraepithelial neoplasia: aspects of the natural history and outcome in 405 women. Obstet Gynecol 2005; 106(6):1319–26.

25. American College of Obstetricians and Gynecologists' Committee on Gynecologic Practice, American Society for Colposcopy and Cervical Pathology (ASCCP). Committee opinion no.675: management of vulvar intraepithelial neoplasia. Obstet Gynecol 2016;128(4):e178–82.

26. McAlpine JN, Kim SY, Akbari A, et al. HPV-independent differentiated vulvar intraepithelial neoplasia (dVIN) is associated with an aggressive clinical course. Int J Gynecol Pathol 2017;36(6): 507–16.

27. Silverberg MJ, Lau B, Justice AC, et al. Risk of anal cancer in HIV-infected and HIV-uninfected individuals in North America. Clin Infect Dis 2012;54(7): 1026–34.

28. Hoots BE, Palefsky JM, Pimenta JM, et al. Human papillomavirus type distribution in anal cancer and anal intraepithelial lesions. Int J Cancer 2009; 124(10):2375–83.

29. Yang EJ, Quick MC, Hanamornroongruang S, et al. Microanatomy of the cervical and anorectal squamocolumnar junctions: a proposed model for anatomical differences in HPV-related cancer risk. Mod Pathol 2015;28(7):994–1000.

30. Palefsky JM, Holly EA, Ralston ML, et al. High incidence of anal high-grade squamous intra-epithelial lesions among HIV-positive and HIV-negative homosexual and bisexual men. AIDS 1998;12(5): 495–503.

31. Berry JM, Jay N, Cranston RD, et al. Progression of anal high-grade squamous intraepithelial lesions to invasive anal cancer among HIV-infected men who have sex with men. Int J Cancer 2014;134(5): 1147–55.

32. Palefsky JM. Screening to prevent anal cancer: current thinking and future directions. Cancer Cytopathol 2015;123(9):509–10.

Cervical Glandular Neoplasia
Classification and Staging

Gulisa Turashvili, MD, PhD, FRCPC[a], Kay J. Park, MD[b],*

KEYWORDS

- Cervical adenocarcinoma • Human papillomavirus • Classification • Staging

Key points

- Endocervical adenocarcinomas can be broadly divided into human papillomavirus (HPV) -driven and non-HPV-driven groups harboring distinct clinicopathologic features and prognosis.
- The International Endocervical Adenocarcinoma Criteria and Classification system integrates morphology, cause/pathogenesis, and biological behavior of these subtypes.
- Clinical staging of endocervical adenocarcinoma is problematic, and accurate pathologic staging is crucial for optimal clinical management and prognostication.
- The pattern-based classification of endocervical adenocarcinoma identifies a subset of patients with good clinical outcomes who could be treated conservatively.

ABSTRACT

Endocervical adenocarcinomas (EAs) account for 25% of all primary cervical carcinomas. Approximately 85% of EAs are driven by high-risk human papillomavirus (HPV) infection, the most common of which is the so-called usual type endocervical adenocarcinomas. Non-HPV-driven subtypes harbor distinct clinicopathologic features and prognosis and have been increasingly recognized in recent years, which has led to efforts to improve classification of EA based on clinically relevant and reproducible criteria. This review discusses a recently proposed classification system, the International Endocervical Adenocarcinoma Criteria and Classification, which uniquely integrates morphology, cause/pathogenesis, and biological behavior of HPV and non-HPV-driven subtypes of EA.

OVERVIEW

Endocervical adenocarcinomas (EAs) account for 25% of all primary carcinomas of the uterine cervix.[1] Although the role of high-risk human papillomavirus (HPV) infection in the pathogenesis of EA is well known,[2–5] increasing recognition of non-HPV-driven subtypes harboring distinct clinicopathologic features and prognosis[6–8] has led to efforts to improve classification of EA based on clinically relevant and reproducible criteria.

The current World Health Organization (WHO) classification of cervical tumors categorizes EAs based on morphologic (predominantly cytoplasmic) features.[3] Its major limitations are bypassing current evidence for different pathogenetic mechanisms in various subtypes, unclear definitions, and questionable reproducibility

Disclosure Statement: The authors have nothing to disclose. This research was funded in part through the NIH/NCI Cancer Center Support Grant P30 CA008748.

[a] Department of Pathology and Laboratory Medicine, Mount Sinai Hospital, University of Toronto, 600 University Avenue, Toronto, Ontario M5G 1X5, Canada; [b] Department of Pathology, Memorial Sloan Kettering Cancer Center, 1275 York Avenue, New York, NY 10065, USA

* Corresponding author.

E-mail address: parkk@mskcc.org

Surgical Pathology 12 (2019) 281–313
https://doi.org/10.1016/j.path.2019.01.002
1875-9181/19/© 2019 Elsevier Inc. All rights reserved.

resulting in a classification system that is not useful for clinical management. In contrast, the International Endocervical Adenocarcinoma Criteria and Classification (IECC) system uniquely integrates morphology, cause/pathogenesis, and biological behavior of EA subtypes.[9] The IECC was based on a cohort 409 EAs from 7 institutions worldwide and sought to differentiate HPV-related EA (HPVA) and HPV unrelated EA (NHPVA) by morphology alone using the presence or absence of HPV-associated features, namely, conspicuous apical mitoses and apoptotic bodies seen at scanning magnification. HPVAs were further subclassified based on cytoplasmic features, whereas NHPVAs were subcategorized based on no or limited HPV features (Table 1). The IECC was validated by immunohistochemistry (IHC) for p16, p53, vimentin, and progesterone receptor (PR), and HPV RNA in situ hybridization (ISH): HPV and p16 were expressed in 95% and 90% of usual type endocervical adenocarcinomas (UEA), and only 3% and 37% of NHPVAs, respectively.[9] Important clinical differences were identified: NHPVA EAs were larger and occurred in older patients compared with HPVA EAs (P<.001).[9]

The IECC system was recently validated on a cohort of 75 EAs by assessing interobserver reproducibility among gynecologic pathologists based on histology and IHC (p16, PR, p53, Napsin-A, vimentin, CDX2, GATA3). The IECC classification was superior to the WHO classification ($\kappa = 0.46$ vs 0.3 for histology; $\kappa = 0.51$ vs 0.33 with IHC). For the IECC, agreement was a majority in 73 (97%; ≥4/7 agreed) and perfect in 42 (56%; 7/7 agreed), compared with a majority in 56 (75%) and perfect in 7 (10%) EAs for the WHO classification. Reproducibility was poor for WHO HPVA subtypes (UEA $\kappa = 0.36$, mucinous not otherwise specified [NOS] $\kappa = 0.13$, intestinal $\kappa = 0.31$, villoglandular $\kappa = 0.21$) and good in NHPVA types (gastric type $\kappa = 0.63$, clear cell $\kappa = 0.81$, mesonephric $\kappa = 0.5$). The IECC showed excellent correlation with HPV status.[10]

Given that the IECC classification allows segregation of EAs into different pathogenetic subcategories that are readily recognizable by morphology, the IECC 2017 classification system will likely replace the 2014 WHO system in the next iteration. This review emphasizes the IECC system with correlates to the WHO wherever applicable.

HUMAN PAPILLOMAVIRUS–ASSOCIATED SUBTYPES

- UEA
- Villoglandular carcinoma (VC)
- HPV-associated mucinous carcinoma
- Invasive stratified mucin-producing carcinoma

Usual Type Endocervical Adenocarcinoma

Definition
UEA is defined by the WHO as the most common form of EA with relative mucin depletion.[3] IECC defines UEA as having HPVA-like features, specifically, conspicuous apical mitotic figures and apoptotic bodies seen at scanning magnification with no more than 50% of tumor cells containing intracytoplasmic mucin; benign squamous metaplasia may also be seen.[9]

Epidemiology
UEA accounts for about 85% to 90% of all EAs, representing the most common subtype in the IECC.[9] It usually presents in the fourth to fifth decade.

Clinical features and macroscopy
Most cases (80%) present with vaginal bleeding and a mass lesion, which is exophytic in 50%. Ulceration or diffuse infiltration of the cervical wall ("barrel-shaped cervix") is less common. Some patients may be asymptomatic with abnormal cervical cytology.

Morphology
Well to moderately differentiated EAs show cribriform, papillary, solid, microglandular or cystic growth patterns composed of round to oval mucin-depleted glands. Poorly differentiated forms show clusters, cords, or single-cell infiltration with desmoplastic or inflammatory stromal reaction. Mucin pools may be present. Tumor cells are pseudostratified with enlarged, elongated, and hyperchromatic nuclei, prominent nucleoli, and apical amphophilic to eosinophilic, mucin-poor cytoplasm with apoptotic bodies and readily identifiable "floating" mitoses on the luminal slide of cells. Grading of UEA is based on the proportion of glandular differentiation; however, its prognostic value is controversial (Fig. 1).

Ancillary studies
UEA is usually but not always diffusely positive for p16 and carcinoembryonic antigen (CEA) with 90% expressing diffuse p16 in the IECC study.[9,11] Vimentin, estrogen receptor (ER), and PR are generally reported to be negative in UEA; however, a recent report on the IECC cases showed vimentin, ER, and PR expression in up to 13%, 5%, and 20% of UEA, respectively.[12,13] ISH for high-risk HPV messenger RNA (mRNA) has been shown to be more sensitive and specific than p16 and is considered superior to p16 in detecting HPV-positive adenocarcinomas.[9] UEA is usually

Table 1
Morphologic features, human papillomavirus status, and immunophenotype of endocervical adenocarcinomas

IECC Subtypes	Morphology[9]	Positive High-Risk HPV (%)[9]	Positive (Diffuse) P16 IHC (%)[9]	Other IHC
HPV-driven EA	Apical mitotic figures and apoptotic bodies seen at scanning magnification	*88*	*82*	*Variable (see below in this table under various subtypes)*
Usual type	0%–50% of cells with intracytoplasmic mucin, with or without benign squamous differentiation	87	83	Pos CEA; neg vimentin, ER, PR
Villoglandular	Usual-type morphology with exophytic long slender papillae	100	50	Pos CEA
Mucinous NOS	Usual-type morphology with >50% of cells containing intracytoplasmic mucin	100	100	Pos CEA, CK7; variable CDX2, CK20; neg ER, PR
Mucinous intestinal	Usual-type morphology with ≥50% of cells with goblet morphology	100	75	Pos CEA, CK7; variable CDX2, CK20; Neg ER, PR
Mucinous signet ring	Usual-type morphology with ≥50% of cells with signet-ring morphology	–	–	Pos CEA, CK7; variable CDX2, CK20; Neg ER, PR
iSMILE	Invasive nests of stratified columnar cells with peripheral palisading and variable intracytoplasmic mucin	100	50	–
Non-HPV-driven EA	No easily identifiable apical mitotic activity and apoptotic bodies at scanning magnification	*3*	*38*	*Variable (see below in this table under various subtypes)*
Gastric	Tumor cells with abundant clear, foamy, or pale eosinophilic cytoplasm, distinct cytoplasmic borders, low nuclear-cytoplasmic ratio, and irregular basally located nuclei, with or without intestinal differentiation; includes MDA	4	33	Pos HIK1083; variable CK7, CK20, CEA; aberrant p53; neg ER, PR

(continued on next page)

Table 1
(continued)

IECC Subtypes	Morphology[9]	Positive High-Risk HPV (%)[9]	Positive (Diffuse) P16 IHC (%)[9]	Other IHC
Mesonephric	Ductal, tubular, papillary, cordlike, or other growth patterns with intraluminal eosinophilic colloidlike material resembling mesonephric remnants	–	100	Pos CKs (pan-CK, EMA, CAM5.2), calretinin, vimentin, CD10 (apical); variable PAX8, TTF1, HNF-1β, androgen receptor, inhibin; neg ER, PR, CK20, CEA
Clear cell	Solid, papillary, and/or tubulocystic architecture with polygonal cells and highly atypical but uniform nuclei	0	29	Pos HNF-1β, napsin-A; neg CD10, CEA, ER, PR; wild-type p53
Endometrioid	"Confirmatory endometrioid features": at least focal low-grade endometrioid type (lined by columnar cells with pseudostratified nuclei) glands, with or without squamous differentiation and/or endometriosis	0	67	Pos CEA, EMA, CK7; neg ER, PR, vimentin
Serous	Papillary and/or micropapillary architecture with diffusely highly atypical nuclei in stratified and pseudostratified cells and relative discohesion	0	50	Variable CEA, CA125, WT1; neg ER, PR; aberrant p53
EA NOS	EA unclassifiable by the above criteria	*83*	*33*	*Variable*

Abbreviation: EMA, epithelial membrane antigen.

cytokeratin (CK) 7 positive, CK20 negative, and at least 75% are PAX8 positive. Tumors with intestinal differentiation can express intestinal markers like CK20 and CDX2.[14] None of these tests should be used in isolation but always as part of a panel.

Precursor
UEA is usually associated with adenocarcinoma in situ (AIS).

Human papillomavirus status
UEA is associated with high-risk HPV (HPV 18 > HPV 16 > other).[2] The IECC study found HPV in 88% of EAs.[9]

Prognosis
Five-year disease-free survival is 77% to 91%, whereas 5-year overall survival is 50% to 65% (stage IA: 93%–100%; stage IB: 83%; stage II: 50%–59%; stage III: 13%–31%; stage IV: 6%).

Villoglandular Carcinoma

Definition
VC is defined by the WHO as a variant of EA with a distinct exophytic, villous-papillary growth,[3] and by the IECC as EA with usual-type morphology and exophytic long slender papillae.[9]

Fig. 1. UEA. (*A*) Cribriform glands with relative mucin depletion, tall columnar cells, easily identifiable apoptotic bodies, and luminal mitoses, resembling endometrioid adenocarcinoma, ×200. (*B*) Numerous floating mitoses and apoptotic bodies, ×600.

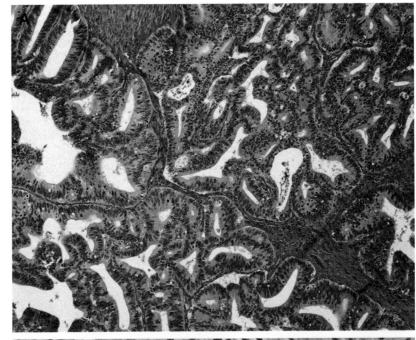

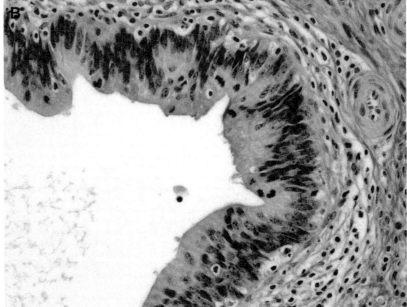

Epidemiology

VC is rare and accounts for less than 1% of EA. The mean age is 35 years (younger compared with UEA).[15] Association with oral contraceptives has been described.

Clinical features and macroscopy

VCs present with an exophytic, papillary, friable mass measuring up to 4 cm, vaginal bleeding, or abnormal cervical cytology.

Morphology

VC is composed of villous fronds of variable thickness and length covered by one to several layers of tall, mucin-poor endocervical or intestinal-type (goblet) cells that typically show mild cytologic atypia with pseudostratification and low mitotic activity. Apoptotic bodies may be present. The stroma in the villous fronds is composed of hypercellular spindle cells and may contain acute and chronic inflammatory cells. Stromal invasion is usually

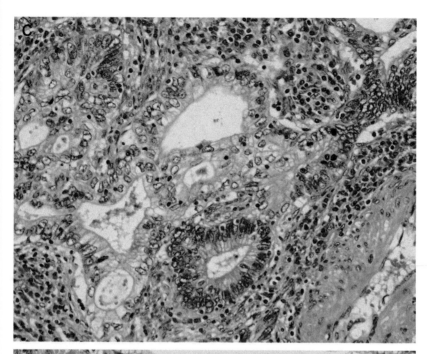

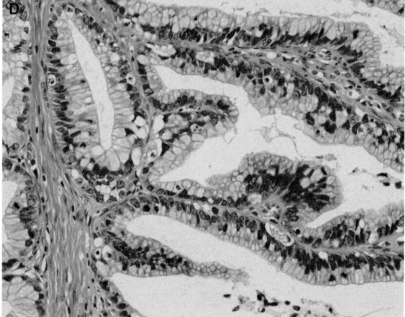

Fig. 1. (*continued*). (*C, D*) UEA with clear cytoplasm mimicking GCA, mitoses, and apoptotic bodies still easily visible, ×400.

absent or superficial. VC should not be diagnosed in small biopsies because the presence of other higher-grade components cannot be assessed. By definition, VC is low grade (**Fig. 2**).

Ancillary studies
VCs are diffusely positive for p16 and CEA.

Precursor
VC is often associated with AIS.

Human papillomavirus status
VC has been shown to be associated with HPV types 16, 18, and 45.[2,16] The IECC study found HPV in 100% of VCs.[9]

Prognosis
Superficially invasive VCs typically have an excellent prognosis. However, association with a high-grade component and positive lymph nodes has been described.[17,18]

Fig. 2. Villoglandular exophytic tumor with long slender papillae: (*A*) whole slide image; (*B*) ×40.

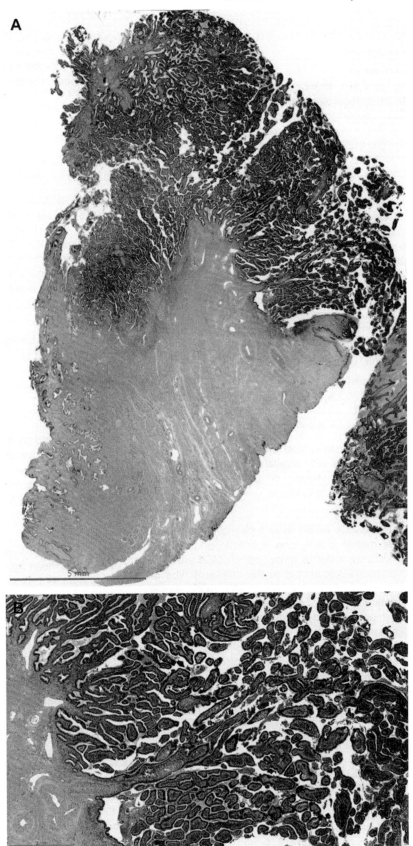

Human Papillomavirus–Associated Mucinous Carcinomas

Definition
In the WHO, mucinous carcinomas are lumped together regardless of HPV status and subclassified according to cytoplasmic features. MC NOS is defined as an adenocarcinoma with mucin production that cannot be classified as any of the specific types of EA: intestinal type with areas of intestinal mucin (goblet cell), signet ring cell type with focal or diffuse signet ring cell differentiation, or gastric type with gastric mucin production.[3] The IECC separates HPV-associated MC from the non-HPV-associated gastric type, with stratification according to the following type of mucin present:

- Mucinous NOS: ≥50% cells with intracytoplasmic mucin in a background of UEA
- Mucinous intestinal: ≥50% cells with goblet morphology in a background of UEA
- Mucinous signet ring: ≥50% cells with signet ring morphology in a background of UEA[9]

Epidemiology
Intestinal MC accounts for 10% to 15% of all EAs and affects women aged 44 to 54 years. In the IECC study, MCs constituted 6% of the cohort.[9]

Clinical features and macroscopy
MCs presents with vaginal bleeding, abdominal discomfort, exophytic or ulcerated mass, or abnormal cervical cytology.

Morphology
All HPVA MCs exhibit usual type morphology with brisk mitotic activity and apoptotic bodies, and variable cytoplasmic mucin. HPVA MCs are then subclassified according to the dominant type of mucin. By IECC definitions, MC NOS shows greater than 50% of cells containing intracytoplasmic mucin without specific features of gastric, intestinal, or signet ring cell–type EA. Intestinal MC shows ≥50% of cells with goblet morphology, sometimes argentaffin and Paneth cells. Signet ring cell MC shows ≥50% of cells with signet ring morphology (abundant cytoplasmic mucin vacuoles displacing the nuclei) and diffuse, trabecular, glandular, and cordlike growth patterns without desmoplastic stroma. Grading of MCs is similar to UEA (Fig. 3).

Ancillary studies
MCs, like UEA, are typically diffusely positive for p16, CK7, and CEA. CDX2 and CK20 staining may be variable with more intestinal-type morphology corresponding to expression of intestinal markers.[14] Whereas up to 13% of UEA can express vimentin, all HPVA MC are vimentin negative, except invasive stratified mucin-producing carcinoma (see later discussion). ER and PR are also generally negative in HPVA mucinous carcinomas. PAX8 is positive in about 50% (except invasive stratified mucin-producing carcinoma [iSMILE]).

Precursor
AIS may be found and may have similar mucinous features as the invasive component.

Human papillomavirus status
Intestinal and signet ring cell MCs are associated with high-risk HPV subtypes.[2,19–21] The IECC study found HPV in 100% of HPVA MC but not in gastric-type mucinous carcinoma. It is clear that mucin-producing carcinomas of the cervix are heterogeneous and include both HPVA and NHPVA subtypes.[9]

Prognosis
The prognosis is similar to UEA and depends on grade, stage, and lymph node status.

Invasive Stratified Mucin-Producing Carcinoma

Definition
iSMILE is defined by the IECC as EA with HPVA-like features that are composed of invasive nests of stratified columnar cells with peripheral palisading and variable intracytoplasmic mucin.[9] It is not recognized as a distinct entity in the current WHO classification.

Epidemiology
In the IECC study, iSMILE constituted 3% of the cohort.[9] The mean age at diagnosis has been reported to be 44 years.[22]

Clinical features
iSMILE presents with vaginal bleeding, cervical mass, or ascites.[22]

Macroscopy
Macroscopy is not well defined, but probably is similar to UEA.

Morphology
Stratified mucin-producing intraepithelial lesion (SMILE) is a variant pattern of AIS thought to arise from pluripotent reserve cells at the cervical transformation zone and is composed of immature metaplastic epithelial cells with intracytoplasmic mucin stratified throughout the entire thickness of the epithelium. Moderate nuclear atypia, hyperchromasia, brisk mitoses, and apoptotic bodies are typical.[23] The invasive counterpart (iSMILE) has been described as a distinct form of invasive

Fig. 3. Mucinous HPV associated. (*A*) Usual type shows numerous luminal mitoses and apoptotic bodies easily visible at scanning magnification with greater than 50% tumor cells showing mucin of no specific type, ×200. (*B*) Intestinal-type goblet cells in usual type with intraluminal villous projection demonstrating tapered tip typical of UEA, ×600.

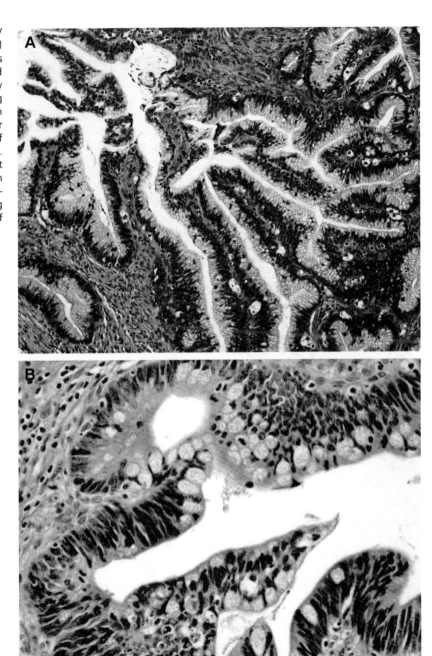

carcinoma with morphologic features resembling SMILE.[22] Unlike conventional adenocarcinomas, iSMILEs do not form conspicuous lumens or well-formed glands. Rather, the tumor cells have intracytoplasmic mucin/microlumens stratified throughout the thickness of the nests. They often have palisading nuclei at the periphery of the nests and are commonly associated with a brisk acute inflammatory infiltrate, including neutrophils and eosinophils. This pattern can be pure or associated with other patterns like UEA, squamous carcinoma, adenosquamous carcinoma, colloid-like carcinoma, and signet ring–like carcinoma, which belies the phenotypic malleability of iSMILE. The tumor can be superficial or deep with depth of invasion ranging from less than 1 to 19 mm.[22] No specific grading system exists (**Fig. 4**).

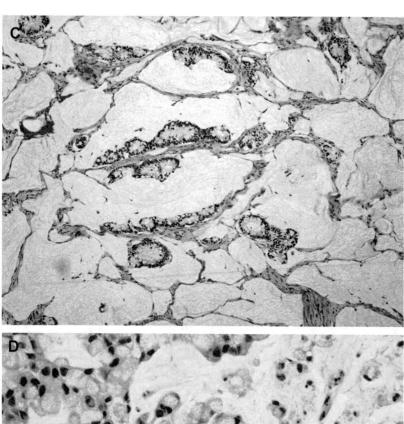

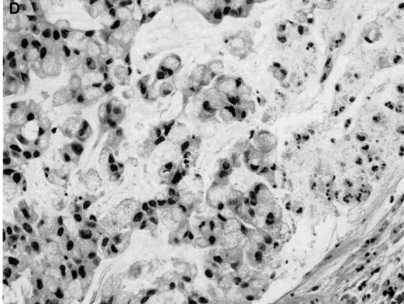

Fig. 3. (continued). (C) Intestinal-type mucinous colloidlike adenocarcinoma with extravasated mucin, ×100. (D) Signet ring mucinous adenocarcinoma, ×600.

Ancillary studies

As with other HPV-associated neoplasms, p16 is typically diffuse and strong with a minority of cases expressing vimentin, ER, and PR (12.5%, 14.2%, and 25%, respectively).[12,22] Unlike UEA, iSMILEs have less frequent PAX8 positivity (14.3% vs 75%) and express the squamous markers p63 (25%), p40 (28.6%), and GATA3 (14.3%).[12] Although only 3.6% of UEA has aberrant p53 staining, 28.6% of iSMILEs showed mutation pattern p53 by IHC.[12]

Precursor

SMILE is thought to arise as a result of high-risk HPV infection in the embryonic/stem cell–like reserve cells of the transformation zone.[23]

Human papillomavirus status

The IECC study found HPV in 100% of iSMILEs.[9]

Prognosis

Metastatic carcinoma was found in 3 of 8 cases (mean follow-up 11 months) in a small study.[22] It

Fig. 4. iSMILE. (*A*) SMILE involving surface endocervical glands–mucin-containing cells are stratified throughout the entire thickness of the epithelium and in areas that appear to lift and displace normal endocervical glands (*center right*) ×100. (*B*) Invasive SMILE with nests of tumor showing peripheral palisading, small lumens, and associated acute inflammatory response, ×100. (*C*) Anastomosing pattern of iSMILE, ×100.

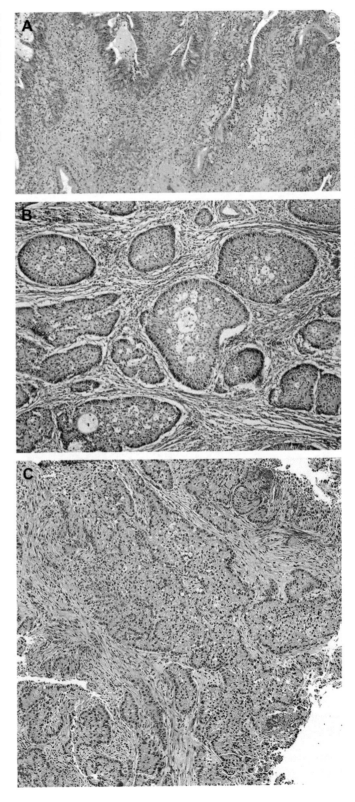

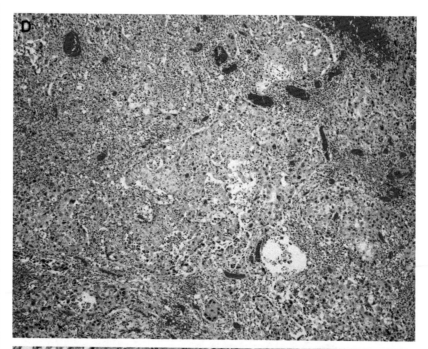

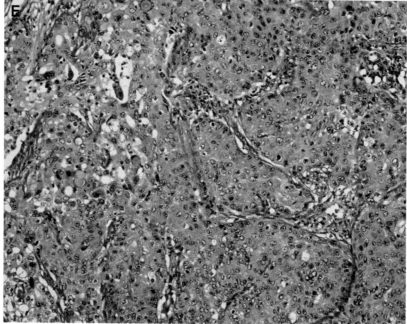

Fig. 4. (*continued*). (*D*) iSMILE with poorly formed nests, exuberant acute inflammatory infiltrate, high nuclear grade, and cell discohesion, ×100. (*E*) Mucin-poor (*right*) adjacent to mucin-rich (*left*) components in same tumor, ×200.

is unclear whether iSMILEs have an inherently worse outcome than UEA when adjusted for stage.

NON-HUMAN PAPILLOMAVIRUS–ASSOCIATED SUBTYPES

- Gastric-type adenocarcinoma
- Mesonephric carcinoma (MNC)
- Clear cell carcinoma (CCC)

- Serous carcinoma (SC)
- Endometrioid adenocarcinoma

All non-HPV-associated EAs as defined by the IECC have an absence of easily identifiable mitotic activity and apoptotic bodies at scanning magnification. Their subclassification is subsequently based on cytoplasmic and architectural features as delineated in later discussion.

Gastric-Type Cervical Adenocarcinoma

Definition
Gastric-type cervical adenocarcinoma (GCA) is defined by the WHO as a subtype of MC with gastric differentiation.[3] By IECC criteria, these tumors are composed of cells with abundant clear, foamy, or pale eosinophilic cytoplasm, distinct cytoplasmic borders, generally low nuclear-cytoplasmic ratios, and irregular basally located nuclei with limited or no HPVA-like features.[9]

Epidemiology
GCA is the second-most common subtype of EA and the most common subtype of NHPVA, accounting for 10% of EA in the IECC (up to 25% in Japanese populations).[9] The mean age at presentation is 42 years. Most cases are sporadic, but GCA can be associated with germline *STK11* mutations (Peutz-Jeghers syndrome).[24-26]

Clinical features and macroscopy
Patients can present with vaginal bleeding, mucoid, watery discharge, or abdominal discomfort, "barrel-shaped" cervix, and firm, indurated masses with tan to yellow, hemorrhagic, friable, or mucoid cut surfaces, abnormal cervical cytology in asymptomatic patients, or ovarian metastases.

Morphology
Tumor cells contain abundant clear, foamy, or pale eosinophilic cytoplasm with distinct cytoplasmic borders. Nuclei are typically basally located and can range from small round/ovoid to markedly enlarged, irregular with vesicular chromatin and prominent nucleoli. The cells usually contain tall apical mucin. Intestinal differentiation may be present. GCAs can vary from the well-differentiated end of the spectrum, so-called minimal deviation adenocarcinoma (MDA) or adenoma malignum to poorly differentiated forms, sometimes all within the same tumor.[27-29] Pure MDA can be underrecognized due to a deceptively bland morphologic appearance; however, adequate sampling should allow for correct diagnosis because there are usually at least focally obvious malignant tumor cells.[30] Grading of GCA is not recommended given that even "well-differentiated"–appearing tumors behave aggressively[31]; thus, GCA is best regarded as inherently high grade. When GCA becomes poorly differentiated, as in most malignancies, the tumor cells can grow as single cells and clusters with high nucleus to cytoplasmic ratios and loss of the abundant cytoplasm. Although these tumors

are called gastric type due to the pyloric gland-type mucin within the cells, they morphologically resemble pancreatobiliary adenocarcinomas with similar immunohistochemical profiles (**Fig. 5**).

Ancillary studies
The neutral gastric/pyloric-type mucin of GCA stains magenta-pink with combined periodic acid Schiff/Alcian blue (PAS/AB), whereas the acidic mucin of normal endocervical glands and UEA stains dark blue/navy. This PAS/AB special stain can be a simple method to detect the presence of gastric mucin, especially because the HIK1083 antibody is not widely available and can be negative in poorly differentiated GCAs.[27,31-33] p16 is usually negative or focally positive, although up to 8.5% have been shown to have diffuse strong expression typical of HPV-associated tumors.[9,32,34] Aberrant p53 expression is common, seen in up to 52% of cases, whereas ER and PR are typically negative with rare exception. CK7 is always positive, whereas markers of intestinal differentiation CK20 and CDX2 can be positive in up to 50% of cases, albeit focally.[32,35] PAX8 is usually positive in GCA (68%–80%) and can be a useful marker in distinguishing from tumors of pancreatobiliary origin.[12,32]

Precursor
Nonobligate precursor lesions include lobular endocervical glandular hyperplasia (LEGH), atypical LEGH, and gastric-type AIS.[36,37] The rate of progression from any of these lesions to GCA is unknown, and it is uncertain whether the presence of nonatypical LEGH requires an excisional procedure of the entire lesion.

Human papillomavirus status
True GCAs are HPV negative. Occasional cases with limited HPV-associated features can resemble gastric-type adenocarcinoma and be HPV positive, demonstrating that there can be some morphologic overlap between HPVA and gastric-type adenocarcinoma.[9,38]

Prognosis
GCA is an aggressive, chemorefractory tumor with a propensity for peritoneal and abdominal spread.[31,35,39,40] Most patients present at advanced stage, but even those presenting at stage I still have a guarded prognosis, with a 62% 5-year disease-specific survival compared with 96% for stage I UEA.[39] The 5-year disease-specific survival for all stages is 32%.[31,39]

Molecular features
In addition to *STK11* mutations in syndromic patients, GCAs show 3q gain and 1p loss,[36]

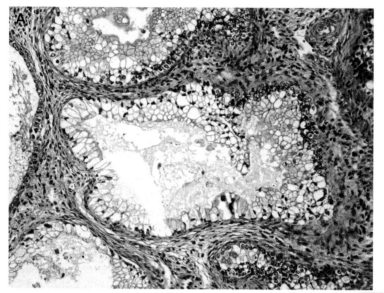

Fig. 5. Gastric-type adenocarcinoma. (*A*) Well-formed glands lined by cells with abundant clear to foamy cytoplasm, tall apical mucin, basally located nuclei that range from small and pyknotic to enlarged with prominent nucleoli, ×200. (*B*) High magnification shows foamy nature of cytoplasm, distinct cell borders, and basally located atypical nuclei with irregular nuclear membranes, open chromatin, and prominent nucleoli, ×600. (*C*) Mucin-rich glands adjacent to mucin-poor glands embedded in hyalinized stroma, ×400.

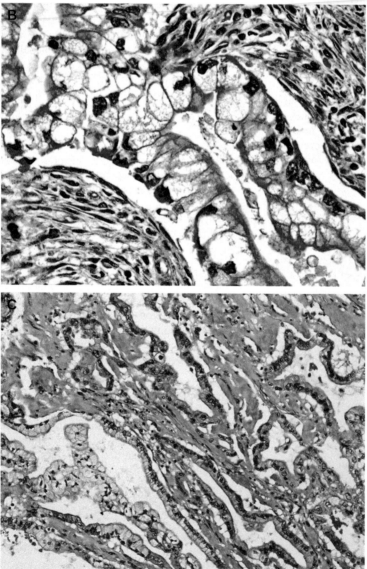

Fig. 5. (continued). (D) Well-formed gland adjacent to single cells and clusters, some of which have a signet ring cell appearance, ×400. (E) Tumor arises in association with LEGH (along the periphery) and has focal intestinal-type goblet cells, ×400. (F) Minimal deviation pattern of gastric type with deep diffuse stromal infiltration by extremely well-differentiated glands without associated desmoplastic response, ×100.

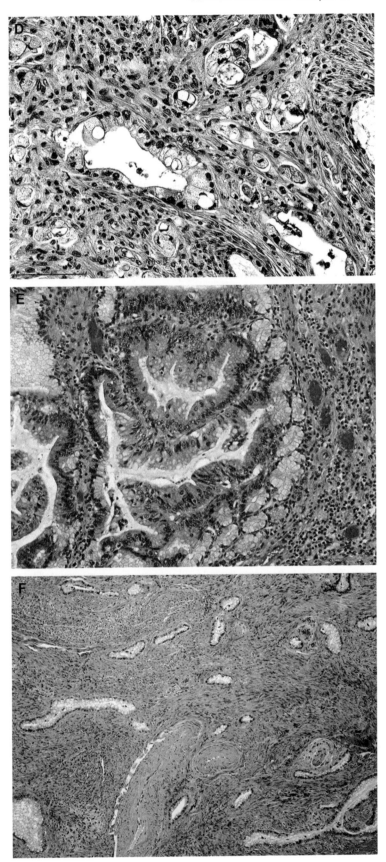

whereas *TP53* mutations are found in almost 50%.[35]

Mesonephric Carcinoma

Definition

MNC of the cervix is defined by the WHO as a tumor arising from mesonephric remnants,[3] and by the IECC as EA with no or limited HPVA-like features and an admixture of growth patterns (ductal, tubular, papillary, cordlike, and others) as well as intraluminal eosinophilic colloidlike material resembling mesonephric remnants.[9]

Epidemiology

MNC accounts for less than 1% of EA. The mean age at presentation is 50 years.[41]

Clinical features and macroscopy

MNC can present with abnormal vaginal bleeding or abnormal cervical cytology. These tumors are often located in the lateral to posterior cervical wall and may be deeply invasive with extension into parametrium. They may also present as a diffusely thickened or "barrel-shaped cervix" without a discrete mass.

Morphology

MNC may arise in a background of mesonephric hyperplasia and can show a variety of growth patterns, including ductal (pseudoendometrioid), tubular, papillary, sex cord–like, solid, spindled, and retiform (branching, slitlike spaces with intraluminal fibrous papillae). The tubular pattern may contain intraluminal eosinophilic colloidlike material typically seen in mesonephric remnants or hyperplasia. Tumor cells are cuboidal to columnar with pale to eosinophilic cytoplasm, mild to moderate cytologic atypia, and mitotic activity that can be brisk. The nuclei often have irregular nuclear membranes, frequent grooving, and nuclear pseudoinclusions reminiscent of papillary thyroid carcinoma. MNC can be differentiated from mesonephric hyperplasia based on degree of gland crowding, infiltrative growth, increased mitotic activity, intraluminal cellular debris, and nuclear atypia. There is no established grading system for MNC. Because of the wide ranging morphologic patterns of MNCs, the differential can be varied depending on the dominant growth pattern. Sometimes the tumor can have a prominent papillary pattern with cuboidal cells containing clear cytoplasm, mimicking CCC. A spindle cell component with heterologous differentiation can also be present, which has been designated malignant mixed mesonephric tumor (now outdated). MNC associated with a small cell carcinoma, not HPV associated, has also been described.[42] Mesonephric-like carcinomas have been described in the uterine corpus and adnexa and can include corded and hyalinized morphology[43,44] (**Fig. 6**).

Ancillary studies

MNCs are positive for CKs, calretinin, vimentin, and CD10 (apical), and negative for ER and PR, CK20, and CEA. PAX8 and hepatocyte nuclear factor-1β (HNF-1β) are typically positive.[45,46] GATA3 has emerged as a robust marker for mesonephric remnants and hyperplasia and can also be present in cervical MNC.[46,47] Thyroid transcription factor 1 (TTF1) has been reported to be positive in mesonephric-like carcinomas of the upper gynecologic tract but tends to be less positive in cervical tumors.[46] p16 is negative or focally positive.[45] Androgen receptor and inhibin can be positive in 30% of cases.[41]

Precursor

MNC is thought to arise from mesonephric remnants and/or hyperplasia.

Human papillomavirus status

MNCs are HPV negative.[35,42,45]

Prognosis

These tumors can be very aggressive, even when low stage, and some pathologic features, such as solid or spindled morphology, may portend a worse prognosis. Late recurrence and metastasis have been described.[41]

Molecular features

Recent studies have shown canonical *KRAS* mutations in most MNCs, with a smaller number harboring *NRAS* mutations. *ARID1A/B* are also commonly mutated. Chromosomal abnormalities, including gain of 1q, loss of 1p, and gain of chromosomes 10 and 12, were common. MNCs are microsatellite stable and do not harbor *PTEN* or *PIK3CA* mutations typical of endometrial endometrioid adenocarcinomas.[48]

Clear Cell Carcinoma

Definition

CCC is defined by the WHO as an EA composed predominantly of clear or hobnail cells the architectural patterns of which are solid, tubulocystic, and/or papillary,[3] and by the IECC as EA with no or limited HPVA-like features composed of solid, papillary, and/or tubulocystic architecture with polygonal cells and highly atypical but uniform nuclei.[9]

Epidemiology

CCC accounts for less than 5% of EA. Its incidence was 3% in the IECC study.[9] CCC can occur sporadically or in association with in utero diethylstilbestrol (DES) exposure.[49,50] It has a bimodal

Fig. 6. Mesonephric carcinoma. (*A*) Gross image of cervix with tan, firm mass involving full thickness of wall. (*B*) Corresponding hematoxylin and eosin (H&E) whole slide image. (*C*) Tubular pattern with diffuse infiltration with focal eosinophilic luminal secretions without desmoplastic response, ×20.

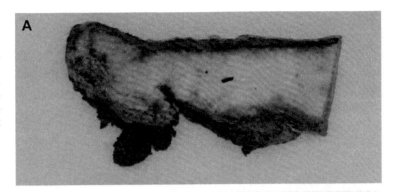

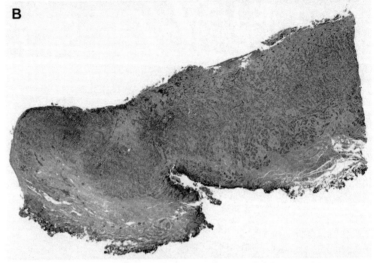

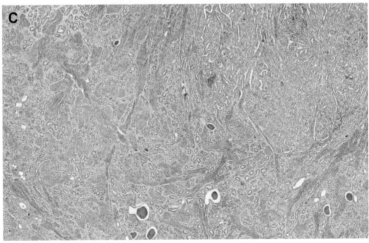

age distribution. DES-associated CCC is rare with peak risk of disease at 19 years. In contrast, the peak age risk for sporadic tumors is wide, ranging from pediatric to postmenopausal populations. A recent 40-year follow-up study in DES-exposed patients showed that the cumulative risk for developing CCC is 1 in 750 in exposed patients, and 1 in 520 when the risk was adjusted to include nonexposed patients within the same birth cohort and year of diagnosis.[51]

Clinical features and macroscopy

DES-associated CCCs are typically ectocervical or in the anterior upper third of the vagina, whereas

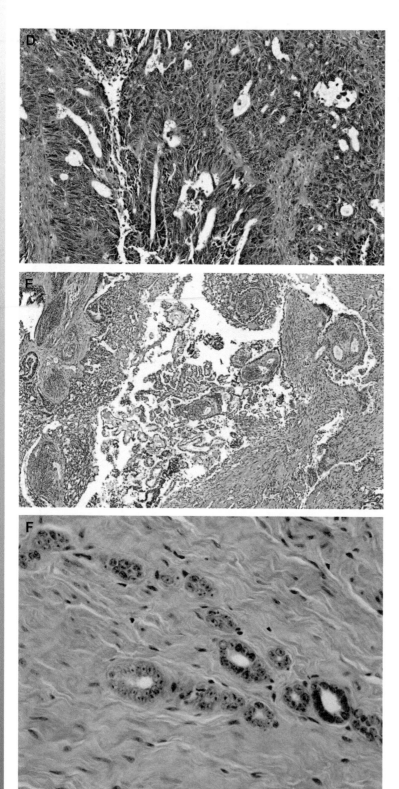

Fig. 6. (continued). (D) Tall columnar cells with endometrioid morphology, ×200. (E) Papillary growth resembling CCC, ×40. (F) Tubular glands with enlarged nuclei, open chromatin, prominent nucleoli, ×400.

Fig. 7. CCC. (*A*) Tubulocystic pattern of CCC, ×40. (*B*) Tubular glands with single layer of flattened, cuboidal, and hobnail cells with eosinophilic to clear cytoplasm, ×200.

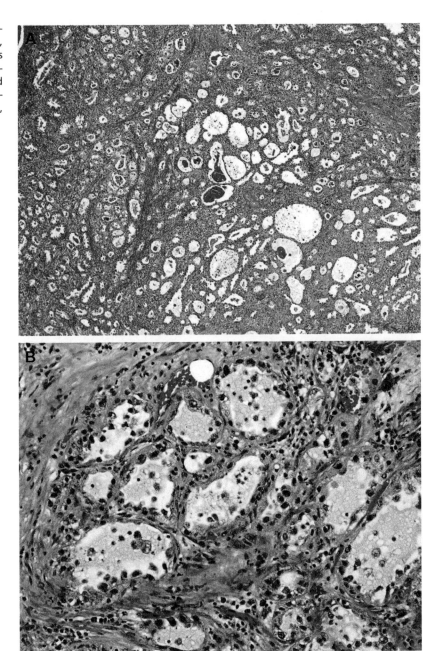

sporadic tumors tend to arise in the endocervix and present similarly to UEA. The most common symptom is vaginal bleeding and/or discharge, with a polypoid or ulcerated, friable mass measuring up to 4 cm or abnormal cytology. Endophytic tumors can be larger.

Morphology

CCC can be composed of any combination of solid, tubulocystic, and papillary architecture with polygonal cells and highly atypical but uniform nuclei. Tumor cells typically contain abundant clear glycogen-rich cytoplasm with or without eosinophilic intracytoplasmic hyaline globules. Papillae often contain dense, hyalinized eosinophilic stroma in the fibrovascular cores. Tumor cells are flat to cuboidal or hobnail with clear or less commonly eosinophilic cytoplasm, uniform atypia, prominent nucleoli, and low mitotic rate.

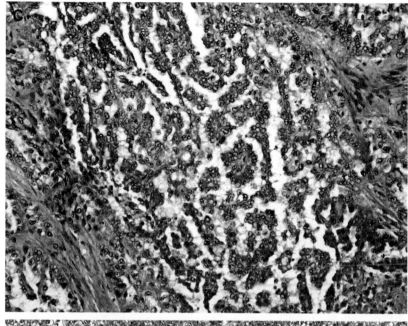

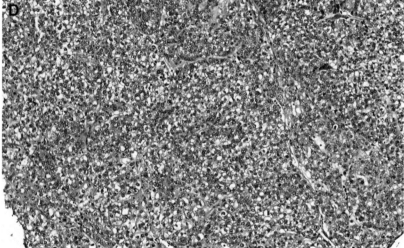

Fig. 7. (continued). (C) Papillary pattern of CCC with uniform nuclei and eosinophilic fibrovascular cores, ×100. (D) Solid pattern of CCC, ×100 (H&E-stained slides).

The oxyphilic variant of CCC is difficult to recognize as such when composed of purely solid growth. Acute inflammatory cells, plasma cells, and psammoma bodies may be present. By definition, CCC is high grade (Fig. 7).

Ancillary studies

CCCs are typically positive for CK7, PAX8, HNF-1β, and Napsin-A. Both p16 and p53 may be positive (aberrant pattern) or negative (wild-type pattern), whereas CD10, ER, and PR are usually, but not always, negative. CEA has been consistently negative in these tumors, which could make it a useful marker to distinguish CCC from gastric type, which can also have abundant clear cytoplasm.

Precursor

There is no known precursor in the cervix.

Human papillomavirus status

CCCs are HPV negative.[9,35]

Prognosis

Low-stage CCCs have excellent survival (90%), whereas advanced tumors recur within 2 to 3 years, typically involving pelvic lymph nodes.[52]

Molecular features

Not much is known regarding the molecular genetics of cervical CCC. One study showed microsatellite instability in all DES-exposed and 50% of non-DES-exposed cases, whereas no mutations in *KRAS*, *HRAS*, *WT1*, *ER*, or *TP53* were found.[53]

Another study evaluating EAs had 1 case of CCC with no evidence of microsatellite instability.[54]

Endometrioid Carcinoma

Definition
EC is defined by the WHO as an EA arising in the cervix that has endometrioid morphologic features.[3] The IECC defines EC as an EA with no or limited HPVA-like features and confirmatory endometrioid features, which consist of at least focally identified low-grade endometrioid glands lined by columnar cells with pseudostratified nuclei demonstrating no more than moderate atypia, ± squamous differentiation, and/or endometriosis.[9]

Epidemiology
Until the IECC, specific diagnostic criteria for cervical endometrioid adenocarcinoma were lacking, leading to great variability in the reporting of its frequency. When strict evaluation for HPV-related features was applied, only 1.1% were classified into this category. Therefore, true endometrioid adenocarcinoma of the cervix is exceedingly rare.

Clinical features and macroscopy
EC has a similar presentation to UEA, most commonly uterine bleeding or vaginal discharge, exophytic or ulcerated mass, or it can be asymptomatic.

Morphology
"Confirmatory endometrioid features" include at least focal round to oval endometrioid-type glands lined by columnar cells with pseudostratified round nuclei with mild to moderate atypia, eosinophilic cytoplasm with no or minimal mucin. Cribriform and papillary patterns, squamous differentiation, and/or endometriosis may be present. Overall, ECs are morphologically similar to endometrial ECs and must be differentiated from direct extension from the corpus. ECs can be graded like endometrial ECs (Fig. 8).

Ancillary studies
Because of the rarity and only recently described strict morphologic criteria for distinguishing ECs from UEA, little is known regarding their immunophenotype. It is likely that these stain similarly to endometrial ECs.

Precursor
True cervical ECs are presumed to arise from endometriosis.

Human papillomavirus status
All 3 ECs in the IECC study were HPV negative.[9]

Prognosis
The prognosis is unknown due to rarity.

Molecular features
The molecular features are unknown due to rarity.

Serous Carcinoma

Definition
SC is defined by the WHO as a rare cervical EA with identical histologic appearance to endometrial or adnexal SC.[3] By the IECC, these tumors show papillary and/or micropapillary architecture with cells showing diffusely distributed highly atypical nuclei in stratified and pseudostratified cells.[9]

Epidemiology
Some investigators doubt the existence of cervical SC, thinking that most cases likely represent either drop metastasis from the uterine corpus or adnexae, or a "high-grade" morphologic variant of UEA. Studies of SCs of the cervix have shown bimodal age distribution (premenopausal and postmenopausal), with the premenopausal cases being HPV positive, WT1 negative, with good overall outcomes, whereas the postmenopausal cases were HPV negative, WT1 positive, with poor outcomes and concurrent serous tubal intraepithelial carcinoma in the fallopian tubes that underwent sectioning and extensively examining the fimbriated end.[55,56] These findings suggest that true SC of the cervix does not exist, and those previously reported as such likely represent metastases in the postmenopausal setting. In the premenopausal setting, cervical SCs may indeed represent a morphologic variant of UEA.

Clinical features and macroscopy
Drop metastases of SC from the corpus or adnexa can present with vaginal bleeding, watery discharge, polypoid or fungating mass, indurated cervix, or abnormal cervical cytology.

Morphology
Drop metastases from the uterine corpus or adnexa will resemble those primary site tumors, papillary and/or micropapillary architecture with slitlike spaces, diffuse highly atypical and pleomorphic nuclei in stratified and pseudostratified cells, brisk mitotic activity, cellular budding, and psammoma bodies. Glandular areas with irregular luminal borders may be present. High-grade papillary or micropapillary variants of usual HPV-associated EA may have a component of more conventional columnar cells with intracytoplasmic mucin[57] (Fig. 9).

Ancillary studies
Tumors will stain like high-grade SC of uterine or adnexal origin depending on the primary site. If the tumor represents a variant of UEA, it will stain like a UEA.

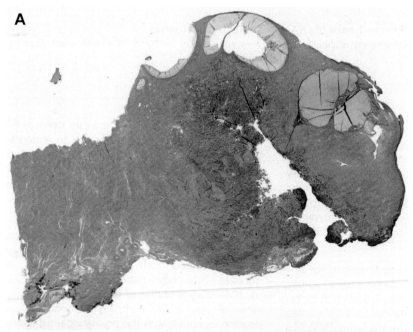

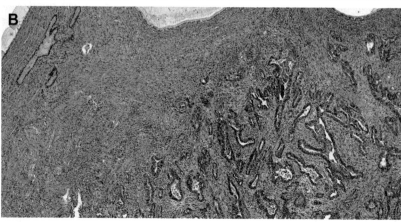

Fig. 8. Endometrioid carcinoma. (*A*) Full-slide view of cervix with adenocarcinoma located in cervical wall extending to deep margin without mucosal involvement. (*B*) Endometrioid-type glands in deep stroma (*right*) with overlying normal endocervical mucosa (*left*), ×100.

Precursor
Adenocarcinoma in situ is typically present adjacent to cervical carcinomas with serous-like growth patterns, lending more support to the idea that serous carcinoma of the cervix is a morphologic variant of UEA.

Human papillomavirus status
All SCs in the IECC study were HPV negative.[9]

Prognosis
For primary UEA with serouslike features, prognosis is dependent on stage and other typical high-risk features.

Molecular features
Older patients with SCs have been shown to harbor *TP53* mutations, similar to endometrial and pelvic SCs.[58]

STAGING OF ENDOCERVICAL ADENOCARCINOMA

Optimal management and prognostication of EA are based on a comprehensive pathology report. EA staging depends primarily on the International Federation of Gynecology and Obstetrics (FIGO) staging system, which is based on the presence or absence of a clinically visible or palpable lesion.[59] The clinically visible mass implies at least stage FIGO IB1, whereas staging of nonclinically visible tumors relies on microscopic measurements ("pathologic staging"): IA1 includes ≤3 mm depth of stromal invasion and ≤7 mm width, whereas IA2 includes greater than 3 mm but less than 5 mm depth and ≤7 mm width.[60]

Fig. 8. (*continued*). (*C*) High power of endometrioid glands with tumor-infiltrating lymphocytes, ×400. (*D*) Endometrial endometrioid adenocarcinoma extending into cervix, ×20.

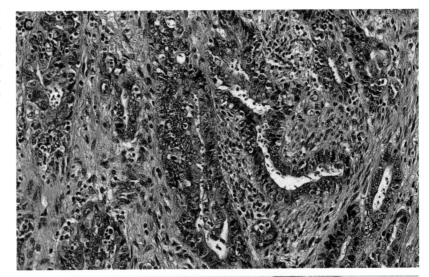

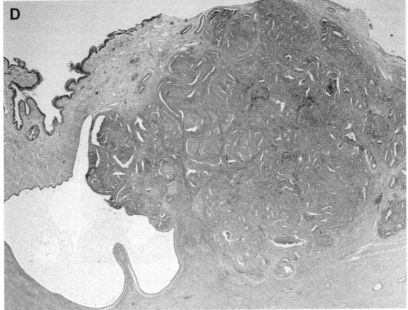

Accurate staging is extremely important because FIGO IA1 tumors are often treated by local excision with clear margins, whereas IA2 and IB1 tumors require radical surgery (radical hysterectomy or trachelectomy). Given that FIGO staging of cervical tumors does not consider variables, such as lymph node status as well as omental, peritoneal, adnexal, pelvic, and abdominal organ involvement, use of the pTNM category by the Union for International Cancer Control and the American Joint Committee on Cancer TNM staging system is recommended.

The International Collaboration on Cancer Reporting, an alliance formed by the Royal Colleges of Pathologists of Australasia and the United Kingdom, the College of American Pathologists, the Canadian Partnership Against Cancer, and the European Society of Pathology, developed a standardized, evidence-based reporting data set based on the 2014 WHO classification[3] and the 2009 FIGO staging system for cervical cancers[59] with "required" and "recommended" elements for EA.[60] **Table 2** summarizes the required and recommended elements from this study.

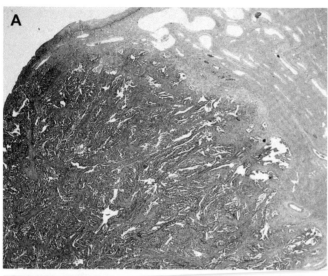

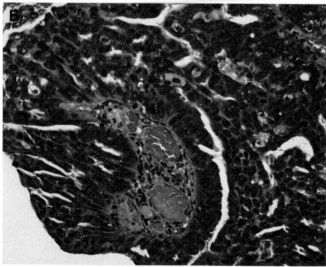

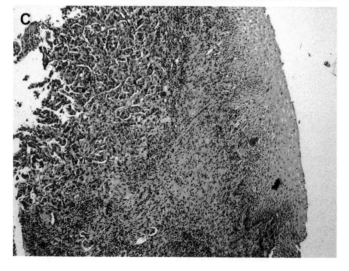

Fig. 9. (*A*) Serous-like EA with complex papillary growth, ×20. (*B*) Slit-like spaces, mitoses, and apoptotic bodies resembling high grade serous carcinoma of adnexa, ×400. (*C*) Micropapillary pattern of UEA, ×200.

Fig. 9. (continued). (*D*) Ovarian HGSC metastasizing to cervix, ×20. (*E*) Metastatic ovarian HGSC with pleomorphic nuclei, prominent nucleoli, slitlike spaces, irregular luminal contours, ×400. (*F*) Pagetoid spread of endometrial SC involving cervical mucosa, ×600.

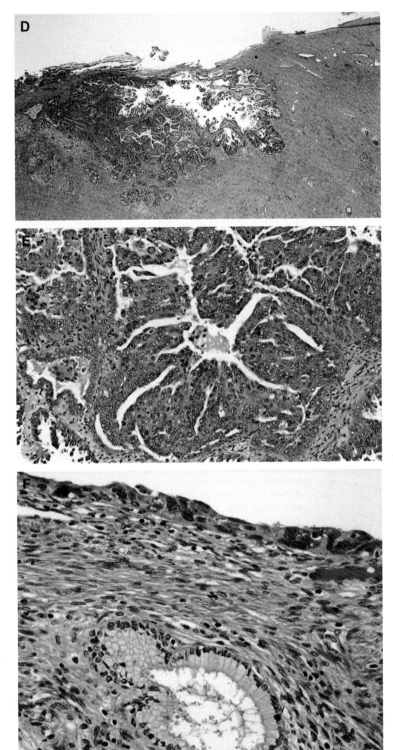

Table 2
Pathology reporting of endocervical adenocarcinoma

Clinical	Type of specimen submitted: • Loop/cone excision • Simple hysterectomy • Radical hysterectomy • Simple trachelectomy • Radical trachelectomy • Pelvic exenteration • Lymph nodes by anatomical groups 　○ Regional (paracervical, parametrial, pelvic: obturator, internal, common or external iliac, presacral, lateral sacral) 　○ Nonregional (para-aortic, inguinal, other) 　○ Sentinel vs nonsentinel • Prior treatment (chemotherapy, radiation, chemoradiation)[a] • Other
Macrocopic	• Number of tissue pieces (loop/cone excision) • Dimensions of each tissue piece (loop/cone excision) • Depth of specimen, ectocervix diameter (2 dimensions), and depth (thickness) (loop/cone excision, trachelectomy, hysterectomy) • Parametrium (radical trachelectomy or hysterectomy) • Vaginal cuff length (minimum, maximum) Tumor: • Location • Number of foci • Dimensions of each focus • Macroscopic appearance (exophytic, ulcerated)[a] Margins: • Distance to margins (invasive, in situ)
Microscopic	Dimensions of tumor: • Horizontal extent (2 measurements) • Depth of invasion or thickness • Size of metastasis[a] • Extranodal extension[a] Extent of invasion of extracervical structures, including uterine corpus Histologic type Grade[a] Lymphovascular invasion Precursor lesion (AIS, SMILE) Lymph node status: • Number examined • Number involved Distant metastases pTNM stage

[a] Recommended elements (all other elements are required).

PATTERN-BASED CLASSIFICATION OF ENDOCERVICAL ADENOCARCINOMA

The current staging system for EA does not provide specific guidelines on how to measure the invasive component which can be problematic because the lack of a defined basement membrane in endocervical glands makes determination of the exact point of origin of invasion difficult. The frequent association with AIS, which can be quite exuberant, and frequently exophytic growth precludes an accurate and consistent measurement of the depth of invasion.[61] In an attempt to prevent overtreatment and morbidities related to unnecessary procedures, such as lymph node dissection in early-stage EA, a risk stratification system has been developed based on the pattern of stromal invasion.[62–65] The system applies only to HPV-associated UEA, and the entire tumor must be examined microscopically to assign the appropriate group. Pattern A UEA is architecturally well to moderately differentiated and lacks destructive stromal invasion and lymphovascular invasion. Pattern B UEA shows focal destructive invasion arising in a background of pattern A glands and may be accompanied by LVI. Pattern C tumors show diffuse destructive invasion with marked desmoplastic reaction (**Fig. 10, Table 3**).

The pattern-based classification has been shown to correlate with the risk of lymph node metastasis and clinical outcome. Pattern A tumors are not associated with lymph node metastasis, limited to stage I, and do not recur, whereas pattern C tumors frequently presented at stage II or higher had positive lymph nodes in 22.5% and recurred in 19.7%; pattern B tumors also presented at stage I, and the few lymph node–positive cases also showed LVI.[62–65] Similar results were reported by multiple subsequent studies.[66–69] Furthermore, given the excellent prognosis of pattern A tumors, this system eliminates the need to differentiate pattern A tumors from AIS, which can be challenging with poor reproducibility.[66,67] Further studies have shown that positive lymph node status is a significantly poor prognostic factor in pattern C tumors, and stratifying these tumors based on the presence of LVI and lymph node status could guide treatment.[63,70] In an attempt to further fine tune morphology to outcomes in pattern C tumors, micropapillary growth pattern was shown to be associated with lymph node metastases compared with no lymph node metastases in tumors showing linear destructive growth; recurrence was associated with diffuse destructive growth (44%) but not seen in tumors with a band-like lymphocytic infiltrate.[71]

Several studies have demonstrated this 3-tiered system to be reproducible among pathologists, with the reported kappa values ranging from fair to almost perfect (k = 0.24–0.84)[68] and moderate (k = 0.65).[66] Another study showed an overall concordance of 74% with kappa values of 0.54, 0.32, and 0.59 for patterns A, B, and C, respectively.[72] Kappa values improved when comparing binarized patterns (A vs B and C).[66,68]

This system is applicable to all resections as invasion pattern on cones, and loop electrosurgical excision procedures (LEEPs) can predict invasion pattern on a subsequent hysterectomy, particularly in pattern B and C tumors.[73] Unfortunately, application in biopsies is suboptimal, particularly in pattern A tumors. Based on the presence or absence of destructive invasion in biopsy material, patients could undergo standard treatment or cone/LEEP procedure, respectively. Destructive invasion in a cone or LEEP would trigger additional surgery.[74]

It should be emphasized that pattern classification applies only to HPV-associated adenocarcinoma and not any of the non-HPV subtypes. In a study by Stolnicu and colleagues,[75] all non-HPV-associated adenocarcinomas were categorized as pattern C.

MOLECULAR ALTERATIONS IN USUAL TYPE ENDOCERVICAL ADENOCARCINOMA

Several studies of UEA have identified prevalent mutations in the members of the PI3K/Akt/mTOR signaling pathway regulating cell cycle, including *PIK3CA* (11%–25%), *KRAS* (18%), and *PTEN* (4%) genes.[76–79] These mutations are promising because they may be amenable to targeted therapy.[80,81] An integrated analysis of 178 samples based on copy number, methylation, mRNA, and microRNA profiling by The Cancer Genome Atlas Research Network demonstrated a unique set of endometrial-like, predominantly HPV-negative, cervical cancers with high frequencies of *KRAS*, *ARID1A*, and *PTEN* mutations. This adenocarcinoma-rich subgroup showed high expression of miR-375 and low expression of miR-205-5p and miR-944.[82] It is likely that these HPV-negative endometrial-like tumors are likely endometrioid adenocarcinomas of the corpus/lower-uterine segment extending to the cervix and erroneously included in the analysis.

Two recent studies correlating pattern of invasion with genetic alterations have given molecular support to this morphologic classification.[69,70] Both studies showed that pattern A tumors had fewer significant tumor suppressor and oncogene abnormalities than pattern B or C. In a study of 20 UEAs interrogating hotspot regions of 50 oncogenes using targeted sequencing, prevalent mutations involving *PIK3CA* (30%), *KRAS* (30%), *MET* (15%), and *RB1* (10%) were detected. *PIK3CA*, *KRAS*, and *RB1* mutations were seen only in patterns B or C, and *KRAS* mutations correlated with advanced stage (at least FIGO stage II). In the second study, 52 cases were evaluated for hotspot mutations in 13 genes and showed mutations in similar genes. Unlike the Hodgson study, 2 (20%) pattern A tumors harbored *KRAS* mutations as well as 5 (29%) pattern B and 5 (20%) pattern C. The remaining pattern A tumors (8) showed no other mutations, whereas patterns B and C showed additional mutations in *PIK3CA*, *PTEN*, *CDKN2A*, *PPP2R1A*, and *FBXW7*.[69] The data suggest that pattern A tumors are indeed biologically distinct from patterns B and C with a possible tumor progression model in which mutations accumulate as the tumor invades the surrounding stroma.[69,70] The pattern-based classification has been advocated to be incorporated into the current FIGO staging system.[83] Of note, 1 case from

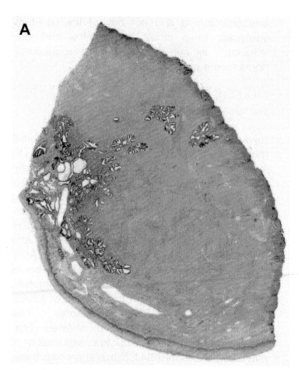

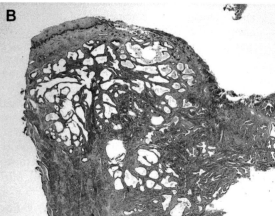

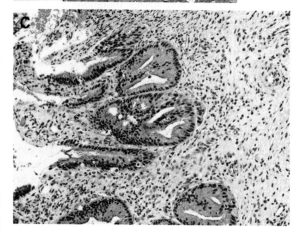

Fig. 10. Pattern-based classification. (*A, B*) Pattern A shows well-rounded, simple to complex glandular growth deep into cervical wall without stromal desmoplasia: whole slide imaging (*A*) and ×20 (*B*). (*C, D*) Pattern B shows single cells and clusters of invasive tumor arising from the base of well-formed glands, ×200.

Fig. 10. (continued). (*E, F*) Pattern C shows diffuse destructive stromal invasion with desmoplasia and complex expansile labyrinthine growth, ×20.

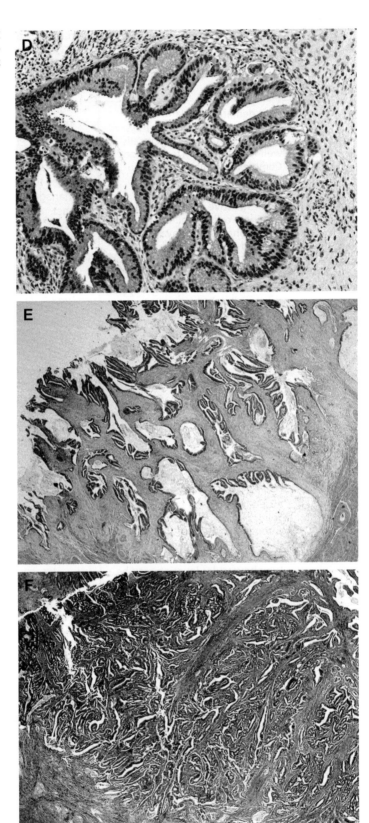

Table 3
Pattern-based classification of usual type endocervical adenocarcinoma

Patterns	Histologic Criteria
Pattern A	• Well-demarcated glands with rounded contours, frequently forming groups (architecturally well-moderately differentiated) • Complex intraglandular (cribriform, papillary) growth acceptable • No destructive stromal invasion • No single cells or cell detachment • No lymphovascular invasion • No solid growth
Pattern B	• Focal destructive stromal invasion arising from pattern A glands, with individual or small groups of tumor cells within desmoplastic or inflamed stroma • Foci of invasion may be single, multiple, or linear at tumor base • Lymphovascular invasion may be present • No solid growth
Pattern C	• Diffuse destructive stromal invasion with diffusely infiltrative glands (angulated, interspersed open glands, or canalicular pattern) and extensive desmoplastic response • Confluent growth filling a 4× field (5 mm) with glands, papillae, or mucin lakes • Solid, poorly differentiated component (architecturally high grade) present; nuclear grade is disregarded • Lymphovascular invasion may be present

Adapted from Roma AA, Mistretta TA, Diaz De Vivar A, et al. New pattern-based personalized risk stratification system for endocervical adenocarcinoma with important clinical implications and surgical outcome. Gynecol Oncol 2016;141(1):37; with permission.

the Spaans study showed loss of PMS2 by IHC. Upon careful review of that case, the investigators concluded that this was misclassification of a lower uterine segment endometrial endometrioid adenocarcinoma (HPV negative) as UEA in a patient who had undergone supracervical hysterectomy 20 years prior.

SUMMARY

EA is a heterogeneous disease comprising both HPV- and non-HPV-associated subtypes that have distinct clinicopathologic features. The IECC system is superior to the WHO classification because it uniquely integrates morphology, cause/pathogenesis, and biological behavior of these subtypes. Pattern-based classification is clinically significant in HPV-associated EAs and should be incorporated in management algorithms. Understanding specific morphologic features, immunophenotype, and limitations of IHC is crucial for accurate classification and pathologic staging of these tumors, which, in turn, guide optimal clinical management and prognostication of patients. Last, clinically relevant classification systems in EA (both IECC and pattern-based classification) will aid in the discovery of novel prognostic and predictive biomarkers as well as identification of therapeutic targets.

REFERENCES

1. Wilbur DC, Colgan TJ, Ferenczy AS, et al. Tumors of the uterine cervix - glandular tumors and precursors. In: Kurman RJ, Carcangiu M-L, Herrington CS, et al, editors. WHO classification of tumours of female reproductive organs. Lyon (France): International Agency for Research on Cancer; 2014. p. 183–94.
2. An HJ, Kim KR, Kim IS, et al. Prevalence of human papillomavirus DNA in various histological subtypes of cervical adenocarcinoma: a population-based study. Mod Pathol 2005;18(4):528–34.
3. Kurman RJ, Carcangiu ML, Herrington CS, et al. WHO classification of tumors of female reproductive organs. 4th edition. IARC. Lyon (France): WHO Press; 2014.
4. Young RH, Clement PB. Endocervical adenocarcinoma and its variants: their morphology and differential diagnosis. Histopathology 2002;41(3):185–207.
5. Andersson S, Rylander E, Larsson B, et al. The role of human papillomavirus in cervical adenocarcinoma carcinogenesis. Eur J Cancer 2001;37(2):246–50.
6. Molijn A, Jenkins D, Chen W, et al. The complex relationship between human papillomavirus and cervical adenocarcinoma. Int J Cancer 2016;138(2):409–16.
7. Holl K, Nowakowski AM, Powell N, et al. Human papillomavirus prevalence and type-distribution in cervical glandular neoplasias: results from a European multinational epidemiological study. Int J Cancer 2015;137(12):2858–68.
8. Pirog EC, Lloveras B, Molijn A, et al. HPV prevalence and genotypes in different histological subtypes of cervical adenocarcinoma, a worldwide analysis of 760 cases. Mod Pathol 2014;27(12):1559–67.
9. Stolnicu S, Barsan I, Hoang L, et al. International endocervical adenocarcinoma criteria and classification (IECC): a new pathogenetic classification for

invasive adenocarcinomas of the endocervix. Am J Surg Pathol 2018;42(2):214–26.

10. Hodgson A, Park KJ, Djordjevic B, et al. International endocervical adenocarcinoma criteria and classification: validation and interobserver reproducibility. Am J Surg Pathol 2019;43(1):75–83.

11. Zielinski GD, Snijders PJ, Rozendaal L, et al. The presence of high-risk HPV combined with specific p53 and p16INK4a expression patterns points to high-risk HPV as the main causative agent for adenocarcinoma in situ and adenocarcinoma of the cervix. J Pathol 2003;201(4):535–43.

12. Stolnicu S, Barsan I, Hoang L, et al. Diagnostic algorithmic proposal based on comprehensive immunohistochemical evaluation of 297 invasive endocervical adenocarcinomas. Am J Surg Pathol 2018;42(8):989–1000.

13. Kalof AN, Cooper K. p16INK4a immunoexpression: surrogate marker of high-risk HPV and high-grade cervical intraepithelial neoplasia. Adv Anat Pathol 2006;13(4):190–4.

14. Park KJ, Bramlage MP, Ellenson LH, et al. Immunoprofile of adenocarcinomas of the endometrium, endocervix, and ovary with mucinous differentiation. Appl Immunohistochem Mol Morphol 2009;17(1):8–11.

15. Young RH, Scully RE. Villoglandular papillary adenocarcinoma of the uterine cervix. A clinicopathologic analysis of 13 cases. Cancer 1989;63(9):1773–9.

16. Jones MW, Silverberg SG, Kurman RJ. Well-differentiated villoglandular adenocarcinoma of the uterine cervix: a clinicopathological study of 24 cases. Int J Gynecol Pathol 1993;12(1):1–7.

17. Fadare O, Zheng W. Well-differentiated papillary villoglandular adenocarcinoma of the uterine cervix with a focal high-grade component: is there a need for reassessment? Virchows Arch 2005; 447(5):883–7.

18. Utsugi K, Shimizu Y, Akiyama F, et al. Villoglandular papillary adenocarcinoma of the uterine cervix with bulky lymph node metastases. Eur J Obstet Gynecol Reprod Biol 2002;105(2):186–8.

19. Sal V, Kahramanoglu I, Turan H, et al. Primary signet ring cell carcinoma of the cervix: a case report and review of the literature. Int J Surg Case Rep 2016;21: 1–5.

20. Balci S, Saglam A, Usubutun A. Primary signet-ring cell carcinoma of the cervix: case report and review of the literature. Int J Gynecol Pathol 2010;29(2): 181–4.

21. Giordano G, Pizzi S, Berretta R, et al. A new case of primary signet-ring cell carcinoma of the cervix with prominent endometrial and myometrial involvement: immunohistochemical and molecular studies and review of the literature. World J Surg Oncol 2012;10:7.

22. Lastra RR, Park KJ, Schoolmeester JK. Invasive stratified mucin-producing carcinoma and stratified mucin-producing intraepithelial lesion (SMILE): 15 cases presenting a spectrum of cervical neoplasia with description of a distinctive variant of invasive adenocarcinoma. Am J Surg Pathol 2016;40(2): 262–9.

23. Park JJ, Sun D, Quade BJ, et al. Stratified mucin-producing intraepithelial lesions of the cervix: adenosquamous or columnar cell neoplasia? Am J Surg Pathol 2000;24(10):1414–9.

24. Kuragaki C, Enomoto T, Ueno Y, et al. Mutations in the STK11 gene characterize minimal deviation adenocarcinoma of the uterine cervix. Lab Invest 2003;83(1):35–45.

25. Lee JY, Dong SM, Kim HS, et al. A distinct region of chromosome 19p13.3 associated with the sporadic form of adenoma malignum of the uterine cervix. Cancer Res 1998;58(6):1140–3.

26. Mikami Y, Hata S, Melamed J, et al. Lobular endocervical glandular hyperplasia is a metaplastic process with a pyloric gland phenotype. Histopathology 2001;39(4):364–72.

27. Mikami Y, McCluggage WG. Endocervical glandular lesions exhibiting gastric differentiation: an emerging spectrum of benign, premalignant, and malignant lesions. Adv Anat Pathol 2013;20(4):227–37.

28. Gilks CB, Young RH, Aguirre P, et al. Adenoma malignum (minimal deviation adenocarcinoma) of the uterine cervix. A clinicopathological and immunohistochemical analysis of 26 cases. Am J Surg Pathol 1989;13(9):717–29.

29. Pirog EC, Park KJ, Kiyokawa T, et al. Gastric-type adenocarcinoma of the cervix: tumor with wide range of histologic appearances. Adv Anat Pathol 2019;26(1):1–12.

30. McCluggage WG, Harley I, Houghton JP, et al. Composite cervical adenocarcinoma composed of adenoma malignum and gastric type adenocarcinoma (dedifferentiated adenoma malignum) in a patient with Peutz Jeghers syndrome. J Clin Pathol 2010; 63(10):935–41.

31. Kojima A, Mikami Y, Sudo T, et al. Gastric morphology and immunophenotype predict poor outcome in mucinous adenocarcinoma of the uterine cervix. Am J Surg Pathol 2007;31(5):664–72.

32. Carleton C, Hoang L, Sah S, et al. A detailed immunohistochemical analysis of a large series of cervical and vaginal gastric-type adenocarcinomas. Am J Surg Pathol 2016;40(5):636–44.

33. Pirog EC. Diagnosis of HPV-negative, gastric-type adenocarcinoma of the endocervix. Methods Mol Biol 2015;1249:213–9.

34. Turashvili G, Morency EG, Kracun M, et al. Morphologic features of gastric-type cervical adenocarcinoma in small surgical and cytology specimens. Int J Gynecol Pathol 2018, [Epub ahead of print].

35. Park KJ, Kiyokawa T, Soslow RA, et al. Unusual endocervical adenocarcinomas: an immunohistochemical analysis with molecular detection of

human papillomavirus. Am J Surg Pathol 2011;35(5): 633–46.

36. Kawauchi S, Kusuda T, Liu XP, et al. Is lobular endo-cervical glandular hyperplasia a cancerous precursor of minimal deviation adenocarcinoma?: A comparative molecular-genetic and immunohisto-chemical study. Am J Surg Pathol 2008;32(12): 1807–15.

37. Talia KL, Stewart CJR, Howitt BE, et al. HPV-negative gastric type adenocarcinoma in situ of the cervix: a spectrum of rare lesions exhibiting gastric and intes-tinal differentiation. Am J Surg Pathol 2017;41(8): 1023–33.

38. Wada T, Ohishi Y, Kaku T, et al. Endocervical adeno-carcinoma with morphologic features of both usual and gastric types: clinicopathologic and immunohis-tochemical analyses and high-risk HPV detection by in situ hybridization. Am J Surg Pathol 2017;41(5): 696–705.

39. Karamurzin YS, Kiyokawa T, Parkash V, et al. Gastric-type endocervical adenocarcinoma: an aggressive tumor with unusual metastatic patterns and poor prognosis. Am J Surg Pathol 2015; 39(11):1449–57.

40. Kojima A, Shimada M, Mikami Y, et al. Chemoresist-ance of gastric-type mucinous carcinoma of the uter-ine cervix: a study of the Sankai Gynecology Study Group. Int J Gynecol Cancer 2018;28(1):99–106.

41. Silver SA, Devouassoux-Shisheboran M, Mezzetti TP, et al. Mesonephric adenocarcinomas of the uterine cervix: a study of 11 cases with immunohistochemical findings. Am J Surg Pathol 2001;25(3):379–87.

42. Cavalcanti MS, Schultheis AM, Ho C, et al. Mixed mesonephric adenocarcinoma and high-grade neuroendocrine carcinoma of the uterine cervix: case description of a previously unreported entity with insights into its molecular pathogenesis. Int J Gynecol Pathol 2017;36(1):76–89.

43. Patel V, Kipp B, Schoolmeester JK. Corded and hy-alinized mesonephric-like adenocarcinoma of the uterine corpus: report of a case mimicking endome-trioid carcinoma. Hum Pathol 2018, [Epub ahead of print].

44. Mirkovic J, McFarland M, Garcia E, et al. Targeted genomic profiling reveals recurrent KRAS mutations in mesonephric-like adenocarcinomas of the female genital tract. Am J Surg Pathol 2018;42(2): 227–33.

45. Kenny SL, McBride HA, Jamison J, et al. Meso-nephric adenocarcinomas of the uterine cervix and corpus: HPV-negative neoplasms that are commonly PAX8, CA125, and HMGA2 positive and that may be immunoreactive with TTF1 and hepatocyte nuclear factor 1-beta. Am J Surg Pathol 2012;36(6):799–807.

46. Pors J, Cheng A, Leo JM, et al. A comparison of GATA3, TTF1, CD10, and calretinin in identifying mesonephric and mesonephric-like carcinomas of the gynecologic tract. Am J Surg Pathol 2018; 42(12):1596–606.

47. Howitt BE, Emori MM, Drapkin R, et al. GATA3 is a sensitive and specific marker of benign and malig-nant mesonephric lesions in the lower female genital tract. Am J Surg Pathol 2015;39(10):1411–9.

48. Mirkovic J, Sholl LM, Garcia E, et al. Targeted genomic profiling reveals recurrent KRAS mutations and gain of chromosome 1q in mesonephric carci-nomas of the female genital tract. Mod Pathol 2015;28(11):1504–14.

49. Herbst AL. Behavior of estrogen-associated female genital tract cancer and its relation to neoplasia following intrauterine exposure to diethylstilbestrol (DES). Gynecol Oncol 2000;76(2):147–56.

50. Kaminski PF, Maier RC. Clear cell adenocarcinoma of the cervix unrelated to diethylstilbestrol exposure. Obstet Gynecol 1983;62(6):720–7.

51. Huo D, Anderson D, Palmer JR, et al. Incidence rates and risks of diethylstilbestrol-related clear-cell adenocarcinoma of the vagina and cervix: update after 40-year follow-up. Gynecol Oncol 2017; 146(3):566–71.

52. Reich O, Tamussino K, Lahousen M, et al. Clear cell carcinoma of the uterine cervix: pathology and prog-nosis in surgically treated stage IB-IIB disease in women not exposed in utero to diethylstilbestrol. Gy-necol Oncol 2000;76(3):331–5.

53. Boyd J, Takahashi H, Waggoner SE, et al. Molecular genetic analysis of clear cell adenocarcinomas of the vagina and cervix associated and unassociated with diethylstilbestrol exposure in utero. Cancer 1996;77(3):507–13.

54. Mills AM, Liou S, Kong CS, et al. Are women with en-docervical adenocarcinoma at risk for lynch syn-drome? Evaluation of 101 cases including unusual subtypes and lower uterine segment tumors. Int J Gynecol Pathol 2012;31(5):463–9.

55. Togami S, Sasajima Y, Kasamatsu T, et al. Immuno-phenotype and human papillomavirus status of se-rous adenocarcinoma of the uterine cervix. Pathol Oncol Res 2015;21(2):487–94.

56. Domfeh AB, Kuhn E, Park KJ, et al. Papillary serous carcinoma of the cervix – two diseases with distinct clinico-pathologic profiles? Mod Pathol 2013; 26(suppl 2):272A.

57. Stewart CJR, Koay MHE, Leslie C, et al. Cervical car-cinomas with a micropapillary component: a clinico-pathological study of eight cases. Histopathology 2018;72(4):626–33.

58. Nofech-Mozes S, Rasty G, Ismiil N, et al. Immunohis-tochemical characterization of endocervical papil-lary serous carcinoma. Int J Gynecol Cancer 2006; 16(Suppl 1):286–92.

59. Pecorelli S, Zigliani L, Odicino F. Revised FIGO stag-ing for carcinoma of the cervix. Int J Gynaecol Ob-stet 2009;105(2):107–8.

60. McCluggage WG, Judge MJ, Alvarado-Cabrero I, et al. Data set for the reporting of carcinomas of the cervix: recommendations from the International Collaboration on Cancer Reporting (ICCR). Int J Gynecol Pathol 2018;37(3):205–28.

61. Zaino RJ. Glandular lesions of the uterine cervix. Mod Pathol 2000;13(3):261–74.

62. Diaz De Vivar A, Roma AA, Park KJ, et al. Invasive endocervical adenocarcinoma: proposal for a new pattern-based classification system with significant clinical implications: a multi-institutional study. Int J Gynecol Pathol 2013;32(6):592–601.

63. Roma AA, Park KJ, Xie H, et al. Role of lymphovascular invasion in pattern C invasive endocervical adenocarcinoma. Am J Surg Pathol 2017;41(9):1205–11.

64. Roma AA, Mistretta TA, Diaz De Vivar A, et al. New pattern-based personalized risk stratification system for endocervical adenocarcinoma with important clinical implications and surgical outcome. Gynecol Oncol 2016;141(1):36–42.

65. Roma AA, Diaz De Vivar A, Park KJ, et al. Invasive endocervical adenocarcinoma: a new pattern-based classification system with important clinical significance. Am J Surg Pathol 2015;39(5):667–72.

66. Parra-Herran C, Taljaard M, Djordjevic B, et al. Pattern-based classification of invasive endocervical adenocarcinoma, depth of invasion measurement and distinction from adenocarcinoma in situ: interobserver variation among gynecologic pathologists. Mod Pathol 2016;29(8):879–92.

67. Douglas G, Howitt BE, Schoolmeester JK, et al. Architectural overlap between benign endocervix and pattern-A endocervical adenocarcinoma: are all pattern-A tumors invasive? Pathol Res Pract 2017;213(7):799–803.

68. Paquette C, Jeffus SK, Quick CM, et al. Interobserver variability in the application of a proposed histologic subclassification of endocervical adenocarcinoma. Am J Surg Pathol 2015;39(1):93–100.

69. Spaans VM, Scheunhage DA, Barzaghi B, et al. Independent validation of the prognostic significance of invasion patterns in endocervical adenocarcinoma: pattern A predicts excellent survival. Gynecol Oncol 2018;151(2):196–201.

70. Hodgson A, Amemiya Y, Seth A, et al. Genomic abnormalities in invasive endocervical adenocarcinoma correlate with pattern of invasion: biologic and clinical implications. Mod Pathol 2017;30(11):1633–41.

71. Alvarado-Cabrero I, Roma AA, Park KJ, et al. Factors predicting pelvic lymph node metastasis, relapse, and disease outcome in pattern C endocervical adenocarcinomas. Int J Gynecol Pathol 2017; 36(5):476–85.

72. Rutgers JK, Roma AA, Park KJ, et al. Pattern classification of endocervical adenocarcinoma: reproducibility and review of criteria. Mod Pathol 2016;29(9): 1083–94.

73. Djordjevic B, Parra-Herran C. Application of a pattern-based classification system for invasive endocervical adenocarcinoma in cervical biopsy, cone and loop electrosurgical excision (LEEP) material: pattern on cone and LEEP is predictive of pattern in the overall tumor. Int J Gynecol Pathol 2016;35(5):456–66.

74. Park KJ, Roma AA. Pattern based classification of endocervical adenocarcinoma: a review. Pathology 2018;50(2):134–40.

75. Stolnicu S, Barsan I, Hoang L, et al. Stromal invasion pattern identifies patients at lowest risk of lymph node metastasis in HPV-associated endocervical adenocarcinomas, but is irrelevant in adenocarcinomas unassociated with HPV. Gynecol Oncol 2018;150(1):56–60.

76. Ojesina AI, Lichtenstein L, Freeman SS, et al. Landscape of genomic alterations in cervical carcinomas. Nature 2014;506(7488):371–5.

77. Wright AA, Howitt BE, Myers AP, et al. Oncogenic mutations in cervical cancer: genomic differences between adenocarcinomas and squamous cell carcinomas of the cervix. Cancer 2013;119(21): 3776–83.

78. Lou H, Villagran G, Boland JF, et al. Genome analysis of Latin American cervical cancer: frequent activation of the PIK3CA pathway. Clin Cancer Res 2015;21(23):5360–70.

79. Tornesello ML, Annunziata C, Buonaguro L, et al. TP53 and PIK3CA gene mutations in adenocarcinoma, squamous cell carcinoma and high-grade intraepithelial neoplasia of the cervix. J Transl Med 2014;12:255.

80. Fruman DA, Rommel C. PI3K and cancer: lessons, challenges and opportunities. Nat Rev Drug Discov 2014;13(2):140–56.

81. Chappell WH, Steelman LS, Long JM, et al. Ras/Raf/ MEK/ERK and PI3K/PTEN/Akt/mTOR inhibitors: rationale and importance to inhibiting these pathways in human health. Oncotarget 2011;2(3): 135–64.

82. Cancer Genome Atlas Research Network, Albert Einstein College of Medicine, Analytical Biological Services, et al. Integrated genomic and molecular characterization of cervical cancer. Nature 2017; 543(7645):378–84.

83. Roma AA. Patterns of Invasion of Cervical Adenocarcinoma as Predicators of Outcome. Adv Anat Pathol 2015;22(6):345–54.

Benign and Premalignant Lesions of the Endometrium

Wesley Daniel Mallinger, DO, Charles Matthew Quick, MD*

KEYWORDS

- EIN • Atypical hyperplasia • Benign hyperplasia • Endometrial metaplasia • Papillary proliferations

---

Key points

- The balance of estrogen in relation to progesterone is a key factor in the development of benign, premalignant, and malignant endometrial lesions.

- Prolonged unopposed or poorly opposed estrogen exposure is associated with the disordered proliferative endometrial pattern as well as benign hyperplasia, and also increases the risk for the development of premalignant and malignant lesions.

- Our current understanding implicates discrete clonal alterations in atypical hyperplasia/endometrioid intraepithelial neoplasia.

- The diagnosis of atypical hyperplasia/endometrioid intraepithelial neoplasia is reliant on the presence of 4 well-defined features as assessed by light microscopy as well as exclusion of benign and malignant mimics.

- Sampling limitations and pitfalls exist, and the pathologist must have knowledge of how to deal with these issues to give the appropriate information to the clinician.

ABSTRACT

In this review, we highlight the benign and premalignant lesions of the endometrium that the pathologist may encounter in daily practice. We begin by detailing our current understanding of excess estrogen in the progression of endometrial neoplasia. We outline the currently accepted terminology to be used when evaluating proliferative endometrial lesions, while highlighting their key features. Attention is then turned to the molecular underpinnings of neoplastic progression and how this can be exploited with immunohistochemical stains when appropriate. Finally, we discuss types of metaplasia and their associations, including so-called papillary proliferations of the endometrium.

Most surgical pathologists encounter a healthy volume of endometrial biopsy/curettage in daily practice. By far, the most common clinical indication for endometrial sampling is abnormal uterine bleeding. There are a myriad of causes for abnormal uterine bleeding that must be considered when reviewing endometrial samples, the most important of which is overt malignancy. Even if a diagnosis of malignancy can be excluded, a number of important benign and premalignant lesions may be present. These lesions may have clinical implications in their own right, and it is important for the pathologist to recognize and appropriately categorize these entities to give the clinician the information they need to properly manage the patient.

In this review, we highlight the important benign and premalignant lesions of the endometrium that

---

Disclosure Statement: The authors do not have any disclosure of a relationship with a commercial company that has a direct financial interest in subject matter or materials discussed in article or with a company making a competing product.
Department of Pathology, University of Arkansas for Medical Sciences, 4301 West Markham Street, Slot 517, Little Rock, AR 72205, USA
* Corresponding author.
E-mail address: QuickCharlesM@uams.edu

Surgical Pathology 12 (2019) 315–328
https://doi.org/10.1016/j.path.2019.01.003
1875-9181/19/© 2019 Elsevier Inc. All rights reserved.

the pathologist may encounter in daily practice. A paramount concept that must be understood is the spectrum of hyperplasia and intraepithelial neoplasia in the evaluation of risk for subsequent development of carcinoma. This topic has been contentious over the past several decades, especially with regard to categorizing features and terminology. We present the currently accepted terminology and salient features that a pathologist must evaluate to provide the appropriate information to the clinician. Often, the differential diagnosis includes various types of benign metaplasias, as well as papillary endometrial proliferations, which is also discussed. Pitfalls and mimics can cause a significant amount of frustration and anxiety and, as such, these entities are approached in a practical manner with regard to diagnosis and proper clinical management.

HORMONAL BALANCE

The effect of estrogen and progesterone on the endometrium cannot be overstated. When evaluating an endometrial sampling, it is extremely important that the pathologist do their due diligence in determining whether there is a clinical cause for an increase in estrogen in relation to progesterone. It has been shown that an increase in the ratio of estrogen to progesterone is a key driver in the progression of endometrial premalignant lesions.[1] There is a proverbial "tug of war" between the proliferative effects of estrogen and the purging effects of progesterone withdrawal in tumorigenesis. If estrogen predominates, then an environment of proliferation will sustain glands with early or "latent" mutations. The link between increased estrogen and endometrial cancer has been well-established.[2,3] With an understanding of these effects, current contraceptives use low-dose estrogen and progesterone in an appropriate balance to mitigate the risk of cancer development. Evidence shows that the use of low-dose, combined contraceptives lowers the risk of endometrial carcinoma regardless of the presence or absence of other risk factors.[4,5] Progestin-only forms of contraceptives are also available and have been shown to reduce risk even more substantially.[6] Tamoxifen therapy is another important consideration when considering premalignant and malignant lesions of the endometrium. Despite its antagonistic action on estrogen receptors within the breast, tamoxifen acts as an agonist on endometrial tissue. The resultant increase in estrogenic activity, especially with a relative lack of progesterone in postmenopausal patients, leads to an increased risk of the development of not only endometrial polyps, but also premalignant and malignant endometrial lesions.[7,8]

In addition to exogenous hormones, there are 2 other important sources of endogenous excess estrogen. The most common is increased adipose tissue leading to peripheral conversion of precursor steroids to estrogen. The patient's weight or body mass index is a useful surrogate for evaluating the amount of adipose tissue and is a key piece of information that should be considered in every case. A second, less common, source of excess estrogen is an estrogen-secreting tumor, such as an ovarian granulosa cell tumor. Alternatively, polycystic ovarian syndrome in adults may lead to poor production of progesterone, and thus relatively unopposed estrogen. When paired with chronic anovulation, this hormonal imbalance may result in endometrial hyperplasia and, ultimately, carcinoma. Any of these sources of excess estrogen, relative to progesterone, can drive the progression of endometrial neoplasia.

PROGRESSION

With the critical role of excess estrogen established, a framework of tumorigenesis can be outlined. Our current understanding includes several distinct entities along a sequence ending with cancer. Despite our need to create distinct categories, the effects are usually seen as a spectrum and indeed may not be entirely linear. Our goal is to set forth criteria that can be used to identify where, in this continuum, the patient's sample falls. The progression generally follows along the path of proliferative to disordered proliferative endometrium, benign hyperplasia, atypical hyperplasia (AH) / endometrioid intraepithelial neoplasia (EIN), and finally carcinoma; however, the development of premalignant and malignant endometrial lesions can also certainly occur in the absence of benign hyperplasia.

COMPLEXITY AND ATYPIA

The majority of pathologists and clinicians are most familiar with the 4 tiered classification scheme of endometrial hyperplasia as outlined by Kurman and colleagues.[9] This is not surprising given the fact that it formed the basis for the World Health Organization (WHO) Blue Book classification of endometrial precancerous lesions from 1994 until the most recent edition in 2014. In this former system, risk stratification was determined based on both glandular complexity and nuclear atypia. Complexity was defined by the density and pattern of glandular architecture, whereas atypia was defined cytologically, based on varying degrees of nuclear atypia and loss of polarity. By assessing complexity and atypia separately, 4 categories were available for classification. Progression to carcinoma was noted in 1% of simple hyperplasia, 3% in complex hyperplasia, 8% in simple hyperplasia with atypia, and 29% in complex hyperplasia with atypia (complex AH).[9] Multiple studies demonstrated poor diagnostic reproducibility.[10–12] Not surprisingly, this finding was most notable with regard to the determination of presence of atypia, the key component for risk stratification. In 2014, the WHO refined the terminology and criteria, largely based on the endometrial intraepithelial neoplasia system developed by Dr George Mutter and colleagues. This resulted in a new, 2-tiered system, which aims to be more reproducible. A particular nomenclature centered nuance should be noted: the term *endometrioid* has been substituted for *endometrial* in the most recent 2014 WHO classification to avoid confusion with endometrial intraepithelial carcinoma, a precursor to uterine serous carcinoma. As we focus on the currently accepted concept of progression, we will touch on similarities between the current and previous classification schemes.

DISORDERED PROLIFERATIVE ENDOMETRIUM

One of the earliest manifestations of excess estrogen in relation to progesterone is disordered proliferative endometrium. In disordered proliferative endometrium, the ratio of glands to stroma is relatively preserved, although a small shift toward more glands may be present. In addition, scattered cystic and sacculated glands, a result of continued epithelial proliferation, are present (**Fig. 1**). Patchy tubal metaplasia is usually present, and may mimic atypia at low magnification. These features are indicative of unopposed, or poorly opposed, estrogen exposure, which in a premenopausal or perimenopausal women may be related to prolonged anovulatory cycles. Importantly, Because this problem is systemic, all fragments of endometrial functionalis in the sample should demonstrate these features, and should not be a focal or discrete finding.

BENIGN HYPERPLASIA

The endometrium may manifest benign ("simple") hyperplasia, evidenced by an increase in the ratio of glands to stroma. Usually, the increased gland to stroma ratio is diffuse and involves the entire sample. Areas of increased proliferation are sometimes patchy, composed of small glands, and punctuated by glands with cystic change, resulting in the somewhat confusing description of "regularly irregular" gland crowding (**Fig. 2**). Additionally, frequent mitotic figures, focal hemorrhage, fibrin thrombi, and stromal breakdown may be present.[13] Importantly, cytologic demarcation (discussed elsewhere in this article) and nuclear atypia should be absent.

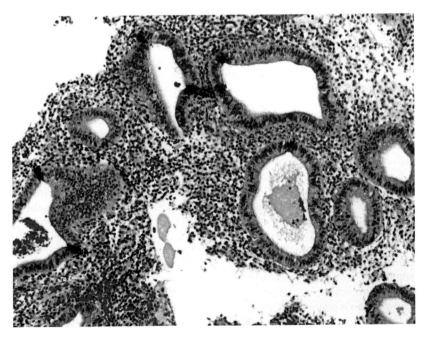

Fig. 1. Disordered proliferative endometrium composed of slightly crowded, sacculated glands with tubal metaplasia (H&E, original magnification ×10).

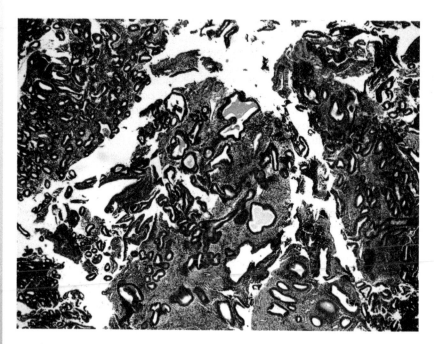

Fig. 2. Benign hyperplasia demonstrating a regularly irregular pattern of small proliferating glands and cystic glands (H&E, original magnification ×4).

ATYPICAL HYPERPLASIA/ENDOMETRIOID INTRAEPITHELIAL NEOPLASIA

Many overlapping histologic features exist between benign hyperplasia and AH/EIN. The key distinguishing feature that separates these entities is cytologic demarcation. Simply stated, cytologic demarcation denotes a population of glands that is distinct from the background glands. The designation atypical, when referring to AH, describes the appearance of the precancerous glands relative to the background. This designation is not the same definition of atypia that was used in the previous hyperplasia classification scheme. In fact, the cytology of AH/EIN can be quite bland, yet still have a distinct appearance compared the background endometrium. Altered cytology, or atypia, is secondary to underlying driver mutations allowed to persist in the environment of hyperplasia, leading to the histologic appearance of a clonal population.[14] These driver mutations are discussed in greater detail elsewhere in this article.

Famously, morphometric analysis was used to aid in the identification of EIN.[14] Fortunately, criteria that can be readily assessed by pathologists using light microscopy have been identified to diagnose EIN.[15] These criteria include a gland to stroma ratio of greater than 55%, cytologic demarcation from the background endometrial epithelium, size greater than 1 mm, and exclusion of benign mimics as well as carcinoma (**Fig. 3**). The size criterion is historic and largely based on computer models; however, there is some usefulness

in its retention because it helps to prevent over-diagnosis based on small areas of crowding. Multiple discontinuous foci should not be added together to fulfill the size criteria. If a diagnosis of definitive EIN is not possible, the pathologist can diagnose focal gland crowding with a comment for the clinician to resample after an appropriate interval of time, usually 3 to 6 months. This consideration is important, because focal gland crowding has shown a significant incidence of subsequent EIN or carcinoma upon additional sampling.[16] Many mimics of AH/EIN exist and are covered throughout the remainder of this review.

ATYPICAL HYPERPLASIA/ENDOMETRIOID INTRAEPITHELIAL NEOPLASIA AND CARCINOMA RISK

In the EIN literature, It has been shown that a diagnosis of AH/EIN carries an approximately 45-fold greater risk of developing endometrioid carcinoma compared with benign hyperplasia.[17] Furthermore, in the AH literature, approximately 30% to 40% of patients may have concurrent carcinoma with around one-third of these being myoinvasive.[18,19] As a result, hysterectomy is recommended for patients with a diagnosis of AH/EIN. An alternative treatment option in younger patients who desire preserved fertility is medical management with high-dose progestins.[20] Studies have shown this to be an effective treatment strategy and, in some patients, may result in various metaplasias, a decrease in gland crowding, and a loss

Fig. 3. A focus of atypical hyperplasia/endometrioid intraepithelial neoplasia (*left*) displaying crowding altered cytology (when compared with the background endometrium on the *right*) and a size greater than 1 mm (H&E, original magnification ×4).

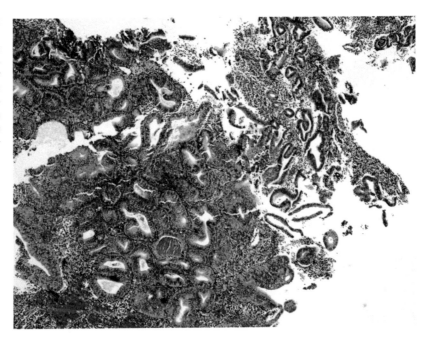

of atypia.[21,22] Several studies have analyzed various biomarkers to predict response to progestins, but results have been conflicting.[23–28]

MOLECULAR AND IMMUNOHISTOCHEMICAL FEATURES

As described, the diagnosis of AH/EIN involves the use of light microscopy and objective criteria to identify a clonal population of glands harboring molecular alterations. While we continue to learn more about the molecular mechanisms of carcinoma progression, several well-defined alterations have been described, which may be exploited as adjunctive studies in difficult cases.

PTEN is a tumor suppressor gene that has been implicated in many human cancers, including endometrial carcinoma.[29] Loss of PTEN nuclear and cytoplasmic expression has been shown to occur in 83% of endometrial carcinomas and 55% of endometrial precancers.[30] However, patchy PTEN loss is common and has been described in as many as 19% of benign hysterectomy specimens, and up to 43% of benign endometrial biopsies.[31,32] *PTEN* alterations are thought to occur as early events in tumorigenesis, and have been shown to act synergistically with other mutations.[33–36] Glands that acquire *PTEN* mutations are periodically shed via menses, but are able to persist in states of anovulation. Owing to the frequency of *PTEN* alterations in benign endometrium and the technical difficulty with

staining and interpretation, PTEN immunohistochemical staining is not a particularly useful tool to aid in the diagnosis of endometrial precancers. Despite its current lack of clinical usefulness, it may have future prognostic value as it relates to patient obesity.[37]

PAX2 is an important gene in the development of the Mullerian and urogenital systems, and shows persistent nuclear expression in the adult endometrium. Normal PAX2 immunostaining displays robust nuclear positivity, which makes it a relatively easy stain to interpret when searching for a loss of normal staining. The finding of a loss of nuclear expression in 71% of endometrial precancers and 77% of cancers has implicated its potential role as a tumor suppressor in the endometrium (**Fig. 4**).[38] It should also be noted that focal loss of expression has been shown in up to 38% of benign endometrial samples.[38] Several studies have evaluated the usefulness of PAX2 as an adjunct in the diagnosis of AH/EIN, including its use in training scenarios.[39–42] The overall opinion is that, when used appropriately, PAX2 can help to support a diagnosis of AH/EIN, although the diagnosis should be based on fulfilling the previously stated histologic criteria. Interestingly, studies have shown a relative increase in PAX2 expression in rare premalignant lesions.[39,43] This finding is curious, and may be related to a compensatory increase in expression similar to that seen in other tumor suppressor genes. The takeaway message is that PAX2 should never be used as a screening tool for

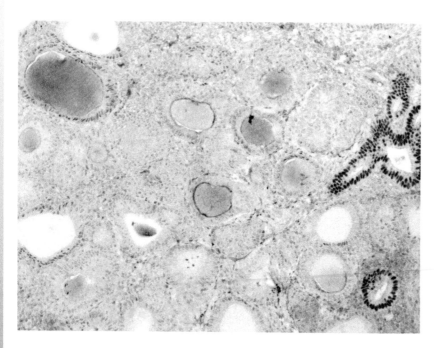

Fig. 4. PAX2 immunohistochemistry showing loss of staining in endometrioid intraepithelial neoplasia with a positive internal control consisting of entrapped normal glands (*right*) (PAX2, original magnification ×10).

evaluating endometrial biopsies, but that loss of staining can help to support a diagnosis of AH/EIN in difficult circumstances.

Microsatellite instability owing to defective mismatch repair is another cause of AH/EIN and endometrial carcinoma. The concept of defective mismatch repair and endometrial carcinoma is well-established, especially in the context of Lynch syndrome. The association with AH/EIN and mismatch repair most commonly centers on sporadic *MLH1* promoter hypermethylation acting as a driver for additional mutations.[44,45] Despite this association, it is not routine practice at this time to evaluate cases of AH/EIN for mismatch repair status.

Additional markers of interest are being evaluated for their usefulness in supporting a diagnosis of AH/EIN including BCL-2 and β-catenin; however, more evidence is needed to support their clinical use.[42,46]

INTERPRETIVE DIFFICULTY AND PITFALLS

A few issues can cause interpretive difficulty when evaluating for AH/EIN. One such issue is tissue fragmentation. This problem is common with endometrial samples, and can complicate the 1-mm size threshold required for a diagnosis of AH/EIN. Ordering additional levels may help to solve this predicament. If the 1-mm size criteria is not met, but there are other features worrisome for AH/EIN, it is prudent to give a descriptive diagnosis (atypical glandular proliferation or focal gland crowding) so that appropriate follow-up sampling can occur. Additionally, separation of the glands and stroma may preclude the evaluation of the gland to stroma ratio, which requires intact endometrium. Again, a descriptive diagnosis and appropriate communication with the clinician can ensure additional sampling, if warranted. When the majority of the sample contains AH/EIN, so-called over-run or extensive EIN, it may be difficult to evaluate cytologic demarcation from the background endometrium. A careful search for background "orphan" benign glands can identify the presence of 2 gland populations; however, normal background endometrial glands are not always present (**Fig. 5**). If this is the case, then other features such as degree of crowding, epithelial cytology, and PAX2 staining may be helpful.

Endometrial polyps may contain glands that are morphologically different from the background nonpolyp endometrium, mimicking cytologic demarcation. To further complicate the issue, AH/EIN can occur in polyps; in this scenario, the cytologic comparison should occur between glands of corresponding tissue (ie, compare AH/EIN involving a polyp with the background polyp glands). The presence of a polyp is important because polyps are more likely to occur in an endometrium with EIN (43.3%) versus benign endometrium (12.9%).[47] Another consideration is metaplastic change, which can mimic AH/EIN, but may also be seen in conjunction with AH/EIN. AH/EIN-associated metaplasia was noted in 37%

Fig. 5. Two over-run, "orphan" glands (*orange arrow*), indicative of the background endometrium may be seen surrounded by atypical hyperplasia/endometrioid intraepithelial neoplasia in this example (H&E, original magnification ×10).

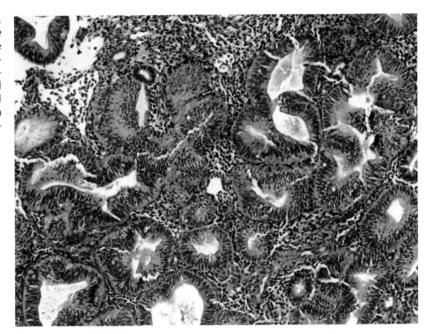

of cases in 1 study.[47] Metaplasias are discussed further in subsequent sections. Occasionally, secretory endometrium may present as a mimic of AH/EIN. Further complicating this issue is the possibility of AH/EIN with secretory change, which is thankfully rare. In the face of these mimics, one should still rely on the previously described criteria, thus comparing the metaplastic or secretory crowded glands with the background endometrium.[48,49]

ENDOMETRIAL METAPLASIA

In addition to benign and premalignant proliferations of the endometrium, the pathologist may encounter altered differentiation in the form of metaplasia. Metaplasia develops as an adaptive mechanism to certain stimuli and is represented by morphologic changes of the cytoplasm and/or nucleus.[50] Some of the most common types are squamous/morular, mucinous, and tubal metaplasia. Less common types include papillary syncytial, secretory, and synovial type metaplasia. In the presence of certain types of metaplasia, associations can be drawn, including morular metaplasia and *CTNNB1* mutations, secretory metaplasia with hormonal influences, and papillary syncytial metaplasia as a reactive change.[50] It is important to note that a diagnosis of metaplasia alone is not useful, because metaplastic changes may be seen in benign, premalignant, and malignant endometrial lesions. To this end, the primary

diagnosis should be first stated and secondarily the presence of metaplasia(s) noted.

SQUAMOUS METAPLASIA

Two types of squamous metaplasia may be encountered in the uterus; however, only one seems to be truly squamous. True squamous (keratinizing) metaplasia of the uterus is rare, and has been termed ichthyosis uteri. This type of squamous metaplasia covers the superficial endometrium with a laminar layer of mature squamous epithelium and is a manifestation of prolonged irritation or chronic inflammation. Much more common is squamous morular metaplasia or morular metaplasia. Morular metaplasia displays some features of squamous metaplasia, namely, a whorling architecture with increased eosinophilic cytoplasm, but does not show a squamous immunophenotype (ie, p63 is commonly negative or minimally positive). Morular change is associated with AH/EIN, and carcinoma and frequently demonstrates β-catenin (nuclear/cytoplasmic), CD10, and CDX2 expression.[51–54] It has been shown that the morular component of lesions showing nuclear β-catenin expression are inert and do not contribute to lesion progression.[51] Several points must be emphasized when dealing with morular metaplasia. The morular component of a lesion should be mentally subtracted when evaluating the gland to stroma ratio when considering a diagnosis of AH/EIN. Additionally, the morular

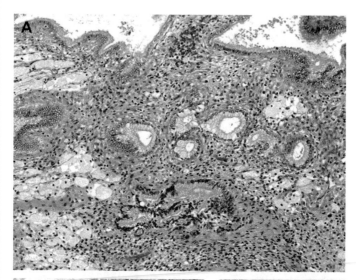

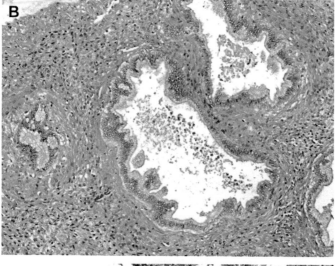

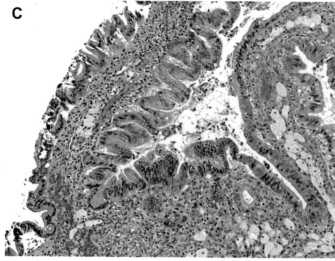

Fig. 6. (*A*) Type A mucinous metaplasia composed of a single layer of bland mucinous epithelium. (*B*) Type B mucinous metaplasia often displays epithelial tufting, yet lacks nuclear atypia. (*C*) Type C mucinous metaplasia displays epithelial architectural complexity as well as nuclear atypia (H&E, original magnification ×10).

component may artificially cause cribriforming and is not indicative of carcinoma. Although morules are not considered neoplastic in their own right, their presence should be noted owing to their association with AH/EIN and endometrioid carcinoma.

TUBAL METAPLASIA

Tubal metaplasia is a common finding within the endometrium and is associated with increased estrogen exposure. The ciliated cells line portions of the glands, especially in disordered proliferative, or anovulatory, endometrium. The endocrine origins of tubal metaplasia are supported by their increased occurrence in patients on tamoxifen.[55] Tubal metaplasia can show cytologic atypia, creating concern for a high-grade intraepithelial lesion. Staining for p53 and TERT have been shown to be of some benefit in supporting the reactive nature of atypia in this instance.[56]

MUCINOUS METAPLASIA

Mucinous metaplasia may be encountered within the endometrium and has been associated with hyperestrogenic states.[57] A classification scheme defining types A, B, and C was originally proposed by Nucci and colleagues[58] and stressed the importance of architectural complexity. Type A lesions showed scattered mucinous glands or small epithelial tufts with no appreciable cytoplasmic atypia or architectural complexity. Type B and C lesions showed increasing levels of epithelial complexity with type C also demonstrating cytologic atypia (**Fig. 6**). Their study was notable in that the incidence of carcinoma in subsequent samples was 0%, 64.7%, and 100% in types A, B, and C lesions, respectively.[58] Additional studies have shown a loss of PAX2 and the presence of *KRAS* mutations in complex mucinous metaplasia, but not in architecturally simple lesions. This finding implies a relationship between acquired genetic alterations and architectural complexity.[59–61] Based on these findings, mucinous metaplasia with simple architectural features may be considered a benign finding, but appreciable architectural complexity in the setting of mucinous differentiation should be noted and prompt additional sampling or consideration of hysterectomy.[57]

PAPILLARY SYNCYTIAL METAPLASIA

So-called papillary syncytial metaplasia is an entity associated with endometrial breakdown and

Fig. 7. Eosinophilic \ papillary metaplasia. Note its superficial location and the presence of abundant neutrophils (H&E, original magnification ×10).

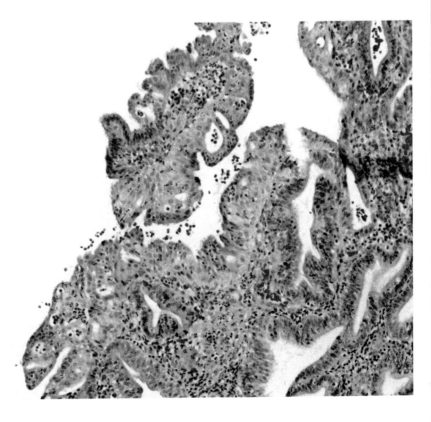

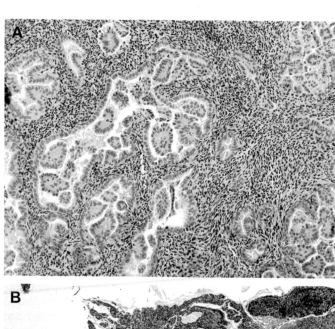

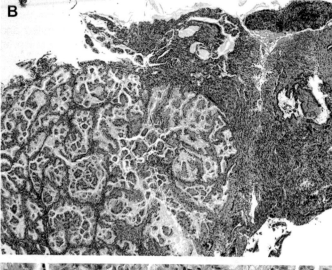

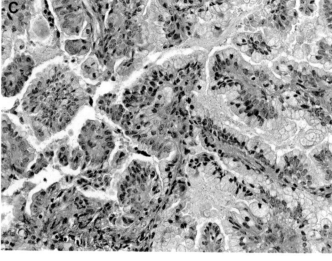

Fig. 8. (*A*) A simple papillary proliferations of the endometrium (PPE) composed of bland cells forming short, intraglandular papillae (H&E, original magnification ×4). (*B*) An example of a complex PPE with mucinous metaplasia and papillae with secondary and tertiary branching (H&E, original magnification ×4). (*C*) Note that the lining of this complex PPE lacks significant nuclear atypia (H&E, original magnification ×10).

repair. The epithelium may show cellular enlargement with eosinophilic cytoplasm with a preserved nuclear to cytoplasmic ratio, and mild to moderate nuclear atypia (**Fig. 7**). Pseudopapillae and neutrophils are often present. These features may prompt consideration of carcinoma, namely serous or clear cell types. The degree of cytologic atypia and nuclear to cytoplasmic ratio are the most helpful features in this distinction. When this possibility arises, immunohistochemical staining with p53, p16, and Ki-67 may be beneficial. Notably, p53 should demonstrate wild-type staining, but in some cases will be increased above expected background levels. Additionally, p16 may also show increased expression, yet still fall short of that associated with serous carcinoma. Ki-67 labeling will be lower than expected when compared with serous carcinoma.[62]

SYNOVIAL-LIKE METAPLASIA

Synovial-like metaplasia has recently been described in 11 patients who had levonorgestrel-releasing intrauterine devices.[63] Synovial-like metaplasia displays cells arranged in a palisading, flat arrangement, perpendicular to the endometrial surface. They can demonstrate patchy CD68 staining, and are negative for estrogen receptor (ER), progesterone receptor (PR), or cytokeratin.[63] The clinical significance of this finding has not been elucidated; however, the pathologist should be aware of this entity, especially in a patient with an intrauterine device.

PAPILLARY PROLIFERATIONS OF THE ENDOMETRIUM

The group of lesions commonly referred to as papillary proliferations of the endometrium (PPE) present as epithelial-lined papillae on the endometrial surface or within endometrial glands. Typically, the lining epithelium shows little to no cytologic atypia. These lesions occur in postmenopausal women and are often associated with endometrial polyps and various types of metaplasia, especially the mucinous type. First described by Lehman and Hart[64] in 2001, PPEs were divided into simple and complex based on the extent of glandular involvement. In their study of 9 cases, they found no association with simple or complex papillary proliferations and carcinoma. In 2013, a larger study of 59 cases defined simple PPEs as having short, predominantly nonbranching stalks, whereas complex PPEs demonstrated longer stalks with secondary and tertiary branching or diffuse filling of cystic spaces with papillae in more than 3 foci[65] (**Fig. 8**). Based on this

schema, 69% of complex PPEs showed progression to or concomitant EIN/carcinoma, compared with only 12% of simple PPEs. Based on those findings, it is rational to use architectural features as a tool in risk stratification of PPEs. Recent studies have aimed to identify immunohistochemical and/or molecular markers to help in the classification of these lesions.[66,67] Despite optimism in this regard, no specific marker has been proven helpful in regard to risk stratification. Further study is needed to add additional tools to the proven usefulness of architectural risk stratification for this uncommon entity.

REFERENCES

1. Parazzini F, La Vecchia C, Bocciolone L, et al. The epidemiology of endometrial cancer. Gynecol Oncol 1991;41(1):1–16.
2. Shapiro S, Kelly JP, Rosenberg L, et al. Risk of localized and widespread endometrial cancer in relation to recent and discontinued use of conjugated estrogens. N Engl J Med 1985;313(16):969–72.
3. Zeleniuch-Jacquotte A, Akhmedkhanov A, Kato I, et al. Postmenopausal endogenous oestrogens and risk of endometrial cancer: results of a prospective study. Br J Cancer 2001;84(7):975–81.
4. Stanford JL, Brinton LA, Berman ML, et al. Oral contraceptives and endometrial cancer: do other risk factors modify the association? Int J Cancer 1993; 54(2):243–8.
5. Collaborative Group on Epidemiological Studies on Endometrial Cancer. Endometrial cancer and oral contraceptives: an individual participant meta-analysis of 27 276 women with endometrial cancer from 36 epidemiological studies. Lancet Oncol 2015;16(9):1061–70.
6. Weiderpass E, Adami HO, Baron JA, et al. Use of oral contraceptives and endometrial cancer risk (Sweden). Cancer Causes Control 1999;10(4):277–84.
7. Cheng WF, Lin HH, Torng PL, et al. Comparison of endometrial changes among symptomatic tamoxifen-treated and nontreated premenopausal and postmenopausal breast cancer patients. Gynecol Oncol 1997;66(2):233–7.
8. Cohen I, Perel E, Flex D, et al. Endometrial pathology in postmenopausal tamoxifen treatment: comparison between gynaecologically symptomatic and asymptomatic breast cancer patients. J Clin Pathol 1999; 52(4):278–82.
9. Kurman RJ, Kaminski PF, Norris HJ. The behavior of endometrial hyperplasia. A long-term study of "untreated" hyperplasia in 170 patients. Cancer 1985; 56(2):403–12.
10. Allison KH, Reed SD, Voigt LF, et al. Diagnosing endometrial hyperplasia: why is it so difficult to agree? Am J Surg Pathol 2008;32(5):691–8.

11. Kendall BS, Ronnett BM, Isacson C, et al. Reproducibility of the diagnosis of endometrial hyperplasia, atypical hyperplasia, and well-differentiated carcinoma. Am J Surg Pathol 1998; 22(8):1012–9.

12. Zaino RJ, Kauderer J, Trimble CL, et al. Reproducibility of the diagnosis of atypical endometrial hyperplasia: a Gynecologic Oncology Group study. Cancer 2006;106(4):804–11.

13. World Health Organization (WHO). WHO classification of tumors of female reproductive organs. Lyon (France): International Agency for Research on Cancer; 2014.

14. Mutter GL, Zaino RJ, Baak JP, et al. Benign endometrial hyperplasia sequence and endometrial intraepithelial neoplasia. Int J Gynecol Pathol 2007;26(2): 103–14.

15. Hecht JL, Ince TA, Baak JP, et al. Prediction of endometrial carcinoma by subjective endometrial intraepithelial neoplasia diagnosis. Mod Pathol 2005; 18(3):324–30.

16. Huang EC, Mutter GL, Crum CP, et al. Clinical outcome in diagnostically ambiguous foci of 'gland crowding' in the endometrium. Mod Pathol 2010; 23(11):1486–91.

17. Lacey JV Jr, Mutter GL, Nucci MR, et al. Risk of subsequent endometrial carcinoma associated with endometrial intraepithelial neoplasia classification of endometrial biopsies. Cancer 2008;113(8): 2073–81.

18. Trimble CL, Kauderer J, Zaino R, et al. Concurrent endometrial carcinoma in women with a biopsy diagnosis of atypical endometrial hyperplasia: a Gynecologic Oncology Group study. Cancer 2006; 106(4):812–9.

19. Giede KC, Yen TW, Chibbar R, et al. Significance of concurrent endometrial cancer in women with a pre-operative diagnosis of atypical endometrial hyperplasia. J Obstet Gynaecol Can 2008;30(10): 896–901.

20. Gultekin M, Diribas K, Dursan P, et al. Current management of endometrial hyperplasia and endometrial intraepithelial neoplasia (EIN). Eur J Gynaecol Oncol 2009;30(4):396–401.

21. Wheeler DT, Bristow RE, Kurman RJ. Histologic alterations in endometrial hyperplasia and well-differentiated carcinoma treated with progestins. Am J Surg Pathol 2007;31(7):988–98.

22. Mentrikoski MJ, Shah AA, Hanley KZ, et al. Assessing endometrial hyperplasia and carcinoma treated with progestin therapy. Am J Clin Pathol 2012; 138(4):524–34.

23. Gunderson CC, Dutta S, Fader AN, et al. Pathologic features associated with resolution of complex atypical hyperplasia and grade 1 endometrial adenocarcinoma after progestin therapy. Gynecol Oncol 2014;132(1):33–7.

24. Upson K, Allison KH, Reed SD, et al. Biomarkers of progestin therapy resistance and endometrial hyperplasia progression. Am J Obstet Gynecol 2012; 207(1):36.e1-8.

25. Ørbo A, Arnes M, Lyså LM, et al. Expression of PAX2 and PTEN correlates to therapy response in endometrial hyperplasia. Anticancer Res 2015;35(12): 6401–9.

26. Qin Y, Yu Z, Yang J, et al. Oral progestin treatment for early-stage endometrial cancer: a systematic review and meta-analysis. Int J Gynecol Cancer 2016; 26(6):1081–91.

27. Wang Y, Wang Y, Zhang Z, et al. Mechanism of progestin resistance in endometrial precancer/cancer through Nrf2-AKR1C1 pathway. Oncotarget 2016; 7(9):10363–72.

28. Zhang H, Yan L, Bai Y, et al. Dual-specificity phosphatase 6 predicts the sensitivity of progestin therapy for atypical endometrial hyperplasia. Gynecol Oncol 2015;136(3):549–53.

29. Mutter GL. PTEN, a protean tumor suppressor. Am J Pathol 2001;158(6):1895–8.

30. Mutter GL, Lin MC, Fitzgerald JT, et al. Altered PTEN expression as a diagnostic marker for the earliest endometrial precancers. J Natl Cancer Inst 2000; 92(11):924–30.

31. Yang HP, Meeker A, Guido R, et al. PTEN expression in benign human endometrial tissue and cancer in relation to endometrial cancer risk factors. Cancer Causes Control 2015;26(12):1729–36.

32. Mutter GL, Ince TA, Baak JP, et al. Molecular identification of latent precancers in histologically normal endometrium. Cancer Res 2001;61(11): 4311–4.

33. Zhou XP, Kuismanen S, Nystrom-Lahti M, et al. Distinct PTEN mutational spectra in hereditary non-polyposis colon cancer syndrome-related endometrial carcinomas compared to sporadic microsatellite unstable tumors. Hum Mol Genet 2002;11(4): 445–50.

34. van der Zee M, Jia Y, Wang Y, et al. Alterations in Wnt-β-catenin and Pten signalling play distinct roles in endometrial cancer initiation and progression. J Pathol 2013;230(1):48–58.

35. Ayhan A, Mao TL, Suryo Rahmanto Y, et al. Increased proliferation in atypical hyperplasia/endometrioid intraepithelial neoplasia of the endometrium with concurrent inactivation of ARID1A and PTEN tumour suppressors. J Pathol Clin Res 2015;1(3): 186–93.

36. Matias-Guiu X, Catasus L, Bussaglia E, et al. Molecular pathology of endometrial hyperplasia and carcinoma. Hum Pathol 2001;32(6):569–77.

37. Westin SN, Ju Z, Broaddus RR, et al. PTEN loss is a context-dependent outcome determinant in obese and non-obese endometrioid endometrial cancer patients. Mol Oncol 2015;9(8):1694–703.

38. Monte NM, Webster KA, Neuberg D, et al. Joint loss of PAX2 and PTEN expression in endometrial pre-cancers and cancer. Cancer Res 2010;70(15): 6225–32.

39. Joiner AK, Quick CM, Jeffus SK. Pax2 expression in simultaneously diagnosed WHO and EIN classification systems. Int J Gynecol Pathol 2015;34(1): 40–6.

40. Quick CM, Laury AR, Monte NM, et al. Utility of PAX2 as a marker for diagnosis of endometrial intraepithelial neoplasia. Am J Clin Pathol 2012;138(5):678–84.

41. Allison KH, Upson K, Reed SD, et al. PAX2 loss by immunohistochemistry occurs early and often in endometrial hyperplasia. Int J Gynecol Pathol 2012;31(2):151–9.

42. Trabzonlu L, Muezzinoglu B, Corakci A. BCL-2 and PAX2 expressions in EIN which had been previously diagnosed as non-atypical hyperplasia. Pathol Oncol Res 2017. https://doi.org/10.1007/s12253-017-0378-0.

43. Kahraman K, Kiremitci S, Taskin S, et al. Expression pattern of PAX2 in hyperplastic and malignant endometrium. Arch Gynecol Obstet 2012;286(1):173–8.

44. Vierkoetter KR, Kagami LA, Ahn HJ, et al. Loss of mismatch repair protein expression in unselected endometrial adenocarcinoma precursor lesions. Int J Gynecol Cancer 2016;26(2):228–32.

45. Djordjevic B, Barkoh BA, Luthra R, et al. Relationship between PTEN, DNA mismatch repair, and tumor histotype in endometrial carcinoma: retained positive expression of PTEN preferentially identifies sporadic non-endometrioid carcinomas. Mod Pathol 2013;26(10):1401–12.

46. Brachtel EF, Sánchez-Estevez C, Moreno-Bueno G, et al. Distinct molecular alterations in complex endometrial hyperplasia (CEH) with and without immature squamous metaplasia (squamous morules). Am J Surg Pathol 2005;29(10):1322–9.

47. Carlson JW, Mutter GL. Endometrial intraepithelial neoplasia is associated with polyps and frequently has metaplastic change. Histopathology 2008; 53(3):325–32.

48. Parra-Herran CE, Monte NM, Mutter GL. Endometrial intraepithelial neoplasia with secretory differentiation: diagnostic features and underlying mechanisms. Mod Pathol 2013;26(6):868–73.

49. Jeffus S, Winham W, Hooper K, et al. Secretory endometrial intraepithelial neoplasia. Int J Gynecol Pathol 2014;33:515–6.

50. Nicolae A, Preda O, Nogales FF. Endometrial metaplasias and reactive changes: a spectrum of altered differentiation. J Clin Pathol 2011;64(2): 97–106.

51. Lin MC, Lomo L, Baak JP, et al. Squamous morules are functionally inert elements of premalignant endometrial neoplasia. Mod Pathol 2009;22(2): 167–74.

52. Saegusa M, Okayasu I. Frequent nuclear beta-catenin accumulation and associated mutations in endometrioid-type endometrial and ovarian carcinomas with squamous differentiation. J Pathol 2001; 194(1):59–67.

53. Chiarelli S, Buriticá C, Litta P, et al. An immunohistochemical study of morules in endometrioid lesions of the female genital tract: CD10 is a characteristic marker of morular metaplasia. Clin Cancer Res 2006;12(14 Pt 1):4251–6.

54. Wani Y, Notohara K, Saegusa M, et al. Aberrant Cdx2 expression in endometrial lesions with squamous differentiation: important role of Cdx2 in squamous morula formation. Hum Pathol 2008;39(7): 1072–9.

55. Di Benedetto L, Giovanale V, Caserta D. Endometrial tubal metaplasia in a young puerperal woman after breast cancer. Int J Clin Exp Pathol 2015;8(6): 7610–3.

56. Simon RA, Peng SL, Liu F, et al. Tubal metaplasia of the endometrium with cytologic atypia: analysis of p53, Ki-67, TERT, and long-term follow-up. Mod Pathol 2011;24(9):1254–61.

57. Turashvili G, Childs T. Mucinous metaplasia of the endometrium: current concepts. Gynecol Oncol 2015;136(2):389–93.

58. Nucci MR, Prasad CJ, Crum CP, et al. Mucinous endometrial epithelial proliferations: a morphologic spectrum of changes with diverse clinical significance. Mod Pathol 1999;12(12): 1137–42.

59. Yoo SH, Park BH, Choi J, et al. Papillary mucinous metaplasia of the endometrium as a possible precursor of endometrial mucinous adenocarcinoma. Mod Pathol 2012;25(11):1496–507.

60. Alomari A, Abi-Raad R, Buza N, et al. Frequent KRAS mutation in complex mucinous epithelial lesions of the endometrium. Mod Pathol 2014;27(5): 675–80.

61. He M, Jackson CL, Gubrod RB, et al. KRAS mutations in mucinous lesions of the uterus. Am J Clin Pathol 2015;143(6):778–84.

62. McCluggage WG, McBride HA. Papillary syncytial metaplasia associated with endometrial breakdown exhibits an immunophenotype that overlaps with uterine serous carcinoma. Int J Gynecol Pathol 2012;31(3):206–10.

63. Stewart CJ, Leake R. Endometrial synovial-like metaplasia associated with levonorgestrel-releasing intrauterine system. Int J Gynecol Pathol 2015;34(6):570–5.

64. Lehman MB, Hart WR. Simple and complex hyperplastic papillary proliferations of the endometrium: a clinicopathologic study of nine cases of apparently localized papillary lesions with fibrovascular stromal cores and epithelial metaplasia. Am J Surg Pathol 2001;25(11):1347–54.

65. Ip PP, Irving JA, McCluggage WG, et al. Papillary proliferation of the endometrium: a clinicopathologic study of 59 cases of simple and complex papillae without cytologic atypia. Am J Surg Pathol 2013; 37(2):167–77.

66. Park CK, Yoon G, Cho YA, et al. Clinicopathological and immunohistochemical characterization of papillary proliferation of the endometrium: a single institutional experience. Oncotarget 2016;7(26): 39197–206.

67. Stewart CJR, Bigby S, Giardina T, et al. An immunohistochemical and molecular analysis of papillary proliferation of the endometrium. Pathology 2018; 50(3):286–92.

Endometrial Carcinoma
Grossing, Frozen Section Evaluation, Staging, and Sentinel Lymph Node Evaluation

Vinita Parkash, MBBS[a],*, Oluwole Fadare, MD[b]

KEYWORDS

- Endometrial carcinoma • Staging • Frozen section • Intraoperative assessment
- Sentinel lymph node evaluation • Grossing

Key points

- The International Society of Gynecological Pathologists guidelines for standardized processing and assessment of endometrial carcinoma are reviewed.
- Recent advances, including processing of sentinel nodes and semiquantitative scoring of extent of lymphovascular space invasion, are discussed.
- Controversial issues such as assessing invasion from adenomyosis and presence of in situ carcinoma in the fallopian tube are discussed.
- A broad discussion of the use of intraoperative frozen section evaluation in endometrial carcinoma is presented.

ABSTRACT

This article gives an overview of the pathologic assessment of resection specimens removed for uterine carcinoma. Areas of controversy and recent developments in pathologic staging are addressed. This includes assessment of myometrial invasion in the setting of adenomyosis, fallopian tube involvement, and vascular invasion. An overview of the role and evaluation of sentinel node assessments in the staging of endometrial carcinoma is provided.

OVERVIEW

Pathologic staging of cancer; that is, assigning an accurate extent, type, and grade to a cancer, assigns risk and determines prognosis for the patient with cancer. It is, therefore, the principal factor that directs therapy for cancer. The reliable and accurate pathologic assessment of resection specimens is essential to accurate pathologic staging. This article covers the generally accepted principles and recommendations for grossing and intraoperative assessment of resection specimens for endometrial carcinoma. Selected challenges and areas of controversy in the pathologic staging of these specimens are highlighted. To do this, the risk groupings for endometrial carcinoma are briefly reviewed because these are pertinent to the discussion.

Briefly, the European Society for Medical Oncology (ESMO) risk stratifies endometrial carcinoma into 3 groupings based on pathologic findings.[1] A similar algorithm is followed by the

---

Conflict of interest and funding disclosures: none.

[a] Department of Pathology and Obstetrics and Gynecology, Yale School of Medicine, PO Box 208070, New Haven, CT 06510, USA; [b] Department of Pathology, Anatomic Pathology Division, University of California San Diego Health, 9300 Campus Point Drive, Suite 1-200, MC 7723, La Jolla, CA 92037, USA

* Corresponding author.

E-mail address: Vinita.parkash@yale.edu

Surgical Pathology 12 (2019) 329–342
https://doi.org/10.1016/j.path.2019.02.002
1875-9181/19/© 2019 Elsevier Inc. All rights reserved.

National Comprehensive Cancer Network (NCCN) and the Japan Society of Gynecologic Oncology Group, with minor modifications.[2,3] Broadly speaking, low-risk endometrial carcinoma is stage 1, grade 1 to 2 endometrioid carcinoma with less than 50% myoinvasion and without lymphovascular invasion. Intermediate-risk carcinoma is either stage 1, grade 1 or grade 2 endometrioid carcinoma with greater than 50% myoinvasion, or stage 1, grade 3 endometrioid carcinoma with less than 50% myoinvasion. High-risk carcinoma includes nonendometrioid carcinoma of any stage and grade 3 endometrioid carcinoma that is more than 50% invasive. The intermediate-risk category is further stratified into a low-intermediate–risk (LIR) group in the absence of additional adverse factors and high-intermediate–risk (HIR) group when these factors are present. These adverse factors differ between classifications. The presence of lymphovascular invasion classifies an intermediate risk carcinoma to the HIR group. In addition, the NCCN guidelines use a combination of other adverse factors, including age, lower uterine segment (LUS) or surface endocervical involvement, and tumor size, to move patients from a low risk or LIR grouping to a HIR grouping.[2] These are also summarized in the recently published consensus recommendations by the International Society of Gynecological Pathologists (ISGyP) Task Force on Endometrial Carcinoma[4].

GROSS ASSESSMENT AND MICROSCOPIC SECTIONS OF HYSTERECTOMY (INCLUDING ADNEXA AND OMENTUM) FOR ENDOMETRIAL CARCINOMA

Formal evidence-based guidelines do not exist for the optimal pathologic evaluation of resection specimens removed for uterine cancer. However, it is generally accepted that a thorough gross examination is essential to an accurate microscopic evaluation. The ISGyP Task Force on Endometrial Carcinoma has proposed consensus guidelines for standardizing the processing and evaluation of uteri with endometrial carcinoma.[5]

GROSS EXAMINATION AND SECTIONING OF THE UTERUS

As with other specimens, the uterus (and adnexa) should be measured, weighed, and fixed as soon as feasible to minimize the downstream effects of ischemia times and autolysis, which can impede histologic assessment and subtyping of tumors by immunohistochemistry or molecular studies.

There is lack of consensus on serosal inking before sectioning; some pathologists think it

beneficial in assessing serosal involvement on microscopy. Nonserosal surfaces and parametria should be inked, especially if a radical hysterectomy is performed for an invasive tumor centered in or involving the LUS and/or endocervix; this aids in the accurate assessment of percentage depth of cervical invasion, which may be required to design radiation treatment.[5]

The uterus should be bivalved in the coronal plane and sectioned at 4 to 5 mm intervals perpendicular to the sagittal plane in the corpus, and parallel to the sagittal plane in the LUS and contiguous cervix (Fig. 1). Sectioning may be parallel to the sagittal plane in the fundus if the tumor is located primarily in the fundus. This method also permits an easier assessment of depth of invasion of cornual tumors.

The minimal recorded information at gross evaluation should include uterine dimensions and weight, the location and estimated extent of the tumor (proximity to landmarks eg, cervix or serosa), and tumor size. Assessing tumor size is admittedly challenging, even in a single dimension, but should be attempted wherever feasible. Some studies document association with increased incidence of nodal involvement with larger tumors and it is among the adverse risk factors considered for upstaging in the NCCN guidelines.[2,5]

The extent of sampling for microscopic evaluation should be tailored to ensure accurate and complete information. It is generally recommended that 3 to 4 sections of tumor are sufficient to achieve this goal.[6] These sections should be taken in areas with maximal gross myometrial invasion (full-thickness endomyometrium), with at least 1 section in proximity to uninvolved endometrium to accurately assess myometrial invasion.

It is recommended that an additional 2 sections each (anterior and posterior) of the LUS and cervix each be submitted for microscopic evaluation.[5] An additional 1 to 2 sections of uninvolved endometrium are also recommended.[5] However, some, including the authors, think that the routine extended evaluation of grossly normal LUS, cervix, and benign endometrium in which a well-defined tumor is present in the fundus or corpus, distant from these landmarks does not offer additional information. As the expense of health care skyrockets, the utility of uncovering nominal amounts of information must be balanced against the expense of the effort. A thoughtful use of resources may allow for a more personalized approach and appropriately allocated effort, with greater resources directed toward cases that do require more detailed and extensive microscopic evaluation, while allowing for limited sectioning for low-risk specimens. The authors suggest that, in the setting of a biopsy-proven low-grade

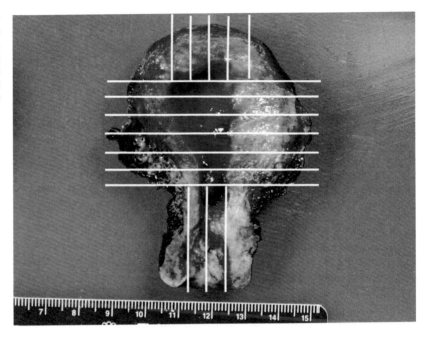

Fig. 1. Method of sectioning the uterus. The corpus is sectioned perpendicular to the sagittal plane, whereas the LUS and contiguous cervix is sectioned parallel to the sagittal plane.

endometrioid carcinoma located in the corpus, deviation from this extended sampling protocol may be reasonable, with a more limited sectioning of uninvolved endometrium, the LUS, and cervix (2 sections total). High-grade endometrioid carcinomas should be subjected to more extended sampling with submission of sections from anterior and posterior LUS and cervix because microscopic tumor may be found in the cervix even in the absence of grossly visualized disease. One study has demonstrated uncovering an additional 24% of cases with cervical involvement when the entire cervix was examined histologically.[7] However, the study was small and skewed toward cases with negative prognostic factors (62.2% cases were high-grade, and 82.75% of cases, including low-grade endometrioid carcinomas, demonstrated lymphovascular space invasion).[7]

GROSS EXAMINATION AND SECTIONING OF THE FALLOPIAN TUBES, OVARIES, AND OMENTUM

It is recommended that fallopian tubes undergo a sectioning and extensively examining the fimbriated end (SEE-FIM) protocol with ovaries sectioned parallel to the sagittal plane at 3 to 5 mm intervals.[5] This protocol calls for the microscopic evaluation of the entire ovary and fallopian tube. There is insufficient evidence to justify this recommendation for all endometrial carcinomas, although it may be warranted for high-grade

endometrioid and nonendometrioid type carcinoma. In a study by 1 of the authors, unsuspected carcinoma in grossly unremarkable ovaries and fallopian tubes was identified in 2.7% and 1.6% of cases.[8] However, this was seen largely in cases with high-grade carcinoma (clear cell, serous), and carcinomas with deep myometrial invasion. Since that study, although we have continued to submit entire adnexa for assessment, we are assessing more carefully the implications of cost on the health care system as a whole (manuscript in preparation), and favor that a more nuanced approach that balances expense against benefit may be more appropriate.

The ISGyP taskforce recommends that 4 blocks with multiple sections be submitted from grossly normal omentum.[5]

THE MORCELLATED UTERUS

As minimally invasive surgery becomes du jour because of clinical benefits, an increasing number of uteri with endometrial carcinoma are received morcellated or fragmented.[9] In most cases, morcellation is done in-bag either intraperitoneally or, more commonly, intravaginally to avoid dissemination.[10] Several techniques exist for dividing the uterus intraoperatively, some more destructive (eg, tissue paper rolling) than others (eg, Pryor technique, bivalving).[11] The authors have asked their clinicians to limit fragmenting the specimen into as few parts as possible and favor bivalving the uterus because it allows for better identification of the endometrial cavity. Morcellation is not recommended for biopsy-proven endometrioid endometrial carcinoma. However, when done, the specimen is received as identifiable fragments with adnexa and cervix amputated but intact, and with the corpus divided or cored. Attempts are made to identify the entire endometrial cavity and sample generously. Some investigators have suggested that injecting methylene blue into the cavity before surgery is of benefit in identifying the endometrium[12] but we have not had to use that technique.

A more challenging scenario is the evaluation of a morcellated uterus in which an unsuspected endometrial carcinoma is discovered in a hysterectomy done for a benign indication, typically leiomyoma. Because these are often morcellated destructively, reconstructing landmarks is difficult. Again, all attempts are made to identify the endometrial cavity and sample generously. In these cases, unlike the previous category of morcellated specimens, the authors append a note communicating the possible limitations of the pathologic evaluation. At least 1 report suggests the possibility of a missed significant finding in a morcellated specimen.[13]

GROSS EVALUATION AND MICROSCOPIC SECTIONING OF PROPHYLACTIC HYSTERECTOMIES DONE FOR GENETIC PREDISPOSITION SYNDROMES (PRIMARILY LYNCH SYNDROME)

The current recommendations are that the entire endometrium, LUS, tubes, and ovaries be submitted for histologic evaluation in the setting of prophylactic hysterectomy. Of 4 studies, in which prophylactic hysterectomy was performed in 134 subjects with Lynch syndrome (median age 48 years),[14–17] endometrial carcinoma was detected in 10 (7.5%) and ovarian carcinoma in 3 (2.2%). Although in most cases tumor was identified grossly, there were some in which the tumors were small or microscopic. Therefore, until more data accrue, submission of the entire specimen is the most prudent, if effort intensive, approach.

FROZEN SECTION EVALUATION IN THE ASSESSMENT OF ENDOMETRIAL CARCINOMA

The role of frozen section evaluation in endometrial carcinoma is practice-specific. The authors recommend developing appropriate-use criteria in collaboration with clinicians to define the process for one's own institution, depending on the favored algorithm and in accordance with the guidelines of The Choosing Wisely campaign from the American Society for Clinical Pathology, which is designed to reduce wasteful use of medical resources.[18] The campaign recommends that frozen section evaluation be performed only if intraoperative assessment influences intraoperative decision making.[18] The following principles apply:

1. Absent an unusual scenario, a frozen section evaluation is unwarranted in cases preoperatively triaged to lymphadenectomy. This typically includes cases of biopsy-proven high-grade endometrial carcinoma. Both the NCCN guidelines and the Mayo algorithm triage such patients to staging, absent a medically inoperable situation.[2,19,20] Although a change in diagnosis from a grade 3 endometrioid to serous carcinoma can influence the extent of lymphadenectomy, the role of frozen section evaluation in accurately assigning type and grade is limited. In a report by 1 of the authors in which grade and type was evaluated, grading was not reported in more than 50% of cases; and the concordance with final grade was only 72%.[21] Additionally, the grade modification on permanent evaluation was more often a downward rather than upward alteration relative to the final grade assignment (33% downgrading vs 9% for upgrading), suggesting that there was greater likelihood of harm to patients from inappropriate extensive surgery for low-risk patients rather than the converse. At institutions following NCCN guidelines, low-grade endometrial adenocarcinoma and, indeed, all endometrial adenocarcinoma are a priori triaged to lymphadenectomy because that is the primary treatment of apparent uterine-confined endometrial carcinoma, which obviates a specific role for intraoperative frozen section evaluation of the uterus.[2]

2. Frozen section evaluation may play a role in 2 settings. It may be warranted in cases in which the preoperative biopsy was suspicious (eg, atypical hyperplasia with extreme complexity). An intraoperative diagnosis of carcinoma in this setting would change intraoperative decision making by triggering a lymphadenectomy. More consistently, it is necessary at institutions following the Mayo algorithm for management of patients with endometrial carcinoma.[19,20,22] Here, the goal is to identify low-risk carcinomas, defined as grade 1 to 2 endometrioid carcinoma on endometrial biopsy, that are less than 2 cm at gross evaluation, and stage 1A, so these can be spared a

lymphadenectomy because of a low risk for nodal disease. The latter 2 elements are evaluated intraoperatively. This model is difficult to replicate in places other than the Mayo Clinic, which has an unusual ability to process a large volume of frozen sections per individual specimen.[22–24] Most institutions limit microscopic intraoperative frozen section evaluation to a single section in an area of maximal gross tumor invasion, which has less than ideal yield for concordance with the final results.[21] A modified protocol is applicable at places other than Mayo Clinic (**Fig. 2**).[22,24] The authors recommend that in the setting of grossly normal ovaries and fallopian tubes, and gross endometrial tumor less than 2 cm, at least 2 sections of endometrium at maximal depth of invasion be frozen.[22,23] One of these should be contiguous with cervix if the tumor approximates this landmark. This allows for accurate triaging of low-risk patients in almost all cases.[22,24] Intraoperatively reported parameters should include gross tumor size, depth of myometrial invasion, cervical involvement if the tumor approximates the cervix, lymphovascular space invasion, and the identification of a high-grade component, if present. Any of these can trigger lymphadenectomy. The authors do not recommend random frozen section evaluation in uteri without a visible lesion because the likelihood of identifying carcinoma is only 15%, even in the setting of biopsy-proven carcinoma.[21]

3. Frozen section evaluation in the setting of atypical endometrial hyperplasia (AEH). The role of frozen section evaluation in the setting of AEH is unclear. The lack of standardization of frozen section methodology, documented high interobserver variability in diagnosing atypical hyperplasia, and small study size are among the factors that limit the accurate prediction of risk of concurrent carcinoma at frozen section evaluation. The risk for concurrent carcinoma in a patient with a preoperative diagnosis of AEH also depends to some extent on volume of disease and complexity of hyperplasia according to a well-conducted larger-size study.[25] Most carcinomas found in patients with AEH are low-risk noninvasive carcinoma.[25–27] That said, it should be noted that several studies have found high-risk carcinoma in subjects with atypical hyperplasia to the extent of 49.5%, which has led some investigators to recommend staging for patients with AEH.[28,29] The authors suggest that, if requested, pathologists apply the general rules for frozen section evaluation; that is, eschew random sampling for grossly normal uteri while selectively examining sections with grossly visible tumor.

4. Frozen section assessments in patients with Lynch syndrome should follow the usual guidelines for frozen section assessment in patients with endometrial disease (ibidem 1–3) if a pathologic condition is diagnosed on screening routine annual or biannual endometrial-biopsy.[30] In patients undergoing interval prophylactic hysterectomy and salpingo-oophorectomy, intraoperative gross evaluation may be prudent due to an increased risk for endometrial carcinoma, with microscopic frozen section assessment limited to scenarios with a grossly visible endometrial lesion.

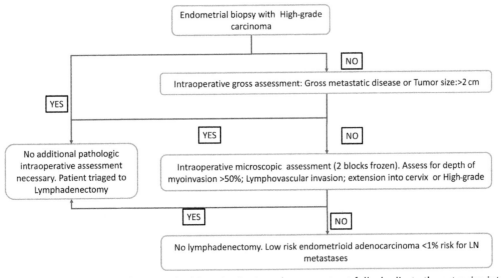

Fig. 2. A modified Mayo algorithm is applicable to institutions that cannot not fully duplicate the extensive intraoperative assessment feasible at the Mayo Clinic.

SELECTED AREAS OF DIFFICULTY AND CONTROVERSY IN THE STAGING OF ENDOMETRIAL CARCINOMA

ASSESSING MYOMETRIAL INVASION

The endomyometrial junction is irregular, often with fibrosis and myoid metaplasia.[31] Therefore, the traditional criterion of a tumor gland next to muscle is insufficient in itself to warrant a diagnosis of invasion.[31] An irregular outline of the tongue of tumor compared with uninterrupted endomyometrial junction elsewhere, presence of desmoplastic stroma, and/or the presence of an inflammatory infiltrate are helpful criteria to make the assessment of myometrial invasion.[31] In general, the authors tend toward conservativism in this setting (Fig. 3A). The tendency to overestimate invasion is higher for generalist pathologists in comparison with subspecialty pathologists.[31] This tendency is further heightened by the College of American Pathologists (CAP) requires reporting depth of invasion in millimeters.[32] This results often in a minimal invasion being listed as 1 mm and computed to 10% myometrial invasion, especially because computer programs have numeric entry fields that reject noninteger entries (postmenopausal myometrial thickness is 10–12 mm on average).[33] In cases in which the endomyometrial junction is not identified, an imaginary line at the presumptive endomyometrial junction is used to measure the depth of invasion.[4,31] Care should be taken to not include the thickness of a polypoid tumor in this assessment.[4,31] Care should also be used to not include muscle bands that often appear to be drawn into a polypoid tumor to assess depth of myometrial invasion (Fig. 3B). Myometrial thickness is assessed in the area of maximal myometrial invasion (including if in the LUS). The myometrial thickness should be inclusive of the leiomyoma if maximal depth of invasion overlies a myoma. Vascular invasion should not be included in estimation of myoinvasive depth.[4]

ASSESSING INVASION IN THE SETTING OF ADENOMYOSIS

Distinguishing tumor colonization of adenomyosis is occasionally challenging. As when assessing myometrial invasion, a combination of characteristics are helpful, including the outline of the focus, the presence of associated benign glands, and the presence of endometrial stroma surrounding the focus (Fig. 4A, B). A careful search for endometrial stroma is warranted because the stroma often demonstrates fibromyxoid eosinophilic metaplasia (Fig. 4C, D). The presence of the usual vascular pattern of endometrial stroma is a helpful in distinguishing myoid stroma from the myometrium, as is the absence of broad myometrial bands that is typical of myometrium.[31] The ISGyP task force recommends measuring depth of invasion from the endomyometrial junction in all cases of invasion from adenomyosis for the purposes of consistency and reproducibility.[4] Although the authors agree that this methodology improves reliability and is applicable in most cases, there are exceptions to the rule. Assessing myometrial invasion from adenomyosis is pertinent to clinical management in 2 scenarios (Fig. 5). In 1 setting, invasive carcinoma with less than 50% myoinvasion elsewhere is associated with a focus of apparent invasion from an adenomyotic focus in the deep myometrium. Here, the authors think that it makes eminent sense to err on the side of caution and assess myoinvasion from the endomyometrial junction (therefore, the tumor would be assessed at >50% myoinvasion). However, in the second setting, in which the patient has tumor wholly limited to the endometrium, with only a single unequivocal focus of invasion from an adenomyotic focus, the depth of invasion should measure from the endomyometrial junction of the adenomyotic focus, with the percentage invasion expressed as a function of myometrial thickness measured from the same adenomyotic focus. This situation is extremely infrequent, and we have seen at most a handful of cases in the setting of extremely small postmenopausal uteri. This situation, the authors think, is more akin to adenocarcinoma arising in adenomyosis rather than the previous scenario in which multifocally invasive adenocarcinoma invades adenomyosis and myometrium.

EVALUATING INVOLVEMENT OF THE LOWER UTERINE SEGMENT

Controversy exists on the implications of LUS involvement (LUSI) in endometrial carcinoma. LUSI is considered an adverse risk factor in the United States[2,4,5] but not by the ESMO.[1] The controversy exists in part because (1) there is no universally accepted definition of the anatomic limits of the LUS, (2) there is no agreement on what involvement by carcinoma means (invasive only or noninvasive also?), and (3) studies may not have distinguished between tumors centered in the LUS and those simply extending into the LUS.[34] The original definition of LUS by Aschoff defined a portion of the uterus between the anatomic internal os and the histologic internal os; however, its existence as a defined anatomic structure remains debatable, save perhaps in pregnancy and labor.[35] The authors use the term

Fig. 3. Assessing myometrial invasion. (*A*) A broad tongue of tumor appears to push deeply below the normal endomyometrial junction. The broad irregular bands of myometrium that invaginate between tongues of tumor (*green arrow*) increase concern for invasion. However, the authors would not call this invasive. The *yellow arrow* points to a benign gland at the edge of the tumor. (*B*) Polypoid tumor showing an edge to a benign endometrium (*yellow arrow*). Note again the broad bands of myometrium that are pulled into the tumor (*green arrow*), a common finding in polypoid tumors (transected in this image), which should not be misconstrued as invasion.

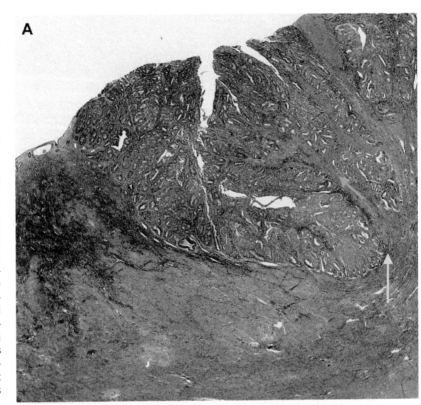

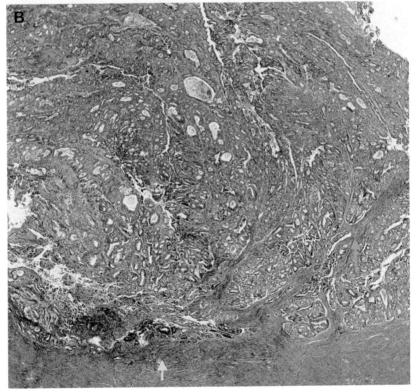

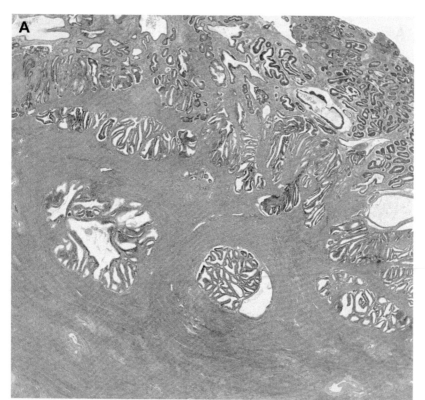

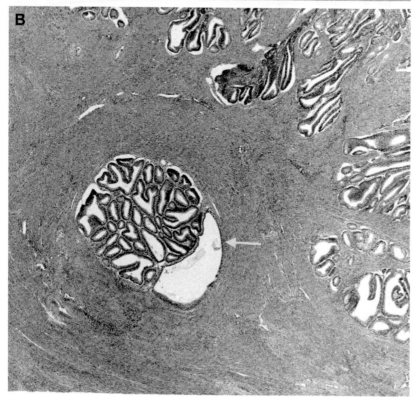

Fig. 4. Tumor involving adenomyosis. (*A*) Tumor has the rounded profile of adenomyosis. Indeed, in many areas this is arguably atypical hyperplasia involving adenomyosis. (*B*) *Arrow* points to dilated benign gland.

Fig. 4. (continued). (C) A different case of adenomyosis involved by endometrial intraepithelial carcinoma. (D) The endometrial stroma shows fibrosis with myoid metaplasia. In this case, it is easily recognizable as adenomyosis. The capillary vascular pattern is also helpful in distinguishing fibrotic and myoid endometrial stroma from true myometrium. (H&E, original magnification [A] ×20, [B] ×40, [C] ×100 [D] ×200).

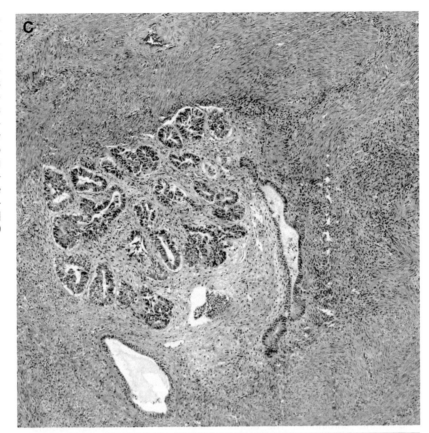

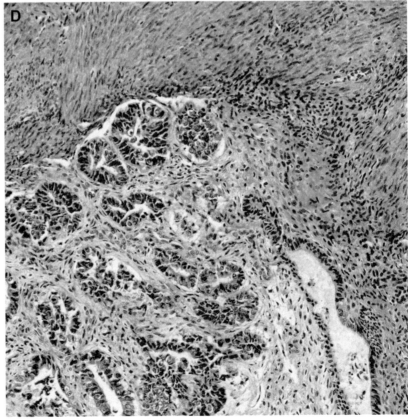

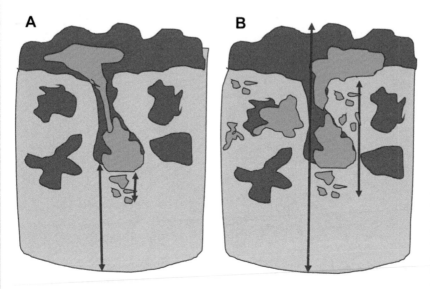

Fig. 5. Cartoon depicting how invasion from adenomyosis should be measured. Brown depicts benign endometrium; gray depicts areas of carcinoma. The depth of invasion (*short double ended arrows*) and myometrial thickness (*long double ended arrows*) are shown. (*A*) Carcinoma is endometrium delimited with focal invasion from a deep adenomyotic foci. We would report this as less than 50% myoinvasive. (*B*) The carcinoma is multifocally invasive. Here, the point of origin of the focus of invasion is difficult to confidently state. We, therefore, measure this from the endomyometrial junction and call this greater than 50% myoinvasive.

occasionally to describe the location of a tumor that involves both the endometrium and upper endocervix but do not report LUSI routinely for endometrial carcinoma. The authors think that LUSI should not be reported as present unless unequivocal invasive carcinoma is identified in the LUS. This interpretation is consistent with the general principles in the staging of endometrial carcinoma. Mucosal cervical stromal involvement does not confer an adverse outcome and that reasonably implies that noninvasive lower uterine tumor would not either.[4]

EVALUATING INVOLVEMENT OF THE FALLOPIAN TUBE

The increased sectioning of the fallopian tubes has led to the discovery of a larger number of cases with endometrial carcinoma in the fallopian tube. Controversy exists in 2 situations: (1) the implication of loose tumor clusters in the fallopian tubes and (2) staging of intraepithelial involvement of the fallopian tube in a patient with endometrial carcinoma. Evidence-based data are lacking on whether the former confers a negative outcome. Although some studies report a negative outcome,[36,37] especially in the setting of serous carcinoma, others with a mixed subset of cases do not.[38,39] The taskforce recommends documenting the finding in the pathologic report, without upstaging.[4]

Perhaps even more controversial is whether noninvasive fallopian tube involvement should

result in staging the patient as stage IIIA. With respect to management (but not staging), the point is somewhat moot in the setting of a carcinoma with other factors that predispose to poor outcome (deep myoinvasion, high tumor grade, presence of lymphovascular invasion) because these cases will necessarily triage to postoperative therapy. The clinical implications are significant in the small subset of cases in which there is isolated intraepithelial tumor in the fallopian tube, in the absence of other factors known to influence poor outcomes. Here, upstaging the patient to stage IIIA results in the recommendation of additional treatment, including possibly external beam radiation therapy or chemotherapy.[2] The authors think that staging these patients as stage IIIA in the absence of convincing data is problematic. Using the principle that mucosa-limited tumor in all other sites does not upstage cancer, the authors think it more prudent to discuss both the possibility of an independent tubal primary and intraepithelial spread, and to communicate the absence of definitive data to drive management decisions. Patient preferences necessarily play a more significant role in management in the setting of uncertainty. This interpretation is also consistent with the recommendation for reporting of ovarian involvement in endometrial carcinoma, in which it is recommended that both the possibility of metastases and synchronous primaries be posited when the clinicopathologic features are nondiagnostic of either scenario.[4]

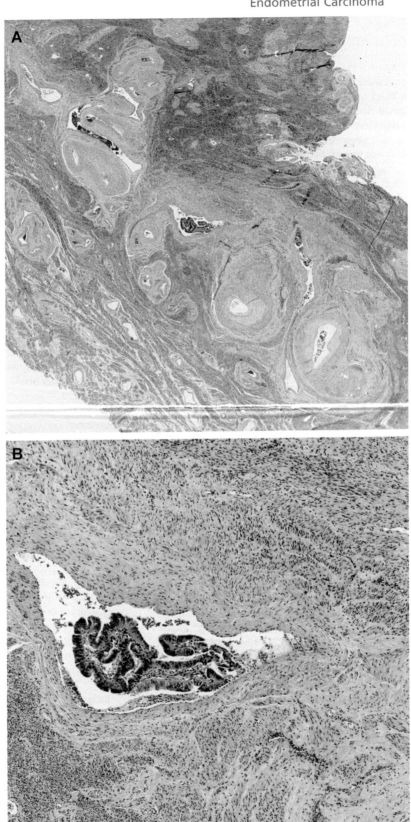

Fig. 6. Vascular pseudoinvasion. (*A*) Large fragments of tumor are present in large caliber vessels. (*B*) On higher magnification, these fragments are associated with stroma, proteinaceous material, and debris that is characteristic of vascular pseudoinvasion. (H&E, original magnification [*A*] ×20; [*B*] ×100).

EVALUATING VASCULAR INVASION

Vascular invasion should be distinguished from so-called pseudovascular invasion, which is an artifact of either surgical technique or processing. Large tissue fragments, often with crush artifact, inflammatory debris, and associated stroma in large-caliber venous channels that do not conform to the shape of the channel, are clues to artifactual tumor displacement into vessels[40](Fig. 6). This is often associated with endomyometrial clefts showing similar displacement of tissue. Of note, the depth of true vascular invasion does not change the stage of the carcinoma.[4] Therefore, a tumor that shows less than 50% myometrial invasion but also shows deeper lymphovascular invasion would be staged as 1A.

An important new recommendation is to score the extent of lymphovascular invasion present in hysterectomy specimens because this has prognostic significance.[4] The recommended system scores on a 3-tier scale, no lymphovascular invasion, focal lymphovascular invasion (few vessels at edge of tumor), and substantial lymphovascular invasion (diffuse or multifocal vascular invasion).[41,42] Substantial lymphovascular space invasion was the strongest independent prognostic indicator of locoregional recurrence, distant metastases and overall survival in the PORTEC (Post Operative Radiation Therapy in Endometrial cancer-trials).[41]

SENTINEL LYMPH NODE PROCESSING

Oncologists are increasingly turning to sentinel lymph node (SLN) mapping to spare endometrial carcinoma patients with low risk for metastatic disease the side effects of a lymphadenectomy. Sentinel node acquisition by the surgeon and processing by the pathologist needs to adhere to specific performance requirements to yield results comparable with or better than traditional systemic lymphadenectomy outcomes[2] with respect to detection of nodal metastases. SLN mapping should be followed by an ultrastaging protocol by pathologic assessment to ensure detection of low-volume metastatic disease.

Sentinel nodes should be described as to size and presence of dye, and the node sectioned at 2 to 3 mm intervals parallel to the long axis.[5] These are then subjected to an extended leveling process (ultrastaging) to ensure detection of metastatic lesions greater than 2 mm.[5] One of 2 protocols are recommended.[5] If the primary slide is negative for carcinoma, the ultrastaging protocol is activated. The Memorial Sloan Kettering Cancer Center protocol applies ultrastaging only if the tumor is myoinvasive or associated with lymphovascular space invasion.[5] All blocks of the SLNs are sectioned with 2 slides at each of 2 levels 50 microns apart (for a total of 4 slides). One slide (hematoxylin-eosin [H&E] stain) at each level (2 H&E stains total) is reviewed for tumor. If tumor is absent, the reserved unstained slide is stained with a pancytokeratin cocktail. The University of Texas at MD Anderson protocol cuts 3 slides 250 microns apart. If the primary slide is negative, then 1 of the remaining 2 slides is stained for pancytokeratin to identify tumor. It remains to be seen whether isolated small-volume disease (isolated tumor cells or micrometastases) confer substantial negative prognosis on patients with endometrial carcinoma.

The ISGyP Task Force follows the CAP–American Joint Committee on Cancer recommendations and advises on staging lymph nodes with isolated tumor cells as negative (pN0(i+)) and documenting micrometastases as (pN1mi).[4] This is, however, at odds with the International Federation of Gynecology and Obstetrics staging system, which stages lymph nodes as positive even with isolated tumor cells present.[42]

Ultimately, it is hoped that standardizing the processing and reporting of endometrial carcinoma will allow patients to get more standardized treatment and allow for the collection of broadscale data on this common carcinoma.

REFERENCES

1. Colombo N, Creutzberg C, Amant F, et al. ESMO-ESGO-ESTRO Consensus Conference on Endometrial Cancer: diagnosis, treatment and follow-up. Ann Oncol 2016;27:16–41.
2. Koh WJ, Abu-Rustum NR, Bean S, et al. Uterine neoplasms, version 1.2018, NCCN clinical practice guidelines in oncology. J Natl Compr Canc Netw 2018;16(2):170–99.
3. Sasada S, Yunokawa M, Takehara Y, et al. Baseline risk of recurrence in stage I–II endometrial carcinoma. J Gynecol Oncol 2018;29(1):e9.
4. Singh N, Hirschowitz L, Zaino R, et al. Pathologic prognostic factors in endometrial carcinoma (other than tumor type and grade). Int J Gynecol Pathol 2019;38(Suppl 1):S93–113.
5. Malpica A, Euscher ED, Hecht JL, et al. Endometrial carcinoma, grossing and processing issues: recommendations of the international society of gynecologic pathologists. Int J Gynecol Pathol 2019; 38(Suppl 1):S9–24.
6. Ganesan R, Singh N, McCluggage WG. Standards and datasets for reporting cancers; dataset for histological reporting of endometrial cancer. The Royal College of Pathologists; 2017. p. 1–39.

7. Syed S, Reed N, Millan D. Adequacy of cervical sampling in hysterectomy specimens for endometrial cancer. Ann Diagn Pathol 2015;19(2):43–4.

8. Fadare O, Khabele D. Salpingo-oophorectomy specimens for endometrial cancer staging: a comparative analysis of representative sampling versus whole tissue processing. Hum Pathol 2013;44(4):643–50.

9. Casarin J, Multinu F, Ubl DS, et al. Adoption of minimally invasive surgery and decrease in surgical morbidity for endometrial cancer treatment in the United States. Obstet Gynecol 2018;131(2):304–11.

10. Taylan E, Sahin C, Zeybek B, et al. Contained morcellation: review of current methods and future directions. Front Surg 2017;4:15.

11. Montella F, Riboni F, Cosma S, et al. A safe method of vaginal longitudinal morcellation of bulky uterus with endometrial cancer in a bag at laparoscopy. Surg Endosc 2014;28:1949.

12. Pavlakis K, Vrekoussis T, Pistofidis G, et al. Methylene blue: how to visualize the endometrium in uterine morcellation material. Int J Gynecol Pathol 2014;33:135–9.

13. Rivard C, Salhadar A, Kenton K. New challenges in detecting, grading, and staging endometrial cancer after uterine morcellation. J Minim Invasive Gynecol 2012;19(3):313–6.

14. Karamurzin Y, Soslow RA, Garg K. Histologic evaluation of prophylactic hysterectomy and oophorectomy in Lynch syndrome. Am J Surg Pathol 2013;37(4):579–85.

15. Downes MR, Allo G, McCluggage WG, et al. Review of findings in prophylactic gynaecological specimens in Lynch syndrome with literature review and recommendations for grossing. Histopathology 2014;65(2):228–39.

16. Tzortzatos G, Andersson E, Soller M, et al. The gynecological surveillance of women with Lynch syndrome in Sweden. Gynecol Oncol 2015;138(3):717–22.

17. Bartosch C, Pires-Luis AS, Meireles C, et al. Pathologic findings in prophylactic and nonprophylactic hysterectomy specimens of patients with lynch syndrome. Am J Surg Pathol 2016;40(9):1177–91.

18. Available at: http://www.choosingwisely.org/clinician-lists/ascp-frozen-section-on-pathology-specimen/. Accessed March 9, 2019.

19. Mariani A, Dowdy SC, Cliby WA, et al. Prospective assessment of lymphatic dissemination in endometrial cancer: a paradigm shift in surgical staging. Gynecol Oncol 2008;109:11–8.

20. Mariani A, Webb MJ, Keeney GL, et al. Low-risk corpus cancer: is lymphadenectomy or radiotherapy necessary? Am J Obstet Gynecol 2000;182:1506–19.

21. Desouki MM, Li Z, Hameed O, et al. Intraoperative pathologic consultation on hysterectomy specimens for endometrial cancer: an assessment of the accuracy of frozen sections, "gross-only"

evaluations, and obtaining random sections of a grossly "normal" endometrium. Am J Clin Pathol 2017;148:345–53.

22. Bogani G, Dowdy SC, Cliby WA, et al. Role of pelvic and para-aortic lymphadenectomy in endometrial cancer: current evidence. J Obstet Gynaecol Res 2014;40:301–11.

23. Parkash V, Rassaei N, Keeney GL, et al. Can we accurately predict high risk endometrial carcinoma preoperatively? Mod Pathol 2010;23:416A–21A.

24. Parkash V, Rassaei N, Fadare O, et al. Inter-institutional differences in frozen section protocols for endometrial carcinoma. Mod Pathol 2010;23:416A–21A.

25. Leitao MM Jr, Han G, Lee LX, et al. Complex atypical hyperplasia of the uterus: characteristics and prediction of underlying carcinoma risk. Am J Obstet Gynecol 2010;203:349.

26. Boyraz G, Başaran D, Salman MC, et al. Does preoperative diagnosis of endometrial hyperplasia necessitate intraoperative frozen section consultation? Balkan Med J 2016;33:657–61.

27. Stephan JM, Hansen J, Samuelson M, et al. Intraoperative frozen section results reliably predict final pathology in endometrial cancer. Gynecol Oncol 2014;133:499–505.

28. Morotti M, Menada MV, Moioli M, et al. Frozen section pathology at time of hysterectomy accurately predicts endometrial cancer in patients with preoperative diagnosis of atypical endometrial hyperplasia. Gynecol Oncol 2012;125:536–40.

29. Whyte JS, Gurney EP, Curtin JP, et al. Lymph node dissection in the surgical management of atypical endometrial hyperplasia. Am J Obstet Gynecol 2010;202:176.e1–-4.

30. Available at: https://www.sgo.org/wp-content/uploads/2012/09/2014-ACOG-bulletin.pdf. Accessed March 9, 2019.

31. Soslow RA. Practical issues related to uterine pathology: staging frozen section, artifacts and Lynch syndrome. Mod Pathol 2016;29(Suppl 1):S59–77.

32. Available at: http://www.cap.org/ShowProperty?nodePath=/UCMCon/Contribution%20Folders/WebContent/pdf/cp-endometrium-17protocol-4000.pdf. Accessed March 9, 2019.

33. Zalud I, Conway C, Schulman H, et al. Endometrial and myometrial thickness and uterine blood flow in postmenopausal women: the influence of hormonal replacement therapy and age. J Ultrasound Med 1993;12:737–41.

34. Fadare O, Gwin K, Quick CM, et al. The boundaries of the lower uterine segment and its assessment by pathologists. Mod Pathol 2018;31:404A–69A, 8.

35. Heller D. Lesions of the lower uterine segment: a review. J Gynecol Surg 2016;32(1):1–5.

36. Snyder MJ, Bentley R, Robboy SJ. Transtubal spread of serous adenocarcinoma of the endometrium: an underrecognized mechanism of metastasis. Int J Gynecol Pathol 2006;25:155–60.

37. Felix AS, Sinnott JA, Vetter MH, et al. Detection of endometrial cancer cells in the fallopian tube lumen is associated with adverse prognostic factors and reduced survival. Gynecol Oncol 2018;150(1):38–43.

38. Favazza L, Soslow R, Leitao M, et al. Clinical outcomes of patients with tumoral displacement into fallopian tubes in patients treated by robotically assisted hysterectomy for newly diagnosed endometrial cancer. USCAP 2018 Abstracts: Modern Pathology 2018;31:404–469A (Abstract No 1173).

39. Albright BB, Black JD, Passarelli R, et al. Associated characteristics and impact on recurrence and survival of free-floating tumor fragments in the lumen of fallopian tubes in Type I and Type II endometrial cancer. Gynecol Oncol Rep 2018;23:28–33.

40. Krizova A, Clarke BA, Bernardini MQ, et al. Histologic artifacts in abdominal, vaginal, laparoscopic, and robotic hysterectomy specimens: a blinded, retrospective review. Am J Surg Pathol 2011;35(1):115–26.

41. Bosse T, Peters EE, Creutzberg CL, et al. Substantial lymph-vascular space invasion (LVSI) is a significant risk factor for recurrence in endometrial cancer–A pooled analysis of PORTEC 1 and 2 trials. Eur J Cancer 2015;51(13):1742–50.

42. Amant F, Mirza MR, Koskas M, et al. Cancer of the corpus uteri. Int J Gynecol Obstet 2018;143(Suppl 2):37–50.

High-Grade Endometrial Carcinomas
Classification with Molecular Insights

Joseph W. Carlson, MD, PhD[a,b,]*, Denis Nastic, MD[a,b]

KEYWORDS

- Endometrial cancer • Molecular pathologic assessment • TCGA • POLE • MSI • p53 • Prognosis

---

Key points

- Pathologic assessment provides key parameters for risk assessment in endometrial carcinoma. Determination of tumor subtype and grade use routine hematoxylin-eosin stain and selected immunohistochemistry (IHC), and will likely incorporate molecular classification in the future.

- Endometrial carcinoma is molecularly heterogeneous. The Cancer Genome Atlas (TCGA) successfully identified 4 molecular subgroups in 2013 (*POLE*-mutated, microsatellite instability [MSI], low copy number, high copy number).

- Several groups have proposed surrogate methods to recapitulate TCGA molecular subgroups using readily available laboratory techniques (*POLE* sequencing, mismatch repair IHC, and p53 IHC).

- Retrospective studies indicate that molecular subtyping adds prognostic value. The current challenge is to validate and explore these molecular subtypes in prospective studies, which are ongoing.

- Beyond prognosis, molecular subtyping is increasingly important for choice of therapy (eg, MSI status and immune checkpoint inhibitor therapy).

ABSTRACT

This article provides an overview of the current diagnosis of endometrial carcinoma subtypes and provides updates, including the most recent molecular findings from The Cancer Genome Atlas and others. Interpretation of relevant immunohistochemistry and critical diagnostic differential diagnosis with pitfalls are discussed.

OVERVIEW

Endometrial carcinoma is the most common gynecologic cancer in developed countries. Most women will survive this cancer and require only surgical management. However, women with high-grade carcinomas are at risk for recurrence and death. Thus, these patients can benefit from additional therapies. The molecular understanding of endometrial cancer has increased greatly in recent years and holds the promise of improving risk prediction and tailoring therapies. Although routine histology with a selected number of immunohistochemical markers is the current gold standard for diagnosis that guides clinical management, integration of molecular status into treatment decision-making is certainly in the future.

High-grade endometrial carcinomas have been the focus of much attention in recent years, given that these are often clinically aggressive, recur,

---

Disclosure Statement: This work was funded by grants from the Radiumhemmets forskningsfonder and Region Stockholm.
[a] Department of Oncology–Pathology, Karolinska Institutet, Stockholm SE-17176, Sweden; [b] Department of Clinical Pathology and Cytology, Karolinska University Hospital, Radiumhemmet P1:02, Stockholm SE-17176, Sweden.
* Corresponding author. Department of Clinical Pathology and Cytology, Karolinska University Hospital, Radiumhemmet P1:02, Stockholm SE-17176, Sweden.
E-mail address: joseph.carlson@ki.se

1875-9181/19/© 2019 Elsevier Inc. All rights reserved.

Abbreviations	
EC	Endometroid carcinoma
EIC	Endometrial intraepithelial carcinoma
EIN	Endometrial intraepithelial neoplasia
ER	Estrogen receptor
FIGO	International Federation of Gynecology and Obstetrics
IHC	Immunohistochemistry
MMR	Mismatch repair
MSI	Microsatellite instability
MSS	Microsatellite stable
P53mut	p53 IHC in a pattern consistent with mutated TP53 gene (either intense nuclear, null, or cytoplasmic)
P53wt	p53 IHC in a pattern consistent with wildtype TP53 gene
POLE	DNA polymerase epsilon catalytic subunit
POLEmut	Pathogenic mutations in the POLE gene
PR	Progesterone receptor
TCGA	The Cancer Genome Atlas

and can lead to patient death. There are significant problems with interobserver reproducibility, even between expert pathologists, in the histologic classification of endometrial carcinoma. A recent study demonstrated that 3 expert gynecologic pathologists had major disagreement in the interpretation 20 out of 56 (35.8%) of cases reviewed.[1] These difficulties in interobserver agreement seem to be related significantly to the molecular characteristics of the tumors.[2] Thus, it is perhaps only the prototypical forms of endometrial carcinoma that can be diagnosed and subtyped with certainty, although more ambiguous forms may, in the future, require a molecular analysis of some kind to provide sufficient prognostic and therapeutic information for patient management.[3]

The pathologist provides 5 critical parameters that are essential for risk prediction.[4] These are (1) tumor cell type, (2) tumor grade, (3) depth of myometrial invasion, (4) cervical stromal invasion, and (5) lymphovascular space invasion. This first part of this article is specifically focused on the first 2 of these parameters. Diagnosis begins with a histologic determination of cell type, followed by, in the case of endometrioid tumors, application of International Federation of Gynecology and Obstetrics (FIGO) grading.[5] The critical classification from a pathologist's standpoint is determining

endometrioid versus nonendometrioid tumor types, and FIGO grade 3 versus FIGO grades 1 to 2 endometrioid tumors. Thus, the primary focus of this article is strategies for separating true low-grade tumors (endometrioid FIGO 1–2) from other types. The secondary focus is determining, when possible, tumor cell type among the high-grade tumors (eg, endometrioid grade 3 vs serous). The second half of this article provides an overview of the current molecular classification of endometrial cancer, with particular focus on clinical translation.

ENDOMETRIOID CARCINOMA: OVERVIEW

Endometrioid carcinomas (ECs) represent the most common subtype of endometrial cancer. These tumors frequently arise from endometrial precancers (endometrioid intraepithelial neoplasia or atypical hyperplasia). Increased or prolonged unopposed estrogen exposure is a risk factor. They are molecularly heterogeneous, characterized by varying numbers and types of somatic mutations. The prognosis of FIGO 1 to 2 endometrioid tumors overall is excellent. The prognosis of endometrioid FIGO 3 tumors is poorer; however, even in high-grade endometrioid tumors, few patients die of their disease and clinical behavior is highly dependent on the molecular context of the tumor.

ENDOMETRIOID CARCINOMA: MORPHOLOGY

Prototypical ECs resemble benign endometrial epithelium, typically in the proliferative phase but sometimes with a secretory appearance. They are most commonly glandular tumors composed of columnar cells with oval nuclei (Fig. 1A). The nuclei are typically basally located, whereas the cytoplasm is often eosinophilic. The luminal contour is smooth, a feature that can be helpful in distinguishing this subtype from other histotypes. Aberrant differentiation is common in endometrioid tumors, with frequent presence of squamous (either keratinizing or morular), mucinous, and/or secretory differentiation, also in keeping with the plasticity of the benign endometrium. Thus, even well-differentiated (ie, FIGO 1–2) endometrioid tumors can show a wide spectrum of appearances.[6]

ECs are characterized by a variety of growth patterns, not only including glandular but also papillary, cribriform, solid, and mazelike patterns. As tumors become more poorly differentiated, they begin to exhibit increasingly solid nonsquamous growth. FIGO grading is the cornerstone of diagnosis in endometrioid tumors (Table 1).

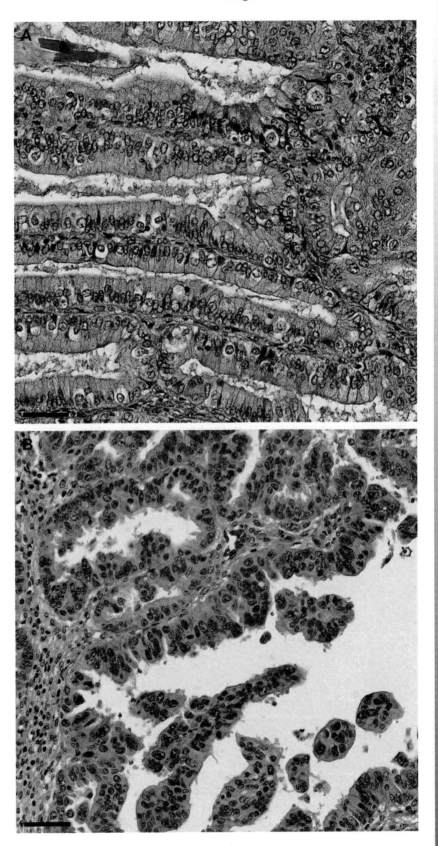

Fig. 1. (*A*) Prototypical EC. (*B*) Serous carcinoma.

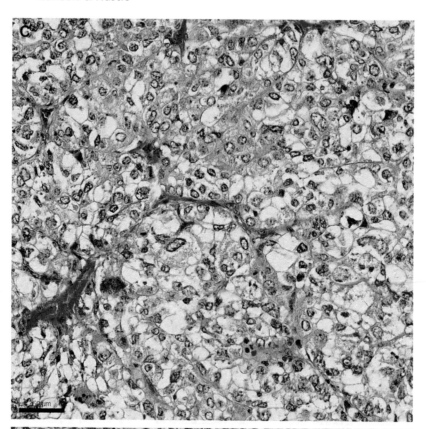

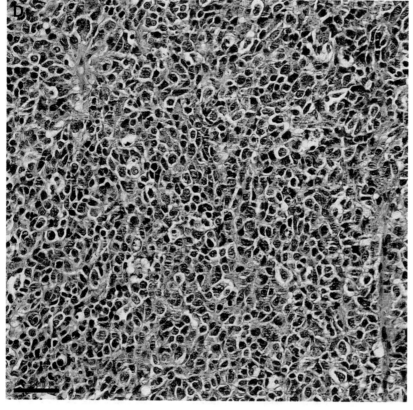

Fig. 1. (continued). (*C*) Clear cell carcinoma. (*D*) Undifferentiated carcinoma.

Table 1
International Federation of Gynecology and Obstetrics grading of endometrioid carcinomas

Grade	Characteristic
1[a]	Up to 5% solid, nonsquamous growth
2[a]	Between 6%–50% solid, nonsquamous growth
3	>50% solid, nonsquamous growth

[a] The presence of grade 3 nuclei in more than 50% of the tumor increases the grade by 1 point.

ENDOMETRIOID CARCINOMA: IMMUNOPHENOTYPE

There is no single specific marker of endometrioid differentiation. Additionally, the immunophenotype varies according to grade and molecular subtype of the tumor. If correctly optimized and interpreted, p53 immunohistochemistry (IHC), has been shown to be 96% sensitive and 99% specific for *TP53* gene mutation status.[7] Identification of an abnormal p53 pattern, indicating an underlying *TP53* mutation in FIGO 1 to 2 tumors, should prompt another review and consensus discussion. This finding is rare. On the other hand, *TP53* mutations are not uncommonly detected in FIGO 3 tumors (see later discussion). Similar to other tumors of the gynecologic tract, these tumors are positive for PAX8, typically positive for estrogen receptor (ER) and progesterone receptor (PR), and show expression of CK7. Approximately 30% show loss of expression of 1 or more mismatch repair (MMR) proteins, primarily loss of MLH1 and PMS2 due to sporadic *MLH1* promoter methylation. Strong, diffuse expression of p16 is unusual in endometrioid endometrial carcinomas but has been described in rare cases.[8] However, patchy p16 expression, with positive expression in 30% to 50% of cells, is quite common. IHC with p16 can thus be useful to help differentiate endometrioid tumors from serous and endocervical adenocarcinomas.

ENDOMETRIOID CARCINOMA: MOLECULAR FEATURES

High-grade ECs commonly (>60%) show *PTEN* (a tumor suppressor gene), *ARID1A* (member of switch–sucrose nonfermenting [SWI-SNF] complex, chromatin regulating), and *PIK3CA* (oncogene) mutations (an endometrioid-like profile). To a lesser extent, they also display *KRAS* (oncogene) and *CTNNB1* (adherence junction, cell division control), mostly in microsatellite instability (MSI)

and microsatellite stable (MSS) tumors, respectively (see later discussion).[9] Roughly 20% to 30% of these tumors also display DNA aneuploidy and *TP53* gene mutations.[10,11]

Key Points
ENDOMETRIOID CARCINOMA

Architecture	Glandular, villoglandular, solid, cribriform, papillary
Cytology	Columnar cells, polarized and oval nuclei
Nuclei	Open chromatin, euchromatic
Additional characteristics	Squamous, mucinous, secretory, tubal differentiation, atypical hyperplasia or endometrial intraepithelial neoplasia background Smooth luminal border
Typical IHC	ER, PR-positive ~30% MMR-deficient FIGO 1-2: p53wt FIGO 3: ~30% p53mut Patchy p16-positive

ENDOMETRIOID CARCINOMA: COMMON DIFFERENTIAL DIAGNOSES WITH PITFALLS

The diagnosis of endometrioid tumors becomes difficult when variant growth patterns and cell differentiation combine to confuse the prototypical morphology (see previous discussion).[6] Variant growth patterns include villoglandular, papillary, micropapillary, intraluminal nonvillous papillae, and other forms of intraluminal complexity. If the cell type is still clearly endometrioid, then the diagnostic difficulty is minimal. However, various forms of altered differentiation or metaplasia can be seen in carcinomas (corresponding to metaplasias seen in the benign endometrium). The altered differentiation can involve the epithelium or, less commonly, stroma. Epithelial differentiation includes squamous (both morular and keratinizing), mucinous, secretory, and tubal or ciliated. The keys to epithelial differentiation are (1) to recognize that the cells are within the spectrum seen for endometrioid type, (2) that the nuclear atypia is low to moderate, and (3) that other high-grade tumor types are excluded, especially serous and clear cell (see later discussion). In fact, the finding of true squamous and overt mucinous differentiation within an endometrial carcinoma is actually a helpful finding to support a diagnosis of endometrioid-type carcinoma. Stromal differentiation can include osteoid formation, spindle cell growth, sex-cord like, and the corded and hyalinized pattern. Importantly, stromal variants should not be diagnosed as carcinosarcoma unless both the epithelial and stromal components are overtly malignant and cytologically high-grade.

EXCLUDING PREDOMINATELY GLANDULAR SEROUS CARCINOMA OR ENDOMETRIAL INTRAEPITHELIAL CARCINOMA FROM ENDOMETRIOID CARCINOMA INTERNATIONAL FEDERATION OF GYNECOLOGY AND OBSTETRICS 1 TO 2 WITH ATYPIA (OR EVEN ATYPICAL HYPERPLASIA OR ENDOMETRIAL INTRAEPITHELIAL NEOPLASIA)

A tumor that at low-power inspection is initially believed to be endometrioid owing to purely glandular growth but on high-power examination reveals high-grade nuclear atypia and brisk mitoses should be regarded as suspicious for serous carcinoma.[12,13] Features that favor endometrioid type are (1) the presence of atypical hyperplasia (AH) or endometrial intraepithelial neoplasia (EIN) in the background, (2) squamous metaplasia, (3) smooth luminal borders, and (4) nuclear polarization. Features that favor serous type are (1) jagged luminal borders; (2) high-grade, hyperchromatic nuclei; (3) cleft formation between cells; and (4) complete loss of polarity, including tufting and release of micropapillary tumor clusters. IHC with p53 can be helpful in this differential because the presence of a *TP53* mutation is common in serous tumors and extremely rare in low-grade endometrioid tumors.

EXCLUDING CLEAR CELL CARCINOMA FROM CLEAR CELL CHANGE IN ENDOMETRIOID TUMORS

Endometrioid tumors can show clear cell change for a variety of reasons.[12] This clear cell appearance can be secondary to secretory differentiation, in which case the tumor cells are columnar and may even impart a piano-key appearance. Clear cell change can be secondary to squamous differentiation, in which case the cytoplasmic clearing arises gradually and is located away from the columnar glandular component. Such squamous clear cell change is also typically seen in multiple foci. Finally, some endometrioid tumors show a clear cell change that is not clearly secretory or squamous. However, the key characteristic and diagnostic features of clear cell carcinoma are

lacking: (1) polygonal cells with centrally located nuclei; (2) a mixture of 2 or more growth patterns, including papillary, tubulocystic, and solid (in the papillary and tubulocystic patterns, cells appear hobnailed); (3) adjacent stroma is typically hyalinized or myxoid; and (4) nuclear atypia is variable but, generally, at least moderate atypia is conspicuous with isolated highly atypical nuclei.

Pitfalls
CLASSIFICATION OF ENDOMETRIOID CARCINOMA

! Pitfall 1: It is important to recognize that endometrioid tumors can grow in villoglandular, papillary, or intraluminal micropapillary patterns. Small atypical micropapillae are believed to represent a form of squamous differentiation. Assess all areas of the tumor, including those removed from the areas of unusual morphology. Nuclear grade and degree of polarization can aid in distinguishing a papillary EC from serous carcinoma.

! Pitfall 2: Overinterpreting squamous differentiation as solid growth: True solid growth typically has nuclear features that resemble the surrounding glandular growth. In contrast, squamous differentiation has eosinophilic to clear cytoplasm with distinct cell borders and cell morphology is typically distinct from the surrounding glands.

! Pitfall 3: Overinterpreting clear cell change as clear cell carcinoma: To establish a diagnosis of clear cell carcinoma, the diagnostic features of clear cell carcinoma must be present. Additionally, squamous differentiation with clear cells is typically admixed with typical squamous and endometrioid areas, and is located more intraluminally. IHC with ER, PR, and NapsinA can assist. Endometrioid tumors are typically ER-positive or PR-positive, and NapsinA-negative.

! Pitfall 4: Overinterpreting solid growth as undifferentiated carcinoma: Undifferentiated carcinomas must show the characteristic features of dyscohesion and lack of a distinct architectural growth pattern. Poorly fixed tumors can make the distinction extremely difficult because autolysis from poor fixation can mimic undifferentiated carcinomas. Proper processing with adequate fixation is critical for accurate assessment of histotype.

SEROUS CARCINOMA: OVERVIEW

Serous carcinomas are the prototypical high-grade carcinoma of the endometrium. Patients are typically older and have a lower body mass index compared with those with endometrioid tumors. They are characterized molecularly by a high degree of chromosomal copy-number alterations and *TP53* mutation. Serous carcinomas are often associated with endometrial polyps and may even be intraepithelial (serous endometrial intraepithelial carcinoma [EIC]). Otherwise their gross features are nonspecific. Serous carcinomas are clinically aggressive.

SEROUS CARCINOMA: MORPHOLOGY

Prototypical serous carcinomas show papillary and micropapillary growth patterns, although these are not required for the diagnosis. They demonstrate high-grade nuclear atypia with hyperchromasia and clumpy, granular chromatin. Nuclei are not polarized but instead show a stratified appearance (**Fig.** 1B). Brisk mitoses are seen. Additionally, serous carcinomas typically show an uneven or jagged luminal boundary, with detachment of atypical cells into the gland lumina.

Serous carcinomas can grow in an intraepithelial fashion, with high-grade carcinoma replacing endometrioid glands without extension beyond the preexisting glandular architecture. This finding can be subtle. This pattern has been termed serous EIC or early serous carcinoma. Importantly, this growth pattern, despite the lack of classic invasion, can be associated with intraabdominal spread and thus requires complete surgical staging.[14]

SEROUS CARCINOMA: IMMUNOPHENOTYPE

Serous endometrial carcinomas, like their high-grade tuboovarian counterparts, characteristically harbor *TP53* mutations and thus display an abnormal p53 staining pattern. They are also diffusely positive for p16. Studies have shown that serous carcinomas primary in the endometrium are typically negative for WT-1 and, when positive, tend to be focal and/or weak.[15] Serous endometrial carcinomas are MMR-intact (ie, positive IHC for MLH1, PMS2, MSH2, and MSH6) and rarely demonstrate loss of PTEN expression.

SEROUS CARCINOMA: MOLECULAR FEATURES

Serous carcinomas are characterized by *TP53* (>90%), a tumor suppressor, and *PPP2R1A*, which controls cell growth and division, mutations.[16,17] They also have numerous copy-number alterations and DNA aneuploidy.[9,17–19]

Key Points	
SEROUS CARCINOMA	
Architecture	Papillary and micropapillary, glandular, solid, jagged luminal border
Cytology	Stratified nuclei, brisk mitotic rate, high Nuclear:Cytoplasmic ratio
Nuclei	High-grade with hyperchromasia, pleomorphism
Additional characteristics	Often associated with endometrial polyp. May be associated with EIC
Typical IHC	p53 abnormal. MMR-intact. ER-positive or PR-positive in 20%–50% of cases[19]. Strong, diffuse p16 positivity

SEROUS CARCINOMA: COMMON DIFFERENTIAL DIAGNOSES WITH PITFALLS

Serous carcinomas that grow in a predominately glandular growth pattern can resemble endometrioid FIGO 1 to 2 tumors and even AH or EIN. See previous discussion of this differential diagnosis.

Serous carcinomas with predominately solid growth have a different differential diagnosis, namely endometrioid FIGO 3, and undifferentiated carcinoma. The presence of a more characteristic morphologic component, even if focal, can assist in subtyping. For example, the presence of focal squamous differentiation in association with carcinoma should result in classification as endometrioid type, whereas the presence of typical serous EIC favors serous. Undifferentiated carcinoma lacks organized architecture and, instead, demonstrates diffuse infiltration through preexisting glands and stroma.

Pitfall

MISCLASSIFICATION OF GLANDULAR SEROUS CARCINOMA

! Favor endometrioid: Smooth luminal contours, mild to moderate nuclear atypia, nuclei are basally located with preservation of polarity, moderate mitotic activity, squamous or other differentiation, p53 wildtype pattern, and p16 nondiffuse pattern

! Favor serous: Jagged luminal contour, high-grade nuclear atypia, stratified nuclei with loss of polarity, clefts, tumor budding or exfoliation of malignant micropapillary tumor aggregates

CLEAR CELL CARCINOMA: OVERVIEW

Clear cell carcinomas are an uncommon subtype of endometrial carcinoma. There are no specific gross features associated with clear cell carcinomas. Clear cell carcinomas are clinically aggressive.

CLEAR CELL CARCINOMA: MORPHOLOGY

Clear cell carcinomas are composed of round to polygonal cells with abundant clear or granular cytoplasm. Nuclei are usually polygonal and centrally located (Fig. 1C). The tumor cells typically grow in a single layer and impart a hobnail appearance. Tall, columnar cell growth is not a feature of clear cell carcinoma. These tumors grow in a mixture of characteristic architectural patterns: papillary, tubulocystic, and solid.[20] Not all 3 patterns are present in every case; however, the presence of at least 2 patterns is helpful in establishing the diagnosis. The adjacent stroma is typically hyalinized or myxoid, leading to the appearance of empty rings. Nuclear atypia is variable and, in many tumors, low to moderate atypia is seen with isolated highly atypical nuclei.

CLEAR CELL CARCINOMA: IMMUNOPHENOTYPE

Clear cell carcinomas are negative for hormone receptors ER and PR; if positive it is in a weak and/or focal fashion.[21] They are positive for NapsinA (~80% of cases, at least focally).[22] Importantly, although clear cell carcinomas typically have a normal or wild-type p53 expression pattern, they can be p53 abnormal in 20% to 30% of cases.[23] The utility of hepatocyte nuclear factor (HNF)-1β has been debated and positivity has been reported in ECs, making it less specific, although it seems to be a highly sensitive marker for clear cell carcinoma.[24]

CLEAR CELL CARCINOMA: MOLECULAR FEATURES

Clear cell carcinomas are genetically heterogenous, sometimes presenting with *TP53* mutations but much less often than their serous counterparts. Much like serous tumors, there is a large portion of *PPP2R1A*-mutated tumors; however, they also display an endometrioid-type profile with 20% to 30% of tumors showing both *PIK3CA* and *ARID1A* mutations. Additionally, some tumors are *POLE*-mutated (5%) or MMR-deficient (ie, negative IHC for 1 or more of MLH1, PMS2,

MSH2, or MSH6).[25] The genetic profile of clear cell carcinomas suggests a highly diverse biology and pathogenesis; importantly, the molecular subgroups within the clear cell carcinomas display different outcomes.[25]

Key Points CLEAR CELL CARCINOMA	
Architecture	Microcystic, papillary, tubulocystic, solid patterns Typically a mixture of at least 2 architectural growth patterns
Cytology	Polygonal cells with abundant clear to granular cytoplasm
Nuclei	Large nuclei, often centrally located
Additional characteristics	Stromal hyalinization or myxoid change Hobnail morphology, often single cell layer thick
Typical IHC	ER-negative, PR-negative NapsinA-positive Can be p53mut but usually p53wt

CLEAR CELL CARCINOMA: COMMON DIFFERENTIAL DIAGNOSES WITH PITFALLS

Clear cell carcinoma must be distinguished from EC with clear cell change, as described previously in the endometrioid section.

Clear cell carcinoma as a component of a mixed carcinoma is another common consideration; however, in reality this is exceedingly rare. For this diagnosis, there should be 2 discrete components and the boundary between the 2 components easily defined. Ideally, there are differing immunohistochemical profiles to support the diagnosis. Admixture or poor circumscription of the 2 components favors a variant morphology or ambiguous carcinoma compared with a true mixed carcinoma.

UNDIFFERENTIATED AND DEDIFFERENTIATED CARCINOMA

The dedifferentiated carcinoma subtype is distinct from endometrioid FIGO 3, both morphologically and molecularly.[26,27] Dedifferentiated carcinomas are undifferentiated carcinomas associated with a well-differentiated (low-grade;

FIGO 1–2) EC. Dedifferentiated carcinomas often contain the undifferentiated component deeper within the endometrium than the well-differentiated component. Thus, the undifferentiated component may only be detected on examination of the hysterectomy specimen. These tumors are aggressive and may be underrecognized. The distinction from FIGO 3 ECs is critical.

UNDIFFERENTIATED CARCINOMA: MORPHOLOGY

Undifferentiated carcinomas are composed of monotonous, solid, dyscohesive small to medium-sized round cells (**Fig.** 1D).[26,28] The cells can focally show a rhabdoid appearance and sometimes can have striking pleomorphism. The tumor grows in a patternless fashion and completely lacks evidence of glandular differentiation.

UNDIFFERENTIATED CARCINOMA: IMMUNOPHENOTYPE

The epithelial nature of undifferentiated tumors can best be demonstrated with EMA (Epithelial Membrane Antigen) and/or keratin, either of which may be positive, typically in a focal or patchy fashion. Strong diffuse keratin expression is not supportive of a diagnosis of undifferentiated carcinoma. Loss of expression of members of the SWI-SNF complex has been demonstrated. Specifically, loss of BRG1 (SMARCA4) (33%), BRM (SMARCA2) (loss in 69% of cases), and INI1 (SMARCB1) (loss in 4% of cases) has been demonstrated.[29] Approximately 50% show loss of MMR protein expression, particularly MLH1 or PMS2.[27]

UNDIFFERENTIATED CARCINOMA: MOLECULAR FEATURES

Undifferentiated or dedifferentiated cancers also display a fairly wide array of genetic profiles, the most common being MSI (~45%) and copy-number low (28%)[30]; however, to a lesser extent, tumors also fall into the other 2 categories as suggested by The Cancer Genome Atlas (TCGA) genomic classification[31] (see later discussion). Of note, undifferentiated carcinomas are thought to arise due to transformation from epithelial cells to mesenchymal-like cells, much like carcinosarcoma, as evidenced by the downregulation of E-cadherin and upregulation of *ZEB1*, *HMGA-2*, and osteonectin.[32]

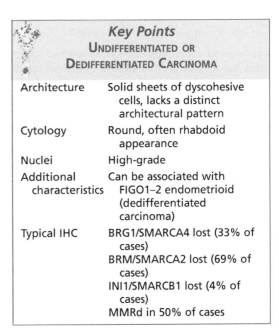

Key Points
UNDIFFERENTIATED OR DEDIFFERENTIATED CARCINOMA

Architecture	Solid sheets of dyscohesive cells, lacks a distinct architectural pattern
Cytology	Round, often rhabdoid appearance
Nuclei	High-grade
Additional characteristics	Can be associated with FIGO1–2 endometrioid (dedifferentiated carcinoma)
Typical IHC	BRG1/SMARCA4 lost (33% of cases) BRM/SMARCA2 lost (69% of cases) INI1/SMARCB1 lost (4% of cases) MMRd in 50% of cases

UNDIFFERENTIATED CARCINOMA: COMMON DIFFERENTIAL DIAGNOSIS WITH PITFALLS

Undifferentiated carcinoma tumors can resemble a solid endometrioid or serous carcinoma. However, the dyscohesive growth and uniformity with lack of other growth patterns favors an undifferentiated carcinoma. Included in the differential of undifferentiated carcinomas are neuroendocrine carcinomas, which are exceedingly rare in the endometrium. Diagnosis of a neuroendocrine carcinoma requires the correct morphology; however, there is admittedly an overlap between large cell neuroendocrine carcinoma and undifferentiated carcinoma. There is uncertainty regarding the distinction of these 2 entities with respect to neuroendocrine marker expression because some experts recommend that expression of neuroendocrine markers in greater than 10% of the tumor should motivate a diagnosis of neuroendocrine carcinoma.[33] However, in the opinion of others, this is too permissive because undifferentiated carcinomas frequently express neuroendocrine markers in a minority of tumor cells.

MIXED CARCINOMA: OVERVIEW

Mixed carcinomas are rare and should only be diagnosed when 2 different, clearly defined histologic types are seen. At least 1 must be a high-grade tumor (ie, so-called type 2).[34] There are no specific gross features.

MIXED CARCINOMA: MORPHOLOGY

If is a mixed carcinoma strongly suspected, diagnosis requires the identification of 2 different tumor histotypes with sufficiently distinct morphology on routine hematoxylin and eosin staining. Molecular studies have demonstrated that true mixed tumors are rare. The diagnosis can be confirmed, if appropriate, by IHC, which should mirror and confirm the morphologic suspicion. Among the most common pitfalls is overinterpretation of clear cell in an EC as a clear cell carcinoma component. The diagnosis of mixed carcinoma should only be made if the morphology is sufficiently clear and distinct, conclusively demonstrating that 2 separate tumor clones are present.[35]

MIXED CARCINOMA: IMMUNOPHENOTYPE

The morphologic appearance of a mixed carcinoma should be confirmed with IHC.

AMBIGUOUS CARCINOMA

Beyond the histologic subtypes (see previous discussion), there exists a group of tumors in which precise subtyping is difficult.[3,12,36] These have been termed ambiguous carcinomas. These tumors are typically high-grade, in which the differential diagnosis stands between EC, FIGO 3, serous carcinoma, or other high-grade subtypes. Thus, the clinical implications of difficulties in subtyping may be minimal in situations in which the precise histologic subtyping does not dictate management. Subtyping can be improved through consensus diagnosis and the use of a panel of immunohistochemical markers (see previous discussion).

CARCINOSARCOMA: OVERVIEW

Carcinosarcomas, also referred to as malignant mixed Müllerian tumors (MMMTs), represent a form of predominately sarcomatous dedifferentiation of an endometrial carcinoma. Carcinosarcomas have no specific gross features but often present with a large, friable intracavitary mass. Carcinosarcomas are highly aggressive.

CARCINOSARCOMA: MORPHOLOGY

Carcinosarcoma is a tumor consisting of both malignant epithelial and mesenchymal components. By definition, both components must be high-grade. Previously, carcinosarcomas were called MMMTs and were divided into homologous and heterologous types based on the nature of the

sarcomatous component. Often the sarcomatous component is intimately admixed with the carcinomatous component, leading to a biphasic morphology.

CARCINOSARCOMA: IMMUNOPHENOTYPE

IHC is not required for the diagnosis of carcinosarcoma. The diagnosis relies on the characteristic mixed carcinoma and sarcoma morphology. Analysis of the epithelial component can confirm that it is high-grade.

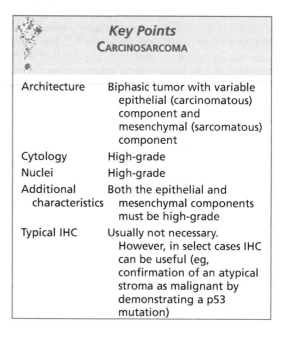

Key Points CARCINOSARCOMA	
Architecture	Biphasic tumor with variable epithelial (carcinomatous) component and mesenchymal (sarcomatous) component
Cytology	High-grade
Nuclei	High-grade
Additional characteristics	Both the epithelial and mesenchymal components must be high-grade
Typical IHC	Usually not necessary. However, in select cases IHC can be useful (eg, confirmation of an atypical stroma as malignant by demonstrating a p53 mutation)

CARCINOSARCOMA: COMMON DIFFERENTIAL DIAGNOSIS WITH PITFALLS

Carcinosarcoma must be distinguished with EC with spindle cell differentiation and the corded and hyalinized EC. In this tumor the endometrioid tumor is low-grade (FIGO 1–2). Additionally, the spindle cell component is cytologically bland, lacking significant nuclear atypia (Fig. 2A, B).

Dedifferentiated carcinomas occasionally contain undifferentiated carcinoma closely admixed with the typical carcinomatous component. Here the undifferentiated component is not sarcomatous but rather dyscohesive, epithelioid, and monotonous. Sarcomatous differentiation tends to be cohesive with spindled morphology. Additionally the carcinomatous component of a carcinosarcoma is high-grade. Undifferentiated carcinomas can be associated with a myxoid stroma, or even a reactive stroma showing some atypia. However, on careful examination, the stroma should not be malignant. Tumor cells

Fig. 2. Histology of a corded and hyalinized EC, which must be distinguished from carcinosarcoma. (*A*) Low-power view. (*B*) High-power view.

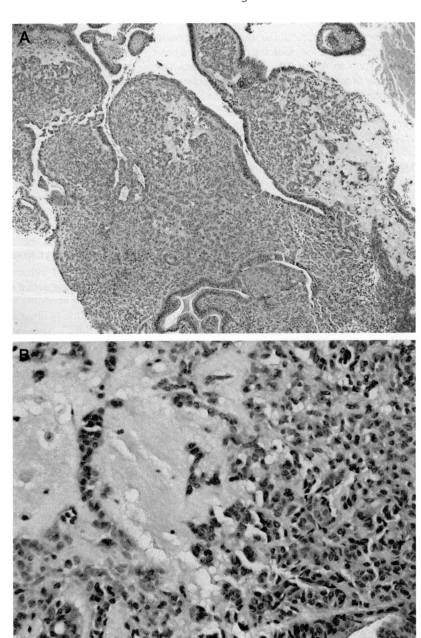

in undifferentiated carcinoma may show rhabdoid differentiation but do not demonstrate rhabdomyosarcomatous features; as such, they are not positive for markers of skeletal muscle differentiation.

MESONEPHRIC-LIKE ADENOCARCINOMA

MESONEPHRIC-LIKE ADENOCARCINOMA: OVERVIEW

Mesonephric-like carcinomas have been described in the endometrium and ovary. They

are morphologically indistinguishable from true mesonephric carcinomas of the cervix. However, they are probably not truly derived from mesonephric remnants given their anatomic location.

MESONEPHRIC-LIKE ADENOCARCINOMA: MORPHOLOGY

Mesonephric-like adenocarcinoma tumors are characterized by a variety of growth patterns, including solid, papillary, retiform, tubular, and glandular. The glands may show dense eosinophilic secretions. Solid foci may show spindled morphology. They lack squamous and mucinous differentiation, and they lack the presence of a precursor, such as AH or EIN. They further lack the presence of mesonephric rests and mesonephric hyperplasia.[37]

MESONEPHRIC-LIKE ADENOCARCINOMA: IMMUNOPHENOTYPE

Mesonephric-like adenocarcinoma tumors are GATA-3, calretinin, and CD10-positive. No p53 mutation is present. The tumors are negative for ER and PR. Expression of TTF-1 is common (approximately 90% of tumors), and can be strong and diffuse (approximately 60% of tumors). Some tumors show an inverse pattern of TTF-1 and GATA3 expression.[38]

MESONEPHRIC-LIKE ADENOCARCINOMA: MOLECULAR FEATURES

Mesonephric-like adenocarcinoma tumors have been shown to harbor activating KRAS mutations and are MSS. They do not have PTEN mutations.[39]

IMMUNOHISTOCHEMISTRY IN ENDOMETRIAL CARCINOMAS

Probably the most studied of immunohistochemical markers is p53. The staining pattern of p53 can either be mutant or wildtype (**Fig. 3**). An abnormal p53 pattern is noted when all tumor cell nuclei are positive (missense mutation, see **Fig. 3**B); when all are negative (null-pattern, nonsense mutation, see **Fig. 3**C); or, rarely, in a recently described pattern, when there is extensive cytoplasmic staining (see **Fig. 3**D).[7] IHC for p53 may be useful in the distinction of endometrioid and serous carcinomas. Most (if not all) serous carcinomas show an aberrant or mutant p53 staining pattern. It should be noted that approximately 30% of FIGO 3 ECs also show a mutant pattern. Thus, an abnormal p53 pattern may not aid in this differential; however, the presence of a wild-type pattern should essentially exclude serous carcinoma, particularly in cases of nonclassic histology. Low-grade, endometrioid FIGO 1 to 2, tumors should be p53 wildtype (p53wt) with rare exception.[11] Another useful area for p53 IHC is confirming distinct components in mixed carcinomas, which often will show a mutant p53 (p53mut) pattern. To differentiate serous and endometrioid tumors, p16 staining can also help. In serous carcinomas, p16 often shows strong reactivity in most (>90%) tumor cells in which endometrioid typically shows a patchy staining pattern.[40,41] However, uncommonly, ECs can show strongly positive p16 staining, so morphologic correlation is essential.

ER is expressed in low-grade ECs, whereas serous and high-grade endometrioid are more likely to be negative.[42] Undifferentiated and clear cell carcinomas are usually ER-negative.[40,43] The use of HNF1β and NapsinA in trying to identify clear cell endometrial carcinomas seems to be less robust than for ovarian counterparts; it seems to be less sensitive and less specific because high-grade endometrioid and serous ECs, to a high degree, also express HNF1β.[24] Besides being negative for ER, PR, and PAX8,[44] undifferentiated and dedifferentiated carcinomas have been found to lose expression of SWI-SNF subunits (INI1/SMARCB1, BRG1/SMARCA4).[28,29,45] A subset of undifferentiated carcinomas harbor mutations in TP53. This suggests a different pathogenic profile (serous-like) in some undifferentiated ECs. Studies of a multitude of other antibodies (eg, PTEN, HER-2, and IMP2) have shown poor sensitivity and specificity. In the case of PTEN, this may be technically challenging with resultant difficulty in interpretation.[10] TCGA study indicated that almost all MSI tumors were of endometrioid type and lacked the extensive copy-number variation seen in serous tumors.

In the context of improving the reproducibility and accuracy of typing (EC), the use of IHC boils down to this: no single marker can be used to identify histotype on its own. Therefore, in practical clinical use, a panel of markers is most useful for IHC to be helpful.[46,47] Problems remain in interpreting discrepant results in panels, as well as selecting the cases in which immunohistochemical panels are appropriate to use.

MOLECULAR CLASSIFICATION OF HIGH-GRADE ENDOMETRIAL CARCINOMAS

THE CANCER GENOME ATLAS GENOMIC CLASSIFICATION OF ENDOMETRIAL CARCINOMAS

The arrival and development of next-generation sequencing has enabled targeted sequencing for use in the clinical setting. In conjunction with morphology and IHC, it adds another objective layer of information to the diagnosis and prognostication of ECs. However, most ECs display a wide spectrum of gene mutations within the same histotype, as well as slightly overlapping gene mutations in different histotypes. The relationship between histotype, immunophenotype, gene mutation profile, and TCGA group is presented in **Table 2**. Tumor heterogeneity is believed to further

Fig. 3. Immunohistochemical evaluation of p53 IHC. Studies have demonstrated that IHC is a sensitive and specific method for evaluating *TP53* gene mutation status. (*A*) p53 wildtype pattern, showing variation in both staining intensity and distribution (ie, mosaic staining). (*B*) p53 mutant pattern of overexpression, with intense nuclear staining in most nuclei. This is the most common pattern.

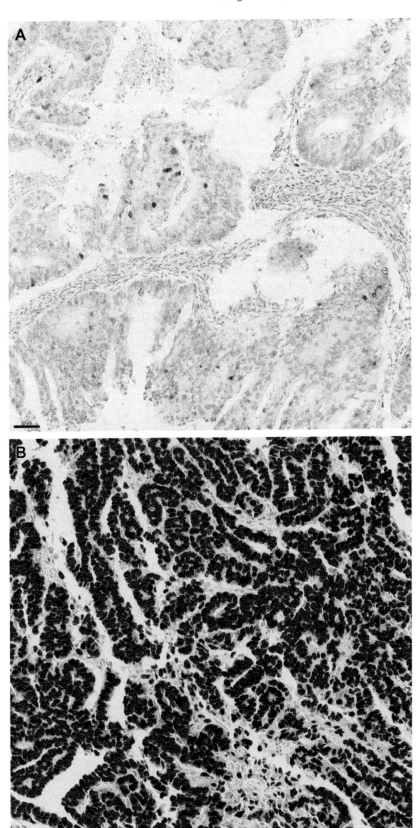

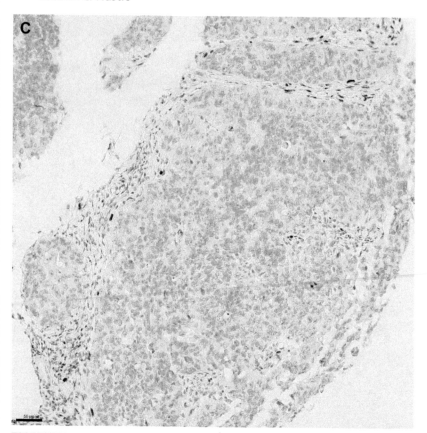

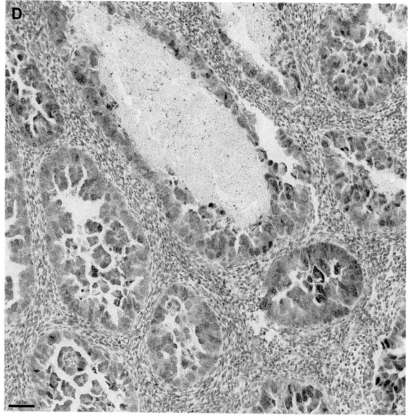

Fig. 3. (continued). (C) p53 mutant pattern, so-called null staining. This pattern is also diagnostic for a TP53 mutation and is characterized by complete lack of staining in all tumor cells. Occasional intratumoral lymphocytes can be positive and must be ignored to correctly evaluate the staining. (D) p53 mutant pattern, cytoplasmic expression only. This is the rarest of the staining patterns but is also diagnostic of a TP53 mutation.

Table 2
Relationship between histotype and immunohistochemical pattern, gene mutation profile, and The Cancer Genome Atlas group associations

Histotype	IHC Pattern	Gene Mutation Profile	TCGA Group
High-grade EC	p53wt (but ~20%–30% are p53mut) ER+/− p16 weak and focal MMRd common	*CTNNB1, PIK3CA, ARID1A, PTEN*	CN-high, POLE-mutated, MSI
Serous carcinoma	p53mut ER −/+ p16 strong	*TP53, PP2R1A*	CN-high
Clear cell carcinoma	p53wt ER− p16 weak and focal	*TP53, PP2R1A, ARID1A* (20%–30%), *PTEN*	All 4 of TCGA molecular groups, most commonly CN-high (47%) and CN-low (34%)
Undifferentiated or dedifferentiated carcinoma	p53wt, BRG1 (SMARCA4) loss may be seen, and less commonly INI-1 (SMARCB1) loss p16 weak and focal	MSI, E-cadherin downregulated	All 4 of TCGA molecular groups, most commonly MSI (45%) and CN-low (28%)

Abbreviations: CN, copy number; mut, mutant; wt, wildtype.

blur the picture because different parts of the tumor may show different alterations (passenger mutations).[48,49] For these reasons, diagnosing and prognosticating ECs based solely on molecular findings is still challenging. There is a need for both prognostic and treatment-specific genetic-based prospective studies, which is currently underway (PORTEC4 study).

In 2013, TCGA[31] proposed a molecular classification of ECs after testing 373 ECs (307 endometrioid, 53 serous, and 13 mixed serous and endometrioid). The classification was based on genomic, transcriptomic, and proteomic analyses, and integrated somatic gene mutations, MSI, and copy-number alterations to produce an integrated genomic classifier instead of specific single gene profile signatures (see previous discussion). This resulted in 4 groups with prognostic implications.

Key Features
MOLECULAR SUBTYPES IDENTIFIED IN THE CANCER GENOME ATLAS STUDY

POLE-ultramutated

ECs characterized by mutations in the *POLE* gene (exonuclease domain, a subunit of DNA polymerase epsilon), very high mutation rates, variable (low to moderate) copy-number variations, and frequent mutation in *PTEN, PIK3CA,* and *KRAS*. This group is associated with favorable clinical outcomes and very few recurrences. A prototypical *POLE* mutated tumor is

shown in **Fig. 4**. Of note, a substantial number of *POLE* mutated tumors also display *TP53* mutations (approximately 30% of cases) and despite this have retrospectively shown favorable outcomes.

MSI or hypermutated

Mostly endometrioid histotype with high mutation rates; MSI-high status mostly due to *MLH1* promoter methylation, few copy-number variations, and frequent *KRAS, PTEN,* and *ARID1A* mutations. Lynch-syndrome tumors represent a minority of MSI tumors. Clinical outcomes were intermediary.

Copy-number low or MSS

Microsatellite-stable endometrioid histotype FIGO 1 and 2 tumors with low overall mutation rates but frequent *CTNNB1* and *PTEN* mutations. Clinical outcomes were intermediary.

Copy-number high or serous-like

High copy-number alterations, low mutation rates with frequent *TP53* and *PPP2R1A* mutations. Most commonly serous histotype with about one-quarter of tumors being high-grade endometrioid. These tumors were prognostically highly unfavorable.

This novel molecular classification is important for both the future construction of EC molecular models but also has important direct clinical and diagnostic implications. The discovery of the *POLE* ultramutated group, which frequently

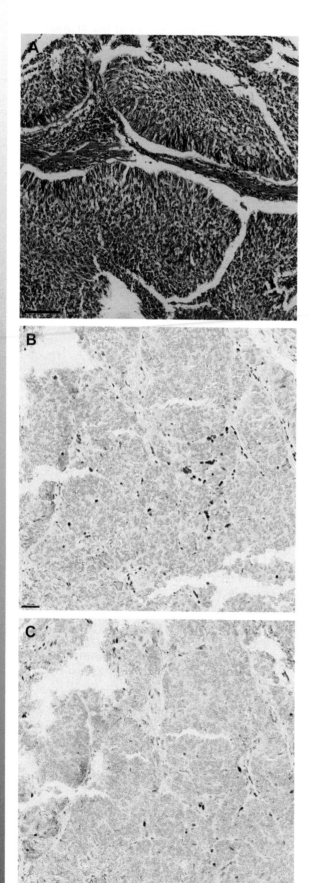

Fig. 4. Histologic features of a *POLE* mutated tumor. (*A*) Note the peritumoral lymphocytic infiltrate, these tumors may be candidates for immunomodulatory therapy; however, the excellent prognosis associated with these tumors brings into question the need for aggressive adjuvant therapy. (*B, C*) Deficient MMR staining in an MSI tumor. This tumor shows negative MSH2 (*B*) and MSH6 (*C*). In the background are scattered positive peritumoral lymphocytes that serve as an internal control.

consisted of high-grade endometrioid ECs, revealed a much better prognosis and fewer recurrences and deaths due to disease.[50,51] It also raised the question of whether *POLE* mutation analysis should be implemented into clinical use sooner rather than later. This analysis might identify a subset of patients with favorable outcomes despite high-grade histology who would otherwise endure adjuvant treatment without added benefit. This favorable outcome for *POLE*-mutated tumors has been reported in several retrospective studies and prospective studies are ongoing.

The MSI group is characterized by similar histologic features as Lynch syndrome tumors, namely intratumoral growth pattern variation, and peritumoral and intratumoral infiltrating lymphocytes. These patterns, combined with a mutational analysis of MMR-related genes or IHC for MMR protein expression (MLH1, MSH2, MSH6, PMS2), may pinpoint patients who are sensitive to adjuvant therapy and thus favorable outcomes.[52] An example of MSH2 and MSH6 loss is shown in **Fig. 4**B, C. In addition, patients with recurrent MSI tumors are candidates for immune-modulating treatments.[53]

Within the high copy number or serous-like genomic group, most tumors were of serous histotype; however, a large subset (35%) showed unequivocal endometrioid histology (almost all high-grade). This points to the value of p53 IHC or *TP53* sequencing because *TP53* mutation in the absence of *POLE* mutation and MSI seems to predict worse outcome independent of histotype.

SURROGATE MODELS OF TUMOR CANCER GENE ATLAS GENOMIC CLASSIFICATION

The methods used by TCGA, such as the use of fresh frozen tissue and whole exome sequencing, are unfortunately too costly, time-consuming, and complicated for practical use in today's clinical setting. Several groups have developed surrogate ways to incorporate TCGA findings into clinical practice. Recent studies from the Vancouver group,[54–56] PORTEC clinical trials,[57,58] and NRG Oncology[59] have independently developed surrogate molecular classifier algorithms for EC cohorts. These have had success in finding clinically applicable molecular-based EC classification models with good predictive results that perform as well as current prognostic tools,[4] and add a new layer of prognostic information within histologic subtypes.

In principle, with slightly different methodologies, these studies have used sequencing of the *POLE* exonuclease domain (corresponding to TCGA *POLE*-mutated group) combined with some form of MSI analysis (often IHC to demonstrate MMRd) and p53 IHC to reproduce TCGA genomic classification groups and survival curves. Tumors that lacked any of these features corresponded to low copy number, MSS, no specific molecular profile TCGA group. In addition, the different genomic groups (p53mut and MSI) remained significant predictors of outcome in multivariable survival analysis when adjusting for histopathological factors.

These results look promising because initial findings suggest that they can be reproduced, used on biopsy samples, and used on formalin-fixed tissue, as well as an add another layer of prognostic information and identify patients for whom adjuvant treatment is appropriate. These retrospective studies have an important limitation, however. Both TCGA and surrogate models have focused on selected patient cohorts, mostly those with high-grade endometrioid and serous tumors. It is not yet clear if these models hold true in other histotypes and/or in a populations in which most tumors are low-grade. Supplementary genomic tests show promise as a part of the EC diagnostic and prognostic future.

REFERENCES

1. Gilks CB, Oliva E, Soslow RA. Poor interobserver reproducibility in the diagnosis of high-grade endometrial carcinoma. Am J Surg Pathol 2013;37(6): 874–81. Available at: http://www.ncbi.nlm.nih.gov/pubmed/23629444. Accessed February 3, 2018.

2. Hoang LN, Kinloch MA, Leo JM, et al. Interobserver agreement in endometrial carcinoma histotype diagnosis varies depending on The Cancer Genome Atlas (TCGA)-based molecular subgroup. Am J Surg Pathol 2017;41(2):245–52. Available at: http://www.ncbi.nlm.nih.gov/pubmed/28079598.

3. Soslow RA. High-grade endometrial carcinomas - strategies for typing. Histopathology 2013;62(1): 89–110.

4. Colombo N, Creutzberg C, Amant F, et al. ESMO-ESGO-ESTRO Consensus Conference on Endometrial Cancer: diagnosis, treatment and follow-up. Ann Oncol 2016;27(1):16–41. Available at: https://academic.oup.com/annonc/article-lookup/doi/10.1093/annonc/mdv484.

5. Kurman RJ, Carcangiu ML, Herrington CS, et al. WHO classification of tumours of female reproductive organs. Lyon (France): IARC Press; 2014. p. 307. Available at: https://books.google.com/books?id=4Tw8ngEACA AJ&pgis=1. Accessed April 13, 2015.

6. Malpica A. How to approach the many faces of endometrioid carcinoma. Mod Pathol 2016;29(S1): S29–44.

7. Köbel M, Piskorz AM, Lee S, et al. Optimized p53 immunohistochemistry is an accurate predictor of TP53 mutation in ovarian carcinoma. J Pathol Clin Res 2016;2(4):247–58. Available at: http://www.ncbi.nlm.nih.gov/pubmed/27840695. Accessed August 14, 2018.

8. Yemelyanova A, Ji H, Shih I-M, et al. Utility of p16 expression for distinction of uterine serous carcinomas from endometrial endometrioid and endocervical adenocarcinomas: immunohistochemical analysis of 201 cases. Am J Surg Pathol 2009;33(10):1504–14.

9. Getz G, Gabriel SB, Cibulskis K, et al. Integrated genomic characterization of endometrial carcinoma. Nature 2013;497(7447):67–73. Available at: http://www.ncbi.nlm.nih.gov/pubmed/23636398. Accessed September 12, 2018.

10. Chiang S, Soslow RA. Updates in diagnostic immunohistochemistry in endometrial carcinoma. Semin Diagn Pathol 2014;31(3):205–15. Available at: http://www.ncbi.nlm.nih.gov/pubmed/24951284. Accessed September 12, 2018.

11. Lax SF, Kendall B, Tashiro H, et al. The frequency of p53, K-ras mutations, and microsatellite instability differs in uterine endometrioid and serous carcinoma: evidence of distinct molecular genetic pathways. Cancer 2000;88(4):814–24. Available at: http://www.ncbi.nlm.nih.gov/pubmed/10679651. Accessed September 10, 2018.

12. Bartosch C, Manuel Lopes J, Oliva E. Endometrial carcinomas: a review emphasizing overlapping and distinctive morphological and immunohistochemical features. Adv Anat Pathol 2011;18(6):415–37. Available at: http://www.ncbi.nlm.nih.gov/pubmed/21993268.

13. Garg K, Soslow RA. Strategies for distinguishing low-grade endometrioid and serous carcinomas of endometrium. Adv Anat Pathol 2012;19(1):1–10.

14. Soslow RA, Pirog E, Isacson C. Endometrial intraepithelial carcinoma with associated peritoneal carcinomatosis. Am J Surg Pathol 2000;24(5):726–32.

15. Al-Hussaini M, Stockman A, Foster H, et al. WT-1 assists in distinguishing ovarian from uterine serous carcinoma and in distinguishing between serous and endometrioid ovarian carcinoma. Histopathology 2004;44(2):109–15.

16. Hoang LN, Mcconechy MK, Meng B, et al. Targeted mutation analysis of endometrial clear cell carcinoma. Histopathology 2015;66(5):664–74.

17. McConechy MK, Ding J, Cheang MC, et al. Use of mutation profiles to refine the classification of endometrial carcinomas. J Pathol 2012;228(1):20–30. Accessed March 5, 2018.

18. Samarnthai N, Hall K, Yeh I-T. Molecular profiling of endometrial malignancies. Obstet Gynecol Int 2010; 2010:162363. Available at: http://www.ncbi.nlm.nih.gov/pubmed/20368795. Accessed September 12, 2018.

19. Gatius S, Matias-guiu X. Practical issues in the diagnosis of serous carcinoma of the endometrium. Mod Pathol 2016;29(S1):S45–58.

20. Fadare O, Zheng W, Crispens M a, et al. Morphologic and other clinicopathologic features of endometrial clear cell carcinoma: a comprehensive analysis of 50 rigorously classified cases. Am J Cancer Res 2013;3(1):70–95. Available at: http://www.pubmedcentral.nih.gov/articlerender.fcgi?artid=3555196&tool=pmcentrez&rendertype=abstract.

21. Hoang LN, Han G, McConechy M, et al. Immunohistochemical characterization of prototypical endometrial clear cell carcinoma-diagnostic utility of HNF-1β and oestrogen receptor. Histopathology 2014;64(4):585–96. Accessed September 9, 2018.

22. Yamashita Y, Nagasaka T, Naiki-Ito A, et al. Napsin A is a specific marker for ovarian clear cell adenocarcinoma. Mod Pathol 2015;28(1):111–7.

23. Fadare O, Gwin K, Desouki MM, et al. The clinicopathologic significance of p53 and BAF-250a (ARID1A) expression in clear cell carcinoma of the endometrium. Mod Pathol 2013;26(8):1101–10.

24. Fadare O, Liang SX. Diagnostic utility of hepatocyte nuclear factor 1-beta immunoreactivity in endometrial carcinomas. Appl Immunohistochem Mol Morphol 2012;20(6):580–7. Available at: http://www.ncbi.nlm.nih.gov/pubmed/22495362. Accessed September 11, 2018.

25. DeLair DF, Burke KA, Selenica P, et al. The genetic landscape of endometrial clear cell carcinomas. J Pathol 2017;243(2):230–41. Available at: http://www.ncbi.nlm.nih.gov/pubmed/28718916. Accessed September 12, 2018.

26. Altrabulsi B, Malpica A, Deavers MT, et al. Undifferentiated carcinoma of the endometrium. Am J Surg Pathol 2005;29(10):1316–21. Available at: http://www.ncbi.nlm.nih.gov/pubmed/16160474.

27. Tafe LJ, Garg K, Chew I, et al. Endometrial and ovarian carcinomas with undifferentiated components: clinically aggressive and frequently underrecognized neoplasms. Mod Pathol 2010;23(6):781–9. Available at: http://www.ncbi.nlm.nih.gov/pubmed/20305618. Accessed January 2, 2015.

28. Stewart CJR, Crook ML. SWI/SNF complex deficiency and mismatch repair protein expression in undifferentiated and dedifferentiated endometrial carcinoma. Pathology 2015;47(5):439–45. Available at: http://linkinghub.elsevier.com/retrieve/pii/S0031302516300812. Accessed September 11, 2018.

29. Ramalingam P, Croce S, McCluggage WG. Loss of expression of SMARCA4 (BRG1), SMARCA2 (BRM) and SMARCB1 (INI1) in undifferentiated carcinoma of the endometrium is not uncommon and is not always associated with rhabdoid morphology. Histopathology 2017;70(3):359–66. Available at: http://doi.wiley.com/10.1111/his.13091. Accessed September 11, 2018.

30. Rosa-Rosa JM, Leskelä S, Cristóbal-Lana E, et al. Molecular genetic heterogeneity in undifferentiated endometrial carcinomas. Mod Pathol 2016;29(11): 1390–8. Available at: http://www.nature.com/doi-finder/10.1038/modpathol.2016.132.

31. Cancer Genome Atlas Research Network, Kandoth C, Schultz N, Cherniack AD, et al. Integrated genomic characterization of endometrial carcinoma. Nature 2013;497(7447):67–73. Available at: http://www.pubmedcentral.nih.gov/articlerender.fcgi?artid=3704730&tool=pmcentrez&rendertype=abstract.

32. Romero-Pérez L, López-García MÁ, Díaz-Martín J, et al. ZEB1 overexpression associated with E-cadherin and microRNA-200 downregulation is characteristic of undifferentiated endometrial carcinoma. Mod Pathol 2013;26(11):1514–24. Available at: http://www.ncbi.nlm.nih.gov/pubmed/23743934. Accessed September 12, 2018.

33. Pocrnich CE, Ramalingam P, Euscher ED, et al. Neuroendocrine carcinoma of the endometrium: a clinicopathologic study of 25 cases. Am J Surg Pathol 2016;40(5):577–86.

34. Bokhman JV. Two pathogenetic types of endometrial carcinoma. Gynecol Oncol 1983;15(1):10–7.

35. Kobel M, Meng B, Hoang LN, et al. Molecular analysis of mixed endometrial carcinomas shows clonality in most cases. Am J Surg Pathol 2016;40(2): 166–80.

36. Soslow RA. Endometrial carcinomas with ambiguous features. Semin Diagn Pathol 2010;27(4): 261–73.

37. Mcfarland M, Quick CM, McCluggage WG. Hormone receptor-negative, thyroid transcription factor 1-positive uterine and ovarian adenocarcinomas: report of a series of mesonephric-like adenocarcinomas. Histopathology 2016;68(7):1013–20.

38. Pors J, Cheng A, Leo JM, et al. A Comparison of GATA3, TTF1, CD10, and calretinin in identifying mesonephric and mesonephric-like carcinomas of the gynecologic tract. Am J Surg Pathol 2018; 42(12):1596–606.

39. Mirkovic J, McFarland M, Garcia E, et al. Targeted genomic profiling reveals recurrent KRAS mutations in mesonephric-like adenocarcinomas of the female genital tract. Am J Surg Pathol 2018;42(2):227–33.

40. Mittal K, Soslow R, McCluggage WG. Application of immunohistochemistry to gynecologic pathology. Arch Pathol Lab Med 2008;132(3):402–23. Available at: http://www.ncbi.nlm.nih.gov/pubmed/18318583. Accessed September 9, 2018.

41. McCluggage WG, Jenkins D. p16 immunoreactivity may assist in the distinction between endometrial and endocervical adenocarcinoma. Int J Gynecol Pathol 2003;22(3):231–5. Available at: https://insights.ovid.com/crossref?an=00004347-200307000-00005. Accessed September 11, 2018.

42. Wei J-J, Paintal A, Keh P. Histologic and immunohistochemical analyses of endometrial carcinomas: experiences from endometrial biopsies in 358 consultation cases. Arch Pathol Lab Med 2013; 137:1574–83. Available at: http://www.ncbi.nlm.nih.gov/pubmed/24168495.

43. Kapucuoglu N, Bulbul D, Tulunay G, et al. Reproducibility of grading systems for endometrial endometrioid carcinoma and their relation with pathologic prognostic parameters. Int J Gynecol Cancer 2008;18(1):790–6.

44. Ramalingam P, Masand RP, Euscher ED, et al. Undifferentiated carcinoma of the endometrium. Int J Gynecol Pathol 2016;35(5):410–8. Available at: http://www.ncbi.nlm.nih.gov/pubmed/26598976. Accessed September 12, 2018.

45. Hoang LN, Lee YS, Karnezis AN, et al. Immunophenotypic features of dedifferentiated endometrial carcinoma??? insights from BRG1/INI1-deficient tumours. Histopathology 2016;69(4):560–9.

46. Nastic D, Shanwell E, Wallin K-L, et al. A selective biomarker panel increases the reproducibility and the accuracy in endometrial biopsy diagnosis. Int J Gynecol Pathol 2017;36(4):339–47. Available at: http://www.ncbi.nlm.nih.gov/pubmed/28244894. Accessed September 10, 2018.

47. Santacana M, Maiques O, Valls J, et al. A 9-protein biomarker molecular signature for predicting histologic type in endometrial carcinoma by immunohistochemistry. Hum Pathol 2014;45(12):2394–403. Available at: http://linkinghub.elsevier.com/retrieve/pii/S004681771400327X. Accessed September 11, 2018.

48. Mota A, Colás E, García-Sanz P, et al. Genetic analysis of uterine aspirates improves the diagnostic value and captures the intra-tumor heterogeneity of endometrial cancers. Mod Pathol 2017;30(1): 134–45. Available at: http://www.ncbi.nlm.nih.gov/pubmed/27586201. Accessed September 12, 2018.

49. Hoang LN, McConechy MK, Köbel M, et al. Histotype-genotype correlation in 36 high-grade endometrial carcinomas. Am J Surg Pathol 2013;37(9): 1421–32. Available at: http://www.ncbi.nlm.nih.gov/pubmed/24076778. Accessed September 9, 2018.

50. Church DN, Briggs SEW, Palles C, et al. DNA polymerase ε and δ exonuclease domain mutations in endometrial cancer. Hum Mol Genet 2013;22(14): 2820–8. Available at: http://www.ncbi.nlm.nih.gov/pubmed/23528559%5Cnhttp://www.pubmedcentral.nih.gov/articlerender.fcgi?artid=PMC3690967.

51. McConechy MK, Talhouk A, Leung S, et al. Endometrial carcinomas with POLE exonuclease domain mutations have a favorable prognosis. Clin Cancer Res 2016;22(12):2865–73.

52. Shikama A, Minaguchi T, Matsumoto K, et al. Clinicopathologic implications of DNA mismatch repair status in endometrial carcinomas. Gynecol Oncol 2016;

140(2):226–33. Available at: http://www.ncbi.nlm.nih.gov/pubmed/26644264. Accessed September 12, 2018.

53. Topalian SL, Hodi FS, Brahmer JR, et al. Safety, activity, and immune correlates of anti–PD-1 antibody in cancer. N Engl J Med 2012;366(26):2443–54. Available at. http://www.ncbi.nlm.nih.gov/pubmed/22658127. Accessed September 12, 2018.

54. Kommoss S, McConechy MK, Kommoss F, et al. Final validation of the ProMisE molecular classifier for endometrial carcinoma in a large population-based case series. Ann Oncol 2018;29(5):1180–8. Available at: https://academic.oup.com/annonc/advance-article/doi/10.1093/annonc/mdy058/4844033. Accessed March 5, 2018.

55. Talhouk A, McConechy MK, Leung S, et al. Confirmation of ProMisE: a simple, genomics-based clinical classifier for endometrial cancer. Cancer 2017; 123(5):802–13.

56. Talhouk A, Hoang LN, McConechy MK, et al. Molecular classification of endometrial carcinoma on diagnostic specimens is highly concordant with final hysterectomy: earlier prognostic information to guide treatment. Gynecol Oncol 2016;143(1):46–53.

57. Stelloo E, Bosse T, Nout RA, et al. Refining prognosis and identifying targetable pathways for high-risk endometrial cancer; a TransPORTEC initiative. Mod Pathol 2015;28:836–44.

58. Stelloo E, Nout RAA, Osse EMM, et al. Improved risk assessment by integrating molecular and clinico-pathological factors in early-stage endometrial cancer - combined analysis of PORTEC cohorts. Clin Cancer Res 2016;22(16):4215–24.

59. Cosgrove CM, Tritchler DL, Cohn DE, et al. An NRG Oncology/GOG study of molecular classification for risk prediction in endometrioid endometrial cancer. Gynecol Oncol 2017;148:174–80. Available at. https://ac.els-cdn.com/S0090825817314592/1-s2.0-S0090825817314592-main.pdf?_tid=8b6203e0-c9c3-4f60-a956-f82e13560a6b&acdnat=1521103822_b00ed8e32f5597a23a104bccfca8bffa. Accessed March 15, 2018.

Uterine Mesenchymal Tumors

Update on Classification, Staging, and Molecular Features

Carlos Parra-Herran, MD[a],*, Brooke E. Howitt, MD[b]

KEYWORDS

- Sarcoma • Uterus • Endometrial stromal sarcoma • Adenosarcoma • PEComa
- Inflammatory myofibroblastic tumor • Rhabdomyosarcoma • Undifferentiated uterine sarcoma

Key points

- Mullerian adenosarcomas can be relatively indolent or highly aggressive; in this regard, high-grade sarcomatous morphology and sarcomatous overgrowth are known poor prognostic factors.
- Recurrent gene abnormalities may play an important role in the diagnosis of uterine sarcomas and our understanding of their biology.
- Other genomic alterations have not only diagnostic potential, but also therapeutic importance.
- Careful examination and generous sampling are key in the diagnosis of uterine sarcomas and exclusion of its mimickers, particularly carcinosarcoma.
- Undifferentiated uterine sarcoma is a diagnosis of exclusion, and as such comprises a heterogeneous group of tumors and may include "dedifferentiated" forms of specific uterine sarcomas.

ABSTRACT

The spectrum of mesenchymal neoplasia in the uterus has expanded in recent years. First, the identification of prevalent, recurrent molecular alterations has led to a more biologically and clinically congruent classification of endometrial stromal tumors. Likewise, the diagnostic criteria of several rare and miscellaneous tumor types have been refined in recent case series (Perivascular Epithelioid Cell tumor, inflammatory myofibroblastic tumor). Pure mesenchymal tumors are still broadly classified based on morphology according to the tumor cell phenotype. Smooth muscle tumors predominate in frequency, followed by tumors of endometrial stromal derivation; the latter are covered in depth in this article with an emphasis on defining molecular alterations and their morphologic and clinical correlates. The remaining entities comprise a miscellaneous group in which cell derivation does not have a normal counterpart in the uterus (eg, rhabdomyosarcoma) or is obscure (eg, undifferentiated uterine sarcoma). This article discusses their clinical relevance, recent insights into their molecular biology, and the most important differential diagnoses. Regarding the latter, immunohistochemistry and (increasingly) molecular diagnostics play a role in the diagnostic workup. We conclude with a few considerations on intraoperative consultation and macroscopic examination, as well as pathologic staging and grading of uterine sarcomas as per the most recent American Joint Cancer Commission and the Fédération Internationale de Gynécologie et d'Obstétrique staging systems.

Disclosure Statement: The authors have no financial disclosures or conflicts of interests to declare pertaining to this work.
[a] Department of Laboratory Medicine, Sunnybrook Health Sciences Centre, University of Toronto, 2075 Bayview Avenue, Toronto, ON, Canada; [b] Department of Pathology, Stanford University, Stanford University School of Medicine, 300 Pasteur Drive H2128E, Stanford, CA 94305-5324, USA
* Corresponding author.
E-mail address: carlos.parraherran@utoronto.ca

surgpath.theclinics.com

INTRODUCTION

A summary of the most salient immunohistochemical and molecular features of the entities discussed in this chapter is presented in **Table 1**.

MÜLLERIAN ADENOSARCOMA

Müllerian adenosarcoma is a mixed lesion with malignant mesenchymal and benign glandular components (**Table 1**). Age at presentation varies greatly (range 13–89 years). Although most patients are postmenopausal, about 30% of patients are of reproductive age.[1–3] The lesion frequently grows on the endometrial surface, mimicking a polyp on clinical and radiologic evaluation.

Macroscopically, adenosarcoma presents as an exophytic mass with variable endophytic growth into the uterine wall. Histologically, the tumor displays a distinct biphasic cellular composition: the glandular component is seen in the form of glands, cysts, and surface lining, all composed of a simple layer of bland Müllerian-type epithelium. Epithelial metaplasia can be appreciated (tubal, squamous, or mucinous); however, architectural complexity or cytologic atypia are absent (with rare exceptions, discussed in Differential Diagnosis). Most glands have narrow lumens, usually compressed by the underlying mesenchymal growth, giving a leaflike appearance. Cystic dilation with rigid contours is common. The stroma around the glands is typically more cellular and atypical; in these cellular areas, 4 or more mitoses/10 high-power fields (HPFs) are counted in the vast majority of cases.[3] The diagnosis of adenosarcoma relies on the identification of the following features (**Fig. 1**A):

- Intraglandular projections and leaflike (phyllodes-like) architecture.
- Stromal cytologic atypia.
- Periglandular stromal condensation.
- Rigid cystic dilation.
- Mitotic activity 2 or more mitoses/10 HPFs.

Original descriptions of this tumor state that the presence of any of these characteristics warrants a diagnosis of adenosarcoma. However, most adenosarcomas have 3 or more. In fact, polyps that display *focally* up to 3 of these features have an indolent outcome and no recurrence or metastases.[4] The term uterine polyp with unusual features has been proposed for such cases. The diagnosis of adenosarcoma is warranted if 2 or more of these findings are present *diffusely throughout the tumor*. Additionally, polyps with bizarre, symplastic type stromal atypia have been described[5]; however, these polyps lack mitotic activity in the atypical cells and also lack other histologic features of adenosarcoma. Similar to uterine polyps with unusual features, these also have a benign clinical behavior.

Adenosarcomas can be classified into clinically and pathologically distinct groups. The high-risk category includes tumors with sarcomatous overgrowth (of any grade) and those with high-grade stromal atypia (regardless of the presence of sarcomatous overgrowth). The low-risk category includes tumors without these adverse features (low-grade adenosarcoma without sarcomatous overgrowth).

1. Low-grade adenosarcoma (**Fig. 1**B). Most adenosarcomas encountered in practice can be classified as low grade. The stromal component resembles the appearance of a low-grade endometrial stromal neoplasm. Atypia is mild and best appreciated under high-power magnification. Stromal cells express CD10, WT1, and hormone receptors.[6,7] Smooth muscle or sex cord stromal differentiation can be noted. Most cases are confined to the uterus (International Federation of Gynecology and Obstetrics [FIGO] stage I). Myometrial invasion, usually superficial, has been reported in 14% of cases.[3] These tumors are considered to have a low malignant potential: vaginal or abdominopelvic recurrence occurs in 25% of cases. Myometrial and vascular space invasion are associated with adverse outcome.[3,8]
2. High-grade adenosarcoma (**Fig. 1**C). Adenosarcomas with a high-grade stromal component have been recently described.[9] High-grade morphology in this context is defined as severe nuclear pleomorphism (nuclei more than twice the size of an endothelial cell nucleus, irregular nuclear membranes, coarse chromatin, prominent nucleoli) identifiable at low-power magnification. High-grade adenosarcoma is usually, but not exclusively, seen in the context of sarcomatous overgrowth. The presence of any high-grade sarcomatous component should be reported, because these lesions are associated with aggressive behavior and rapid widespread recurrence.[9]
3. Adenosarcoma with sarcomatous overgrowth (**Fig. 2**). A minority (approximately 10%) of adenosarcomas contain areas of pure sarcoma representing 25% or more of the tumor. These have been described in the literature as adenosarcoma with sarcomatous overgrowth.[10] The sarcoma can be homologous or heterologous

Table 1
Immunohistochemical and molecular characteristics of primary uterine mesenchymal neoplasms

	Immunohistochemistry	Molecular Features
Mullerian adenosarcoma	ER, PR, CD10 ++ p53 wt (low grade) p53 abnormal (high grade) Myoglobin, MyoD1 ++ (w/ rhabdomyosarcomatous differentiation)	*FGFR2, KMT2C,* and *DICER1* mutations *MDM2/CDK4/HMGA2* and *TERT* amplification *NCOA2/3* fusion Sarcomatous overgrowth: chromosomal instability, chromothripsis, high copy number variation, *MYBL1* amplification, *ATRX* mutations High-grade tumors: *TP53* pathway alterations (67%)
Endometrial stromal nodule Low-grade endometrial stromal sarcoma	ER, PR, CD10 +++ (>90%) SMA, desmin, caldesmon +/− Cyclin D1, BCOR +/− Ki67 <5%	Alterations in 50%–65% of cases: *JAZF1 – SUZ12* (80%), *JAZF1 – PHF1* (6%), *EPC1 – PHF1* (4%), *MEAF6 – PHF1* (3%), *MBTD1 – Cxorf67* (2%)
YWHAE-NUTMN2 high-grade endometrial stromal sarcoma	ER, PR, CD10 +/− SMA, desmin, caldesmon +/− Cyclin D1, BCOR +++ Ki67 ≥5%	*YWHAE-NUTM2A/B* fusion
BCOR-altered high grade endometrial stromal sarcoma	CD10 +++ (*BCOR* fusion) CD10+/− (*BCOR* ITD) ER, PR +/− SMA, desmin, caldesmon +/− Cyclin D1 +++ BCOR ± Ki67 ≥5%	*ZC3H7B – BCOR* fusion *BCOR* internal tandem duplication
Undifferentiated uterine sarcoma	CD10 +++/− ER, PR - SMA, desmin, caldesmon - Keratin, EMA - Ki67 ≥10%	Complex karyotype *NTRK* fusions in subset
SMARCA4-deficient uterine sarcoma	SMARCA4 loss Keratins/EMA – or rare cells +	*SMARCA4* deleterious mutations No other genetic alterations
Uterine tumor resembling ovarian sex cord stromal tumors	Inhibin, calretinin, SF1, WT1 ++ Keratin, EMA ++/− SMA, desmin, caldesmon +/−	*ESR1-NCOA3, ESR1-NCOA2, GREB1-NCOA2,* or *GREB1-CTNNB1* fusions
Perivascular epithelioid cell tumor (PEComa)	HMB45++ Melan-A, MiTF ++ Desmin, caldesmon ++ Cathepsin-K, C-KIT ++	*TSC1/TSC2* mutations *TFE3* or *RAD51B* rearrangements
Inflammatory myofibroblastic tumor	ALK +++ SMA, desmin, caldesmon ++/−	*ALK* rearrangements: *ALK-IGFBP5, ALK-THBS1,* and *ALK-TIMP3*
Rhabdomyosarcoma	Desmin, myoglobin, MyoD1 +++	*DICER1* mutations in embryonal type *PAX3-FKHR* and *PAX7-FKHR* fusions in alveolar type

Abbreviations: ER, estrogen receptor; PR, progesterone receptor; SMA, smooth muscle actin; wt, wild type.

(rhabdomyosarcomatous being the most frequent), and typically are high grade. Sarcomatous overgrowth is highly associated with extrauterine spread at presentation and high rates of recurrence and death.[10,11] Importantly, aggressive behavior in the context of sarcomatous overgrowth is independent of the histologic grade (about 30% of adenosarcomas with

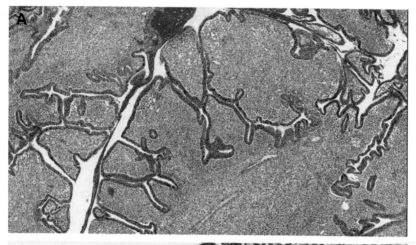

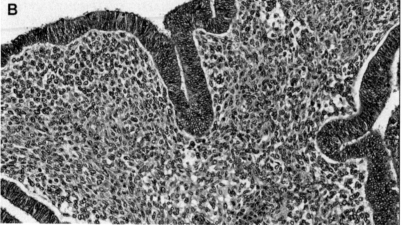

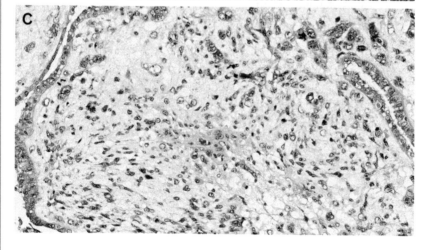

Fig. 1. Müllerian adeno-sarcoma. Biphasic lesion with a benign epithelial component overlying a malignant stromal prolif-eration. The latter pro-trudes into the glandular lumens with a character-istic broad front (leaflike architecture) (A). Low-grade Müllerian adeno-sarcoma is characterized by a relatively mono-tonous stromal com-ponent with only mild cytologic atypia (B). In contrast, high-grade Müllerian adenosarcoma shows significant pleo-morphism and large irregular nuclei with con-spicuous mitoses, in-cluding atypical forms (upper right aspect) (C). Images B and C were taken at the same original magnification (×20).

sarcomatous overgrowth are low grade). Thus, the presence of sarcomatous overgrowth must be always reported.

Müllerian adenosarcoma harbors a number of somatic gene alterations that are exclusive to the mesenchymal component, supporting the theory that this lesion is primarily a mesen-chymal neoplasm. These include *FGFR2*, *KMT2C*, and *DICER1* mutations (11% each), *MDM2/CDK4/HMGA2* amplification (26%),

TERT amplification (21%), and *NCOA2/3* gene fusions (11%).[12,13] Adenosarcomas with sarcomatous overgrowth have a higher number of copy number variations, *MYBL1* amplification, and *ATRX* mutations.[13] In addition, global chromosomal instability and chromothripsis are more common in cases with sarcomatous overgrowth.[11] In contrast with low-grade adenosarcoma, high-grade adenosarcoma frequently harbors *TP53* pathway alterations.[9]

The differential diagnosis of adenosarcoma includes benign and malignant conditions. Endometrial and endocervical polyps can display features suggestive of adenosarcoma, as mentioned. Benign polyps tend to be small. Moreover, periglandular condensation, leaflike architecture, atypia, and mitotic activity, when present, are focal and not fully developed. Carcinosarcoma may enter in the differential, but unlike adenosarcoma, the epithelial component is by definition malignant and high grade. A recently described phenomenon is carcinoma arising in the epithelial component of an adenosarcoma.[14] In this setting, carcinoma is typically low-grade endometrioid, and is found focally within the lesion; in other words, other parts of the tumor retain the classic adenosarcoma morphology with a benign epithelial component. The outcome of these cases, at least in a small series of 20 cases, is more indolent compared with the aggressive behavior of carcinosarcoma.[14] Last, adenosarcoma with sarcomatous overgrowth and high-grade adenosarcoma may mimic a pure uterine sarcoma, especially in small specimens. Thorough tissue sampling and microscopic examination are key in this differential.

Key Features
ADENOSARCOMA

- Biphasic tumor with malignant stromal component and benign epithelial component.

- Leaflike phyllodes architecture with associated stromal condensation under epithelium.

- Stromal component may demonstrate mild to moderate atypia ("low grade") or striking atypia with pleomorphism ("high grade").

- Epithelial component often displays metaplastic changes and may also demonstrate variable atypia.

- Sarcomatous overgrowth is defined as pure sarcoma comprising 25% or more of the tumor.

- Heterologous differentiation may be present (the most common is rhabdomyosarcoma).

- Stage, grade, and presence of sarcomatous overgrowth are the important prognostic factors.

Differential Diagnosis
ADENOSARCOMA

- "Low-grade" adenosarcoma should be distinguished from benign or atypical uterine polyps; in the latter, the characteristic features of adenosarcoma tend to be subtle.

- "High-grade" adenosarcoma should be distinguished from other high-grade uterine sarcomas; identification of the classical architectural features (phyllodes architecture and stromal condensation around epithelial component) is important.

- Some carcinosarcomas may contain "adenosarcoma-like" areas; thus, it is critical to carefully evaluate the epithelial component—although some atypia is permitted in adenosarcoma, overtly malignant cytology and/or architecture should raise high suspicion for carcinosarcoma.

ENDOMETRIAL STROMAL NEOPLASMS

The classification of endometrial stromal neoplasms, and in particular stromal sarcomas, has undergone significant change over the past decade with our increased understanding of molecular alterations (most commonly gene fusions) underlying these tumors. Low-grade endometrial stromal neoplasms by definition have cytologic features typical of nonneoplastic proliferative phase endometrial stroma. Specifically, the neoplastic cells are ovoid to fusiform and bland with no or minimal cytologic atypia. There is conspicuous concentric growth around spiral-arteriole–like vessels. Both endometrial stromal nodule (ESN) and low-grade endometrial stromal sarcoma (LGESS) comprise this low-grade stromal tumor category and share similar molecular alterations, namely translocations resulting in gene fusions, most typically involving the *JAZF1* gene (*JAZF1-SUZ12*); other well-described translocations involve *PHF1* with a variety of fusion partners.[15–22] Together, one of these alterations is found in up to 55% to 90% of low-grade endometrial stromal neoplasms.[23,24] High-grade endometrial stromal sarcomas (HGESS) have distinct

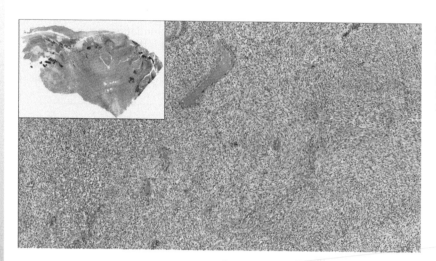

Fig. 2. Müllerian adenosarcoma with sarcomatous overgrowth. Sarcoma represents more than 25% of the tumor volume (see scanning view in inset).

clinical, morphologic, immunophenotypic, and molecular features.

ENDOMETRIAL STROMAL NODULE

ESNs macroscopically present as solitary, well-defined, yellow myometrial masses, often with a softer consistency compared with the very common leiomyoma. Microscopically, ESNs lack lymphovascular invasion and have well-circumscribed borders, with no more than 3 foci of irregular-appearing borders, with each focus of irregularity measuring less than 3 mm (**Fig. 3**).[25–28] ESNs are benign tumors and do not recur when completely excised. There are 3 main differential diagnostic considerations for ESN: low-grade endometrial stromal sarcoma, uterine tumor resembling sex cord stromal tumor (UTROSCT), and leiomyoma, the latter being more commonly confused with stromal nodules when highly cellular.

1. ESN versus LGESS: Microscopically, the neoplastic cells of ESN and LGESS are identical in that they closely resemble nonneoplastic proliferative endometrium. The distinction between ESN and LGESS is made based on the presence or absence of lymphovascular invasion as well as the nature of the borders of the lesion. Thus, a diagnosis of ESN can only be made on complete excision with evaluation of the entire lesion and surrounding myometrium. Neither immunohistochemistry nor molecular analysis will aid in the distinction of ESN from LGESS. Both can have identical immunophenotypes and are associated with the same gene fusions. In some (rare) cases, there is minimal infiltration of the surrounding myometrium, but exceeds that permitted in ESN; for these tumors, one may use the term, "endometrial stromal tumor with limited infiltration."[27] The precise clinical behavior of these rare lesions is unclear.

2. ESN versus (highly cellular) leiomyoma: Both ESN and highly cellular leiomyomas appear blue on low-power examination and are well-circumscribed. Morphologic features suggestive of leiomyoma include intratumoral thick-walled vessels and prominent clefting (**Fig. 4**A). Additionally, in leiomyoma the cells tend to have a more fascicular arrangement (**Fig. 4**B) compared with the perivascular whorling of ESN (see **Fig. 3**B). Immunohistochemistry can be helpful, if muscle markers are positive and CD10 is negative; however, some highly cellular leiomyomas may express CD10 and lack strong smooth muscle marker expression. In contrast, ESNs can harbor smooth muscle differentiation, which express smooth muscle markers. Molecular analysis, although generally not required because both entities are clinically benign, may be useful if a *JAZF1* or *PHF1* rearrangement is identified (supporting the diagnosis of ESN).

3. ESN with sex cord differentiation versus UTROSCT: These 2 tumors may have a significant amount of morphologic overlap, and classification is generally determined by the presence or absence of classical endometrial stromal-type morphology. Molecular testing will potentially be useful because these tumors seem to have distinctly different genetic profiles (see Uterine Tumor Resembling Sex Cord Tumor).

Key Features
ENDOMETRIAL STROMAL NODULE

- Well-circumscribed nodule composed of endometrial stromal–type cells.

- Lymphovascular invasion should be absent.

- Positive for CD10; may also demonstrate smooth muscle marker positivity if smooth muscle differentiation is present.

- A definitive diagnosis of ESN can generally only be made in hysterectomy specimens, because a complete assessment of the border of the tumor is required to exclude low-grade endometrial stromal sarcoma. However, if preservation of fertility is desired, a more conservative approach to complete excision can be considered.

LOW-GRADE ENDOMETRIAL STROMAL SARCOMA

LGESS is often recognized at the time of gross examination of a hysterectomy specimen because the tumor has a characteristic tonguelike penetration into the endometrium and may plug up numerous vessels, imparting a "wormlike" appearance macroscopically. As mentioned, LGESS is composed of neoplastic cells resembling proliferative phase endometrium at high magnification.[28,29] The diagnosis of LGESS is an architectural one, requiring the typical tonguelike pattern of invasion (**Fig. 5**A) and frequent vascular invasion. LGESS is characterized by CD10 (**Fig. 5**B), IFITM1, estrogen receptor (ER), and PR positivity.[30–35] The presence of altered differentiation, such as smooth muscle (**Fig. 6**A), or the presence of non-conventional elements including sex cord, fibromyxoid, and glandular elements can lead to a wide variety of immunophenotype; thus, it is critical to consider the morphologic appearance when interpreting immunohistochemistry and considering the differential diagnoses. Moreover, it is important to note that altered differentiation may take over most of the tumor, and classic endometrial stromal morphology may be very focal.[36] The pattern of myometrial invasion can aid in the distinction of LGESS from leiomyosarcoma, because the latter typically shows destructive infiltration of surrounding tissue, whereas LGESS rarely shows this pattern. One smooth muscle tumor that can mimic the infiltrative pattern of LGESS is intravascular leiomyomatosis. Noting the morphologic features of smooth muscle differentiation, including thick-

walled vessels and clefting, can be helpful. In addition, immunohistochemistry and molecular testing can be performed in challenging cases (see also J Kenneth Schoolmeester's article, "Smooth Muscle Neoplasia of the Female Genital Tract," in this issue for additional details on smooth muscle neoplasms). Similar to smooth muscle tumors, endometrial stromal neoplasms can have significant collagen bands or plaques (**Fig. 6**B). When prominent sex cord differentiation is present (**Fig. 6**C), the principal diagnostic consideration before making a diagnosis of LGESS is UTROSCT. In LGESS, there should be typical areas of overt endometrial stromal differentiation and the classical pattern of invasion, whereas in UTROSCT, a clear endometrial stromal component is lacking or minimal. Glandular elements may also be seen in LGESS (**Fig. 6**D), raising the possibility of adenosarcoma. This is usually easily resolved because the glandular elements of LGESS appear as entrapped normal endometrial glands and lack the architectural features of adenosarcoma, and also lack the malignant characteristics of a carcinosarcoma. Fibromyxoid LGESS (**Fig. 6**E) requires distinction from HGESS with BCOR alterations (more conspicuous nuclear atypia, extensive necrosis, lack of conventional LGESS areas), myxoid leiomyosarcoma (overt atypia and tissue infiltration), and inflammatory myofibroblastic tumor (prominent inflammatory component, ALK expression). Other forms of differentiation (including skeletal muscle, adipocytic, cartilaginous) may be seen in LGESS but are uncommon.

Key Features
LOW-GRADE ENDOMETRIAL STROMAL SARCOMA

- Malignant tumor composed of endometrial stromal-type cells.

- Often prominent tonguelike infiltration into surrounding myometrium with frequent vascular invasion that is grossly evident.

- Positive for CD10; may also demonstrate smooth muscle marker positivity if smooth muscle differentiation is present or sex cord marker positivity in the presence of sex cord differentiation.

- The most common molecular alteration is rearrangement of the *JAZF1* gene, followed by *PHF1*. These may be diagnostically useful tests to confirm the diagnosis.

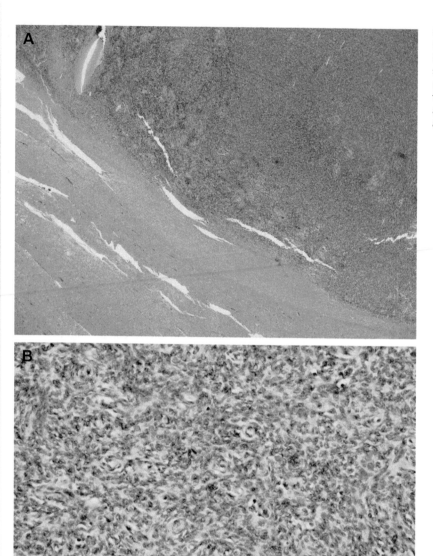

Fig. 3. Endometrial stromal nodule. The tumor is typically well-circumscribed (*A*) and composed of bland fusiform to spindle cells arranged around small spiral arteriole-like vessels (*B*).

HIGH-GRADE ENDOMETRIAL STROMAL SARCOMA

HGESS were included as a new distinct entity in the 2014 World Health Organization classification, and at that time were characterized by t(10;17) resulting in *YWHAE-NUTM2A/B* gene fusions.[28,37,38] Since then, other high-grade uterine sarcomas of possible endometrial origin have been described that harbor alterations in the gene *BCOR*.[39–41] Although these HGESS are much less common than LGESS, they are important to recognize because they are associated with more aggressive behavior and a worse overall clinical outcome. Additionally, specifically in the case of *YWHAE*-altered HGESS, there may be variable portions of the tumor displaying morphologic and immunophenotypic features virtually

Fig. 4. Highly cellular leiomyoma. In contrast with endometrial stromal nodule, which is commonly considered in the differential diagnosis, leiomyoma contains thick-walled vessels (A) and demonstrates a more fascicular growth pattern (B).

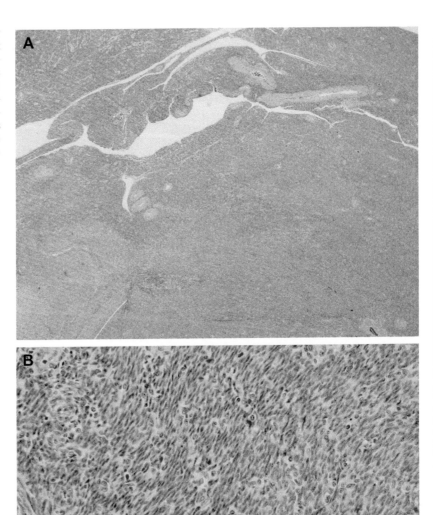

indistinguishable from LGESS.[38,42–44] Molecular testing is often performed to confirm the diagnosis. Macroscopically, HGESS may appear similar to LGESS with finger-like permeation into the myometrium, but also may show destructive invasion. The morphologic, immunophenotypic, and molecular features of HGESS depends on the primary gene alteration and, as such, they will be independently discussed.

YWHAE-ALTERED ENDOMETRIAL STROMAL SARCOMAS

This form of HGESS is characterized microscopically by uniform epithelioid cells arranged in nests encased by a delicate branching vascular network (Fig. 7A, B). Occasionally, nuclei may demonstrate some degree of increased pleomorphism (Fig. 7C), but marked pleomorphism and bizarre

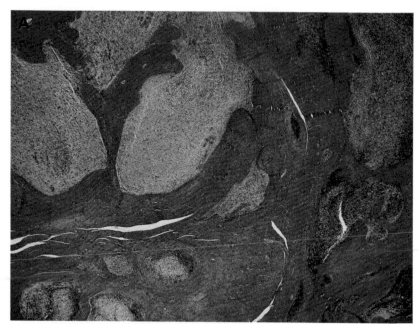

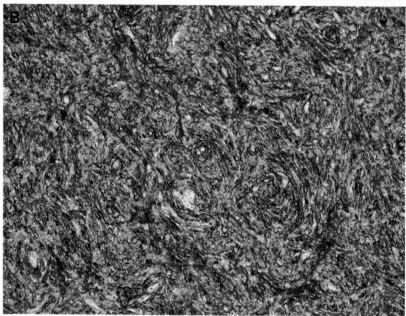

Fig. 5. Low-grade endometrial stromal sarcoma. This lesion has cytologic features similar to endometrial stromal nodule, but invades the myometrium, often extensively, with finger-like processes (A). Strong CD10 positivity (B) is typical of low-grade endometrial stromal neoplasms.

atypia should not be present. Mitoses are generally conspicuous. These tumors may have the HGESS appearance throughout, be associated with distinct nodules of HGESS occurring in what would otherwise morphologically be considered LGESS (Fig. 7D), or be associated with numerous tiny foci of epithelioid nests embedded within areas indistinguishable from LGESS (Fig. 7E). In very rare cases, the high-grade component is minimal and largely masked by the low-grade population. CD10, ER, and PR may highlight the

low-grade foci, but are absent or only focal in the high-grade foci (Fig. 7F). Cyclin D1 is strongly and diffusely (>70% of tumor nuclei) positive in the morphologically high-grade areas of HGESS (Fig. 7G), although this finding is not specific for YWHAE-altered HGESS (discussed elsewhere in this article). Importantly, BCOR immunohistochemistry is often positive and unrelated to BCOR aberrations.[40] As mentioned, these tumors have a t(10;17) resulting in YWHAE-NUTM2A/B gene fusions; the translocation is readily

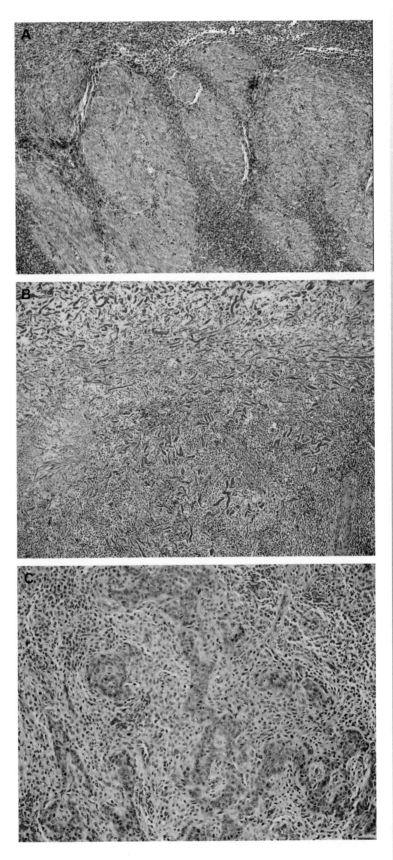

Fig. 6. Variant differentiation in low-grade endometrial stromal neoplasms. Changes can be focal or extensive, and include smooth muscle differentiation (*A*), collagen bands and plaques (*B*), sex cord differentiation (*C*),

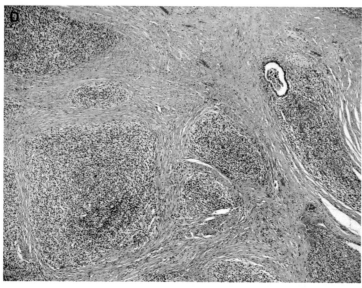

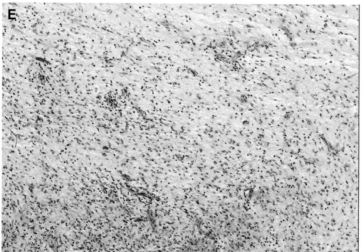

Fig. 6. (*continued*). glandular differentiation (*D*), and fibromyxoid change (*E*).

identifiable upon conventional karyotype and additionally, fluorescence in-situ hybridization (FISH) for breakapart of the *YWHAE* locus can be performed on formalin-fixed paraffin embedded tumor tissue. It is important to note that the morphology of the tumor is important to keep in mind when selecting the tumor block to perform immunohistochemistry, but for molecular analysis, any block is suitable because the genetic alteration is uniform throughout, even with variable low-grade and high-grade morphology.

BCOR-ALTERED SARCOMAS

This is a recently described entity and evidence suggests that it represents a second form of HGESS. Within this group, there are 2 principal types of molecular alterations, one consisting of *BCOR* gene fusions (*ZC3H7B-BCOR*) and the other containing internal tandem duplications (ITD) in *BCOR*. Whether or not the type of alteration is clinically relevant remains to be elucidated, but similar to *YWHAE*-altered HGESS, *BCOR* fusion HGESS have a more aggressive clinical course when compared with LGESS. *BCOR* ITD sarcomas have been reported in smaller numbers, but seem to occur in a younger population and might be associated with a slightly more favorable or indolent clinical course.[45] Otherwise, the macroscopic findings are nondistinct. Microscopically, they have an LGESS-like pattern of invasion (**Fig. 8**A) and are composed of spindled cells

(Fig. 8B) with a variably prominent myxoid stroma (Fig. 8C). The *BCOR* ITD sarcomas may also have a striking round cell component (Fig. 8D). In contrast with *YWHAE*-altered HGESS, *BCOR*-altered HGESS have not to date been described in association with low-grade ESS morphology. Immunohistochemically, *BCOR* fusion sarcomas strongly express both Cyclin D1 and CD10, whereas *BCOR* ITD sarcomas express focal/patchy CD10 positivity (see Fig. 7E) and may in fact be negative for CD10, but are also strongly positive for Cyclin D1 (see Fig. 7F). *BCOR*-associated HGESS may display a limited amount of positivity for ER/PR. Interestingly, immunohistochemical expression of BCOR is only seen in about half of *BCOR*-altered sarcomas.[40,41] Pertinent to the distinction of *BCOR*-associated HGESS from *YWHAE*-altered HGESS, BCOR immunohistochemistry is typically positive in *YWHAE*-altered HGESS. Thus, BCOR positivity is not useful in the distinction between these 2 types of HGESS.

Key Features
HIGH-GRADE ENDOMETRIAL STROMAL SARCOMAS

High-Grade Endometrial Stromal Sarcoma, *YWHAE* Type	High-Grade Endometrial Stromal Sarcoma, *BCOR* Type
t(10;17) reflecting gene fusion involving *YWHAE*	*ZC3H7B-BCOR* gene fusions or internal tandem duplication (ITD) in *BCOR*
May be associated with typical LGESS morphology	Not associated with LGESS component
Epithelioid, nested and uniform appearance with delicate vasculature	Myxoid background; spindled and round cell morphology
Cyclin D1, BCOR +	Cyclin D1 +
CD10, ER/PR − (except in areas of LG morphology)	BCOR +/−
	CD10 +/−
	ER/PR +/−
Clinically aggressive	*BCOR* fusion HGESS clinically aggressive
	BCOR ITD HGESS may be more indolent, but small number of studied cases

Differential diagnosis
HIGH-GRADE ENDOMETRIAL STROMAL SARCOMA

- Low-grade ESS: lacks any "high-grade" foci. Molecular testing useful in this diagnostic consideration.

- Undifferentiated or solid high-grade carcinoma: May also be Cyclin D1 and/or CD10+. Generally less uniform with greater nuclear atypia and pleomorphism. Undifferentiated carcinomas lack the finger-like permeative pattern of invasion seen in ESS. Keratin expression can be seen, although often focally. Molecular testing in questionable cases.

- Epithelioid leiomyosarcoma (vs *YWHAE*-altered HGESS): Smooth muscle marker positivity. May also be associated with more conventional spindled leiomyosarcoma (LMS) morphology, which is a helpful diagnostic clue. Molecular testing in questionable cases.

- Myxoid LMS (vs *BCOR*-altered HGESS): Severe nuclear atypia with hyperchromasia. Strong and diffuse smooth muscle marker positivity. Association with fascicular LMS areas. Molecular testing in questionable cases.

UNDIFFERENTIATED UTERINE SARCOMA

This term is reserved for neoplasms with a diffuse high-grade appearance and the absence of obvious differentiation (smooth muscle, endometrial stromal, or other). Previously classified as part of the spectrum of endometrial stromal neoplasia (and formerly known as undifferentiated endometrial sarcoma), it is known that not all tumors arise in the endometrial surface,[44] and its histogenesis and cell of origin remain obscure; hence, the currently preferred term.

Macroscopically, undifferentiated uterine sarcoma presents as a large (>10 cm), infiltrative, and fleshy tumor with necrosis and hemorrhage filling the endometrial cavity. Microscopically, it is composed of large cells with a high nuclear-to-cytoplasmic ratio, appreciable at low-power magnification (Fig. 9A). Most tumors show brisk pleomorphism, although a subset shows more uniform nuclear morphology. The distinction between pleomorphic and uniform morphologies has no clinical relevance.[46] Nuclei have irregular contours and prominent nucleoli (Fig. 9B). The mitotic rate frequently exceeds 10 per 10 HPFs and tumor cell necrosis is seen consistently. By definition, the tumor lacks any specific mesenchymal lineage or epithelial differentiation. Consequently, smooth

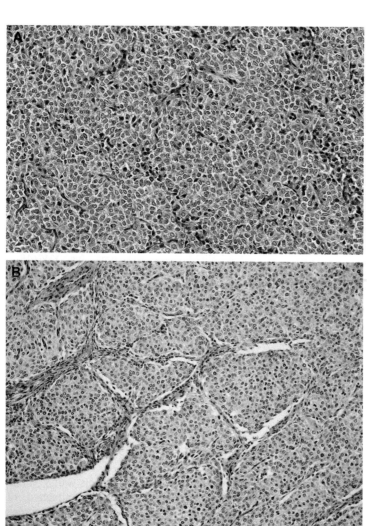

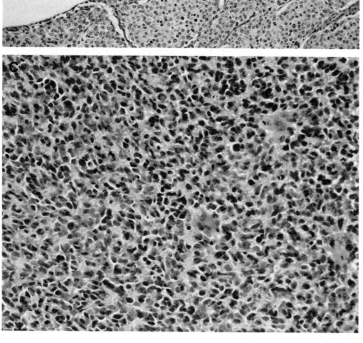

Fig. 7. High-grade endometrial stromal sarcoma with *YWHAE-NUTM2* fusion. Large epithelioid cells arranged in sheets or nested architecture are enveloped by delicately branching thin-walled vasculature (*A*, *B*). Sometimes these sarcomas may demonstrate some moderate pleomorphism (*C*).

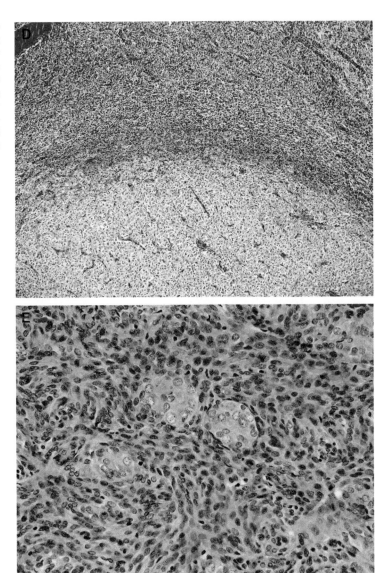

Fig. 7. (*continued*). High-grade endometrial stromal sarcoma with YWHAE-NUTM2 fusion may present as nodules of high-grade morphology(*D*, lower portion) within a tumor that otherwise seems to be low grade (*D*, upper portion). Occasionally, the high-grade foci are limited to small nests of large epithelioid cells throughout the tumor (*E*)

muscle and epithelial immunohistochemical markers are negative. CD10, as well as hormone receptors, can be positive (see **Fig. 9B**). In contrast with endometrial stromal sarcomas, undifferentiated uterine sarcoma lacks specific translocations. This tumor shows a complex karyotype,[47] as well as *TP53* mutations and abnormal p53 expression in some cases.[48]

The diagnosis of undifferentiated uterine sarcoma is one of exclusion: the pathologist must first rule out leiomyosarcoma, HGESS, rhabdomyosarcoma, carcinosarcoma, and, importantly, undifferentiated or dedifferentiated endometrial carcinoma. Thorough sampling usually allows identification of areas of differentiation diagnostic for these entities. Most (approximately 77%)

undifferentiated and dedifferentiated endometrial carcinomas express pan-cytokeratin and low-molecular-weight keratin, which can aid in the differential; conversely, PAX8 is negative in both undifferentiated carcinoma and undifferentiated uterine sarcoma, limiting its value.[49] Significant expression of smooth muscle markers is not expected in undifferentiated uterine sarcoma and should prompt consideration for leiomyosarcoma.

Undifferentiated uterine sarcomas are aggressive. Surgical resection is the only potentially effective treatment, because chemotherapy and hormonal therapy modalities have poor response. Unfortunately, more than 60% have extrauterine spread at the time of presentation.[50] One-third of patients, however, survived for at least 5 years in

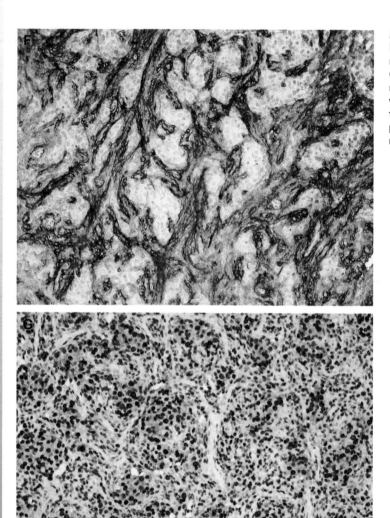

Fig. 7. (*continued*). (*F*) will high-light the low-grade areas, but is negative in the high-grade nests. Cyclin D1 is a very sensitive but not a specific marker for HGESS with *YWHAE* fusions and is typically strongly and diffusely positive (*G*) (CD10, original magnification).

a recent study in which brisk mitotic activity (defined as >25 mitoses in 10 HPFs) was associated with significantly worse 5-year survival.[51] No other independent clinical or pathologic prognostic factor has been validated for this aggressive disease, including stage.[52,53]

SMARCA4-DEFICIENT UTERINE SARCOMA

Recently, a series of undifferentiated uterine sarcomas with recurrent mutations in *SMARCA4* has been described.[54] These lesions are composed of large atypical epithelioid cells, some with rhabdoid morphology, highly reminiscent of the large

cell variant of the so-called small cell carcinoma of the ovary, hypercalcemic type (**Fig. 10**A). Biallelic inactivation of the *SMARCA4* gene correlates with loss of nuclear SMARCA4 (BRG1) expression by immunohistochemistry (**Fig. 10**B), which is the characteristic molecular alteration of this subset of uterine sarcoma. Like undifferentiated uterine sarcomas, SMARCA4-deficient uterine sarcomas are negative to only weakly positive for keratins and epithelial membrane antigen (EMA). Prognosis is equally poor, with a median overall survival of only 7 months.[54] It is important to note that SMARCA4 loss is characteristic of ovarian small cell carcinoma hypercalcemic type, and has also

Fig. 8. High-grade endometrial stromal sarcoma with *ZC3H7B-BCOR* fusion (*A, B*) or with internal tandem duplications (ITD) in *BCOR* (*C, D*).

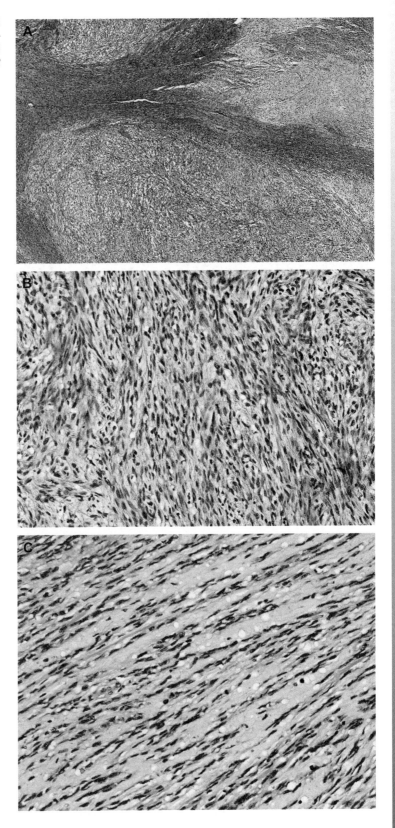

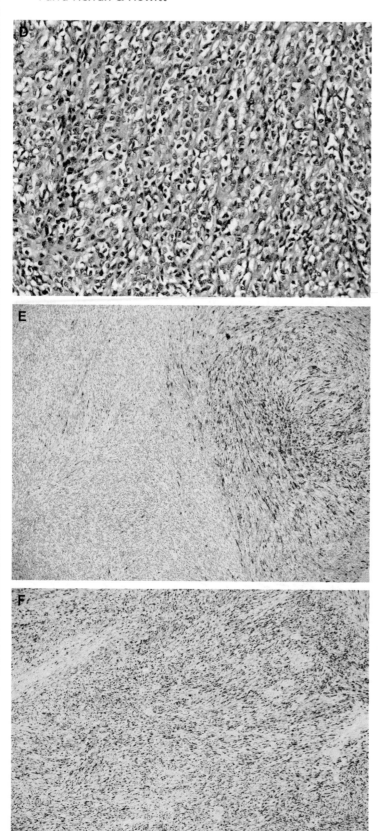

Fig. 8. (*continued*). CD10 is variably positive in ITD BCOR sarcomas (*E*) and similar to other high-grade endometrial stromal sarcomas, also demonstrates strong cyclin D1 positivity (*F*).

been reported in a subset of endometrial undifferentiated carcinomas.[49,55] Unlike undifferentiated carcinomas, which tend to be genetically complex, SMARCA4-deficient uterine sarcomas harbor none to very few genomic alterations other than *SMARCA4* loss.

Key Features
UNDIFFERENTIATED UTERINE SARCOMA

- Large size (>10 cm).
- Large tumor cell population, either pleomorphic or uniform in size.
- High N:C ratio and prominent nucleoli.
- Absence of any definitive homologous or heterologous sarcomatous differentiation.
- SMARCA4 loss characterizes a subset of undifferentiated uterine sarcomas.

Differential Diagnosis
UNDIFFERENTIATED UTERINE SARCOMA

- Undifferentiated carcinoma: Keratin expression (which is usually focal).
- Dedifferentiated carcinoma: Distinct carcinoma areas of endometrioid type.
- Leiomyosarcoma: Fascicular, myxoid of epithelioid areas; smooth muscle marker expression.
- Carcinosarcoma: Biphasic growth with high-grade carcinomatous areas; often heterologous sarcomatous differentiation.
- HGESS: Tonguelike infiltration, areas of low-grade endometrial stromal morphology (*YWHAE*-associated), prominent myxoid change with at most moderate atypia (*BCOR* associated).

UTERINE SARCOMAS WITH NTRK FUSIONS

A subset of tumors originally considered to be undifferentiated uterine sarcomas with spindled morphology harbor *NTRK* (*NTRK1* or *NTRK3*) gene fusions.[56] These sarcomas all had similar fascicular growth and are believed to represent a type of fibrosarcoma in the uterus. Immunohistochemically, they are characterized by desmin negativity and positivity for pan-Trk. Importantly,

identifying these tumors may have clinical implications for targeted therapy. The morphologic features of these tumors overlap with those designated as "endocervical neurofibrosarcoma" by Mills and colleagues,[57] which are further characterized by CD34 and S100 positivity, at least focally.

UTERINE TUMOR RESEMBLING OVARIAN SEX CORD STROMAL TUMOR

As discussed elsewhere in this article, endometrial stromal neoplasms can display sex cord stromal differentiation in variable amounts. Uterine tumors exclusively composed of sex cord stromal-like elements are rare, but well-documented. These, termed UTROSCT, are currently regarded as separate from the endometrial stromal neoplasm category given their significantly lower rates of extrauterine spread and recurrence,[58] and the absence of the *JAZF1* and *PHF1* rearrangements classic of low-grade endometrial stromal neoplasms.[59,60] Moreover, they lack *FOLX2* and *DICER1* mutations, which are characteristic of ovarian adult-type granulosa cell tumors and Sertoli-Leydig cell tumors, respectively.[61,62] Further evidence in support of UTROSCT as a separate diagnostic entity comes from the recent discovery of recurrent fusions involving *NCOA2/3* (either *ESR1-NCOA3*, *ESR1-NCOA2*, or *GREB1-NCOA2*) in a series of 4 UTROSCTs.[63] These genes are involved in steroid hormone expression, and the fusions seem to lead to dysregulation of the nuclear receptor coactivator domain of *NCOA2/3*. Additionally, there is 1 reported case of UTROSCT harboring a *GRB1-CTNNB1* fusion.[64] The cell of origin for UTROSCT remains unknown.

UTROSCT are rare neoplasms affecting women in the third to fifth decades of life.[65] The lesion may be discovered incidentally or present with abnormal uterine bleeding and/or abdominal pain. Clinically, it is frequently mistaken by a leiomyoma, and definitive diagnosis is only made on histopathologic grounds. The lesion is usually well circumscribed with a median size of 6 cm (range, 1–15 cm). Microscopically, UTROSCT displays the same variety of architectural patterns seen in ovarian sex cord stromal tumors, including cords (plexiform pattern), trabeculae, nests, glandlike elements, tubules, and retiform structures (**Fig. 11A**). Tumor cells are monomorphic, with scant cytoplasm and round to ovoid nuclei with uniform chromatin. By immunohistochemistry, UTROSCT characteristically expresses sex cord stromal markers (inhibin, calretinin, CD99, WT1, SF1, Melan-A, FOXL2); indeed, it has been

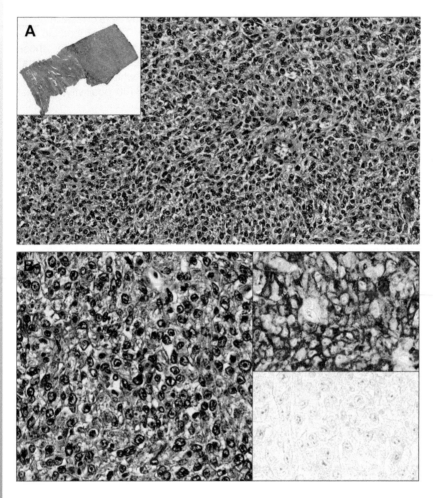

Fig. 9. Undifferentiated uterine sarcoma. Markedly atypical epithelioid and spindled population with nuclear pleomorphism and abundant mitoses. Note the absence of definitive epithelial or mesenchymal (smooth muscle, endometrial stromal, other) differentiation (*A*). Nuclei have coarse chromatin and prominent nucleoli (*B*). Tumor cells can be positive for CD10 (intensely positive in this case, *B* upper right), but should be negative for smooth muscle and skeletal muscle markers (desmin, *B* lower right), epithelial markers, and other lineage-specific markers.

postulated that the diagnosis of UTROSCT requires expression of calretinin (most sensitive marker, positive in 95% of cases) plus at least 1 other sex cord stromal marker[66] (**Fig. 11B**). UTROSCT can also express smooth muscle (desmin, smooth muscle actin, Caldesmon) and epithelial (cytokeratins, EMA) markers.[67,68]

The differential diagnosis of UTROSCT includes a low-grade endometrial stromal neoplasm with sex cord differentiation, in which case areas of classic endometrial stromal morphology should be appreciated. However, this may be difficult to identify reliably in a biopsy or curettage specimen. Thus, biopsy samples that do not allow for a definitive diagnosis of UTROSCT versus low-grade ESS with sex cord elements will need deferral to diagnosis on hysterectomy. Endometrioid carcinoma is another consideration in the differential diagnosis of UTROSCT, because it sometimes can harbor

foci of sex cord differentiation; in this scenario, the glandular component is usually prominent and overtakes the endometrial surface; in contrast, UTROSCT tends to be intramural, lacks squamous differentiation, and the glandlike pattern is not the predominant one. The presence of clusters of luteinized-like cells with abundant eosinophilic cytoplasm is also a clue in favor of UTROSCT.[69]

The clinical course of most patients with UTROSCT is indolent. However, extrauterine spread has been documented in 23.5% of patients, and fatality in 8.8% according to the largest case series published to date.[70] Tumor cell necrosis and high mitotic activity seems to correlate with an adverse outcome. Given these relatively small but significant adverse events, UTROSCT is now considered a neoplasm of low malignant potential; hysterectomy followed by long-term follow-up is recommended.

Key Features
UTERINE TUMOR RESEMBLING OVARIAN SEX CORD STROMAL TUMOR

- Tumor of low malignant potential (indolent clinical behavior in most cases).

- Composed entirely of sex cord elements with widely variable morphology akin to the types of sex cord stromal tumors seen in the ovary.

- Can express sex cord markers (inhibin, calretinin, CD99, WT1, SF1, Melan-A, FOXL2), epithelial markers (keratins, EMA), as well as smooth muscle markers (desmin, smooth muscle actin, Caldesmon).

- May harbor *NCOA2/3* gene fusions, but lack alterations that characterize ovarian sex cord stromal tumors (*FOXL2, DICER1* mutation) or endometrial stromal tumors (*JAZF1, PHF1* rearrangements).

△△ Differential Diagnosis
UTERINE TUMOR RESEMBLING OVARIAN SEX CORD STROMAL TUMOR

- Low-grade endometrial stromal tumor with sex cord stromal differentiation: Areas of conventional endometrial stromal morphology, permeative growth (in LGESS).

- Endometrioid carcinoma: Prominent glandular component, squamous differentiation.

PERIVASCULAR EPITHELIOID CELL TUMOR

The *Perivascular Epithelioid Cell* tumor (commonly known as PEComa) family comprises several lesions composed of cells with a mixed myomelanocytic immunophenotype. Although the uterus is the most common extrarenal location of PEComa (not otherwise specified), only a few series accounting for less than 150 cases have been reported.[71–75] Patient age at presentation is wide, with a peak of incidence around the fourth decade of life.[76] Clinically, the mass is usually mistaken for a smooth muscle tumor.

Microscopically, PEComas tend to have a solid, nested, and/or vaguely fascicular architecture and are cellular with very scant intervening stroma (**Fig. 12A**). A network of uniformly dispersed small capillaries is characteristic. Condensation of tumor cells around vessels is frequent and serves as a useful diagnostic clue. Two distinct patterns can be recognized in varying proportions:

- Epithelioid pattern (in 100% of cases)[72]: polygonal cells with clear to granular eosinophilic cytoplasm, usually positive for melanocytic markers (HMB45, Melan-A, MITF; **Fig. 12B, C**).

- Spindle cell pattern (in 37% of cases)[72]: fusiform cells with less abundant cytoplasm, arranged in fascicles, commonly positive for smooth muscle markers (desmin, caldesmon).

Evaluation of worrisome malignant features is important in PEComas. Nuclear atypia in PEComas is assessed as low (minimal variation in nuclear size), intermediate ($\leq$2-fold variation), and high (>2 fold-variation). Mitotic activity is counted in 50 HPFs. Invasion into the surrounding myometrium can be permeative (ESS-like), or less commonly frankly infiltrative. Geographic tumor cell necrosis is similar to that seen in leiomyosarcoma.

Immunohistochemistry is usually required to confirm the diagnosis. HMB45 and Catepsin-K are the most sensitive markers, being positive in 99% to 100% of uterine PEComas.[72,77] Other markers with less frequent expression include MiTF (66%), Melan-A (46%), smooth muscle actin (80%), desmin (63%), and caldesmon (77%).[77] Importantly, staining for any of these markers is frequently focal (<50% of cells).

Although the classic morphology described predominates in the uterus, the following morphologic variants of PEComa have also been described, some with important molecular correlates:

- Sclerosing PEComa: usually seen in the retroperitoneum. In this variant, the typical epithelioid cells are organized in cords within a densely fibrotic matrix.

- PEComatosis: multiple PEComa nodules in different gynecologic organs and pelvis. They are frequently associated with tuberous sclerosis complex (TSC), a disorder secondary to mutations in *TSC1* or *TSC2*. These genes encode proteins that intrinsically inhibit the mammalian target of rapamycin (mTOR) pathway. Thus, mutations lead to an abnormally activated pathway that can be targeted pharmacologically with mTOR inhibitors.

- Lymphangioleiomyomatosis (LAM)-like PEComa: commonly associated with TSC, these rare tumors resemble LAM in other anatomic locations.

- PEComa with *TFE3* rearrangement: these tumors have a predominant epithelioid morphology; consequently, the have consistent staining for HMB45 and cathepsin-K, but only rare and weak expression of smooth muscle markers.[74] TFE3 protein expression is

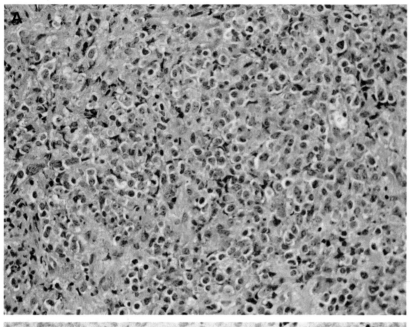

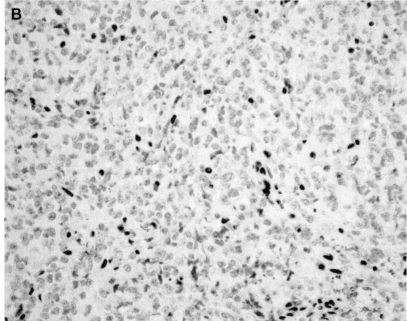

Fig. 10. SMARCA4-deficient uterine sarcoma. This tumor is characterized by large atypical epithelioid cells, some with rhabdoid morphology, reminiscent of large cell variant of small cell carcinoma, hypercalcemic type of the ovary (A). Loss of SMARCA4 (BRG1) nuclear expression is seen in tumor cells, representing the recurrent alteration in this tumor, SMARCA4 inactivation (B). (Courtesy of Dr David Kolin, Brigham and Women's Hospital, Boston, Massachusetts, United States.)

nonspecific; thus, in situ hybridization for TFE3 fusion should be considered to identify this variant. This variant lacks TSC1 and TSC2 gene mutations, and therefore mTOR pathway activation does not play a role in its pathogenesis.

- PEComa with RAD51B rearrangement: only 4 cases have been described, all with an aggressive clinical course.[72,78] They have an indistinct morphology compared with conventional PEComa.

The differential diagnosis mainly includes uterine smooth muscle tumors, particularly those displaying epithelioid morphology. The presence of a vasculature varying in size and including thick-walled vessels, and the absence of melanocytic marker expression are features in favor of a

Fig. 11. Uterine tumor resembling ovarian sex cord stromal neoplasms. This example exhibits a prominent trabecular (cordlike) growth, resembling an adult-type granulosa cell tumor of the ovary (*A*). Tumor cells are positive for pancytokeratin (*B*, left) and calretinin (*B*, right).

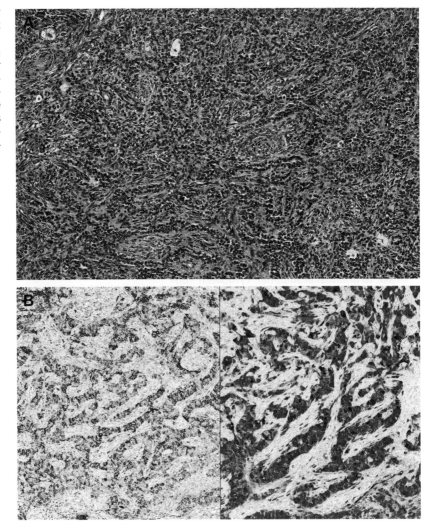

smooth muscle tumor. Conversely, a thin capillary vascular network and diffuse staining for HMB-45, Cathepsin-K and/or Melan-A are in keeping with a PEComa. *YWHAE*-associated HGESS also features round cells, but these contain scant cytoplasm, instead of the abundant clear to eosinophilic cytoplasm of PEComa cells. Melanoma involving the uterus is also an important differential; unlike PEComa, melanoma displays striking nuclear atypia and prominent nucleoli and pigmentation; in addition, it is frequently positive for S100 (only approximately 10% of PEComas are positive) and negative for smooth muscle markers.

The evaluation of malignant potential in PEComa has been the subject of recent investigation. The currently proposed systems are outlined in **Table 2**. The system proposed by

Schoolmeester and colleagues[73] for uterine PEComa has a higher threshold for malignancy compared with the traditional Folpe criteria, and therefore higher specificity for a malignant diagnosis. Bennett and colleagues[72] recently validated Schoolmeester's criteria and suggested reducing the number of features required for malignancy from 4 to 3 to increase the sensitivity of the system. An alternative method is the modified Folpe criteria, postulated by Conlon and colleagues[77] based on outcomes data from 78 uterine PEComas reported in the English literature. It categorizes a PEComa as malignant if it has necrosis or 2 or more worrisome features. Because this approach has greater sensitivity, and therefore a higher chance to capture tumors with potential for aggressive behavior, we recommend using the modified Folpe criteria first, and then note if the tumor meets the more stringent Schoolmeester-Bennett criteria, in which case the risk of early recurrence is higher.[77]

The management of uterine PEComa is primarily complete surgical resection. The addition of chemotherapy and radiation is controversial but has been contemplated in tumors with high-risk features (malignant and uncertain malignant potential). Treatment with mTOR inhibitors has been attempted in patients with advanced-stage disease with promising results.[79]

Key Features
PERIVASCULAR EPITHELIOID CELL TUMOR

- Tumor composed of polygonal cells with clear to granular eosinophilic cytoplasm, usually positive for melanocytic markers.

- A subset contains spindle cells in fascicles and positive for smooth muscle markers.

- Positivity for melanocytic and smooth muscle markers: HMB45, Catepsin-K, MiTF, Melan-A, smooth muscle actin, desmin, and caldesmon.

 ## Differential Diagnosis
PERIVASCULAR EPITHELIOID CELL TUMOR

- Epithelioid smooth muscle tumor: thick vessels, absence of melanocytic marker expression, absence of clear cells.

- HGESS: round cells with very scant cytoplasm, absence of melanocytic and smooth muscle marker expression.

- Melanoma involving the uterus: prominent nuclear atypia, pigmentation, positivity for S100 (rare in PEComa), and absence of smooth muscle marker expression.

INFLAMMATORY MYOFIBROBLASTIC TUMOR

This rare tumor is categorized as of intermediate biologic potential given its risk for local recurrence, seen in approximately 25% of patients.[80,81] Primary uterine involvement is rare with less than 60 cases reported,[82–84] although misdiagnosis as a smooth muscle tumor is frequent and its true frequency may be higher than currently estimated. It affects women of all ages (range, 6–78 years), but predominantly adult, reproductive age women (average age, approximately 45 years). It is usually

seen in hysterectomy specimens with a clinical impression of fibroid(s). On occasion, it can be detected in endometrial curettage or myomectomy specimens. Macroscopically, the tumor is typically indistinguishable from a leiomyoma; however, fleshy and soft areas can be appreciated.

Microscopically, inflammatory myofibroblastic tumor displays 2 morphologic patterns:

- Myxoid pattern, composed of spindle individually dispersed in an abundant myxoid matrix imparting a fasciitis or tissue culturelike appearance. Tumor cell nuclei are elongated and plump, have a wavy appearance, and open chromatin. A mixed inflammatory infiltrate is consistently present in variable amounts: it can be, on occasion, focal (Fig. 13A).
- Fascicular pattern, more cellular compared with myxoid areas, and with a less abundant, more collagenous extracellular matrix. Cells are grouped in intersecting fascicles and have eosinophilic cytoplasm, highly resembling smooth muscle. Nuclei appear wavy and relatively hypochromatic similar to myxoid areas (Fig. 13B).
- Fibromatosis-like pattern, hypocellular but composed mostly of a dense collagenous matrix, with little to no myxoid stroma, less prominent inflammation, and less conspicuous tumor cells.

Uterine inflammatory myofibroblastic tumor consistently (>90%) harbors rearrangement of the *Anaplastic Lymphoma Kinase (ALK)* gene located at 2p23.[85,86] Most *ALK* fusion rearrangements involve the transmembrane domain; *IGFBP5*, *THBS1*, and *TIMP3* are the most common fusion partner genes.[87] Fusion rearrangements can be detected by FISH or RNA sequencing assays. This alteration is associated with diffuse and intense nuclear ALK expression by immunohistochemistry (Fig. 13C).[88]

The main differential diagnosis of inflammatory myofibroblastic tumor of the uterus is a smooth muscle neoplasm of conventional or myxoid type. Indeed, it is conceivable that many indolent inflammatory myofibroblastic tumors are diagnosed as leiomyoma, whereas those with aggressive behavior are misclassified as myxoid leiomyosarcoma, as demonstrated in a published series.[83] In the presence of a predominantly myxoid tumor, attention to the nuclear morphology is helpful: myxoid smooth muscle tumors have cells arranged in fascicles with tapered-end and hyperchromatic nuclei, contrasting with the more individually dispersed ("tissue culture"-like), wavy,

Fig. 12. Perivascular epithelioid tumor. Cellular neoplasm composed of nested epithelioid cells surrounded by fascicles of spindled cells (*A*). Epithelioid cells have indistinct borders, a polygonal shape, and clear to vaguely eosinophilic cytoplasm; notice the aggregation of tumor cells around vessels (*B*). Cells are focally positive for HMB45 (*C*, left) and diffusely positive for smooth muscle actin (*C*, right).

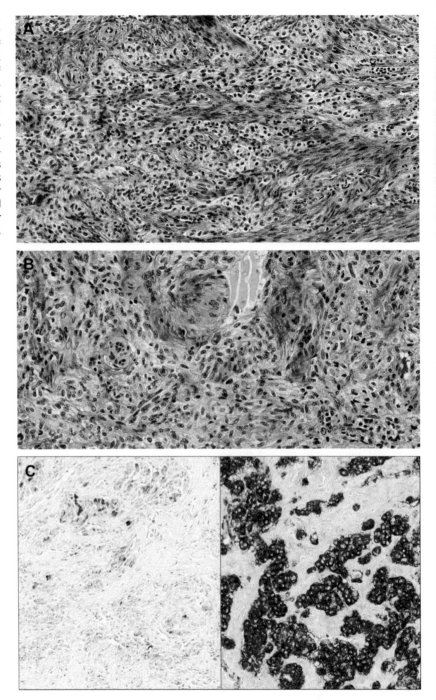

and open vesicular nuclei of inflammatory myofibroblastic tumor. If the tumor has a predominantly fascicular pattern, distinction can be very difficult to make. It is advisable to consider ancillary testing for ALK in a uterine mesenchymal tumor with any myxoid component, particularly if the cytologic features suggest an inflammatory myofibroblastic tumor. Diffuse and strong nuclear ALK expression by immunohistochemistry is consistent with inflammatory myofibroblastic tumor. Ideally, the diagnosis should be confirmed with FISH or RNA sequencing, because some myxoid leiomyosarcomas can show ALK staining.[89] Immunohistochemistry for p53 and p16 can also be considered

Table 2
Classification of perivascular epithelioid cell tumors

	Schoolmeester et al,[73] 2014	Bennett et al,[72] 2018	Revised Folpe Criteria (2015)
Benign	<4 features: Size ≥5 cm Severe atypia Necrosis Vascular invasion Mitoses ≥1/50 HPFs	<3 features: Size ≥5 cm Severe atypia Necrosis Vascular invasion Mitoses ≥1/50 HPFs	≤1 feature: Invasive edge Size ≤5 to <10 cm 2–3 mitoses/50 HPFs Vascular invasion
Unknown malignant potential			1 feature: Atypia size ≥10 cm mitoses ≥4/50 HPFs
Malignant	≥4 features	≥3 features	Necrosis or ≥2 worrisome features

Abbreviation: HPF, high-power field.

if leiomyosarcoma is suspected; inflammatory myofibroblastic tumor has normal expression for these markers; conversely, approximately 50% of uterine leiomyosarcomas show abnormal p53 and p16 expression patterns.[90] A subset of myxoid leiomyosarcomas harbor *PLAG1* gene fusions, and demonstrate PLAG1 expression by immunohistochemistry.[91] Smooth muscle markers (desmin, smooth muscle actin, Caldesmon) are frequently positive in inflammatory myofibroblastic tumor, limiting their role in this differential. Other diagnostic considerations include sarcomatous overgrowth of an adenosarcoma as well as fibromyxoid LGESS (**Fig. 13D**). The identification of an intimally admixed benign epithelial component in the former, or the classic permeative architecture and uniform cytomorphology in the latter, will indicate the right diagnosis. ALK testing can also be of help.

Formerly considered an indolent tumor, recent series have reported tumor recurrence, metastases, and death in patients with uterine inflammatory myofibroblastic tumor.[83,84] Certain morphologic features seem to be associated with an aggressive outcome including necrosis, large tumor size (>7 cm), moderate to severe atypia, high mitotic activity (>10 per 10 HPFs) and infiltrative borders.[83,84] Thus, close follow-up is advisable when making this diagnosis, particularly if any of the worrisome features listed are observed. The presence of *ALK* gene alterations has not only diagnostic but potential therapeutic applications, because it can be targeted with tyrosine kinase inhibitors (crizotinib). This therapeutic approach has been applied successfully to nongynecologic patients with unresectable and/or recurrent tumors, especially in the pediatric population.[92–95]

Key Features
INFLAMMATORY MYOFIBROBLASTIC TUMOR

- Morphologic patterns: myxoid, fascicular, and fibromatosis-like.

- Variable amounts of mixed chronic inflammatory infiltrate.

- May be well-circumscribed or infiltrative.

- Variable tumor size, atypia, mitoses, and necrosis; clinical behavior varies widely based on the presence or absence of worrisome histologic features.

- Positive for ALK by immunohistochemistry, but also may be positive for CD10 and smooth muscle markers.

- *ALK* gene fusions can be detected by RNA sequencing, or inferred by FISH assay.

Differential diagnosis
UTERINE MYXOID NEOPLASMS

Myxoid smooth muscle tumors
- Spindle cells arranged in fascicles and bundles.

- Elongated hyperchromatic nuclei with tapered tips (cigar shape).

- Variable vascularity (which includes thick blood vessels).

- H-Caldesmon expression (can be focal) and negative *ALK* testing.

- Myxoid leiomyosarcoma has infiltrative tumor borders and abnormal p53 and p16 expression (approximately 50%).

- A subset of myxoid leiomyosarcoma express PLAG1 by immunohistochemistry and harbor *PLAG1* gene fusions.

Inflammatory myofibroblastic tumor

- Spindle and epithelioid cells, mostly individually dispersed (fasciitis or tissue culture-like appearance); variable fascicular component (usually minor).

- Oval, pale vesicular nuclei.

- Positive ALK staining and *ALK* fusion/rearrangement, normal p53 and p16 staining.

Myxoid endometrial stromal sarcoma

- Uniform vascular network of small-caliber vessels.

- Low-grade tumors: monotonous ovoid to short spindled cells without significant atypia; sex cord, glandular differentiation; *JAZF1-SUZ12*, *JAZF1-PHF1*, and *MEAF6-PHF1* translocations.

- High-grade tumors: moderate or severe atypia, frequent mitoses and absence of low-grade areas; *ZC3H7B-BCOR* fusion or *BCOR* ITD.

Adenosarcoma with myxoid changes

- Benign epithelial component; lack of ALK expression.

RHABDOMYOSARCOMA

Gynecologic tumors with pure malignant skeletal muscle differentiation are rare in adults. They are more common in children; in this population, embryonal rhabdomyosarcoma is the most common sarcoma of the lower genital tract. In adults, embryonal, pleomorphic, and alveolar types have been described[96]; most patients are postmenopausal and present with vaginal bleeding. The majority of cases have widespread extrauterine dissemination at the time of diagnosis.

Morphologically, embryonal rhabdomyosarcoma appears as edematous and hypocellular with a typical hypercellular zone underneath the epithelium (so-called cambium layer; Fig. 14). Tumor cells have high nuclear-to-cytoplasmic ratios and enlarged hyperchromatic nuclei. Rarely, rhabdomyoblasts are observed; these appear as cells with globoid cytoplasm. Pleomorphic rhabdomyosarcoma contains large hyperchromatic

cells with scant eosinophilic cytoplasm and significant variation in nuclear size and shape. Alveolar rhabdomyosarcoma is composed of sheets of noncohesive small round hyperchromatic cells, separated by fibrous septa, and forming saccular spaces between them (hence, the "alveolar" appearance). By immunohistochemistry, tumor cells are positive for desmin, myogenin, and myo-D1.[96] Hormone receptors are negative.[97]

Recurrent inactivating mutations in *DICER1* have been described in embryonal rhabdomyosarcoma. These can be germline (in the setting of familial pleuropulmonary blastoma predisposition syndrome) or somatic.[98–100] *PAX3-FKHR* or *PAX7-FKHR* gene fusions have been reported in alveolar rhabdomyosarcomas, the latter associated with better prognosis.[101]

The diagnosis of uterine rhabdomyosarcoma first requires the exclusion of carcinosarcoma and adenosarcoma with rhabdomyosarcomatous differentiation. Adequate sampling and a thorough examination are usually sufficient for this purpose. The cambium layer often observed in embryonal rhabdomyosarcoma may mimic the periglandular condensation pattern seen in adenosarcoma; for the latter, it is important to look for an intimally admixed and uniformly distributed glandular component. Distinction between pleomorphic rhabdomyosarcoma and leiomyosarcoma can be challenging and necessitates the use of immunohistochemistry; in this setting, myogenin and caldesmon are the most useful markers for skeletal and smooth muscle differentiation, respectively.

Although most tumors show response to chemotherapy, the overall prognosis remains poor. In the gynecologic tract, the median progression-free survival is 9 months, and the 5-year overall survival is only 29%.[102] Nonembryonal types are more aggressive with significantly shorter progression-free intervals.[102]

STAGING AND GRADING OF UTERINE SARCOMAS

Uterine sarcoma is a new chapter in the eighth edition of the American Joint Committee on Cancer (AJCC) Cancer Staging Manual.[103] In this edition, tumor grade is not necessary for leiomyosarcoma, because all are considered high grade. The grading of endometrial stromal sarcoma and adenosarcoma should follow a 2-tier system of low grade and high grade, following the definitions provided in this article. Undifferentiated uterine sarcoma, rhabdomyosarcoma, and SMARCA4-deficient tumors are, by definition, high grade.

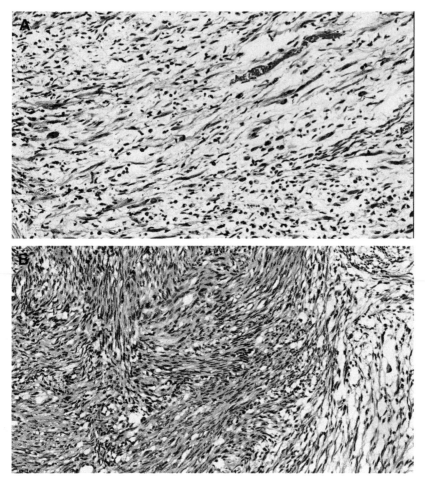

Fig. 13. Inflammatory myofibroblastic tumor (IMT). Myxoid areas contain abundant pale extracellular matrix, which separates the neoplastic cells imparting a tissue culture-like appearance. Cells are elongated and have homogeneous chromatin. Note the mixed inflammatory component throughout (*A*). Fascicular areas highly resemble uterine smooth muscle, but also contain inflammatory cells and merge imperceptibly with conventional myxoid areas, which are usually present (*B*).

UTROSCT, inflammatory myofibroblastic tumor, and PEComa do not require grading.

The latest AJCC Cancer Staging Manual maintains the previous staging definitions as per the FIGO and TNM systems. It is important to note that staging criteria for adenosarcoma are different from those for leiomyosarcoma, endometrial stromal sarcoma, and others. The premise for this is that adenosarcomas arise (mostly) in the endometrium, and risk stratification relies on the presence and depth of myometrial invasion. Conversely, leiomyosarcoma and endometrial stromal sarcoma are inherently myoinvasive, and it is tumor size that determines the stage. Measuring tumor size can be difficult if the specimen is received fragmented or distorted; correlation with imaging and intraoperative findings is imperative, and at least estimation of whether the tumor is greater or less than 5 cm should be attempted. Last, the

AJCC recommends reporting features that do not affect the stage but have prognostic value: this is the case for sarcomatous overgrowth in adenosarcoma and lymphovascular space invasion in leiomyosarcoma.

INTRAOPERATIVE CONSULTATION AND GROSS EXAMINATION CONSIDERATIONS

On occasion, the surgeon may request intraoperative consultation on a uterine tumor if it is deemed suspicious for malignancy on clinical, radiologic, or intraoperative examination. Intraoperative diagnosis of sarcoma may prompt total hysterectomy (if initial resection is only a myomectomy) and/or removal of the ovaries and fallopian tubes. In this situation, the pathologist must carefully examine the tumor, sectioning at 5- to 10-mm intervals

Fig. 13. (*continued*). The extracellular matrix is myxoid, which is high-lighted on Alcian blue stain at pH2.5 (*C*, left). Tumor cells characteristically show strong ALK immunohistochemical expression (*C*, right). The differential diagnosis for IMT is broad and can include not only myxoid smooth muscle neoplasms, but also myxoid endometrial stromal neoplasms, such as this low-grade endometrial stromal sarcoma with JAZF1 rearrangement confirmed by fluorescence in-situ hybridization (*D*).

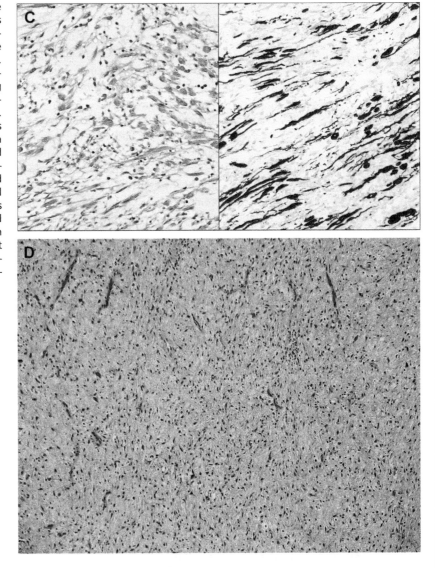

and looking for suspicious features: soft consistency, extensive hemorrhage, necrosis, infiltrative borders, and growth into vascular spaces. Sampling should include viable tissue, ideally at the interface with necrotic tissue and with the surrounding uterine wall. Two to 3 initial sections are recommended, with consideration for further sampling if necessary. Overtly malignant features such as mitoses, cytologic atypia, and necrosis can be identified intraoperatively, supporting a diagnosis of sarcoma. Further classification is not advisable in general, because it requires extensive tumor sampling and it does not affect intraoperative management. For instance, a tumor with undifferentiated uterine sarcoma features on frozen section may indeed be a carcinosarcoma or a leiomyosarcoma after proper sampling, or one with initial UTROSCT features be an endometrial stromal tumor with sex cord stromal differentiation.

Any uterine mass with suspicious features for malignancy should be thoroughly sampled at a rate of 1 section per each centimeter of the tumor's greatest dimension. Sampling should represent all the changes seen grossly, as well as the relation of the tumor with adjacent structures (endometrium, myometrium, serosa, cervix, etc). It is important to prepare the specimen promptly and ensure proper fixation. If molecular testing requires fresh tissue (depending on the institution), this should be obtained immediately after the specimen is received.

Staging of Uterine Sarcomas (Excluding Adenosarcoma)

TNM	FIGO	Definition
T1	I	Tumor confined to the uterus
T1a	IA	Tumor is 5 cm or less in greatest dimension
T1b	IB	Tumor is more than 5 cm in greatest dimension
T2	II	Tumor extends beyond the uterus, within the pelvis
T2a	IIA	Tumor involves adnexa
T2b	IIB	Tumor involves other pelvic tissue
T3	III	Tumor involves abdominal tissues or regional lymph nodes
T3a	IIIA	Tumor extends to 1 abdominal site
T3b	IIIB	Tumor extends to more than 1 abdominal site
N1	IIIC	Tumor involves reginal lymph nodes
T4	IVA	Tumor invades bladder or rectal mucosa
M1	IVB	Distant metastases (liver, lung, bone)

Staging of Uterine Adenosarcomas

TNM	FIGO	Definition
T1	I	Tumor confined to the uterus
T1a	IA	Tumor is limited to the endometrium/endocervix
T1b	IB	Tumor invades less than one-half of the myometrium
T1c	IC	Tumor invades one-half or more of the myometrium
T2	II	Tumor extends beyond the uterus, within the pelvis
T2a	IIA	Tumor involves adnexa
T2b	IIB	Tumor involves other pelvic tissues
T3	III	Tumor involves abdominal tissues
T3a	IIIA	Tumor extends to one abdominal site or regional lymph nodes
T3b	IIIB	Tumor extends to more than 1 abdominal site
N1	IIIC	Tumor involves reginal lymph nodes
T4	IVA	Tumor invades bladder or rectal mucosa
M1	IVB	Distant metastases (liver, lung, bone)

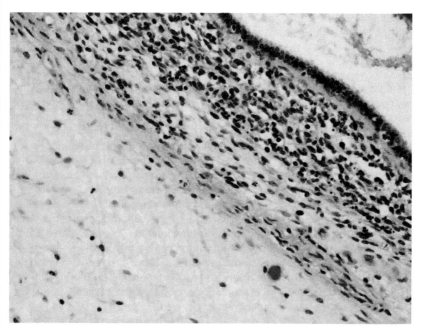

Fig. 14. Rhabdomyosarcoma, embryonal type. The sarcomatous tumor cells condense beneath benign epithelium, forming the cambium layer. Cytologically the cells are hyperchromatic, with a high nuclear to cytoplasmic ratio and conspicuous mitoses and apoptotic bodies.

REFERENCES

1. Kerner H, Lichtig C. Müllerian adenosarcoma presenting as cervical polyps: a report of seven cases and review of the literature. Obstet Gynecol 1993; 81(5 Pt 1):655–9.

2. Jones MW, Lefkowitz M. Adenosarcoma of the uterine cervix: a clinicopathological study of 12 cases. Int J Gynecol Pathol 1995;14(3):223–9.

3. Clement PB, Scully RE. Mullerian adenosarcoma of the uterus: a clinicopathologic analysis of 100 cases with a review of the literature. Hum Pathol 1990;21(4):363–81.

4. Howitt BE, Quade BJ, Nucci MR. Uterine polyps with features overlapping with those of Müllerian adenosarcoma: a clinicopathologic analysis of 29 cases emphasizing their likely benign nature. Am J Surg Pathol 2015;39(1):116–26.

5. Tai LH, Tavassoli FA. Endometrial polyps with atypical (bizarre) stromal cells. Am J Surg Pathol 2002; 26(4):505–9.

6. Amant F, Schurmans K, Steenkiste E, et al. Immunohistochemical determination of estrogen and progesterone receptor positivity in uterine adenosarcoma. Gynecol Oncol 2004;93(3):680–5.

7. Amant F, Steenkiste E, Schurmans K, et al. Immunohistochemical expression of CD10 antigen in uterine adenosarcoma. Int J Gynecol Cancer 2004;14(6):1118–21.

8. Kaku T, Silverberg SG, Major FJ, et al. Adenosarcoma of the uterus: a Gynecologic Oncology Group clinicopathologic study of 31 cases. Int J Gynecol Pathol 1992;11(2):75–88.

9. Hodgson A, Amemiya Y, Seth A, et al. High-grade Müllerian adenosarcoma: genomic and clinicopathologic characterization of a distinct neoplasm with prevalent tp53 pathway alterations and aggressive behavior. Am J Surg Pathol 2017;41(11):1513–22.

10. Clement PB. Müllerian adenosarcomas of the uterus with sarcomatous overgrowth. A clinicopathological analysis of 10 cases. Am J Surg Pathol 1989;13(1):28–38.

11. Lee J-C, Lu T-P, Changou CA, et al. Genomewide copy number analysis of Müllerian adenosarcoma identified chromosomal instability in the aggressive subgroup. Mod Pathol 2016;29(9):1070–82.

12. Piscuoglio S, Burke KA, Ng CKY, et al. Uterine adenosarcomas are mesenchymal neoplasms. J Pathol 2016;238(3):381–8.

13. Howitt BE, Sholl LM, Dal Cin P, et al. Targeted genomic analysis of Müllerian adenosarcoma. J Pathol 2015;235(1):37–49.

14. El Hallani S, Lin D, Masback A, et al. Endometrioid adenocarcinoma arising from Mullerian adenosarcoma of the uterus and ovary: clinico-pathologic characterization with emphasis on its distinction from carcinosarcoma. Mod Pathol 2018;98(S3): 418.

15. Koontz JI, Soreng AL, Nucci M, et al. Frequent fusion of the JAZF1 and JJAZ1 genes in endometrial stromal tumors. Proc Natl Acad Sci U S A 2001;98(11):6348–53.

16. Stewart CJR, Leung YC, Murch A, et al. Evaluation of fluorescence in-situ hybridization in monomorphic endometrial stromal neoplasms and their histological mimics: a review of 49 cases. Histopathology 2014;65(4):473–82.

17. Nucci MR, Harburger D, Koontz J, et al. Molecular analysis of the JAZF1-JJAZ1 gene fusion by RT-PCR and fluorescence in situ hybridization in endometrial stromal neoplasms. Am J Surg Pathol 2007; 31(1):65–70.

18. Micci F, Panagopoulos I, Bjerkehagen B, et al. Consistent rearrangement of chromosomal band 6p21 with generation of fusion genes JAZF1/PHF1 and EPC1/PHF1 in endometrial stromal sarcoma. Cancer Res 2006;66(1):107–12.

19. Huang H-Y, Ladanyi M, Soslow RA. Molecular detection of JAZF1-JJAZ1 gene fusion in endometrial stromal neoplasms with classic and variant histology: evidence for genetic heterogeneity. Am J Surg Pathol 2004;28(2):224–32.

20. Oliva E, de Leval L, Soslow RA, et al. High frequency of JAZF1-JJAZ1 gene fusion in endometrial stromal tumors with smooth muscle differentiation by interphase FISH detection. Am J Surg Pathol 2007;31(8):1277–84.

21. D'Angelo E, Ali RH, Espinosa I, et al. Endometrial stromal sarcomas with sex cord differentiation are associated with PHF1 rearrangement. Am J Surg Pathol 2013;37(4):514–21.

22. Micci F, Gorunova L, Gatius S, et al. MEAF6/PHF1 is a recurrent gene fusion in endometrial stromal sarcoma. Cancer Lett 2014;347(1):75–8.

23. Chiang S, Ali R, Melnyk N, et al. Frequency of known gene rearrangements in endometrial stromal tumors. Am J Surg Pathol 2011;35(9):1364–72.

24. Lee C-H, Nucci MR. Endometrial stromal sarcoma–the new genetic paradigm. Histopathology 2015; 67(1):1–19.

25. Tavassoli FA, Norris HJ. Mesenchymal tumours of the uterus. VII. A clinicopathological study of 60 endometrial stromal nodules. Histopathology 1981;5(1):1–10.

26. Fekete PS, Vellios F. The clinical and histologic spectrum of endometrial stromal neoplasms: a report of 41 cases. Int J Gynecol Pathol 1984; 3(2):198–212.

27. Dionigi A, Oliva E, Clement PB, et al. Endometrial stromal nodules and endometrial stromal tumors with limited infiltration: a clinicopathologic study of 50 cases. Am J Surg Pathol 2002;26(5):567–81.

28. Kurman R, Carcangiu M, Herrington C, et al. World Health Organization classification of tumours of female reproductive organs. 2014. International Agency for Research on Cancer, Lyon France. p. 135–150.

29. Chang KL, Crabtree GS, Lim-Tan SK, et al. Primary uterine endometrial stromal neoplasms. A clinicopathologic study of 117 cases. Am J Surg Pathol 1990;14(5):415–38.

30. McCluggage WG, Sumathi VP, Maxwell P. CD10 is a sensitive and diagnostically useful immunohistochemical marker of normal endometrial stroma and of endometrial stromal neoplasms. Histopathology 2001;39(3):273–8.

31. Chu P, Arber DA. Paraffin-section detection of CD10 in 505 nonhematopoietic neoplasms. Frequent expression in renal cell carcinoma and endometrial stromal sarcoma. Am J Clin Pathol 2000;113(3):374–82.

32. Chu PG, Arber DA, Weiss LM, et al. Utility of CD10 in distinguishing between endometrial stromal sarcoma and uterine smooth muscle tumors: an immunohistochemical comparison of 34 cases. Mod Pathol 2001;14(5):465–71.

33. Toki T, Shimizu M, Takagi Y, et al. CD10 is a marker for normal and neoplastic endometrial stromal cells. Int J Gynecol Pathol 2002;21(1):41–7.

34. Nascimento AF, Hirsch MS, Cviko A, et al. The role of CD10 staining in distinguishing invasive endometrial adenocarcinoma from adenocarcinoma involving adenomyosis. Mod Pathol 2003;16(1):22–7.

35. Parra-Herran CE, Yuan L, Nucci MR, et al. Targeted development of specific biomarkers of endometrial stromal cell differentiation using bioinformatics: the IFITM1 model. Mod Pathol 2014;27(4):569–79.

36. Yilmaz A, Rush DS, Soslow RA. Endometrial stromal sarcomas with unusual histologic features: a report of 24 primary and metastatic tumors emphasizing fibroblastic and smooth muscle differentiation. Am J Surg Pathol 2002;26(9):1142–50.

37. Lee C-H, Ou W-B, Mariño-Enriquez A, et al. 14-3-3 fusion oncogenes in high-grade endometrial stromal sarcoma. Proc Natl Acad Sci U S A 2012;109(3):929–34.

38. Lee C-H, Mariño-Enriquez A, Ou W, et al. The clinicopathologic features of YWHAE-FAM22 endometrial stromal sarcomas: a histologically high-grade and clinically aggressive tumor. Am J Surg Pathol 2012;36(5):641–53.

39. Hoang LN, Aneja A, Conlon N, et al. Novel high-grade endometrial stromal sarcoma: a morphologic mimicker of Myxoid Leiomyosarcoma. Am J Surg Pathol 2017;41(1):12–24.

40. Chiang S, Lee C-H, Stewart CJR, et al. BCOR is a robust diagnostic immunohistochemical marker of genetically diverse high-grade endometrial stromal sarcoma, including tumors exhibiting variant morphology. Mod Pathol 2017;30(9):1251–61.

41. Lewis N, Soslow RA, Delair DF, et al. ZC3H7B-BCOR high-grade endometrial stromal sarcomas: a report of 17 cases of a newly defined entity. Mod Pathol 2017;31(4):674–84.

42. Sciallis AP, Bedroske PP, Schoolmeester JK, et al. High-grade endometrial stromal sarcomas: a clinicopathologic study of a group of tumors with heterogenous morphologic and genetic features. Am J Surg Pathol 2014;38(9):1161–72.

43. Lee C-H, Ali RH, Rouzbahman M, et al. Cyclin D1 as a diagnostic immunomarker for endometrial stromal sarcoma with YWHAE-FAM22 rearrangement. Am J Surg Pathol 2012;36(10):1562–70.

44. Aisagbonhi O, Harrison B, Zhao L, et al. YWHAE rearrangement in a purely conventional low-grade endometrial stromal sarcoma that transformed over time to high-grade sarcoma: importance of molecular testing. Int J Gynecol Pathol 2018;37(5):441–7.

45. Mariño-Enriquez A, Lauria A, Przybyl J, et al. BCOR internal tandem duplication in high-grade uterine sarcomas. Am J Surg Pathol 2018;42(3):335–41.

46. Conklin CMJ, Longacre TA. Endometrial stromal tumors: the new WHO classification. Adv Anat Pathol 2014;21(6):383–93.

47. Halbwedl I, Ullmann R, Kremser M-L, et al. Chromosomal alterations in low-grade endometrial stromal sarcoma and undifferentiated endometrial sarcoma as detected by comparative genomic hybridization. Gynecol Oncol 2005;97(2):582–7.

48. Kurihara S, Oda Y, Ohishi Y, et al. Endometrial stromal sarcomas and related high-grade sarcomas: immunohistochemical and molecular genetic study of 31 cases. Am J Surg Pathol 2008;32(8):1228–38.

49. Ramalingam P, Masand RP, Euscher ED, et al. Undifferentiated carcinoma of the endometrium: an expanded immunohistochemical analysis including PAX-8 and basal-like carcinoma surrogate markers. Int J Gynecol Pathol 2016;35(5):410–8.

50. Leath CA, Huh WK, Hyde J, et al. A multi-institutional review of outcomes of endometrial stromal sarcoma. Gynecol Oncol 2007;105(3):630–4.

51. Hardell E, Josefson S, Ghaderi M, et al. Validation of a mitotic index cutoff as a prognostic marker in undifferentiated uterine sarcomas. Am J Surg Pathol 2017;41(9):1231–7.

52. Pautier P, Nam EJ, Provencher DM, et al. Gynecologic Cancer InterGroup (GCIG) consensus review for high-grade undifferentiated sarcomas of the uterus. Int J Gynecol Cancer 2014;24(9 Suppl 3):S73–7.

53. Gadducci A, Sartori E, Landoni F, et al. Endometrial stromal sarcoma: analysis of treatment failures and survival. Gynecol Oncol 1996;63(2):247–53.

54. Kolin DL, Dong F, Baltay M, et al. SMARCA4-deficient undifferentiated uterine sarcoma (malignant rhabdoid tumor of the uterus): a clinicopathologic entity distinct from undifferentiated carcinoma. Mod Pathol 2018;31(9):1442–56.

55. Hoang LN, Lee Y-S, Karnezis AN, et al. Immunophenotypic features of dedifferentiated endometrial carcinoma - insights from BRG1/INI1-deficient tumours. Histopathology 2016;69(4):560–9.

56. Chiang S, Cotzia P, Hyman DM, et al. NTRK fusions define a novel uterine sarcoma subtype with features of fibrosarcoma. Am J Surg Pathol 2018; 42(6):791–8.

57. Mills AM, Karamchandani JR, Vogel H, et al. Endocervical fibroblastic malignant peripheral nerve sheath tumor (neurofibrosarcoma): report of a novel entity possibly related to endocervical CD34 fibrocytes. Am J Surg Pathol 2011;35(3): 404–12.

58. Blake EA, Sheridan TB, Wang KL, et al. Clinical characteristics and outcomes of uterine tumors resembling ovarian sex-cord tumors (UTROSCT): a systematic review of literature. Eur J Obstet Gynecol Reprod Biol 2014;181:163–70.

59. Staats PN, Garcia JJ, Dias-Santagata DC, et al. Uterine tumors resembling ovarian sex cord tumors (UTROSCT) lack the JAZF1-JJAZ1 translocation frequently seen in endometrial stromal tumors. Am J Surg Pathol 2009;33(8):1206–12.

60. Nucci MR, Schoolmeester JK, Sukov W, et al. Uterine tumors resembling ovarian sex cord tumor (UTROSCT) lack rearrangement of PHF1 by FISH. Mod Pathol 2014;27:298A.

61. Croce S, de Kock L, Boshari T, et al. Uterine tumor resembling ovarian sex cord tumor (UTROSCT) commonly exhibits positivity with sex cord markers FOXL2 and SF-1 but lacks FOXL2 and DICER1 mutations. Int J Gynecol Pathol 2016;35(4):301–8.

62. Chiang S, Staats PN, Senz J, et al. FOXL2 mutation is absent in uterine tumors resembling ovarian sex cord tumors. Am J Surg Pathol 2015;39(5):618–23.

63. Dickson BC, Childs TJ, Colgan TJ, et al. Uterine tumor resembling ovarian sex cord tumor: a distinct entity characterized by recurrent NCOA2/3 gene fusions. Am J Surg Pathol 2019;43(2):178–86.

64. Croce S, Lesluyes T, Delespaul L, et al. GREB1-CTNNB1 fusion transcript detected by RNA-sequencing in a uterine tumor resembling ovarian sex cord tumor (UTROSCT): a novel CTNNB1 rearrangement. Genes Chromosomes Cancer 2018; 58(3):155–63.

65. Pradhan D, Mohanty SK. Uterine tumors resembling ovarian sex cord tumors. Arch Pathol Lab Med 2013;137(12):1832–6.

66. Irving JA, Carinelli S, Prat J. Uterine tumors resembling ovarian sex cord tumors are polyphenotypic neoplasms with true sex cord differentiation. Mod Pathol 2006;19(1):17–24.

67. de Leval L, Lim GSD, Waltregny D, et al. Diverse phenotypic profile of uterine tumors resembling ovarian sex cord tumors: an immunohistochemical study of 12 cases. Am J Surg Pathol 2010;34(12): 1749–61.

68. Hurrell DP, McCluggage WG. Uterine tumour resembling ovarian sex cord tumour is an immunohistochemically polyphenotypic neoplasm which exhibits coexpression of epithelial, myoid and sex cord markers. J Clin Pathol 2007;60(10):1148–54.

69. Murray SK, Clement PB, Young RH. Endometrioid carcinomas of the uterine corpus with sex cord-like formations, hyalinization, and other unusual morphologic features: a report of 31 cases of a neoplasm that may be confused with carcinosarcoma and other uterine neoplasms. Am J Surg Pathol 2005;29(2):157–66.

70. Moore M, McCluggage WG. Uterine tumour resembling ovarian sex cord tumour: first report of a large series with follow-up. Histopathology 2017;71(5): 751–9.

71. Fadare O. Perivascular epithelioid cell tumor (PEComa) of the uterus: an outcome-based clinicopathologic analysis of 41 reported cases. Adv Anat Pathol 2008;15(2):63–75.

72. Bennett JA, Braga AC, Pinto A, et al. Uterine PEComas: a morphologic, immunohistochemical, and molecular analysis of 32 tumors. Am J Surg Pathol 2018;42(10):1370–83.

73. Schoolmeester JK, Howitt BE, Hirsch MS, et al. Perivascular epithelioid cell neoplasm (PEComa) of the gynecologic tract: clinicopathologic and immunohistochemical characterization of 16 cases. Am J Surg Pathol 2014;38(2):176–88.

74. Schoolmeester JK, Dao LN, Sukov WR, et al. TFE3 translocation-associated perivascular epithelioid cell neoplasm (PEComa) of the gynecologic tract: morphology, immunophenotype, differential diagnosis. Am J Surg Pathol 2015;39(3):394–404.

75. Folpe AL, Mentzel T, Lehr H-A, et al. Perivascular epithelioid cell neoplasms of soft tissue and gynecologic origin: a clinicopathologic study of 26 cases and review of the literature. Am J Surg Pathol 2005;29(12):1558–75.

76. Musella A, De Felice F, Kyriacou AK, et al. Perivascular epithelioid cell neoplasm (PEComa) of the uterus: a systematic review. Int J Surg 2015;19: 1–5.

77. Conlon N, Soslow RA, Murali R. Perivascular epithelioid tumours (PEComas) of the gynaecological tract. J Clin Pathol 2015;68(6):418–26.

78. Agaram NP, Sung Y-S, Zhang L, et al. Dichotomy of genetic abnormalities in PEComas with therapeutic implications. Am J Surg Pathol 2015;39(6):813–25.

79. Starbuck KD, Drake RD, Budd GT, et al. Treatment of advanced malignant uterine perivascular epithelioid cell tumor with mTOR inhibitors: single-institution experience and review of the literature. Anticancer Res 2016;36(11):6161–4.

80. Gleason BC, Hornick JL. Inflammatory myofibroblastic tumours: where are we now? J Clin Pathol 2008;61(4):428–37.

81. Kovach SJ, Fischer AC, Katzman PJ, et al. Inflammatory myofibroblastic tumors. J Surg Oncol 2006;94(5):385–91.

82. Rabban JT, Zaloudek CJ, Shekitka KM, et al. Inflammatory myofibroblastic tumor of the uterus: a clinicopathologic study of 6 cases emphasizing distinction from aggressive mesenchymal tumors. Am J Surg Pathol 2005;29(10):1348–55.

83. Parra-Herran C, Quick CM, Howitt BE, et al. Inflammatory myofibroblastic tumor of the uterus: clinical and pathologic review of 10 cases including a subset with aggressive clinical course. Am J Surg Pathol 2015;39(2):157–68.

84. Bennett J, Nardi V, Rouzbahman M, et al. Inflammatory myofibroblastic tumor of the uterus: a clinico-pathological, immunohistochemical, and molecular analysis of 13 cases highlighting their broad morphologic spectrum. Mod Pathol 2017;30: 1489–503.

85. Coffin CM, Watterson J, Priest JR, et al. Extrapulmonary inflammatory myofibroblastic tumor (inflammatory pseudotumor). A clinicopathologic and immunohistochemical study of 84 cases. Am J Surg Pathol 1995;19(8):859–72.

86. Fuehrer NE, Keeney GL, Ketterling RP, et al. ALK-1 protein expression and ALK gene rearrangements aid in the diagnosis of inflammatory myofibroblastic tumors of the female genital tract. Arch Pathol Lab Med 2012;136(6):623–6.

87. Haimes JD, Stewart CJR, Kudlow BA, et al. Uterine inflammatory myofibroblastic tumors frequently harbor ALK fusions with IGFBP5 and THBS1. Am J Surg Pathol 2017;41(6):773–80.

88. Mohammad N, Haimes JD, Mishkin S, et al. ALK is a specific diagnostic marker for inflammatory myofibroblastic tumor of the uterus. Am J Surg Pathol 2018;42(10):1353–9.

89. Parra-Herran C, Schoolmeester JK, Yuan L, et al. Myxoid leiomyosarcoma of the uterus: a clinicopathologic analysis of 30 cases and review of the literature with reappraisal of its distinction from other uterine myxoid mesenchymal neoplasms. Am J Surg Pathol 2016;40(3):285–301.

90. Schaefer I-M, Hornick JL, Sholl LM, et al. Abnormal p53 and p16 staining patterns distinguish uterine leiomyosarcoma from inflammatory myofibroblastic tumour. Histopathology 2017;70(7):1138–46.

91. Arias-Stella JA, Benayed R, Oliva E, et al. Novel PLAG1 gene rearrangement distinguishes a subset of uterine myxoid leiomyosarcoma from other uterine myxoid mesenchymal tumors. Am J Surg Pathol 2018, [Epub ahead of print].

92. Tothova Z, Wagner AJ. Anaplastic lymphoma kinase-directed therapy in inflammatory myofibroblastic tumors. Curr Opin Oncol 2012;24(4): 409–13.

93. Butrynski JE, D'Adamo DR, Hornick JL, et al. Crizotinib in ALK-rearranged inflammatory myofibroblastic tumor. N Engl J Med 2010;363(18):1727–33.

94. Kelleher FC, McDermott R. The emerging pathogenic and therapeutic importance of the anaplastic lymphoma kinase gene. Eur J Cancer 2010;46(13): 2357–68.

95. Mossé YP, Voss SD, Lim MS, et al. Targeting ALK with crizotinib in pediatric anaplastic large cell lymphoma and inflammatory myofibroblastic tumor: a children's oncology group study. J Clin Oncol 2017;35(28):3215–21.

96. Pinto A, Kahn RM, Rosenberg AE, et al. Uterine rhabdomyosarcoma in adults. Hum Pathol 2018; 74:122–8.

97. Li RF, Gupta M, McCluggage WG, et al. Embryonal rhabdomyosarcoma (botryoid type) of the uterine corpus and cervix in adult women: report of a case series and review of the literature. Am J Surg Pathol 2013;37(3):344–55.

98. Dehner LP, Jarzembowski JA, Hill DA. Embryonal rhabdomyosarcoma of the uterine cervix: a report of 14 cases and a discussion of its unusual clinicopathological associations. Mod Pathol 2012;25(4): 602–14.

99. Doros L, Yang J, Dehner L, et al. DICER1 mutations in embryonal rhabdomyosarcomas from children with and without familial PPB-tumor predisposition syndrome. Pediatr Blood Cancer 2012;59(3):558–60.

100. de Kock L, Rivera B, Revil T, et al. Sequencing of DICER1 in sarcomas identifies biallelic somatic DICER1 mutations in an adult-onset embryonal rhabdomyosarcoma. Br J Cancer 2017;116(12): 1621–6.

101. Sorensen PHB, Lynch JC, Qualman SJ, et al. PAX3-FKHR and PAX7-FKHR gene fusions are prognostic indicators in alveolar rhabdomyosarcoma: a report from the children's oncology group. J Clin Oncol 2002;20(11):2672–9.

102. Ferguson SE, Gerald W, Barakat RR, et al. Clinicopathologic features of rhabdomyosarcoma of gynecologic origin in adults. Am J Surg Pathol 2007;31(3):382–9.

103. Amin MB, Edge S, Greene F, et al, editors. AJCC cancer staging manual. 8th edition. Switzerland: Springer International Publishing; 2017.

Smooth Muscle Tumors of the Female Genital Tract

Kelly A. Devereaux, MD, PhD[a], J. Kenneth Schoolmeester, MD[b],*

KEYWORDS

- Smooth muscle tumors • Leiomyoma • Leiomyosarcoma • Uterus • Vagina • Ovary • Vulva

ABSTRACT

Smooth muscle tumors are the most common mesenchymal tumors of the female genital tract. However, awareness of tumor variants and unconventional growth patterns is critical for appropriate classification and patient management. For example, recognition of fumarate hydratase–deficient leiomyomas allows pathologists to alert providers to the potential for hereditary leiomyomatosis and renal cell carcinoma. Furthermore, myxoid and epithelioid smooth muscle tumors have different thresholds for malignancy than spindled tumors and should be classified by criteria specific to these variants. This article provides an overview of smooth muscle tumors of each major organ of the gynecologic tract and discusses diagnostic challenges.

OVERVIEW

This review of smooth muscle tumors (SMTs) of the female genital tract complements the 2014 edition of the World Health Organization (WHO) Classification of Tumors of the Female Reproductive Organs and is similarly organized by anatomic site.[1] The typical clinical presentation, gross appearance, microscopic features, and prognosis are reviewed for each entity. In addition, major diagnostic issues and differential considerations are discussed.

SMOOTH MUSCLE TUMORS OF THE UTERINE CORPUS

LEIOMYOMAS

Spindled (Conventional, Usual) Leiomyoma

Leiomyomas are the most common SMT of the uterus. The cumulative incidence of leiomyomas by age 50 years is estimated to be 70% for white women and greater than 80% for black women.[2] Although leiomyomas can occur at any age throughout adulthood, most women are perimenopausal or in their fourth to fifth decade at diagnosis. In addition, most women with leiomyomas are asymptomatic and only 20% to 50% experience symptoms.[3] Clinical presentation and symptoms tend to depend on the quantity, size, and distribution of tumors. Some women present with menorrhagia, abnormal uterine bleeding, polycythemia, ascites, pelvic pain or pressure, enlarged uterus, and/or infertility.[3,4] In addition, leiomyomas can potentially complicate pregnancy and/or delivery.[3]

Gross features

Tumors occur at intramural, submucosal, or subserosal locations; are typically round, well-circumscribed nodules; and are often multiple. On cut surface, the nodules are tan-white, whorled, and solid, and protrude or bulge relative to the background myometrium. Although most tumors are solid and firm, some examples show hemorrhage, cystic degeneration, discoloration, or softening (**Fig. 1**). In addition, some may be

Disclosure: The authors have no conflicts of interest to disclose.
a Department of Pathology, Stanford University School of Medicine, 300 Pasteur Drive, L235, Stanford, CA 94305, USA; b Department of Laboratory Medicine and Pathology, Mayo Clinic, 200 First Street, Southwest, Rochester, MN 55905, USA
* Corresponding author.
E-mail address: schoolmeester.j@mayo.edu

Surgical Pathology 12 (2019) 397–455
https://doi.org/10.1016/j.path.2019.02.004
1875-9181/19/© 2019 Elsevier Inc. All rights reserved.

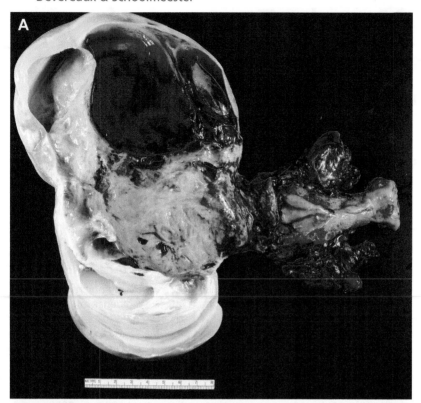

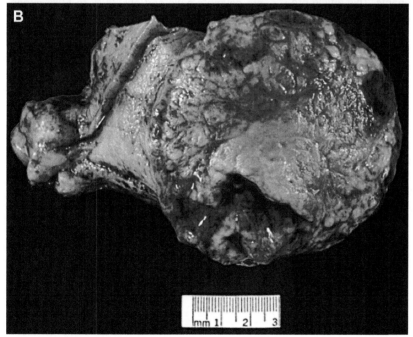

Fig. 1. (*A, B*) Aside from forming prototypical solid masses with a white, whorled cut surface, SMTs originating in the gynecologic tract have an increased tendency to develop various degrees of intratumoral edema, cystic change, and extracellular hyalinization.

calcified. Leiomyomas can range in size from less than 1 cm to greater than 20 cm.

Microscopic features

Conventional leiomyomas have cytologically bland spindled cells with eosinophilic cytoplasm and blunt-ended elongated nuclei that are arranged in intersecting fascicles (Fig. 2). Intermixed thick-walled blood vessels are often prominent. Cytologic atypia is usually mild at most and mitotic figures, if present, are infrequent or mildly increased

Fig. 2. (*A, B*) Most conventional or spindled leiomyomas are composed of fascicles of spindle cells with ample eosinophilic cytoplasm and tubular nuclei and mitotic activity is infrequent.

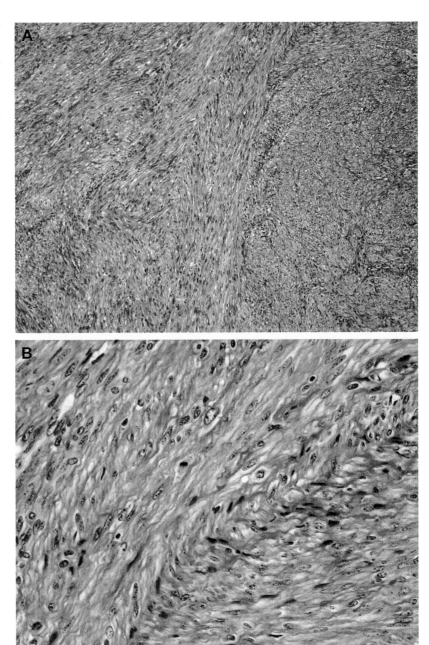

(generally 0–3 mitotic figures per 10 high-power fields [HPFs], but can be up to 10 mitotic figures per 10 HPFs). Although most tumors are well circumscribed, some have irregular borders and/or interdigitate with adjacent myometrium. Various quantities of edema, hyalinization, and macrocysts or microcysts can develop in gynecologic leiomyomas (**Fig. 3**). Infarct or hyaline-type necrosis is a common finding and has a distinct zonation pattern seen as a band of granulation tissue and/ or organizing fibrosis at the interface between the inner nonviable and outer viable tumors cells (**Fig. 4**). Hemorrhage may also be present in the necrotic areas. Early ischemic change can be challenging to distinguish from incipient tumor cell necrosis (**Fig. 5**) because the former can lack defined zonation and have an abrupt transition from viable and nonviable tumor. In cases with equivocal forms of necrosis, consideration of other microscopic features, such as the degree of

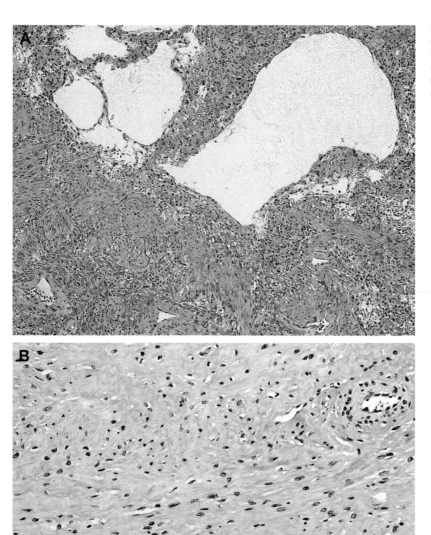

Fig. 3. (*A, B*) In some conventional leiomyomas, macrocysts or microcysts can occur and stromal hyalinization can be prominent.

cytologic atypia and mitotic index, may assist in favoring one type of necrosis over the other. One recent study proposed use of reticulin and trichrome stains to aid in the classification of necrosis from differences in extracellular matrix composition. A honeycomb pattern of reticulin fibers was maintained around nonviable individual tumor cells in 91% of cases of leiomyosarcoma in contrast with 39% of leiomyomas. Trichrome highlighted dense collagen within nonviable regions of 100% of leiomyomas, whereas 36% of leiomyosarcomas had dense collagen in necrotic areas. It was noted that the cases of leiomyosarcoma that had dense collagen in nonviable areas had a retained honeycomb reticulin network.[5]

Awareness of prior therapeutic interventions for leiomyomas is helpful because some features are associated with various forms of treatment.

Fig. 4. Ischemic or hyaline-type necrosis is characterized by a gradient of viable to nonviable tumor, sometimes with a trickling or tendril-like deposition of hyalinization (*A*) and sometimes with a sharply demarcated border (*B*). A granulation tissue–like response can be found bordering this type of necrosis and can be modest or focal

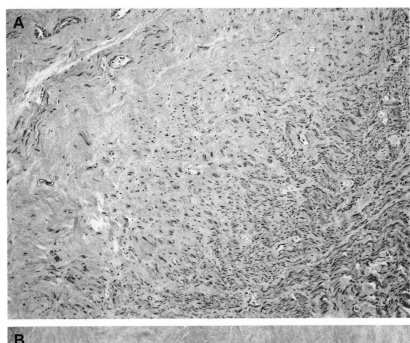

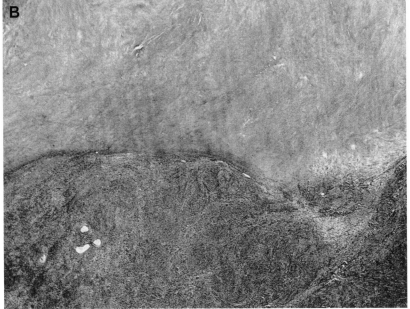

Leiomyomas that undergo embolization may show intravascular or extravascular foreign material, foreign body giant cell reaction, hyaline necrosis, thrombosis, and/or vessel destruction.[6,7] Leiomyomas treated with gonadotropin-releasing hormone agents may have fibrinoid degeneration of vessel walls, decreased number and size of vessels, focal hypercellularity, focal infarcts, hyalinization, and a lymphocytic infiltrate.[8–10] Antifibrinolytic agents such as tranexamic acid can cause thrombosis or infarction, which may mimic tumor cell necrosis.[11]

Prognosis

Leiomyomas are benign with a range of clinical presentations that largely depend on size, quantity, and location. The type and severity of

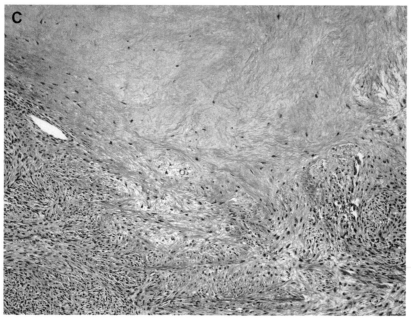

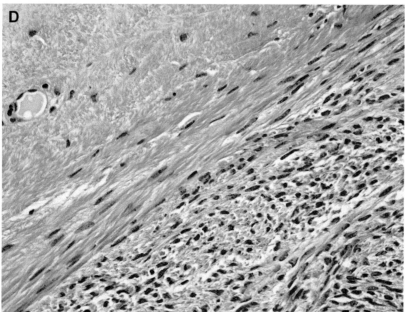

Fig. 4. (continued). (C) or prominent forming a circumferential ring. However, a transition from nonviable to viable tumor is usually seen in all examples of ischemic or hyaline-type necrosis (D).

symptoms often determine the choice of therapy. More conservative uterine-sparing treatments include myomectomy, medical (eg, tranexamic acid, levonorgestrel-releasing intrauterine device, gonadotropin-releasing hormone), and interventional (eg, embolization) options. Hysterectomy is curative and remains the definitive treatment option for women who have completed childbearing.[4]

MORPHOLOGIC VARIANTS

Mitotically Active Leiomyoma

The 2014 edition of the WHO Classification of Tumors of the Female Reproductive Organs defines mitotically active as an otherwise spindled leiomyoma with a mitotic index of greater than 10 mitotic figures per 10 HPFs.[1,12] Women with mitotically active leiomyomas are often reproductive

Fig. 5. (*A, B*) In contrast with ischemic or hyaline-type necrosis, tumor cell necrosis or coagulative necrosis has an abrupt transition from viable to nonviable tumor that lacks a significant inflammatory response or fibrotic response. In some examples, viable islands of tumor can be found within pools of necrosis.

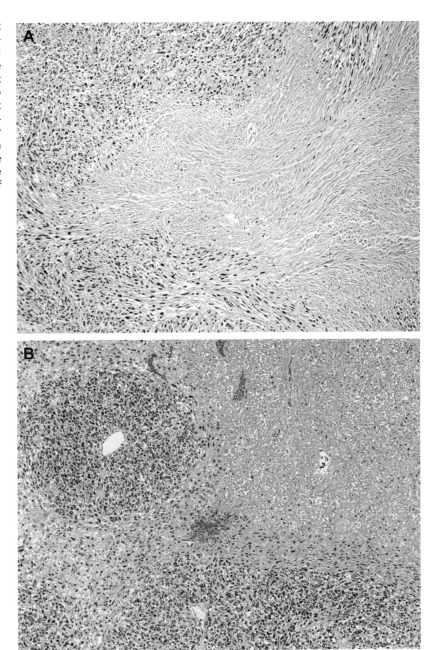

age at diagnosis and present with symptoms similar to conventional leiomyomas.[13,14] This variant has been associated with pregnancy, exogenous progestin use, and secretory endometrium, corroborating the hypothesis that progesterone may have a mitogenic effect.[13]

Gross features

Tumors appear similar to conventional leiomyomas, range in size from 1.3 to 10 cm (mean 5 cm), and are frequently submucosal.[13,14]

Microscopic features

Mitotically active leiomyomas are formed of variable cellular spindle cells with uniformly mild cytologic atypia (**Fig. 6**). Increased mitotic activity (>10 mitotic figures per 10 HPFs) may be diffuse, regional, or focal. Atypical mitotic figures should not be present. Infarct-type necrosis may be seen.[12,13]

Differential Diagnosis

Smooth muscle tumor of uncertain malignant potential

- There is limited experience with otherwise cytologically bland SMTs that have a mitotic index of greater than or equal to 15 mitotic figures per 10 HPFs.[12] The current 2014 WHO lists such SMTs as SMTs of uncertain malignant potential (STUMP) and some studies have suggested designating such proliferative SMTs as STUMPs.[1,15] Others prefer classification as mitotically active leiomyoma with a note explaining currently limited data and recommend patient follow-up.

Spindled (conventional) leiomyosarcoma

- Classification of spindled SMT as leiomyosarcoma generally requires 2 of 3 features: (1) significant cytologic atypia, (2) mitotic index of greater than or equal to 10 mitotic figures per 10 HPFs, (3) tumor cell necrosis. Thorough sampling is important in all SMTs with atypical features.

Prognosis

Prognosis and management of mitotically active leiomyomas are the same as for conventional leiomyomas.[13,14]

Leiomyoma with Bizarre Nuclei (Symplastic Leiomyoma, Atypical Leiomyoma)

Several descriptors have been used for leiomyomas with moderate to severe cytologic atypia, including leiomyoma with bizarre nuclei, symplastic leiomyoma, bizarre leiomyoma, and pleomorphic leiomyoma. The 2014 WHO classification endorses leiomyoma with bizarre nuclei for this variant.[1] Although atypical leiomyoma has been used, this diagnosis can cause confusion with SMT of uncertain malignant potential (STUMP), which has different prognostic significance.

Women are typically reproductive to postmenopausal age (mean, 42.5 years) at diagnosis and present with symptoms identical to conventional leiomyomas.[16]

Gross features

Tumors appear similar to conventional leiomyomas and range in size from 0.7 to 14 cm (mean, 6.8 cm).[16]

Microscopic features

Leiomyomas with bizarre nuclei are characterized by focally, multifocally, or diffusely distributed cells with moderate to severe cytologic atypia (**Fig. 7**). These cells are enlarged, pleomorphic, and contain nuclei that are hyperchromatic, multilobated, and/or multinucleated. Chromatin may appear coarse or smudged. No increased mitotic activity (<4 mitotic figures per 10 HPFs) or tumor cell necrosis is seen. Bizarre chromatin abnormalities, pyknotic nuclei, and karyorrhectic debris may resemble atypical mitotic figures, but, to prevent miscounting these mimics, standard mitotic spindle forms should comprise some component of mitotic activity. Infarct-type necrosis, edema, cystic change, and hyalinization may be present.[16,17]

Differential Diagnosis

Fumarate hydratase–deficient leiomyoma

- Distinguishing leiomyomas with bizarre nuclei from leiomyomas with features of fumarate hydratase (FH) deficiency can be challenging because both variants can have prominent eosinophilic nucleoli with perinucleolar halos, eosinophilic cytoplasmic inclusions, staghorn vessels, and pseudoalveolar edema. Loss of FH expression by immunohistochemistry can be helpful to identify FH-deficient tumors, but it is not entirely sensitive for all genetic alterations of *FH* (discussed later).[18,19]

Smooth muscle tumors of uncertain malignant potential

- Significant cytologic atypia may raise concern for STUMP. Compiled data from in the 2014 WHO classification found that SMTs with focal or multifocal moderate to severe cytologic atypia and a mean mitotic index of 4 figures per 10 HPFs (range, 3–5) recurred in 13.6% of reported cases (3 of 22 cases). SMTs with diffuse moderate to severe cytologic atypia and a mean mitotic index of 4 figures per 10 HPFs (range, 2–9) recurred in 10.4% of reported cases (7 of 67 cases).[1] If tumor cell necrosis is identified with any quantity of significant cytologic atypia, a diagnosis of leiomyosarcoma should be considered.

Leiomyosarcoma

- Significant cytologic atypia may raise concern for leiomyosarcoma, but either a mitotic index of greater than or equal to 10 mitotic figures per 10 HPFs or tumor cell necrosis must be present.

Fig. 6. (*A, B*) Mitotically active leiomyoma is defined by the most recent WHO Classification of Tumors of the Female Reproductive Organs as an otherwise typical leiomyoma with a mitotic index greater than 10 mitotic figures per 10 HPFs.

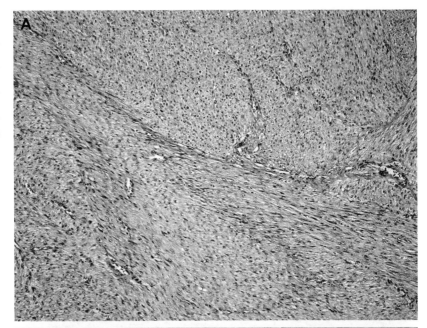

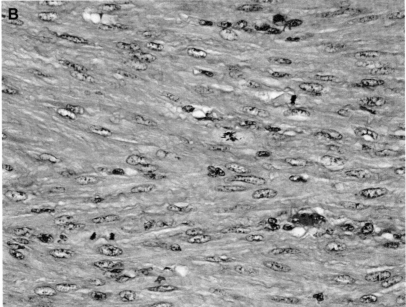

Prognosis

Leiomyomas with bizarre nuclei are benign. Rare cases have recurred if incompletely excised.[16] Recommended management includes complete removal of the lesion either by myomectomy or hysterectomy to limit risk of recurrence as well as to permit comprehensive evaluation of the tumor because SMTs can be morphologically heterogeneous.

Cellular/Hypercellular Leiomyoma

Cellular/hypercellular leiomyomas are defined as SMTs that are significantly more cellular than background myometrium. Women range from reproductive to postmenopausal age (mean, 46 years) at diagnosis and experience symptoms similar to conventional leiomyomas.[20]

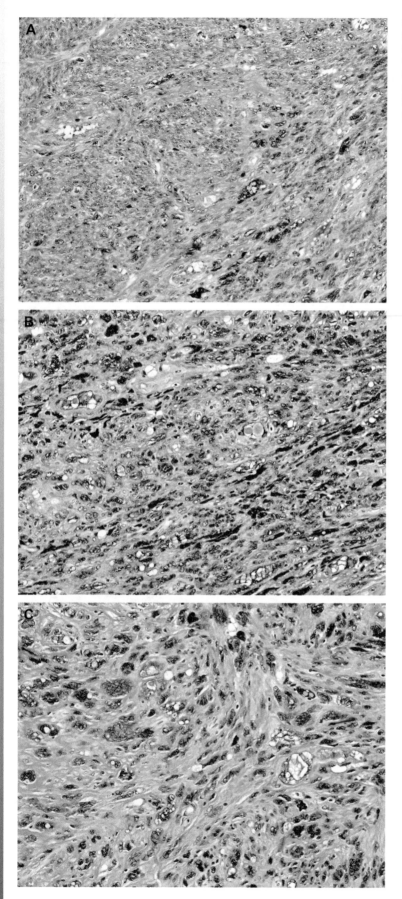

Fig. 7. Leiomyoma with bizarre nuclei has a focal (*A*), multifocal or diffuse (*B*) distribution of cells with markedly pleomorphic nuclei characterized by multinucleation, multilobation, and/or hyperchromasia (*C*). Nuclear pseudoinclusions are common.

Gross features

Tumors appear tan, pink, yellow, or gray and a subset have a soft consistency (**Fig.** 8A). They range in size from 0.5 to 15 cm (mean, 4.6 cm).[20]

Microscopic features

Cellular/hypercellular leiomyomas have considerably increased cellular density relative to background myometrium (**Fig.** 8B, C). Some distinguish hypercellular leiomyomas from cellular leiomyomas by the former having dense cellularity comparable with endometrial stromal neoplasms (**Fig.** 8D, E). Prominent large thick-walled vessels with or without mural hyalinization are present. The tumor cells are spindled and contain variable amounts of eosinophilic cytoplasm. Cytologic atypia is no greater than mild and mitotic activity is low level. Cellular/hypercellular leiomyomas may have irregular borders that interdigitate with myometrium. Artifactual cleftlike spaces or retraction may be found. In some instances, there are cellular seedling leiomyomas in myometrium adjacent to the dominant leiomyoma.[20,21]

Differential Diagnosis

Endometrial stromal nodule/low-grade endometrial stromal sarcoma

- Cellular/hypercellular leiomyomas have overlapping features with endometrial stromal tumors. However, cellular/hypercellular leiomyomas have fascicular architecture and larger thick-walled vessels in contrast with endometrial stromal tumors, which tend to have a haphazard or less organized architecture and smaller thin-walled vessels. In addition, the growth pattern of low-grade endometrial stromal sarcoma is characterized by infiltrative, permeative projections into myometrium and vascular invasion (**Fig.** 8F).[21]

- A panel of antibodies that includes CD10, desmin, and h-caldesmon may be helpful in difficult cases. However, there is overlap in expression of these markers. Cellular/hypercellular leiomyomas can be CD10 positive, whereas endometrial stromal tumors can be variably positive for desmin and h-caldesmon, particularly in tumors with smooth muscle differentiation.[22–24]

Prognosis

Prognosis and management of cellular/hypercellular leiomyomas do not differ from conventional leiomyomas.

Hydropic Leiomyoma

Hydropic leiomyomas have extensive accumulation of edematous fluid secondary to degeneration. Women are usually in their fourth to fifth decade (mean, 45 years) at diagnosis.[25]

Gross features

Tumors can be submucosal, intramural, or subserosal and range in size from 3 to 10 cm (mean, 6.1 cm).[25] The gross appearance depends on the degree of hydropic change but varies from white to yellow to red edematous or gelatinous fluid (**Fig.** 9A). Cystic degeneration may be present.[25] Pedunculated masses can develop adhesions and adhere to adnexal structures.[26]

Microscopic features

Hydropic leiomyomas are characterized by well-circumscribed to poorly circumscribed pools of edema within a conventional, cellular, or, more rarely, epithelioid leiomyoma. The degree of hydropic change can range from mild (10%) to near replacement (95%) of the tumor. Hydropic areas consist of predominately clear-pale edematous to eosinophilic proteinaceous fluid with scattered fibroblasts and thin bundles of collagen (**Fig.** 9B). The hydropic regions are largely devoid of tumor cells but, when present, they are arranged in cords or small nests (**Fig.** 9C). The vasculature of the tumor is often accentuated with a mixture of prominent capillaries and larger muscular vessels.[25]

Perinodular hydropic change describes a pattern whereby small islands or nodules of tumor cells and associated blood vessels are surrounded by hydropic connective tissue (**Fig.** 9D, E). Occasional retraction artifact can occur around these tumor nodules and mimic intravascular growth.[25,26]

Differential Diagnosis

Intravenous leiomyomatosis

- Perinodular hydropic change with artifactual stromal retraction can simulate vascular invasion and mimic intravenous leiomyomatosis. Endothelial markers can be helpful to identify vascular spaces.

Myxoid smooth muscle tumor

- In some cases, myxoid matrix and hydropic change can morphologically overlap. Alcian blue and colloidal iron stains can be helpful to distinguish them because both are positive in myxoid matrix and negative or weakly positive in hydropic change.

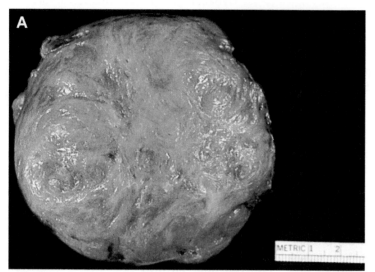

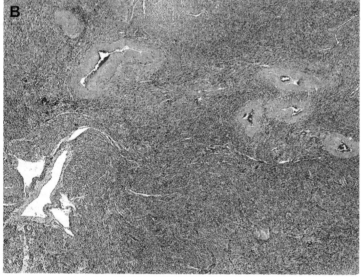

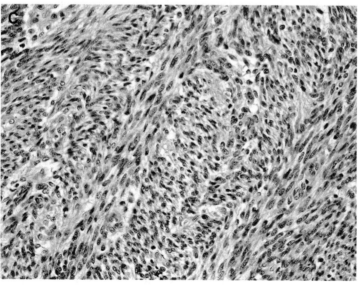

Fig. 8. Cellular and hypercellular leiomyomas often are grossly yellow-tan with a soft consistency (*A*). Cellular and hypercellular leiomyomas have significantly increased cellular density relative to background myometrium (*B*, *C*). Some distinguish a subset of leiomyomas as hypercellular leiomyomas because of even greater cell density that resembles endometrial stromal tumors

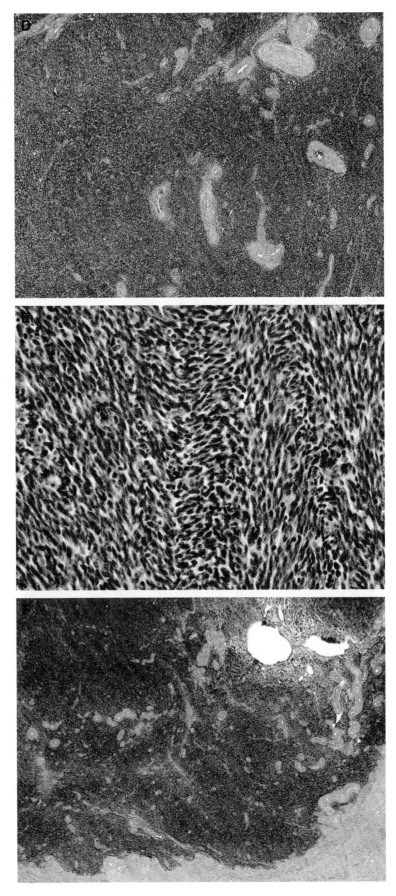

Fig. 8. (continued). (D, E). Although cellular and hypercellular leiomyomas can have mild border irregularities between tumor and myometrium (*F*), they lack an overtly permeative growth found in low-grade endometrial stromal sarcomas.

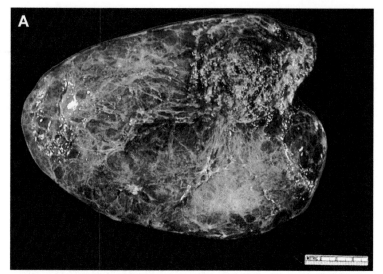

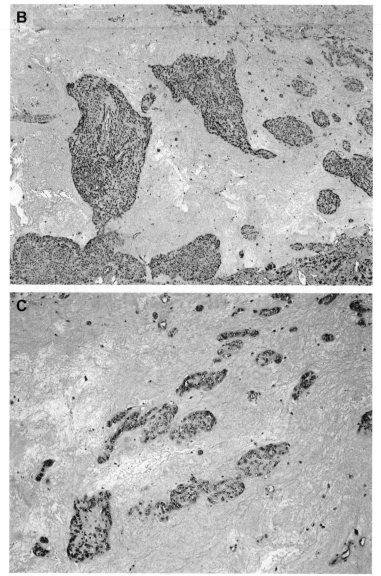

Fig. 9. Hydropic leiomyomas contain macroscopic quantities of edematous, mucoid, or gelatinous fluid that result in a boggy consistency (*A*). Microscopically, regions of clear-pale edematous to eosinophilic proteinaceous fluid (*B*) contain aggregates of tumor that form cords or small nests (*C*). Some examples of hydropic leiomyoma form a nodular architecture

Fig. 9. (*continued*). (*D*) that can result in a corded or plexiform growth of tumor cells (*E*).

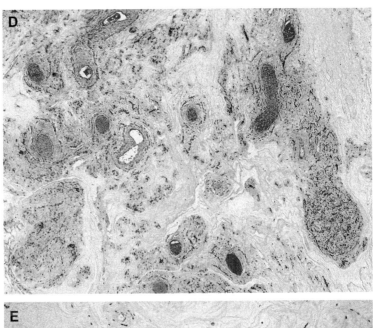

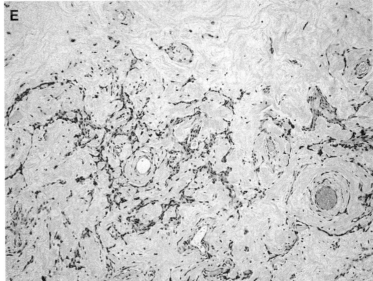

Prognosis

Prognosis and management of hydropic leiomyomas are similar to conventional leiomyomas.

Myxoid Leiomyoma

Myxoid leiomyomas have a prominent myxoid extracellular matrix that is rich in proteoglycans and glycosaminoglycans (eg, hyaluronic acid).[27,28] Accordingly, the myxoid matrix can be highlighted by Alcian blue and colloidal iron stains. A limited quantity of myxoid stroma may be present in otherwise conventional leiomyomas.

Gross features

Tumors often have a soft consistency and exude a mucoid or gelatinous fluid on cut surface.

Microscopic features

Myxoid leiomyomas are characterized by extensive basophilic and pale-staining myxomatous extracellular matrix that exceeds 50% of the overall tumor volume. Spindled or stellate cells are splayed apart by the myxomatous stroma to impart a hypocellular appearance. Myxoid stroma may extend into adjacent areas of more conventional leiomyoma and emulate myometrial invasion, but the periphery of the tumor should remain generally well defined and noninfiltrative.[29] Myxoid leiomyomas should have no greater than mild cytologic atypia, a mitotic index of fewer than 2 mitotic figures per 10 HPFs, and no tumor cell necrosis.[30]

tumors can be negative for desmin and h-caldesmon and positive for keratins.[34,35] Histone deacetylase 8 (HDAC8), a marker of smooth muscle differentiation, is consistently positive in epithelioid SMTs.[35]

 Differential Diagnosis

Myxoid leiomyosarcoma
- Myxoid leiomyosarcomas can be cytologically bland; therefore, thorough sampling is required of myxoid SMTs. Two of 3 features are suggested to classify a myxoid SMT as leiomyosarcoma: (1) significant cytologic atypia, (2) mitotic index greater than or equal to 2 mitotic figures per 10 HPFs and (3) tumor cell necrosis (discussed in relation to myxoid leiomyosarcoma).[30,31]

Hydropic leiomyoma
- Distinguishing hydropic change from myxoid matrix is often difficult because both splay tumor cells and create a hypocellular appearance. Alcian blue or colloidal iron can be helpful in difficult cases.

Differential Diagnosis

Epithelioid leiomyosarcoma
- In contrast with epithelioid leiomyomas, leiomyosarcomas have some combination of significant cytologic atypia, at least 3 to 4 mitotic figures per 10 HPFs, and tumor cell necrosis (see discussion of epithelioid leiomyosarcoma).[32]

Perivascular epithelioid cell tumor
- Perivascular epithelioid cell tumors (PEComas), like epithelioid SMTs, are composed of epithelioid cells typically arranged in a nested architecture and associated with a thin-walled vascular network. Although both SMTs and PEComas express smooth muscle markers and HMB45, PEComas often express melan-A, whereas SMTs usually do not.[36–38]

Poorly differentiated carcinoma
- Poorly differentiated carcinomas are negative for smooth muscle markers and should have more robust immunoreactivity to keratins than epithelioid SMTs.

Prognosis

Prognosis and management of myxoid leiomyomas are the same as conventional leiomyomas.

Epithelioid Leiomyoma

Epithelioid leiomyomas are entirely or predominately (>50% overall tumor volume) composed of epithelial-like tumor cells. Women range from reproductive to postmenopausal age at diagnosis and have clinical presentations identical to those of conventional leiomyomas.[32,33]

Gross features

Tumors are generally grossly similar to conventional leiomyomas and can measure up to 12.5 cm in diameter.[32,33]

Microscopic features

Epithelioid leiomyomas are composed of sheets and/or nests of round to polygonal cells with abundant eosinophilic or clear cytoplasm. Nuclei may be centrally or eccentrically located and round or angulated.[32,33] By definition, there should not be significant cytologic atypia, increased mitotic activity, or tumor cell necrosis.

The immunophenotype of epithelioid leiomyomas diverges from other uterine SMTs in that

Prognosis

Prognosis and management of epithelioid leiomyomas are no different than for conventional leiomyomas.

Plexiform Tumorlet

Plexiform tumorlets are proliferations of epithelioid cells with smooth muscle differentiation that are typically no larger than 1 cm. These lesions are most commonly incidental in women in their third to fifth decade of life (mean, 45 years).[39] Several cases have been associated with leiomyomas and adenomyosis; however, this observation may be coincidental because these are frequent indications for undergoing hysterectomy.[40,41] The cell of origin of plexiform tumorlets has been controversial, with hypotheses varying from endometrial stromal cells, perivascular cells, to myofibroblasts. Microscopic, immunohistochemical, and ultrastructural studies found that plexiform tumorlets are of smooth muscle origin.[39,41]

Gross features

Tumorlets are rarely identified during gross inspection. When macroscopic, their appearance is comparable with that of conventional leiomyomas.[39]

Microscopic features

Plexiform tumorlets are found in either endometrium or myometrium but typically are intramural. Although tumorlets are often solitary, they can be multifocal. Tumorlets have uniform oval to polygonal cells with moderate to scant eosinophilic cytoplasm, round central nuclei and vesicular chromatin arranged in small nests, branching trabecula, and/or cords that are separated by hyalinized stroma, giving the lesion plexiform architecture (Fig. 10). Several cases of tumorlets adjacent to or admixed with adenomyosis have been reported. No increase in mitotic activity, significant cytologic atypia, or necrosis should be present.[39–42]

Differential Diagnosis

Uterine tumor resembling ovarian sex cord tumor
- Uterine tumors resembling ovarian sex cord tumors often grow in cords, nests, and trabeculae and can have a plexiform pattern. In contrast with plexiform tumorlets, they are frequently positive for keratins and sex cord markers.[43–46]

Prognosis

Plexiform tumorlets are benign. No recurrence or metastasis has been reported.[39–42]

Lipoleiomyoma

Lipoleiomyomas comprise a small subset (approximately 0.35%–2.1%) of all uterine leiomyomas and show an admixture of smooth muscle and adipose tissue.[47,48] Women range from reproductive to postmenopausal age (mean, 54 years) at diagnosis and present with symptoms akin to conventional leiomyomas.[48] Although the source of the lipomatous elements in the uterus is unclear, several possibilities have been proposed, including metaplasia, ectopic adipocytes, and iatrogenic displacement.[49,50]

Gross features

Tumors are well-circumscribed nodules that range in size from 0.3 to 35.5 cm (mean, 4.6 cm) and vary in appearance based on extent of the adipocytic component.[48] Tumors with fewer adipocytes have single or multiple soft, yellow foci on cut surface. Adipocyte-rich tumors tend to be more lobulated, soft, and yellow, resembling lipomas.[48]

Microscopic features

Lipoleiomyomas are composed of both smooth muscle and mature adipocytes (Fig. 11A, B). The quantity of adipocytes varies from scattered single cells and small aggregates to extensive sheets.[48,51] Lipoleiomyomas lack cytologic atypia in both smooth muscle and adipocytic components, significant mitotic activity, and tumor cell necrosis (Fig. 11C). Lipoblasts are not present in conventional lipoleiomyomas but can be seen in bizarre lipoleiomyomas in which the scattered lipoblasts have enlarged, scalloped, and hyperchromatic nuclei. However, mitotic activity is absent in bizarre lipoleiomyomas.[52,53] Rare lipoleiomyomatous tumors can resemble hibernomas when containing a brown fat–like component.[54]

Differential Diagnosis

Angiomyolipoma
- Angiomyolipomas of the uterus are very uncommon and contain a mixture of smooth muscle, mature adipose tissue, and dysmorphic blood vessels. They are positive for HMB45 (which can also be seen in lipoleiomyomas) and melan-A (not expected in lipoleiomyomas).[47] Some angiomyolipomas are associated with tuberous sclerosis.[55]

Lipoleiomyosarcoma
- Lipoleiomyosarcomas of the uterus are also rare, typically present in postmenopausal women as large masses, and show frankly malignant features, including cytologic atypia, increased mitoses, and tumor cell necrosis.

Prognosis

Prognosis and management of lipoleiomyomas are identical to that of conventional leiomyomas. Rare instances of liposarcoma arising in a lipoleiomyoma have been reported.[56]

Apoplectic Leiomyoma

Apoplectic leiomyomas occur in women of reproductive to postmenopausal age (mean, 41 years) and are associated with exposure to progesterone or synthetic analogues (progestogens or progestins).[57,58] Most women have a history of leiomyomas and are using oral or intrauterine contraceptives, or are pregnant or postpartum at diagnosis.[57–60] Rare cases of rupture and hemoperitoneum have been reported.[59]

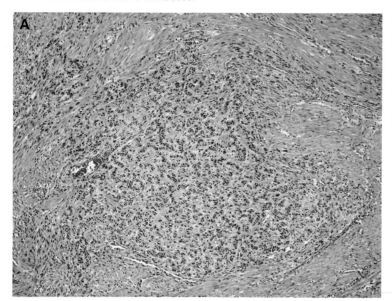

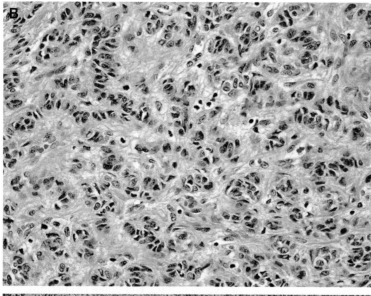

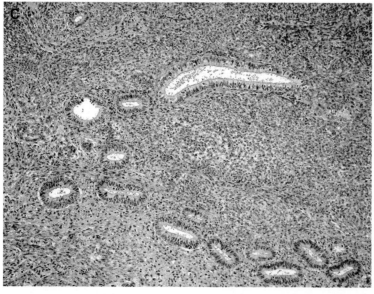

Fig. 10. Plexiform tumorlets are usually incidental intramural proliferations of uniformly oval to polygonal cytologically bland cells arranged in small nests, branching trabeculae, and/or cords, giving the lesion plexiform architecture (*A, B*). Some cases can involve endometrium (*C*). Microscopic, immunohisto-chemical, and ultrastructural studies support a smooth muscle origin for these lesions.

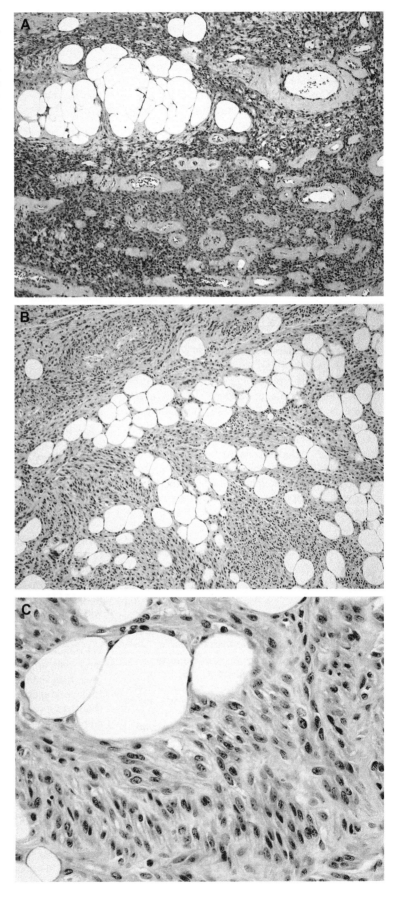

Fig. 11. Lipoleiomyomas are heterogeneous in their content of mature adipose tissue. Some tumors have only focal aggregates of adipocytes such as this cellular example (*A*), whereas others have a more extensive distribution (*B*). Smooth muscle tumor cells and adipocytes are cytologically bland (*C*).

Gross features

In most cases, the uterus is enlarged and contains multiple tan-white nodules that range in size from 0.2 to 15.9 (mean, 6 cm).[57] The cut surface shows varying amounts of congestion and hemorrhage that are often centrally located in the tumor.[59] Tumors may also show some combination of necrosis, cystic change, and/or discoloration (eg, yellow, green, dark brown).[57–60]

Microscopic features

The first indication of the influence of progestins or progesterone may be inactive endometrial glands within (pseudo)decidualized stroma (if nonneoplastic endometrium is present). Apoplectic leiomyomas show ovoid to stellate-shaped areas of central hemorrhage and necrosis (Fig. 12A). A rim of viable tumor cells often located around the hemorrhagic areas is notable for dense aggregates of spindled to epithelioid cells, several with pyknotic nuclei and associated mitotic activity (mean, 3 mitotic figures per 10 HPFs; range, 0–14 figures per 10 HPFs) (Fig. 12B, C).[57] Increased mitotic activity is typically localized to the periphery of these apoplectic zones.[58] When cystic change is present, cystlike structures may be devoid of content or contain hyaline or myxoid material.[57] Abnormal vascular findings have also been documented, including dilated venous channels, hyperplastic arterioles, thick-walled small vessels, myxoid or edematous intimal swelling, and intimal fibrosis.[59,60] Apoplectic alterations affect multiple leiomyomas in most (66%) cases.[57]

⚠ Differential Diagnosis

Spindled smooth muscle tumor of uncertain malignant potential or leiomyosarcoma

- Although necrosis and increased mitotic activity in apoplectic leiomyomas may be concerning, awareness of exogenous hormonal therapy or recent hormonal influence secondary to pregnancy is helpful to prevent misinterpretation as STUMP or leiomyosarcoma. In apoplectic leiomyomas, mitotic activity tends to be limited to the rim of viable cells encircling necrotic centers, and this feature is seen in multiple leiomyomas. STUMP or leiomyosarcoma should have greater cytologic atypia and increased mitotic activity in portions of the tumor distant from necrosis. Furthermore, STUMP and leiomyosarcoma tend to be solitary tumors or are large and predominant.

Prognosis

Prognosis and management of apoplectic leiomyomas are the same as for conventional leiomyomas.

Fumarate Hydratase–Deficient Leiomyoma

A small subset (approximately 0.4%–2.6%) of leiomyomas are associated with alterations of fumarate hydratase (FH).[61–63] FH encodes an enzyme that catalyzes conversion of fumarate to malate in the citric acid or tricarboxylic acid cycle.[64] Biallelic inactivation of FH by somatic alterations or germline alterations in hereditary leiomyomatosis and renal cell cancer (HLRCC) syndrome causes low levels of, or absent, FH and subsequent accumulation of fumarate.[18,62,65–67] Metabolic dysregulation and tumorigenesis ensue, but their mechanisms are incompletely defined.[68–71] FH-deficient leiomyomas have distinctive morphologic features that allow their recognition to subsequently identify patients at risk for HLRCC.

HLRCC is an autosomal dominant disorder that predisposes to developing cutaneous and uterine leiomyomas as well as aggressive forms of renal cell carcinoma.[70,72] Uterine leiomyomas occur in 98% of women with HLRCC and are diagnosed at a mean age of 30 years (approximately 10 years before most conventional leiomyomas are diagnosed). Patients present with multiple leiomyomas, some of which are large and cause severe symptoms, prompting early-age surgical intervention in most cases.[73]

Gross features

In patients with known HLRCC, the uterus almost always has multiple leiomyomas. Tumors can measure from less than 2 to 17 cm.[67] The cut surface of FH-deficient tumors appears tan to brown with a soft consistency.[61,67,73]

Microscopic features

FH-deficient leiomyomas have epithelioid to spindled cells arranged in fascicles or vague nodules (Fig. 13A). Some cells contain eosinophilic intracytoplasmic globules or inclusions. Many cells have round to ovoid nuclei that contain large nucleoli with perinucleolar clearing. Multinucleated cells and cells with bizarre nuclear features may be present (Fig. 13B). Pseudoalveolar edema, defined as splaying of tumor cells to resemble alveoli of the lung, is frequent, at least focally (Fig. 13C). Tumor vasculature is distinctive because of scattered thin-walled vessels that have a staghornlike or hemangiopericytic configuration.[18,61,63,74–77]

FH immunohistochemistry shows granular cytoplasmic staining in conventional leiomyomas, whereas FH-deficient leiomyomas lack expression

Fig. 12. Apoplectic leiomyoma is typically found in patients receiving progestin therapy and classically has a central zone of hemorrhagic necrosis with an accentuated periphery of increased cellularity. Other examples include a centrally located or multifocal stellate zone of necrosis (*A*) with an immediate border of edema (*B*), inflammation, pyknosis (*C*), and mitotic activity.

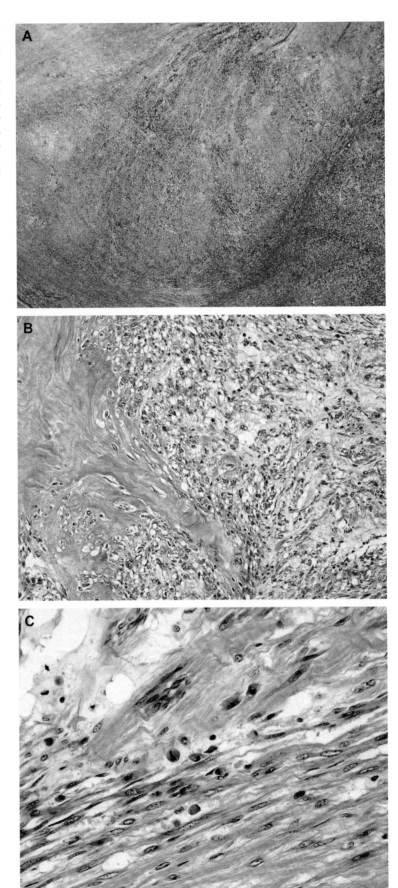

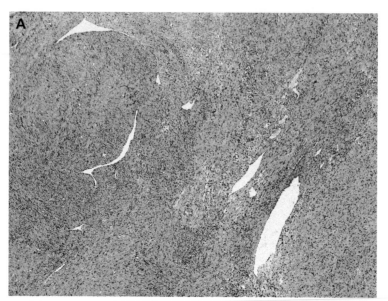

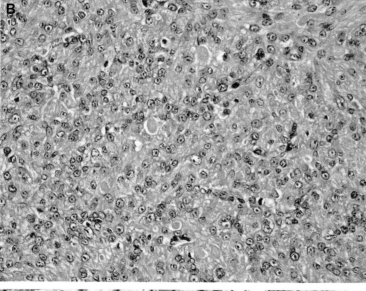

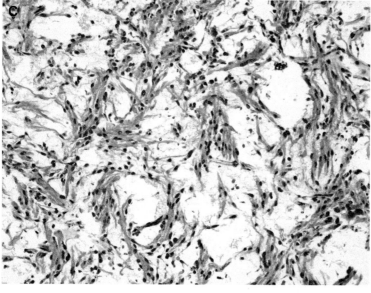

Fig. 13. FH-deficient leiomyoma has a spectrum of features, including epithelioid to spindled cells arranged in fascicles or nodules with intermixed hemangiopericytic vessels (*A*). The cells have round to ovoid nuclei that contain large nucleoli with perinucleolar clearing (*B*). Scattered cells have intracytoplasmic eosinophilic inclusions (*B*). Pseudoalveolar edema, whereby edema causes separation of tumor cells imparting resemblance to alveoli of the lung, is frequent, at least focally (*C*).

of FH. However, retained FH expression does not exclude the possibility of an FH-deficient tumor because some missense mutations produce a nonfunctional but immunoreactive protein. Alternatively, because accumulated fumarate modifies cysteine to produce S-(2-succino)-cysteine (2SC) by succination, detection of 2SC by immunochemistry is an effective marker of FH function and results in granular cytoplasmic staining in FH-deficient tumors.[75,78–81]

HLRCC leiomyomas and leiomyomas with somatic inactivation of *FH* are morphologically and immunohistochemically indistinguishable.[18,62,65,66] Germline genetic testing is currently the most reliable modality to identify patients with HLRCC.[66]

Differential Diagnosis

Leiomyoma with bizarre nuclei

- Leiomyomas with bizarre nuclei show morphologic overlap with FH-deficient leiomyomas. A recent study comparing the morphologic and genetic features of leiomyomas with bizarre nuclei and FH-deficient leiomyomas found considerable morphologic overlap among these tumors. Multivariate analysis identified staghorn vasculature as the only statistically significant feature predictive of an abnormal FH/2SC immunophenotype.[18] FH immunohistochemistry can assist in confirming an FH-deficient tumor, but the stain is not entirely sensitive for all alterations of *FH*.[18,19,67]

Prognosis

Recognition of FH-deficient tumors, with or without confirmation by immunohistochemistry, is important to alert providers to the possibility of HLRCC. Based on clinical risk factors, patients can then be referred for genetic counseling and confirmatory genetic testing as appropriate. Patients with HLRCC may benefit from early screening and surveillance.[18,62,65,66,73] The relationship between FH-deficient leiomyomas and true leiomyosarcomas is not well defined, and only rare examples of FH-deficient uterine leiomyosarcomas have been reported.[82,83]

HETEROLOGOUS ELEMENTS

Although mature adipose tissue is the most common heterologous element associated with leiomyomas (see the discussion of lipoleiomyoma), other heterologous elements may be present.

There have been rare reports of leiomyomas showing:

- Skeletal muscle differentiation[84,85]
- Cartilaginous or chondroid differentiation (Fig. 14)[86,87]
- Bone or osseous differentiation[88]

GROWTH PATTERN VARIANTS

A subset of uterine smooth muscle neoplasms have a distinctive or unusual growth that can cause more severe symptoms and potential for complications and recurrence.

Diffuse Uterine Leiomyomatosis

Diffuse uterine leiomyomatosis is a rare condition characterized by numerous small, benign smooth muscle nodules that enlarge the uterus. Women are of reproductive age at diagnosis and tend to present with more severe symptoms than those produced by conventional leiomyomas.[89,90] The pathogenesis of diffuse uterine leiomyomatosis is unclear, but X-inactivation studies performed on different nodules from the same patient suggested a nonclonal relationship.[91]

Gross features

The uterus is enlarged with a bosselated serosal surface and the myometrium is diffusely distorted by tan-white whorled nodules that measure less than 1 to 3 cm. The nodules often blend into surrounding myometrium or merge with adjacent nodules.[89,90]

Microscopic features

The myometrium is largely overrun by poorly defined, coalescing leiomyomatous nodules. The nodules are often cellular. Myometrial vessels can be compressed or deformed, resulting in long vascular channels that abut and conform to the nodules and can resemble intravascular growth.[89,90]

Differential Diagnosis

Intravenous leiomyomatosis

- Diffuse uterine leiomyomatosis can resemble intravenous leiomyomatosis when nodules compress myometrial vessels. However, this finding is usually focal, and immunohistochemistry for endothelial markers can be helpful to more clearly outline vascular spaces. In contrast with diffuse uterine leiomyomatosis, intravenous leiomyomatosis shows intravascular wormlike plugs of tumor that are seen grossly and microscopically.

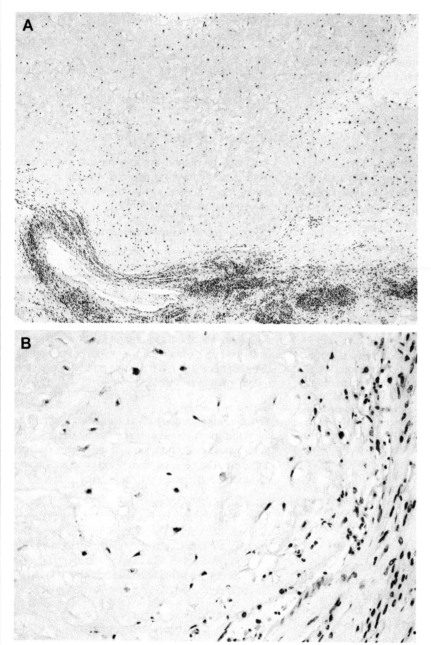

Fig. 14. (*A*, *B*) Leiomyomas with heterologous differentiation can have a range of elements, including adipocytes, skeletal muscle, bone, and cartilage.

Prognosis
Diffuse uterine leiomyomatosis is a benign condition. Hysterectomy is curative and may be performed for symptomatic relief.

Cotyledonoid Dissecting Leiomyoma

Cotyledonoid dissecting leiomyoma is a dissecting variant that infiltrates beyond the confines of the uterus to produce an exophytic mass that grossly resembles placental cotyledons. Women are reproductive age or perimenopausal at diagnosis and present with a pelvic mass, pelvic pain, and/or menorrhagia.[92–94]

Gross features
A bulky exophytic mass (or masses) protrudes from the uterus and is multinodular, red-brown, and congested. In most examples, the exophytic component is contiguous with an intramural

component. The intramural tumor is typically tan-white, solid, and has an ill-defined or vaguely nodular growth pattern within the myometrium. Rare cases have been reported that lack an intramural component.[93,95] Although most dissecting leiomyomas are solid, some have a softer consistency secondary to hydropic or cystic change.[96,97]

Microscopic features
Both extrauterine and intrauterine tumor components have poorly defined nodules of bland tumor cells. The extrauterine component is often hydropic with prominent congested and/or dilated vessels. The intrauterine component has sinuous projections that irregularly dissect background myometrium and occasionally vessels, leading to focal intravascular growth.[92–94,98] Although most examples are a variation of spindled leiomyoma, epithelioid and adipocytic dissecting variants have been reported.[98–101]

Differential Diagnosis

Intravenous leiomyomatosis
- Cotyledonoid dissecting leiomyomas can focally dissect into vessels and mimic intravenous leiomyomatosis. However, intravenous leiomyomatosis has more extensive intravascular growth observable grossly and microscopically and does not produce a cotyledonoid mass.

Prognosis
Cotyledonoid dissecting leiomyomas are benign and hysterectomy is curative. There has been 1 reported recurrence after partial resection.[102]

LEIOMYOMA WITH FOCAL VASCULAR INVASION

A focus of myometrial vascular invasion can occasionally be identified in uterine leiomyomas that lack the gross characteristics of intravenous leiomyomatosis. One study hypothesized that this finding may be a precursor to intravenous leiomyomatosis and metastasizing leiomyoma.[103] However, the 2014 WHO Classification of Tumors of the Female Reproductive Organs states that focal vascular invasion is a phenomenon without prognostic significance.[1]

Intravenous Leiomyomatosis

Intravenous leiomyomatosis is defined as intravascular growth of cytologically bland smooth muscle

outside the confines of a leiomyoma. Women are of reproductive to postmenopausal age at time of diagnosis (mean, 46 years).[104] Clinical presentation depends on the extent of growth, but, in most examples, patients are asymptomatic, experience symptoms of uterine leiomyomas, or present with a pelvic mass.[104–106] In severe cases, growth may extend into the inferior vena cava and right heart, causing cardiopulmonary insufficiency.[107–109]

Gross features
The uterus has multiple convoluted wormlike extensions that infiltrate myometrial and/or parametrial vessels. Tumors may span up to 14 cm in diameter and generally appear similar to conventional leiomyomas; however, some examples are poorly circumscribed.[104] The uterine veins can be distended by tumor plugs, which can then track into veins of the broad ligament, ovary, cervix, and vagina. Association with a leiomyoma may or may not be seen.[104–106,110]

Microscopic features
Intravenous leiomyomatosis is characterized by intravenous growth of histologically benign smooth muscle (**Fig. 15**A). Although most cases coexist with intrauterine leiomyomas, some examples are predominately or entirely intravenous.[104,110] Intravenous tumor may be detached and free floating or show minimal to broad-based attachment to the intima. Nodules of intravenous tumor are notable for rich vascularity and frequent clefting or retraction. Mitotic activity should be absent to infrequent. Hyalinization and hydropic change may be present (**Fig. 15**B). The intravenous tumor usually resembles a spindled leiomyoma of varying cellularity, but epithelioid, myxoid, and lipoleiomyomatous (**Fig. 15**C) forms have been reported.[104,105,110,111]

Differential Diagnosis

Low-grade endometrial stromal sarcoma
- Low-grade endometrial stromal sarcomas permeate the myometrium but typically do not have extensive grossly observable vascular invasion. Although intravenous leiomyomatosis can be cellular, low-grade endometrial stromal sarcoma does not have numerous large, thick-walled vessels or hydropic change. Furthermore, smooth muscle markers can be helpful to differentiate difficult cases if the endometrial stromal tumor does not show smooth muscle differentiation (see the discussion of immunohistochemistry in relation to differential diagnosis of cellular/hypercellular leiomyoma).

Diffuse uterine leiomyomatosis

- Tumor nodules in diffuse uterine leiomyomatosis can compress myometrial vessels and simulate intravascular growth. Endothelial immunohistochemistry can be helpful to define vascular spaces.

Hydropic leiomyoma

- Hydropic leiomyomas, particularly those with perinodular change, can emulate intravenous leiomyomatosis because of retraction artifact. Endothelial markers can assist in outlining vascular structures.

Leiomyosarcoma

- Florid lymphovascular invasion by leiomyosarcoma can microscopically resemble intravenous leiomyomatosis. However, gross evidence of pluglike myometrial growth is absent in leiomyosarcoma and, in contrast with intravenous leiomyomatosis, frankly malignant features should be present.

Myometrial artery protruding into a vein

- Myometrial arteries can protrude into veins, creating a vessel-within-a-vessel phenomenon. Single or multiple lumens of thick-walled arteries appear free floating within an endothelial-lined venous channel and can mimic intravenous leiomyomatosis. This finding is often associated with a history of menorrhagia.[112]

Prognosis

Complete resection by hysterectomy and removal of involved veins yields a low rate of recurrence. Extensive venous infiltration or incomplete excision may lead to persistent intravenous growth and/or recurrence years later.[104–109]

Smooth Muscle Tumor of Uncertain Malignant Potential

STUMPs are a heterogeneous group of SMTs with features that preclude classification as unequivocally benign or malignant. Women are typically in their third to fifth decade (mean, 44.8 years) at diagnosis, which is approximately 10 years before most leiomyosarcomas are diagnosed.[113]

Gross features

Tumors are grossly variable, resembling typical leiomyomas or variants, or can have gross attributes of leiomyosarcoma. Reported STUMPs range in size from 2.5 to 12.2 cm (mean, 7.2 cm).[113]

Microscopic features

A diagnosis of STUMP is reserved for SMTs that have ambiguous features or features that are worrisome, but subdiagnostic, for malignancy.

Diagnostic challenges can arise when there is uncertainty in the type of necrosis or some combination of significant cytologic atypia and increased mitotic activity or a markedly increased mitotic index in an otherwise leiomyoma, among other combinations.[1,114,115]

Scenarios cited in the 2014 WHO classification that should prompt consideration of an SMT as STUMP include:[1]

- SMTs with focal/multifocal or diffuse significant cytologic atypia that lack tumor cell necrosis but have a mitotic index that ranges from 2 to 9 mitotic figures per 10 HPFs (tumors that recurred had a mean index of 4.3 figures per 10 HPFs).
- Cytologically bland SMTs with a mitotic index fewer than 10 mitotic figures per 10/HPFs but that have tumor cell necrosis.
- Cytologically bland SMTs with a mitotic index greater than or equal to 15 mitotic figures per 10 HPFs but without tumor cell necrosis.

A recent review of 22 cases of uterine STUMP found other features were associated with adverse outcomes, including infiltrative or irregular margins, epithelioid differentiation, vascular involvement, and atypical mitoses, and proposed incorporation of these findings when considering a diagnosis of STUMP.[113]

 Differential Diagnosis

Inflammatory myofibroblastic tumor

- Similar to STUMPs, inflammatory myofibroblastic tumors may have a combination of cytologic atypia, increased mitotic activity, tumor cell necrosis, and infiltrative borders, and can be variably positive for smooth muscle markers. At least 50% of inflammatory myofibroblastic tumors and most reported uterine cases to date have an underlying *ALK* rearrangement. Immunohistochemical screening for anaplastic lymphoma kinase (ALK) expression with or without confirmatory fluorescence in situ hybridization or RNA sequencing–based fusion methods can be helpful.[116,117]

Prognosis

The most consistent predictors of STUMP recurrence include the presence of focal/multifocal or diffuse moderate to severe cytologic atypia (13.6% and 10.4% recurrence rate, respectively) or tumor cell necrosis (26.7% recurrence

Fig. 15. Intravenous leiomyomatosis is an intravenous growth of histologically benign smooth muscle that may be detached and free floating or attached to the intima, and frequently has clefting (*A*). Intravenous leiomyomatosis can be hyalinized (*B*) or have various quantities of lipoleiomyomatous differentiation (*C*).

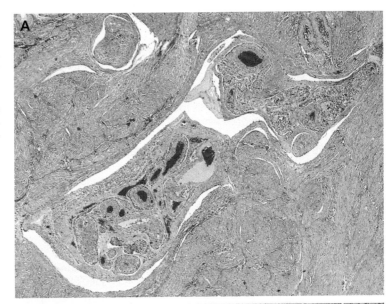

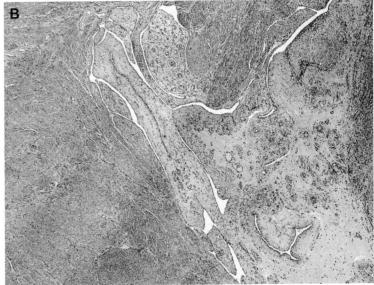

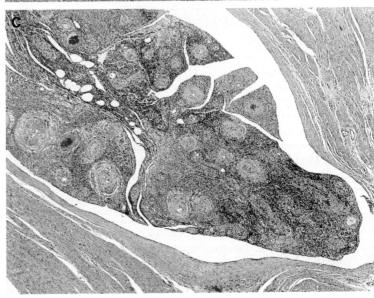

rate).[1,12,15,118–122] Long-term follow-up is recommended for all women diagnosed with STUMP. Many patients with uterine STUMPs are cured by complete resection; however, recurrence or metastasis has been reported in 7% to 36.4% of cases, often after a prolonged period.[15,113,123,124] Predicting which tumors are at an increased risk for aggressive behavior by morphology continues to be a challenge. Some investigators have developed genomic profiling protocols to better predict potential for aggressive behavior.[125,126]

LEIOMYOSARCOMA

Leiomyosarcomas account for 1% to 2% of uterine malignancies.[127] The major histologic types include spindled (conventional), epithelioid, and myxoid, which have differing diagnostic thresholds. When an SMT has features of more than 1 type, overall classification is generally based on the predominant type.

Spindled (Conventional) Leiomyosarcoma

Conventional leiomyosarcomas are the most common uterine sarcoma. Most are diagnosed in women older than 50 years.[127,128] Patients present with nonspecific symptoms, including abnormal uterine bleeding, pelvic pain, or sometimes a palpable pelvic mass.[127,129] Approximately one-half of women present with extrauterine disease.[1] Cases of leiomyosarcoma arising in a leiomyoma have been reported.[130,131]

Gross features

Tumors are typically a singular or predominant mass greater than 5 cm.[127] On cut surface, tumors appear soft and fleshy and range in color from tan to yellow to brown (**Fig. 16**). Tumors may have irregular borders, necrosis, and hemorrhage. Background leiomyomas may be present.[1]

Microscopic features

Conventional leiomyosarcomas are composed of fascicles of spindled cells (**Fig. 17A**). The cells contain abundant eosinophilic cytoplasm with longitudinal fibrils and fusiform nuclei with coarse, sometimes hyperchromatic, chromatin and large nucleoli. Tumor cell nuclei may be markedly pleomorphic, multinucleated, or multilobated (**Fig. 17B**). Moderate to severe cytologic atypia is usually seen focally, multifocally, or diffusely. When present, tumor cell necrosis shows a distinct and abrupt transition from an area of viable, sometimes perivascular, tumor to nonviable tumor (**Fig. 17C**). Distinguishing tumor cell necrosis from early infarct-type necrosis is challenging, with only fair interobserver agreement.[5,132] Leiomyosarcoma commonly infiltrates into myometrium, but this feature is not essential for this diagnosis (**Fig. 17D**).

Conventional leiomyosarcoma is diagnosed when at least 2 of 3 features are present: moderate to severe cytologic atypia, mitotic index greater than or equal to 10 mitotic figures per 10 HPFs, and tumor cell necrosis.[12] When assessing mitotic activity, counts tend to be higher and more reliable when performed in hypercellular areas and parallel to fascicles rather than perpendicular to them.[133] Areas immediately adjacent to necrosis should be avoided for mitotic counts because they are often more mitotically active and can artificially increase the mitotic index. Atypical figures are frequently identified. Osteoclastlike giant cells are found in some leiomyosarcomas.[134] Immunohistochemical studies suggest they are derived from macrophages and likely reactive.[135]

Tumors should not be graded because there is no universally accepted grading system and the utility of grading is controversial.[115] Leiomyosarcomas of the uterus are considered intrinsically high grade.[1]

Conventional leiomyosarcomas are positive for smooth muscle immunohistochemical stains (desmin, h-caldesmon, and smooth muscle actin). Approximately 40% to 50% of tumors are positive for estrogen receptor and progesterone receptor.[136,137] Cell cycle markers such as p16 and p53 are positive in leiomyosarcomas; however, these stains are neither sensitive nor specific for leiomyosarcoma because leiomyomas with bizarre nuclei are also positive for these markers.[138–141] Leiomyosarcomas can be immunoreactive to CD117 (KIT) and DOG1,[142,143] and may also be positive for HMB45.[144]

△△ Differential Diagnosis

Leiomyoma variants including leiomyoma with bizarre nuclei and mitotically active leiomyoma

- Some leiomyoma variants have singular features of leiomyosarcoma, such as severe cytologic atypia or increased mitotic activity. Because SMTs can be heterogeneous, thorough sampling of variants is critical to confidently exclude malignant features (see discussion of leiomyoma variants).

Smooth muscle tumor of uncertain malignant potential

- STUMP is reserved for tumors that show ambiguous or worrisome features but do not meet criteria for leiomyosarcoma (see discussion of STUMP).

Rhabdomyosarcoma

- Rhabdomyosarcoma is rare as a pure tumor of the uterus. Embryonal, spindle cell/sclerosing, and pleomorphic variants have been described. Unlike leiomyosarcoma, rhabdomyosarcoma has cross-striations and is positive for skeletal muscle markers, including myogenin and myoD1.[145] In rare instances, rhabdomyosarcoma and leiomyosarcoma coexist in a single uterine tumor.[146]

Undifferentiated uterine sarcoma

- Undifferentiated uterine sarcomas are high-grade tumors without evidence of a line of differentiation. Undifferentiated tumors are negative for smooth muscle stains.

Carcinosarcoma

- Carcinosarcoma can resemble spindled leiomyosarcoma when there is fascicular architecture of the sarcomatous component. Extensive sampling may be necessary to identify a carcinomatous component. Biopsy or curettage specimens may be particularly challenging because of limited tissue available for evaluation.

Prognosis

Despite aggressive therapy, recurrence and/or metastasis typically occurs within 2 years of diagnosis. Prognosis is best predicted by stage. The overall 5-year survival rate is 15% to 25%, whereas survival rate for stage I and II tumors is 40% to 70%.[1,128,147–154] Tumors confined to the uterus, especially those tumors less than 5 cm, are associated with improved patient survival.[1,151,155–158]

Epithelioid Leiomyosarcoma

Epithelioid leiomyosarcoma is a variant predominantly composed (>50%) of epithelioid cells.[32,33] This variant most commonly occurs in perimenopausal and postmenopausal women.[32,159] Patients present with symptoms akin to conventional leiomyosarcomas.[32,159]

Gross features

Tumors appear grossly similar to conventional leiomyosarcomas and can range in size from 4 to 13 cm.[32,155,159]

Microscopic features

Epithelioid leiomyosarcomas are predominately (>50%) to entirely composed of polygonal to round cells with abundant eosinophilic to clear cytoplasm (**Fig. 18A, B**). Tumor cells are arranged in sheets, nests, and/or cords (**Fig. 18C, D**).[159]

Stromal hyalinization or edema may be present.[32] In addition, rhabdoid cells, osteoclastlike giant cells, and sex cord–like elements have been reported in epithelioid leiomyosarcomas.[32,160,161]

An epithelioid SMT is classified as leiomyosarcoma when at least 2 of 3 features are present: moderate to severe cytologic atypia, mitotic index of at least 3 or 4 mitotic figures per 10 HPFs, and tumor cell necrosis.[32] When only 1 of these features is identified, a diagnosis of epithelioid STUMP may be considered.

The immunophenotype of epithelioid SMTs can be different from conventional SMTs. Epithelioid SMTs can be negative for desmin and h-caldesmon and positive for keratins.[34,35] HDAC8 is a marker of smooth muscle differentiation and has been shown to be consistently positive in epithelioid SMTs.[35]

Differential Diagnosis

ΔΔ

Epithelioid smooth muscle tumor of uncertain malignant potential

- Epithelioid STUMP, although poorly defined, should be reserved for tumors that do not satisfy criteria for epithelioid leiomyosarcoma.

Poorly differentiated carcinoma

- Poorly differentiated carcinomas are negative for smooth muscle markers and should have more robust immunoreactivity to keratins than epithelioid SMTs.

Malignant perivascular epithelioid cell tumor

- Malignant PEComas are composed of epithelioid cells typically arranged in a nested architecture and can have significant cytologic atypia, increased mitotic activity, and tumor cell necrosis similar to epithelioid leiomyosarcomas.[162,163] Both SMTs and PEComas express smooth muscle markers and HMB45; however, PEComas often express melan-A, but SMTs usually do not.[36–38]

Alveolar soft part sarcoma

- Alveolar soft part sarcoma is composed of polygonal cells with eosinophilic, granular cytoplasm and often prominent cytoplasmic membranes arranged in nests. In contrast with epithelioid leiomyosarcoma, alveolar soft part sarcoma does not express smooth muscle markers and is positive for TFE3 secondary to *TFE3-ASPL* gene fusion found in all tumors. Genetic testing for *TFE3* rearrangement or *TFE3-ASPL* fusion can be helpful in challenging cases.

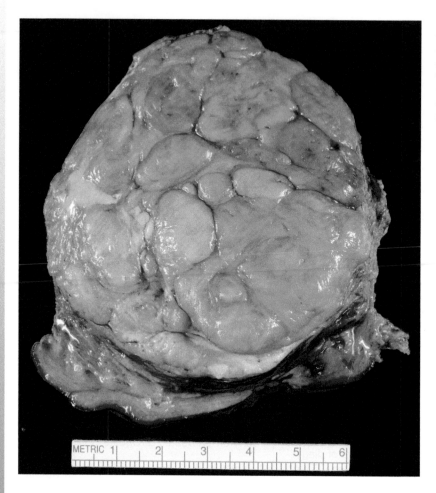

Fig. 16. Spindled or conventional leiomyosarcoma typically presents a solitary mass with a soft, fleshy cut surface that may or may not have gross evidence of necrosis.

Prognosis

Epithelioid leiomyosarcomas are aggressive and are associated with a poor prognosis.

Myxoid Leiomyosarcoma

Myxoid leiomyosarcoma is a variant of leiomyosarcoma with an extensively myxoid matrix. Women are typically postmenopausal at diagnosis and present with similar symptoms to conventional leiomyosarcomas.[31,164,165]

Gross features

Tumors are solitary, large masses that range from 3 to 33 cm (mean, 10.8 cm).[31] On cut surface, they are tan to yellow to gray and vary from firm to rubbery to soft. Mucoid and/or gelatinous material is frequently exuded when the tumor is sectioned. Necrotic or hemorrhagic foci may be present.[31,165]

Microscopic features

Myxoid leiomyosarcomas are malignant SMTs with abundantly myxoid stroma (**Fig. 19**A). The quantity of myxoid matrix necessary to classify a leiomyosarcoma as myxoid varies because studies have used different minimums, from greater than or equal to 30% to greater than or equal to 60%.[30,31,164] Areas with copious myxoid stroma appear hypocellular with sparsely arranged spindled to oval to stellate-shaped cells set in abundant pale-staining, eosinophilic to basophilic stroma (**Fig. 19**B). Other areas with less myxoid stroma may have more fascicular architecture and appear more cellular. Most myxoid leiomyosarcomas have an irregular interface with projections into myometrium and/or frank infiltration.[31]

Like other uterine SMTs, cytologic atypia, mitotic index, and tumor cell necrosis are considered for classification of myxoid SMTs. Of these features, 2 of 3 are required to designate a myxoid SMT as leiomyosarcoma.[30,31,164] Importantly, the mitotic index for myxoid SMTs is lowered to greater than or equal to 2 mitotic figures per 10 HPFs.[30] When only 1 feature is present, classification as myxoid STUMP should be considered.

Fig. *17.* Morphologic criteria to classify a spindled SMT (*A*) as leiomyosarcoma require at least 2 of 3 features: (1) moderate to severe cytologic atypia (*B*), (2) mitotic index greater than or equal to 10 mitotic figures per 10 HPFs, (3) tumor cell necrosis

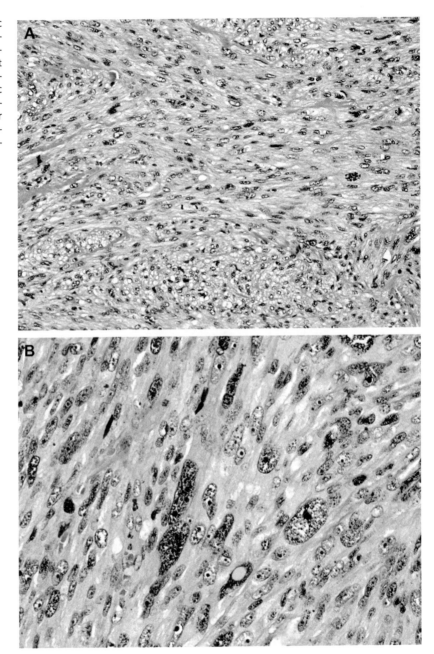

Myometrial infiltration may be a prognostically significant finding in myxoid leiomyosarcoma. Most myxoid leiomyosarcomas have infiltrative borders, but well-circumscribed myxoid SMTs that satisfy criteria for leiomyosarcoma have been reported. In these studies, no patient with a well-circumscribed myxoid leiomyosarcoma experienced recurrence or metastasis. Some investigators have suggested that a designation of STUMP may be more appropriate for well-circumscribed myxoid SMTs meeting criteria for leiomyosarcoma until more data are available.[31,164]

Myxoid leiomyosarcomas are positive for smooth muscle markers by immunohistochemistry, with smooth muscle actin being most sensitive. Estrogen receptor is positive in only a minority (29.4%) of myxoid leiomyosarcomas.[31] Alcian blue and colloidal iron stains can be used to confirm myxoid matrix.

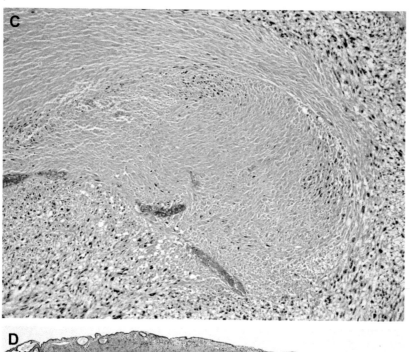

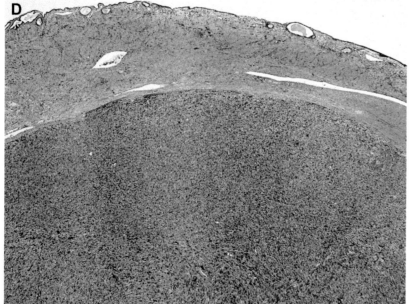

Fig. 17. (continued). (C). Infiltration into myometrium is common but not essential for a diagnosis of leiomyosarcoma; this example of uterine leiomyosarcoma is well circumscribed *(D).*

 Differential Diagnosis

Myxoid leiomyoma

- Thorough sampling is critical in myxoid SMTs because myxoid leiomyoma is essentially a diagnosis of exclusion. Myxoid leiomyoma should be diagnosed when an SMT is well circumscribed, has mild cytologic atypia, fewer than 2 mitotic figures per 10 HPFs, and lacks tumor cell necrosis.

Myxoid smooth muscle tumor of uncertain malignant potential

- The diagnosis of myxoid STUMP should be considered when tumors have 1 of 3 features of malignancy (significant cytologic atypia, mitotic index of $\geq$2 figures per 10 HPFs, tumor cell necrosis). This diagnosis may also be considered in atypical and mitotically active myxoid SMTs that are well circumscribed.

Inflammatory myofibroblastic tumor

- Inflammatory myofibroblastic tumors have myxoid stroma, infiltrative borders, and expression of smooth muscle markers. Most reported uterine inflammatory myofibroblastic tumors have an underlying *ALK* rearrangement. ALK immunohistochemistry with or without genetic confirmation can be helpful in difficult cases.[31]

BCOR-associated high-grade endometrial stromal sarcomas

- High-grade endometrial stromal sarcomas with *ZC3H7B-BCOR* fusion or *BCOR* internal tandem duplication have myxoid features, myometrial infiltration, and lymphovascular invasion.[166,167] Molecular genetic testing for *BCOR* alterations is currently the most reliable method to identify these tumors. BCOR immunohistochemistry identifies a subset of *BCOR*-altered high-grade endometrial stromal sarcomas, but is also consistently expressed by *YWHAE-NUTM2* high-grade endometrial stromal sarcomas.[168]

Prognosis

Patients diagnosed with infiltrative myxoid leiomyosarcoma have a poor prognosis. Although data are limited, overall outcome and survival seem more favorable than for conventional leiomyosarcomas.[127]

Lipoleiomyosarcoma

Lipoleiomyosarcomas are high-grade tumors with smooth muscle and adipocytic differentiation. Women diagnosed with lipoleiomyosarcomas are typically perimenopausal to postmenopausal age and present with symptoms similar to conventional leiomyosarcomas.[169]

Gross features

Tumors are large, with some reported up to 16 cm in diameter.[169] On cut surface, they are tan to yellow and may be gelatinous, necrotic, and/or hemorrhagic.[169–171]

Microscopic features

Lipoleiomyosarcomas have a mixture of cytologically atypical smooth muscle cells and mature adipocytes, and a variable quantity of lipoblasts (**Fig. 20**A–C). Although the lipomatous and smooth muscle components can vary in proportion, the SMT cells predominate and resemble conventional leiomyosarcomas. Mature adipocytes are the next most frequent component. Lipoblasts, either typical or atypical, are the least common component and have scalloped, enlarged hyperchromatic nuclei and vacuolated cytoplasm (**Fig. 20**D). Although there are no defined criteria for lipoleiomyosarcomas, reported cases satisfy criteria for conventional leiomyosarcomas. Immunohistochemically, the spindled cells are positive for smooth muscle markers and adipocytes, and lipoblasts are positive for S100 protein.[169,170]

Differential Diagnosis

Liposarcoma

- Myxoid/round cell, pleomorphic, and well-differentiated liposarcomas have been described in the uterus and can be seen in association with conventional leiomyosarcomas, lipoleiomyosarcomas, conventional leiomyomas, and lipoleiomyomas.[172]

Prognosis

Lipoleiomyosarcomas are aggressive tumors with a poor prognosis.[169,170]

DISSEMINATED OR METASTATIC GROWTH PATTERNS

Cytologically bland and mitotically inactive SMTs of the female genital tract may disseminate, metastasize, or have a distinct growth pattern that can be particularly worrisome in patients with a history of SMTs and raise concern for previous misclassification of prior tumors. Importantly, these entities do not fit the morphologic criteria for a leiomyosarcoma and have an indolent clinical course.

Disseminated Peritoneal Leiomyomatosis

Disseminated peritoneal leiomyomatosis (DPL) is characterized by widespread tumors and/or tumorlets (tens to hundreds) involving pelvic and abdominal peritoneal surfaces. Women are usually of reproductive age and asymptomatic but, depending on the size or distribution, can experience symptoms of pain or pressure. In some patients, tumorlets are found incidentally in the

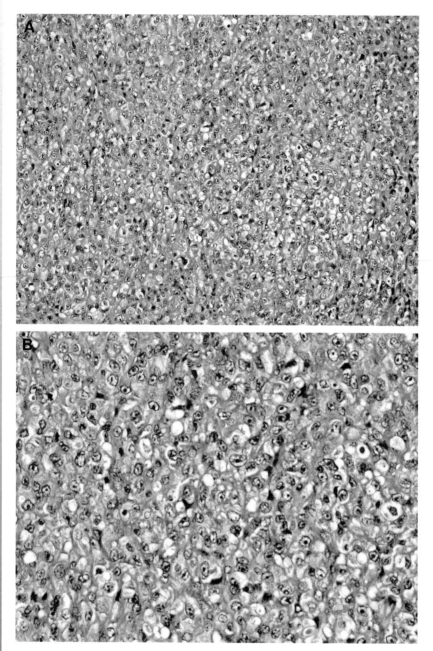

Fig. 18. Epithelioid leiomyosarcomas are predominately (>50%) to entirely composed of polygonal to round cells with abundant eosinophilic to clear cytoplasm (*A, B*). Some tumors have sheetlike architecture (*B*) or are nested and/or corded

work-up or treatment of an unrelated condition. DPL is frequently associated with a history of uterine leiomyomas.[173–176] Some cases have a familial pattern of inheritance.[177]

Although the cause of DPL is unclear, there is a strong association with increased hormonal stimulation. Several cases have been reported during pregnancy or after long-term exogenous estrogen exposure, such as from oral contraceptives, or endogenously increased estrogen production, such as from a fibrothecoma or adult granulosa cell tumor.[176,178–180] Whether these lesions are derived from subperitoneal mesenchyme or a metastatic process is

Fig. 18. (*continued*). (*C, D*). An epithelioid SMT should be classified as leiomyosarcoma when at least 2 of 3 features are present: (1) moderate to severe cytologic atypia, (2) mitotic index of at least 3 or 4 mitotic figures per 10 HPFs, (3) tumor cell necrosis. Infiltration is an important feature of myxoid leiomyosarcoma.

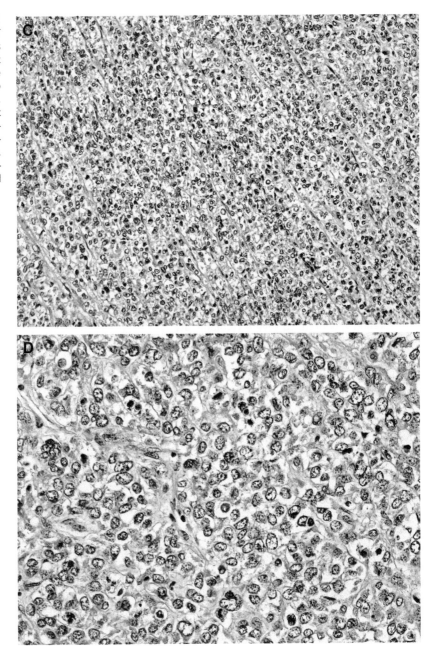

uncertain; however, X-inactivation studies suggest DPL may be a clonal neoplastic process.[181]

Gross features

Tumors and tumorlets are superficially located on peritoneal surfaces and appear similar to conventional leiomyomas grossly. Most lesions are small, ranging from microscopic to less than 5 cm (but they can be larger).[175,176]

Microscopic features

Tumors and tumorlets are well circumscribed and morphologically resemble conventional leiomyomas (**Fig. 21**A). Cytologic atypia and mitotic activity are minimal (**Fig. 21**B).[175] Endometriosis and/or endosalpingiosis can be seen abutting or admixed with these lesions (**Fig. 21**C), and foci of epithelioid cells that may resemble sex cord–like elements can be found.[176,182–185]

Differential Diagnosis

Peritoneal carcinomatosis

- Peritoneal carcinomatosis and DPL have overlapping clinical features. Given that DPL is often discovered incidentally during surgery or cesarean section, an intraoperative frozen section can be helpful to exclude carcinomatosis.

Iatrogenic pelvic leiomyomatosis

- Iatrogenic pelvic leiomyomatosis occurs in patients with a history of laparoscopic myomectomy or morcellated hysterectomy (discussed in relation to iatrogenic peritoneal leiomyomatosis).

Metastatic leiomyosarcoma

- Metastatic leiomyosarcoma can spread multifocally within the abdominopelvic cavity and should show frankly malignant features, including moderate to severe cytologic atypia, increased mitotic index, and/or tumor cell necrosis.

Metastasizing leiomyoma

- Metastasizing leiomyomas typically have significantly fewer nodules and most commonly involve the lung.

Nodular and diffuse peritoneal decidual reaction/ectopic decidua

- Women with a history of cesarean section can develop multiple small peritoneal nodules at the site of surgical incision that clinically mimic DPL. However, these nodules are composed of aggregates of decidualized cells.[186]

Prognosis

Most women with DPL are asymptomatic. Complications related to mechanical obstruction can occur, including bowel obstruction and hydronephrosis. Although there is no standard management of DPL, surgical excision can be performed to achieve symptomatic relief.[187] Stasis in growth or regression of nodules can result after cessation or removal of the hormonal stimulus. In contrast, recurrence can develop with return of the hormonal stimulus, such as pregnancy or hormone replacement therapy.[175,176,188] Treatment with gonadotropin-releasing hormone agonists may be considered.[189]

Iatrogenic Peritoneal Leiomyomatosis

Iatrogenic peritoneal leiomyomatosis, sometimes considered synonymous with DPL, occurs in women with a history of uterine leiomyomas who underwent surgical myomectomy or morcellated hysterectomy. Fragmentation of tumor can lead to dispersal of fragments onto peritoneal surfaces. Iatrogenic peritoneal leiomyomatosis may be diagnosed months to years after surgery. Depending on the size and location of the tumors, women may or may not experience symptoms. Increased awareness of iatrogenic peritoneal leiomyomatosis has prompted modifications of surgical technique to prevent tumor dissemination.[190–193]

Gross features

Tumor distribution and gross appearance often resembles those of DPL.

Microscopic features

Iatrogenic peritoneal leiomyomas are characterized by peritoneal surface involvement by leiomyomatous tumors.[191]

Differential Diagnosis

Disseminated peritoneal leiomyomatosis

- DPL typically occurs in reproductive-aged women exposed to increased hormonal stimulation, whereas iatrogenic peritoneal leiomyomatosis is a mechanical process associated with a history of laparoscopic myomectomy or morcellated hysterectomy.

Prognosis

Iatrogenic peritoneal leiomyomatosis is a benign condition. If symptomatic, tumors can be managed by surgical excision.[190,191]

Other tumor types have been reported to disseminate by similar mechanisms, including endometrial stromal sarcomas, STUMPs, and leiomyosarcomas. Peritoneal seeding should be considered as a possibility in patients with a history of surgical procedures for uterine tumors.[190,191]

Metastasizing Leiomyoma

Metastasizing leiomyomas occur at extrauterine sites in premenopausal and perimenopausal women with a concurrent or antecedent history of leiomyoma. Women may have undergone hysterectomy years to decades before presentation with extrauterine lesions. Patients are often asymptomatic and the finding is often discovered incidentally in the work-up of an unrelated issue. Most examples involve the lung and/or pleura as multiple bilateral

Fig. 19. (*A*, *B*) Myxoid leiomyosarcomas have abundant pale-staining, eosinophilic to basophilic stroma that results in a hypocellular appearance from separation of tumor cells into individual cells or small nests or cords. Current recommendations to classify a myxoid SMT as myxoid leiomyosarcoma are that at least 2 of 3 features be present: (1) significant cytologic atypia, (2) mitotic index of greater than or equal to 2 mitotic figures per 10 HPFs, (3) tumor cell necrosis.

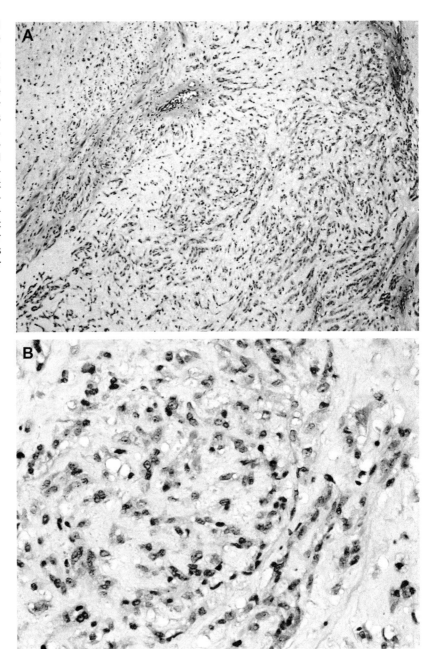

nodules; however, some cases are unilateral and/or solitary.[194–196] Less common sites of involvement include appendix, rib, vertebrae, heart, and retroperitoneum.[197]

Metastasizing leiomyomas were initially thought to be primary tumors of the lung and were classified as fibrous hamartomas.[198] Follow-up studies found a strong association with a history of uterine leiomyomas as well as morphologic and immunophenotypic similarities (including hormone receptor expression) of these lung tumors to uterine leiomyomas.[199] Recent molecular data support a possible clonal relationship between uterine leiomyomas and metastasizing leiomyomas, suggesting spread by lymphovascular dissemination.[200,201] In addition, recurrent cytogenetic abnormalities, specifically 19q and 22q terminal deletions, have been

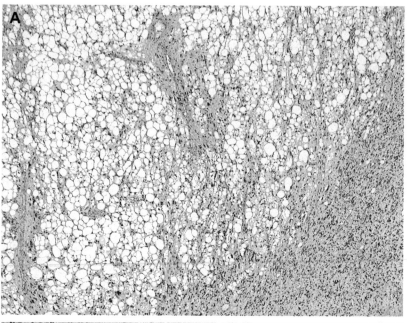

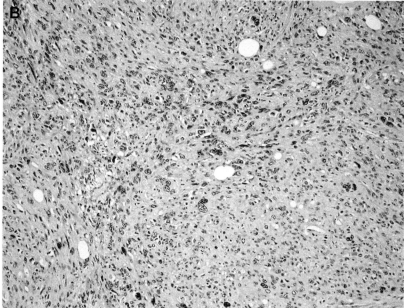

Fig. 20. (A–D) Lipoleio-myosarcomas have a mixture of atypical smooth muscle cells, mature adipocytes, and lipoblasts. Although the lipomatous and smooth muscle components can vary in proportion, the SMT component predominates and resembles conventional leiomyosarcoma. Although there are no defined criteria for lipoleiomyosarcomas, reported cases satisfy criteria for conventional leiomyosarcomas.

reported.[202] These same cytogenetic findings have been observed in 3% of uterine leiomyomas, suggesting that a specific subset are prone to metastasizing.[202,203]

Gross features

Gross features resemble conventional leiomyomas of the uterus, with some lung lesions developing cystic change.[196,204]

Microscopic features

Metastasizing leiomyomas are predominantly spindled tumors that have no significant cytologic atypia or mitotic activity and lack tumor cell necrosis (**Fig. 22**A, B). Lung lesions can entrap bronchoalveolar epithelium or present as small, inconspicuous interstitial nodules (**Fig. 22**C).[204] A metastasizing lipoleiomyoma variant has also been described.[205]

Fig. 20. (continued).

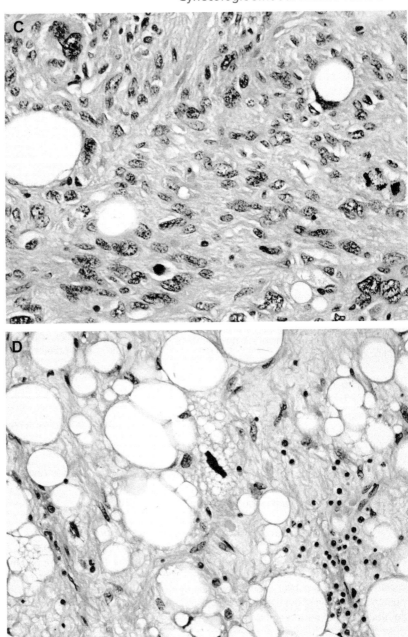

Differential Diagnosis

Metastatic leiomyosarcoma

- Metastatic leiomyosarcoma should have some combination of moderate to severe cytologic atypia, increased mitotic activity, and tumor cell necrosis.

Lymphangioleiomyomatosis

- Unlike metastasizing leiomyoma, lymphangioleiomyomatosis (LAM) results in progressive destruction of lung parenchyma. Smooth muscle cells of metastasizing leiomyoma and perivascular epithelioid cells of LAM are both positive for smooth muscle markers and HMB45 but LAM expresses melan-A, whereas metastasizing leiomyoma generally does not.[206]

Pulmonary hamartoma

- In contrast with metastasizing leiomyoma, pulmonary hamartomas contain disordered proliferations of cartilage, smooth muscle, adipocytes, and vessels.[207]

Epstein-Barr virus–associated primary SMTs

- Epstein-Barr virus–associated primary SMTs of the lung occur in the setting of immunosuppression or immunodeficiency. The Epstein-Barr encoding region can be detected by in situ hybridization.[208]

Prognosis

Metastasizing leiomyoma generally has an indolent clinical course. Resection can be curative in patients with an isolated lesion or limited quantity of lesions, but multifocality may preclude resection. There are no standard management guidelines for metastasizing leiomyoma. Long-term surveillance is warranted when residual nodules are present. Hormonal suppression may be considered to prevent progression, which has been reported in 8.3% to 30% of cases involving the lung.[209–211] Regression has been observed following menopause, delivery if pregnant, or surgical or chemical castration.[210,212]

EXTRAUTERINE SMOOTH MUSCLE TUMORS

Extrauterine SMTs of the female genital tract are rare, resulting in limited understanding of their underlying biology, morphologic spectrum, and clinical course. More recently, the 2014 WHO tumor nomenclature and risk stratification criteria for uterine SMTs have been applied to and validated for SMTs of the ovary, broad ligament, vagina, and vulva.[213–215]

SMOOTH MUSCLE TUMORS OF THE OVARY

SMTs of the ovary account for less than 1% of all ovarian neoplasms. Ovarian SMTs have been speculated to arise from hilar blood vessels, smooth muscle metaplasia of ovarian stroma, smooth muscle metaplasia of endometriotic stroma, or smooth muscle from mature cystic teratomas.[216–219]

Ovarian Leiomyoma

Ovarian leiomyomas occur in women of reproductive to postmenopausal age, but largely occur in premenopausal women.[213,220] Most tumors are asymptomatic and discovered incidentally, but some present with symptoms of a pelvic mass.[213,220] In rare examples, Meigs syndrome can develop or tumor rupture can occur.[213,221] Leiomyomas are typically unilateral, although reports of bilateral cases have been described.[213,220,222,223] Ovarian leiomyomas are often associated with synchronous uterine leiomyomas.[213,224] Cases concomitant with intravenous leiomyomatosis or DPL have been reported.[176,213]

Gross features

Tumors are grossly similar to uterine leiomyomas and range in size from less than 1 cm to greater than 20 cm.[213,220,224] In one series, cellular leiomyomas were larger on average (mean, 10 cm) than conventional leiomyomas (mean, 5.2 cm).[213]

Microscopic features

Ovarian leiomyomas have analogous histologic features to their uterine counterparts. Conventional leiomyomas are most common, but cellular, bizarre nuclei, mitotically active, myxoid, epithelioid, and lipoleiomyoma variants have also been reported.[213,220,222,225,226] Edema, infarct-type necrosis, hyalinization, hydropic change, and cyst formation may be present. Pregnancy-associated tumors tend to have increased cellularity, mitotic activity, and infarct-type necrosis.[213]

⚠️ **Differential Diagnosis**

Fibroma/cellular fibroma/mitotically active cellular fibroma

- Fibromas are common fibroblastic stromal tumors that often have intersecting fascicles resembling SMTs, but their occasional storiform arrangement, more prominent collagen production, and slightly wavy nuclei allow morphologic differentiation from SMTs. Fibromas are positive for sex cord markers, including inhibin (variable), calretinin (variable), and SF-1 (consistently positive), whereas SMTs are negative for these markers. Fibromas can be positive for smooth muscle actin, but are generally negative for desmin.[227]

Sclerosing stromal tumor

- Sclerosing stromal tumors are most common in young women and have zonation or pseudolobules of cellular spindled cells that alternate with acellular edematous and sclerotic areas. Dilated and branching thin-walled vasculature is a frequent feature. Sclerosing stromal tumors are positive for inhibin, calretinin, and SF1 immunohistochemical stains, whereas SMTs are negative.[228]

Low-grade endometrial/endometrioid stromal sarcoma

- Metastatic low-grade endometrial and primary low-grade endometrioid stromal sarcomas may resemble SMTs, especially those that are hypercellular (discussed in relation to cellular/hypercellular uterine leiomyomas). Metastatic low-grade endometrial stromal sarcomas should have a history of a uterine primary. Primary ovarian low-grade endometrioid stromal sarcomas are often associated with endometriosis.[229,230]

Prognosis

Ovarian leiomyomas are benign. When complete resection is performed, it is curative.[213,222]

Ovarian Smooth Muscle Tumor of Uncertain Malignant Potential

STUMPs of the ovary are rare. The few reported examples occurred in women in their fourth to seventh decade (mean, 57 years) who were either asymptomatic or presented with pelvic pain.[213]

Gross features

Tumors are grossly similar to uterine STUMPs and range in size from 4 to 10.3 cm (mean, 6 cm).[213]

Microscopic features

The few described cases had spindled and/or epithelioid differentiation and moderate to severe cytologic atypia without significant mitotic activity and tumor cell necrosis, and did not meet criteria for leiomyoma or leiomyosarcoma.[213]

Prognosis

The prognosis of ovarian STUMP is unknown because of limited data. Long-term follow-up is recommended.

Ovarian Leiomyosarcoma

Women diagnosed with leiomyosarcoma of the ovary are usually postmenopausal and present with pelvic pain or symptoms related to an adnexal mass.[213,231,232]

Gross features

Conventional, myxoid, or epithelioid leiomyosarcomas have been described and show similar gross features to those of the uterus.[213,233,234] Ovarian leiomyosarcomas are large and range in size from 4 to 35 cm.[213] Capsular rupture, adhesions, and/or infiltration into the adjacent structures can occur.[213] Normal ovarian tissue may be difficult to identify because of tumor overgrowth.

Microscopic features

Conventional, myxoid, and epithelioid leiomyosarcomas have analogous morphologic features to

uterine sarcomas, and the same diagnostic criteria for uterine leiomyosarcomas are valid for ovarian leiomyosarcomas.[213]

Differential Diagnosis

Metastatic leiomyosarcoma

- Leiomyosarcomas originating from the uterus can present with extrauterine spread. Before assigning a leiomyosarcoma as primary of the ovary, a uterine primary should be excluded.

Prognosis

In a study of 21 patients with leiomyosarcoma of the ovary, 71% developed recurrent disease after an average of 19 months and more than half died of disease after an average of 24 months.[213]

SMOOTH MUSCLE TUMORS OF THE CERVIX

Malignant mesenchymal cervical tumors constitute less than 1% of all malignancies of this site.[235] Of all cervical mesenchymal tumors, rhabdomyosarcoma is most common, with SMTs being the next most common.[236]

Leiomyoma

Cervical leiomyomas are uncommonly reported and their true incidence is unclear. In a series of 661 consecutive hysterectomy specimens, only 4 cervical leiomyomas were identified or 0.6% of specimens.[237] It is possible that their incidence may be higher because smaller cervical leiomyomas can be subclinical and therefore are undiagnosed.[236] Cervical leiomyomas occur in prepubertal to postmenopausal patients but are usually diagnosed in women in their second to fifth decade of life.[235] Smaller leiomyomas can be asymptomatic, but larger tumors can cause symptoms of vaginal bleeding, obstetric complications, prolapse, urinary retention, or sepsis.[236,238–243]

Gross features

Tumors are grossly similar to leiomyomas of the corpus and range in size from 0.3 to 14 cm.[237,244]

Microscopic features

Most cervical leiomyomas are spindled.[235,237] A rare case of a leiomyoma with bizarre nuclei has been reported.[235] Leiomyomas of the cervix may be exophytic and show superficial ulceration, inflammation, and necrosis.

Differential Diagnosis

Myofibroblastoma (superficial myofibroblastoma, superficial cervicovaginal myofibroblastoma)
- Myofibroblastomas most frequently occur in the vagina but can also develop in the cervix and vulva. Tumors range in cellularity and are composed of bland spindled, ovoid, or stellate cells arranged in vague fascicles with myxoid or collagenous stroma. The small, bland cells of myofibroblastoma differ from the plump spindle cells of SMTs.[244,245]

Endocervical-type adenomyoma
- Endocervical adenomyoma presents as an intramural or exophytic polypoid mass. Although they often show a prominent smooth muscle proliferation, adenomyomas have benign glandular component that is often associated with endometrial stroma.

Differential Diagnosis

Adenosarcoma with sarcomatous overgrowth
- Although sarcomatous overgrowth of adenosarcoma may overrun most of the tumor, at least some portion should have more characteristic phyllodelike architecture with periglandular condensation. Identification of a biphasic neoplasm excludes leiomyosarcoma.

Embryonal rhabdomyosarcoma
- In contrast with leiomyosarcoma, embryonal rhabdomyosarcoma should have subepithelial condensation (cambium layer), alternating hypocellularity and hypercellularity, cross-striations, and occasional intermixed cartilage. Rhabdomyosarcoma, unlike leiomyosarcoma, is positive for skeletal muscle markers myogenin and myoD1.[145]

Prognosis
Cervical leiomyomas are benign and surgical excision is curative.

SMOOTH MUSCLE TUMOR OF UNCERTAIN MALIGNANT POTENTIAL

There have been no reported cases of cervical STUMP.

Leiomyosarcoma

Leiomyosarcomas of the cervix occur in women in their fourth to sixth decade of life and cause abnormal vaginal bleeding and/or abdominopelvic pain.[235,246] On clinical examination, tumors may protrude from the cervix as an exophytic, polypoid mass or circumferentially expand the cervix, causing thickening and distension.[246]

Gross features
Tumors can measure as much as 30 cm in diameter.[247] Spindled, epithelioid, and myxoid leiomyosarcomas have been reported as primary cervical tumors and have identical gross features to uterine corpus leiomyosarcomas.[246–253]

Microscopic features
Classification criteria for cervical spindled, epithelioid, and myxoid leiomyosarcomas are presumably the same as corpus sarcomas, although this has not been formally evaluated.[246–253] Similar to leiomyosarcomas of the corpus, osteoclastlike giant cells have been reported in cervical tumors.[254,255]

Prognosis
In the largest series of 8 patients with leiomyosarcoma of the cervix, 6 (75%) patients died of disease, of whom 4 (75%) died of complications secondary to distant hematogenous metastasis.[246]

SMOOTH MUSCLE TUMORS OF THE BROAD LIGAMENT

SMTs of the broad ligament are the most common mesenchymal tumors of this site.[256] Before designating a tumor as a broad ligament primary, secondary involvement by a uterine or ovarian SMT must be excluded.

Leiomyoma

Of the various visceral ligaments of the endopelvic fascia, the broad ligament is the most commonly involved (**Fig. 23**).[215,257] Women vary from premenopausal to postmenopausal when diagnosed (mean, 55 years) and are usually asymptomatic, with tumors discovered incidentally by radiologic imaging or intraoperatively for an unrelated condition.[215] Larger tumors can cause symptoms of abdominopelvic pain, abdominal distension, or Meigs syndrome.[258–260]

Gross features
Leiomyomas of these sites are grossly similar to uterine leiomyomas but can develop various degrees of edema and cystic degeneration. They range in size from 0.5 to 30.3 cm (mean, 7.5 cm).[215]

Microscopic features

In a series of 57 SMTs of the adnexal and uterine visceral ligaments and adnexal connective tissue, almost all were spindled leiomyomas.[215] Variants are rare, with isolated reports of lipoleiomyoma.[257,260,261]

Differential Diagnosis

Endometriosis with smooth muscle metaplasia

- Endometriosis frequently involves adnexal tissues, and smooth muscle metaplasia can be induced from endometriotic stroma. Even when florid, if smooth muscle is intermixed with endometriosis it is likely metaplastic.[262,263]

Prognosis

Leiomyomas are cured by complete resection.

Smooth Muscle Tumor of Uncertain Malignant Potential

A total of 3 cases of STUMP have been reported (2 broad ligament and 1 adnexal connective tissue). Women ranged from 45 to 70 year old (mean, 61 years) and presented with pelvic pain.[215,264]

Gross features

STUMPs have identical gross findings to uterine STUMPs and range from 7.5 to 12.9 cm (mean, 10.8 cm) (**Fig. 24**).[215,264]

Microscopic features

The few reports of STUMPs were conventional and showed tumor cell necrosis alone, moderate cytologic atypia with a mitotic index of 3 mitotic figures per 10 HPFs, or a combination of moderate cytologic atypia with a mitotic index of 1 mitotic figure per 10 HPFs and tumor cell necrosis.[215,264]

Prognosis

Long-term follow-up is recommended. In 2 cases, neither patient experienced recurrence or metastasis after follow-up of 126 and 178 months.[215]

Leiomyosarcoma

Women are typically perimenopausal or postmenopausal at time of diagnosis (mean, 67 years).[215] Patient symptoms include abdominopelvic pain, abdominal distension, a palpable mass, vaginal bleeding, and/or mechanical obstruction of adjacent organs when the mass is bulky or infiltrative.[265–267] A case of leiomyosarcoma arising in a leiomyoma of the broad ligament has been reported.[268]

Gross features

Tumors vary in size from 3.2 to 21 cm (mean, 10.6 cm) and have analogous gross features to uterine leiomyosarcomas. In the largest case series of 8 cases, 6 (75%) originated from the broad ligament and 2 (25%) originated from the adnexal connective tissue.[215] Other reported sites of origin include the round ligament and parametrium.[257,269,270]

Microscopic features

Leiomyosarcomas of the visceral ligaments have similar histomorphologic features to uterine leiomyosarcomas and may be classified using uterine criteria.[215] A rare case with osteoclastlike giant cells and rhabdoid cells was reported in the broad ligament.[271]

Differential Diagnosis

Metastatic leiomyosarcoma

- Patients with uterine leiomyosarcomas can present with extrauterine disease. Because broad ligament leiomyosarcomas are much less common than uterine leiomyosarcomas, metastasis should first be excluded.

Gastrointestinal stromal tumor

- Gastrointestinal stromal tumors (GISTs) tend to have more fusiform cells arranged in a less overtly fascicular architecture. GISTs and leiomyosarcomas can both be positive for DOG-1 and CD117. A significant number of GISTs are positive for muscle markers.[272] Knowledge of the specific location of the mass and whether there is continuity with the gastrointestinal tract are generally the most helpful findings.

Prognosis

Leiomyosarcomas of the broad ligament are high-grade, aggressive tumors. In patients with leiomyosarcomas of these tissue sites, 6 of 8 patients (75%) experienced recurrence and died of disease 3 to 111 months following diagnosis.

SMOOTH MUSCLE TUMORS OF THE VAGINA

SMTs are the most common mesenchymal neoplasms of the vagina.[1]

Leiomyoma

Vaginal leiomyomas occur in premenopausal to postmenopausal women (mean, 50 years) and can be asymptomatic or cause symptoms such as dyspareunia, vaginal bleeding, a sensation of prolapse, and/or urinary tract pressure.[214,273–275]

Gross features

Tumors are grossly identical to uterine leiomyomas and range in size from 0.6 to 7 cm (mean, 2.6 cm).[214]

Microscopic features

Most vaginal leiomyomas are spindled.[214] Mitotically active leiomyoma and leiomyoma with bizarre nuclei have been described as primary vaginal tumors, but variants at this site are infrequent.[214,276,277]

 Differential Diagnosis

Myofibroblastoma (superficial myofibroblastoma, superficial cervicovaginal myofibroblastoma)

- Myofibroblastomas are composed of bland spindled, ovoid, or stellate cells arranged in vague fascicles with myxoid or collagenous stroma. The small, bland cells of myofibroblastoma differ from plump spindle cells of SMTs.[244,245]

Postoperative spindle cell nodule

- Women who have undergone a recent surgical procedure may develop a reactive nodule of mitotically active spindled cells growing in fascicles.[278] Spindle cell nodules should not show significant cytologic atypia or tumor cell necrosis and are negative for smooth muscle markers by immunohistochemistry.

Prognosis

Vaginal leiomyomas are benign. Complete surgical removal is curative.

SMOOTH MUSCLE TUMOR OF UNCERTAIN MALIGNANT POTENTIAL

There have been no reported cases of STUMP arising in the vagina.

Leiomyosarcoma

Leiomyosarcomas usually develop in premenopausal to postmenopausal women (mean, 53 years) and patients present with symptoms of abdominopelvic pain and/or abnormal vaginal bleeding. On physical examination, tumors may appear as a raised submucosal mass that can clinically resemble a cyst.[214,279–282] Some women have a history of pelvic irradiation.[283]

Gross features

Vaginal leiomyosarcomas are grossly similar to leiomyosarcomas of the uterus. In one series, 11 conventional leiomyosarcomas ranged in size from 3.5 to 9 cm (mean, 5.9 cm) and 1 myxoid leiomyosarcoma measured 4 cm.[214]

Microscopic features

Spindled leiomyosarcomas are the most frequent primary vaginal tumors, but individual cases of myxoid leiomyosarcoma and lipoleiomyosarcoma have been reported.[214,284]

The rarity of vaginal leiomyosarcoma has made development of risk stratification criteria challenging. Vaginal SMT criteria were first proposed in 1979 and required that moderate to severe cytologic atypia and a mitotic index of greater than or equal to 5 mitotic figures per 10 HPFs were necessary to classify an SMT as malignant. Infiltrative margins alone were also a sufficient finding for a diagnosis of leiomyosarcoma.[274] Application of these and the 2014 WHO uterine SMT criteria to a large series of vaginal SMTs found WHO uterine SMT criteria were more sensitive (88.9% vs 100%) and specific (90.2% vs 100%) in predicting malignant potential of conventional SMTs.[214,274] It was recommended that the WHO uterine criteria be adopted for the classification of vaginal SMTs.[214]

Vaginal myxoid and epithelioid SMTs are infrequent and there has yet to be a large series to assess validity of uterine SMT criteria for these tumors. The 1 reported case of myxoid leiomyosarcoma had significant cytologic atypia, more than or equal to 2 mitotic figures per 10 HPFs, and tumor cell necrosis as well as infiltrative borders, satisfying uterine criteria for myxoid leiomyosarcoma.[214]

 Differential Diagnosis

Melanoma

- Melanoma can be spindled or epithelioid, and may or may not contain melanin pigment. By immunohistochemistry, melanoma expresses melanocytic markers (S100 protein, HMB45, melan-A, SOX10) and is negative for smooth muscle markers. Leiomyosarcomas can express HMB45 but generally in a focal to patchy distribution. A panel of markers is ideal when melanoma is a differential consideration.

Prognosis

In 11 patients diagnosed with conventional leiomyosarcoma of the vagina, 8 (73%) experienced disease recurrence and 4 died of disease (36%) over an interval of 2 to 234 months. The 1 patient with vaginal myxoid leiomyosarcoma experienced multiple pelvic recurrences before eventually dying of disease.[214]

SMOOTH MUSCLE TUMORS OF THE VULVA

SMTs are the most common mesenchymal neoplasms of the vulva.[1]

Leiomyoma

Vulvar leiomyomas occur in premenopausal to postmenopausal women (mean, 52 years).[214] Patients present with a slow-growing, painless mass that has developed over many years. Alternatively, the mass can cause pain, pruritus, and/or erythema. Tumors arising in the vulva are often clinically interpreted as various cysts.[282]

Vulvar leiomyomatosis is a condition characterized by multinodular proliferations of smooth muscle affecting the vulva. When the clitoris is involved, clitoral hypertrophy can occur. Patients can also synchronously or metachronously develop numerous smooth muscle neoplasms of the esophagus.[282,285] The pathogenesis of vulvar leiomyomatosis is unknown, but there is an association with Alport syndrome.[286]

Gross features

Tumors are well-circumscribed masses with cut surfaces identical to uterine counterparts. Vulvar leiomyomas range in size from 0.5 to 11.2 cm (mean, 4 cm).[214]

Microscopic features

Most vulvar leiomyomas are conventional leiomyomas.[214,287] Myxoedematous matrix and/or hyaline change can be present.[282] Leiomyoma variants of the vulva are rare but have been reported.[287–290]

 Differential Diagnosis

Aggressive angiomyxoma

- Aggressive angiomyxomas are large, deeply located, and poorly delineated tumors. They are hypocellular with stellate to spindle cells in a myxoedematous matrix and contain medium-walled to thick-walled large vessels that frequently have mural hyalinization.[291] Aggressive angiomyoxoma is hypocellular compared with SMTs and lacks fascicular growth.

Cellular angiofibroma

- Cellular angiofibromas have spindled cells arranged in fascicles with a rich vasculature that often has hyalinized vessel walls.[292] Cellular angiofibromas are negative for desmin and strongly positive for CD34.[293]

Angiomyofibroblastoma

- Angiomyofibroblastomas comprise alternating hypocellular and hypercellular areas and contain bland spindled to plasmacytoid cells in a myxoedematous or fibrocollagenous matrix. Unlike SMTs, angiomyofibroblastoma contains smaller, thin-walled vessels, and tumor cells tend to have a perivascular arrangement. Tumors are consistently positive for desmin and are usually negative for smooth muscle actin.[245]

Solitary fibrous tumor

- Solitary fibrous tumors have bland fibroblastic spindle cells that grow in a storiform architecture with hyalinized stroma and ectatic, branched, thin-walled vessels. Solitary fibrous tumors are positive for STAT6, whereas SMTs are negative.[294]

Prognosis

Vulvar leiomyomas are benign. Complete excision is curative.

Smooth Muscle Tumor of Uncertain Malignant Potential

Few examples of vulvar STUMP have been reported. Women are in their fourth to fifth decade of life.[214]

Gross features

Described tumors have been 6 to 8.5 cm in diameter.[214]

Microscopic features

Conventional and myxoid STUMPs have been described and classified as such by uterine criteria for each respective type.[214]

Prognosis

The 2 reported cases had follow-up of 9 and 19 months and neither patient experienced recurrence or metastasis. Long-term follow-up is recommended for these tumors.[214]

Leiomyosarcoma

Women diagnosed with leiomyosarcoma of the vulva are typically postmenopausal.[214,295] Patients present with mass-related symptoms, but their onset is generally more noticeable because of rapid tumor growth.[214,295]

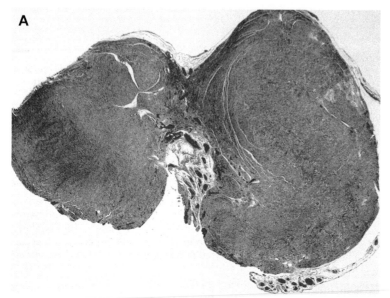

Fig. 21. DPL forms well-circumscribed tumors and tumorlets involving pelvic and abdominal peritoneal surfaces (*A*) that morphologically resemble conventional leiomyomas (*B*). Endometriosis and/or endosalpingiosis can be seen abutting or admixed with these lesions (*C*).

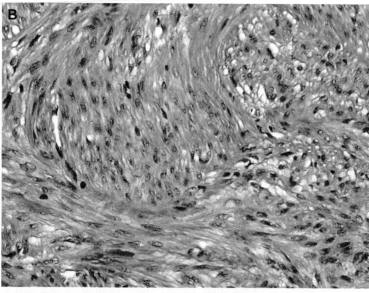

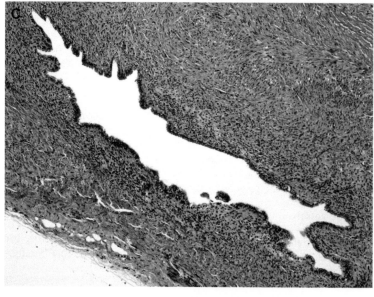

Fig. 22. Metastasizing leio-myoma classically involves the lung as a unilateral, solitary nodule but may present as multiple unilateral or bilateral nodules (*A*). Metastasizing leiomyoma is usually spindled and the cells lack cytologic atypia and significant mitotic activity (*B*). Bronchoalveolar epithelium can be entrapped in lung tumors (*C*).

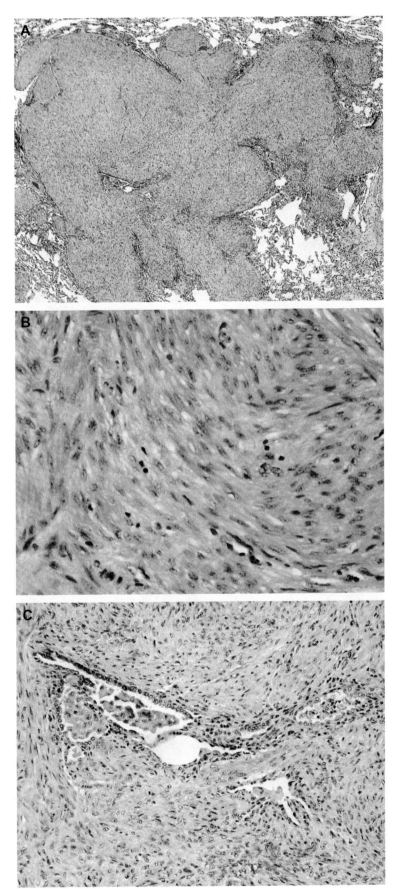

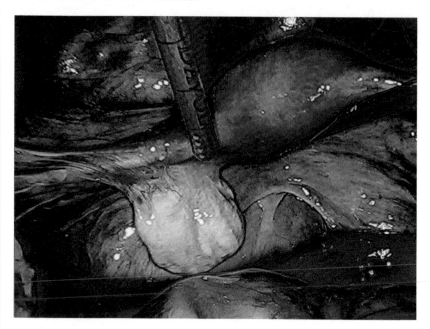

Fig. 23. Laparoscopic view of a leiomyoma involving the broad ligament.

Gross features

Tumors are well-circumscribed to poorly circumscribed and range in size from 5.5 to 13.5 cm.[214]

Microscopic features

Spindled, myxoid, and epithelioid leiomyosarcomas have been reported as primary vulvar tumors and are grossly similar to their uterine counterparts.[214,296–299]

Like vaginal SMTs, the infrequency of vulvar SMTs has complicated the development of risk assessment criteria. The first criteria proposal for vulvar SMTs were published in 1979 and required

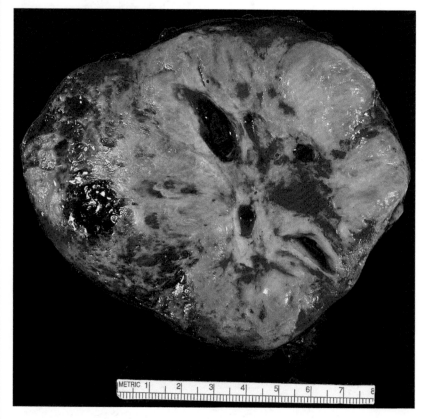

Fig. 24. A STUMP that arose from the broad ligament. The tumor has a fleshy cut surface with cyst formation, edema, and zones of necrosis.

2 of the following features to diagnose low-grade leiomyosarcoma and 3 features to diagnose leiomyosarcoma: (1) size greater than or equal to 5 cm, (2) greater than or equal to 5 mitotic figures per 10 HPFs, (3) infiltrative margins.[274] In 1996, criteria were modified, requiring that at least 3 of the following features be present to diagnose leiomyosarcoma: (1) size greater than or equal to 5 cm, (2) moderate to severe cytologic atypia, (3) greater than or equal to 5 mitotic figures per 10 HPFs, (4) infiltrative margins.[287] When these criteria and 2014 WHO uterine SMT criteria were evaluated in a large series of vulvar SMTs, the sensitivity for a diagnosis of leiomyosarcoma was the same for all criteria sets (100%). However, WHO uterine SMT criteria were most specific (100%), followed by 1996 criteria (93.5%) and 1979 criteria (86.7%).[214] It was therefore proposed that WHO uterine SMT criteria be used in classification of vulvar spindled SMTs.[214]

Similar to the vagina, myxoid and epithelioid SMTs are infrequently encountered in the vulva and the validity of proposed uterine criteria for these leiomyosarcoma variants has not been evaluated in a large series.

ΔΔ **Differential Diagnosis**

Fibrosarcomatous transformation of dermatofibrosarcoma protuberans

- Fibrosarcomatous transformation of dermatofibrosarcoma protuberans has a herringbone arrangement of atypical spindle cells associated with brisk mitotic activity. These tumors usually have a recognizable component of classic dermatofibrosarcoma protuberans if thoroughly sampled. Classic dermatofibrosarcoma protuberans and fibrosarcomatous transformation are negative for desmin and smooth muscle actin.[300–302] Identification of *PDGFB* gene rearrangement can be helpful in diagnostically difficult cases.[300]

Prognosis

All 3 reported patients with vulvar leiomyosarcoma classified by uterine criteria died of disease (4, 36, and 56 months following diagnosis).[214]

REFERENCES

1. Kurman RJ, Herrington CS, Young RH, et al. World Health Organization classification of tumours of female reproductive organs. Lyon (France): International Agency for Research on Cancer (IARC); 2014.
2. Baird DD, Dunson DB, Hill MC, et al. High cumulative incidence of uterine leiomyoma in black and white women: ultrasound evidence. Am J Obstet Gynecol 2003;188:100–7.
3. Buttram VC Jr, Reiter RC. Uterine leiomyomata: etiology, symptomatology, and management. Fertil Steril 1981;36:433–45.
4. Stewart EA. Uterine fibroids. Lancet 2001;357:293–8.
5. Yang EJ, Mutter GL. Biomarker resolution of uterine smooth muscle tumor necrosis as benign vs malignant. Mod Pathol 2015;28:830–5.
6. Weichert W, Denkert C, Gauruder-Burmester A, et al. Uterine arterial embolization with tris-acryl gelatin microspheres: a histopathologic evaluation. Am J Surg Pathol 2005;29:955–61.
7. McCluggage WG, Ellis PK, McClure N, et al. Pathologic features of uterine leiomyomas following uterine artery embolization. Int J Gynecol Pathol 2000;19:342–7.
8. Colgan TJ, Pendergast S, LeBlanc M. The histopathology of uterine leiomyomas following treatment with gonadotropin-releasing hormone analogues. Hum Pathol 1993;24:1073–7.
9. Demopoulos RI, Mesia AF. Effects of leuprolide acetate on treatment of leiomyomata–clues to mechanisms of action. Adv Anat Pathol 1998;5:129–36.
10. Sreenan JJ, Prayson RA, Biscotti CV, et al. Histopathologic findings in 107 uterine leiomyomas treated with leuprolide acetate compared with 126 controls. Am J Surg Pathol 1996;20:427–32.
11. Ip PP, Lam KW, Cheung CL, et al. Tranexamic acid-associated necrosis and intralesional thrombosis of uterine leiomyomas: a clinicopathologic study of 147 cases emphasizing the importance of drug-induced necrosis and early infarcts in leiomyomas. Am J Surg Pathol 2007;31:1215–24.
12. Bell SW, Kempson RL, Hendrickson MR. Problematic uterine smooth muscle neoplasms. A clinicopathologic study of 213 cases. Am J Surg Pathol 1994;18:535–58.
13. Prayson RA, Hart WR. Mitotically active leiomyomas of the uterus. Am J Clin Pathol 1992;97:14–20.
14. Perrone T, Dehner LP. Prognostically favorable "mitotically active" smooth-muscle tumors of the uterus. A clinicopathologic study of ten cases. Am J Surg Pathol 1988;12:1–8.
15. Ip PP, Cheung AN, Clement PB. Uterine smooth muscle tumors of uncertain malignant potential (STUMP): a clinicopathologic analysis of 16 cases. Am J Surg Pathol 2009;33:992–1005.
16. Ly A, Mills AM, McKenney JK, et al. Atypical leiomyomas of the uterus: a clinicopathologic study of 51 cases. Am J Surg Pathol 2013;37:643–9.

17. Downes KA, Hart WR. Bizarre leiomyomas of the uterus: a comprehensive pathologic study of 24 cases with long-term follow-up. Am J Surg Pathol 1997;21:1261–70.

18. Bennett JA, Weigelt B, Chiang S, et al. Leiomyoma with bizarre nuclei: a morphological, immunohistochemical and molecular analysis of 31 cases. Mod Pathol 2017;30:1476–88.

19. Zhang Q, Poropatich K, Ubago J, et al. Fumarate hydratase mutations and alterations in leiomyoma with bizarre nuclei. Int J Gynecol Pathol 2018;37: 421–30.

20. Oliva E, Young RH, Clement PB, et al. Cellular benign mesenchymal tumors of the uterus. A comparative morphologic and immunohistochemical analysis of 33 highly cellular leiomyomas and six endometrial stromal nodules, two frequently confused tumors. Am J Surg Pathol 1995;19:757–68.

21. Oliva E. Cellular mesenchymal tumors of the uterus: a review emphasizing recent observations. Int J Gynecol Pathol 2014;33:374–84.

22. Oliva E, Young RH, Amin MB, et al. An immunohistochemical analysis of endometrial stromal and smooth muscle tumors of the uterus - A study of 54 cases emphasizing the importance of using a panel because of overlap in immunoreactivity for individual antibodies. Am J Surg Pathol 2002;26: 403–12.

23. Nucci MR, O'Connell JT, Huettner PC, et al. h-Caldesmon expression effectively distinguishes endometrial stromal tumors from uterine smooth muscle tumors. Am J Surg Pathol 2001;25:455–63.

24. Rush DS, Tan JY, Baergen RN, et al. h-caldesmon, a novel smooth muscle-specific antibody, distinguishes between cellular leiomyoma and endometrial stromal sarcoma. Am J Surg Pathol 2001;25: 253–8.

25. Clement PB, Young RH, Scully RE. Diffuse, perinodular, and other patterns of hydropic degeneration within and adjacent to uterine leiomyomas. Problems in differential diagnosis. Am J Surg Pathol 1992;16:26–32.

26. Coad JE, Sulaiman RA, Das K, et al. Perinodular hydropic degeneration of a uterine leiomyoma: a diagnostic challenge. Hum Pathol 1997;28:249–51.

27. Busca A, Parra-Herran C. Myxoid mesenchymal tumors of the uterus: an update on classification, definitions, and differential diagnosis. Adv Anat Pathol 2017;24:354–61.

28. Willems SM, Wiweger M, van Roggen JF, et al. Running GAGs: myxoid matrix in tumor pathology revisited: what's in it for the pathologist? Virchows Arch 2010;456:181–92.

29. Busca A, Gulavita P, Parra-Herran C, et al. IFITM1 outperforms CD10 in differentiating low-grade endometrial stromal sarcomas from smooth muscle neoplasms of the uterus. Int J Gynecol Pathol 2018; 37:372–8.

30. Atkins KA, Bell S, Kempson RL. Myxoid smooth muscle tumors of the uterus. Mod Pathol 2001;14: 132A.

31. Parra-Herran C, Schoolmeester JK, Yuan L, et al. Myxoid leiomyosarcoma of the uterus: a clinicopathologic analysis of 30 cases and review of the literature with reappraisal of its distinction from other uterine myxoid mesenchymal neoplasms. Am J Surg Pathol 2016;40:285–301.

32. Prayson RA, Goldblum JR, Hart WR. Epithelioid smooth-muscle tumors of the uterus: a clinicopathologic study of 18 patients. Am J Surg Pathol 1997; 21:383–91.

33. Kurman RJ, Norris HJ. Mesenchymal tumors of the uterus. VI. Epithelioid smooth muscle tumors including leiomyoblastoma and clear-cell leiomyoma: a clinical and pathologic analysis of 26 cases. Cancer 1976;37:1853–65.

34. Rizeq MN, van de Rijn M, Hendrickson MR, et al. A comparative immunohistochemical study of uterine smooth muscle neoplasms with emphasis on the epithelioid variant. Hum Pathol 1994;25: 671–7.

35. de Leval L, Waltregny D, Boniver J, et al. Use of histone deacetylase 8 (HDAC8), a new marker of smooth muscle differentiation, in the classification of mesenchymal tumors of the uterus. Am J Surg Pathol 2006;30:319–27.

36. Schoolmeester JK, Dao LN, Sukov WR, et al. TFE3 translocation-associated perivascular epithelioid cell neoplasm (PEComa) of the gynecologic tract: morphology, immunophenotype, differential diagnosis. Am J Surg Pathol 2015; 39:394–404.

37. Schoolmeester JK, Howitt BE, Hirsch MS, et al. Perivascular epithelioid cell neoplasm (PEComa) of the gynecologic tract: clinicopathologic and immunohistochemical characterization of 16 cases. Am J Surg Pathol 2014;38:176–88.

38. Howitt BE, Schoolmesster JK, Quade BJ. Immunohistochemical analysis of HMB-45, MelanA, CathepsinK in a series of 35 uterine leiomyosarcomas. Mod Pathol 2013;26:279A.

39. Kaminski PF, Tavassoli FA. Plexiform tumorlet: a clinical and pathologic study of 15 cases with ultrastructural observations. Int J Gynecol Pathol 1984; 3:124–34.

40. Cera PJ Jr. Plexiform tumorlet of the uterus: report of two cases. Am J Clin Pathol 1973;59:263–6.

41. Balaton AJ, Vuong PN, Vaury P, et al. Plexiform tumorlet of the uterus: immunohistological evidence for a smooth muscle origin. Histopathology 1986; 10:749–54.

42. Patchefsky AS. Plexiform tumorlet of the uterus: report of a case. Obstet Gynecol 1970;35:592–6.

43. de Leval L, Lim GS, Waltregny D, et al. Diverse phenotypic profile of uterine tumors resembling ovarian sex cord tumors: an immunohistochemical study of 12 cases. Am J Surg Pathol 2010;34: 1749–61.

44. Baker RJ, Hildebrandt RH, Rouse RV, et al. Inhibin and CD99 (MIC2) expression in uterine stromal neoplasms with sex-cord-like elements. Hum Pathol 1999;30:671–9.

45. Hurrell DP, McCluggage WG. Uterine tumour resembling ovarian sex cord tumour is an immuno-histochemically polyphenotypic neoplasm which exhibits coexpression of epithelial, myoid and sex cord markers. J Clin Pathol 2007;60:1148–54.

46. Irving JA, Carinelli S, Prat J. Uterine tumors resembling ovarian sex cord tumors are polyphenotypic neoplasms with true sex cord differentiation. Mod Pathol 2006;19:17–24.

47. Aung T, Goto M, Nomoto M, et al. Uterine lipoleiomyoma: a histopathological review of 17 cases. Pathol Int 2004;54:751–8.

48. Wang X, Kumar D, Seidman JD. Uterine lipoleiomyomas: a clinicopathologic study of 50 cases. Int J Gynecol Pathol 2006;25:239–42.

49. Fadare O, Khabele D. Pleomorphic liposarcoma of the uterine corpus with focal smooth muscle differentiation. Int J Gynecol Pathol 2011;30:282–7.

50. Brandfass RT, Everts-Suarez EA. Lipomatous tumors of the uterus; a review of the world's literature with report of a case of true lipoma. Am J Obstet Gynecol 1955;70:359–67.

51. Jacobs DS, Cohen H, Johnson JS. Lipoleiomyomas of the uterus. Am J Clin Pathol 1965;44:45–51.

52. Fukunaga M, Ushigome S. Uterine bizarre lipoleiomyoma. Pathol Int 1998;48:562–5.

53. Brooks JJ, Wells GB, Yeh IT, et al. Bizarre epithelioid lipoleiomyoma of the uterus. Int J Gynecol Pathol 1992;11:144–9.

54. Chen KT. Uterine leiomyohibernoma. Int J Gynecol Pathol 1999;18:96–7.

55. Lim GS, Oliva E. The morphologic spectrum of uterine PEC-cell associated tumors in a patient with tuberous sclerosis. Int J Gynecol Pathol 2011;30:121–8.

56. McDonald AG, Dal Cin P, Ganguly A, et al. Liposarcoma arising in uterine lipoleiomyoma: a report of 3 cases and review of the literature. Am J Surg Pathol 2011;35:221–7.

57. Bennett JA, Lamb C, Young RH. Apoplectic leiomyomas a morphologic analysis of 100 cases highlighting unusual features. Am J Surg Pathol 2016; 40:563–8.

58. Boyd C, McCluggage WG. Unusual morphological features of uterine leiomyomas treated with progestogens. J Clin Pathol 2011;64:485–9.

59. Norris HJ, Hilliard GD, Irey NS. Hemorrhagic cellular leiomyomas ("apoplectic leiomyoma") of the uterus associated with pregnancy and oral contraceptives. Int J Gynecol Pathol 1988;7: 212–24.

60. Myles JL, Hart WR. Apoplectic leiomyomas of the uterus. A clinicopathologic study of five distinctive hemorrhagic leiomyomas associated with oral contraceptive usage. Am J Surg Pathol 1985;9: 798–805.

61. Siegler L, Erber R, Burghaus S, et al. Fumarate hydratase (FH) deficiency in uterine leiomyomas: recognition by histological features versus blind immunoscreening. Virchows Arch 2018;472:789–96.

62. Harrison WJ, Andrici J, Maclean F, et al. Fumarate hydratase-deficient uterine leiomyomas occur in both the syndromic and sporadic settings. Am J Surg Pathol 2016;40:599–607.

63. Joseph NM, Solomon DA, Frizzell N, et al. Morphology and immunohistochemistry for 2SC and FH aid in detection of fumarate hydratase gene aberrations in uterine leiomyomas from young patients. Am J Surg Pathol 2015;39:1529–39.

64. Lehtonen HJ. Hereditary leiomyomatosis and renal cell cancer: update on clinical and molecular characteristics. Fam Cancer 2011;10:397–411.

65. Alsolami S, El-Bahrawy M, Kalloger SE, et al. Current morphologic criteria perform poorly in identifying hereditary leiomyomatosis and renal cell carcinoma syndrome-associated uterine leiomyomas. Int J Gynecol Pathol 2014;33:560–7.

66. Martinek P, Grossmann P, Hes O, et al. Genetic testing of leiomyoma tissue in women younger than 30 years old might provide an effective screening approach for the hereditary leiomyomatosis and renal cell cancer syndrome (HLRCC). Virchows Arch 2015;467:185–91.

67. Miettinen M, Felisiak-Golabek A, Wasag B, et al. Fumarase-deficient uterine leiomyomas: an immunohistochemical, molecular genetic, and clinicopathologic study of 86 cases. Am J Surg Pathol 2016;40:1661–9.

68. Gross KL, Panhuysen CI, Kleinman MS, et al. Involvement of fumarate hydratase in nonsyndromic uterine leiomyomas: genetic linkage analysis and FISH studies. Genes Chromosomes Cancer 2004;41:183–90.

69. Mroch AR, Laudenschlager M, Flanagan JD. Detection of a novel FH whole gene deletion in the propositus leading to subsequent prenatal diagnosis in a sibship with fumarase deficiency. Am J Med Genet A 2012;158a:155–8.

70. Tomlinson IP, Alam NA, Rowan AJ, et al. Germline mutations in FH predispose to dominantly inherited uterine fibroids, skin leiomyomata and papillary renal cell cancer. Nat Genet 2002;30:406–10.

71. Vanharanta S, Pollard PJ, Lehtonen HJ, et al. Distinct expression profile in fumarate-hydratase-deficient uterine fibroids. Hum Mol Genet 2006; 15:97–103.

72. Launonen V, Vierimaa O, Kiuru M, et al. Inherited susceptibility to uterine leiomyomas and renal cell cancer. Proc Natl Acad Sci U S A 2001;98: 3387–92.

73. Toro JR, Nickerson ML, Wei MH, et al. Mutations in the fumarate hydratase gene cause hereditary leiomyomatosis and renal cell cancer in families in North America. Am J Hum Genet 2003;73:95–106.

74. Sanz J, Teller L, Vockes C. Genetic alterations of uterine fibroids in hereditary leiomyomatosis and renal cancer (HLRCC) syndrome. Mod Pathol 2008;21:223A.

75. Reyes C, Karamurzin Y, Frizzell N, et al. Uterine smooth muscle tumors with features suggesting fumarate hydratase aberration: detailed morphologic analysis and correlation with S-(2-succino)-cysteine immunohistochemistry. Mod Pathol 2014;27:1020–7.

76. Garg G, Mohanty SK. Uterine angioleiomyoma a rare variant of uterine leiomyoma. Arch Pathol Lab Med 2014;138:1115–8.

77. Sanz-Ortega J, Vocke C, Stratton P, et al. Morphologic and molecular characteristics of uterine leiomyomas in hereditary leiomyomatosis and renal cancer (HLRCC) syndrome. Am J Surg Pathol 2013;37:74–80.

78. Bardella C, El-Bahrawy M, Frizzell N, et al. Aberrant succination of proteins in fumarate hydratase-deficient mice and HLRCC patients is a robust biomarker of mutation status. J Pathol 2011;225:4–11.

79. Chen YB, Brannon AR, Toubaji A, et al. Hereditary leiomyomatosis and renal cell carcinoma syndrome-associated renal cancer: recognition of the syndrome by pathologic features and the utility of detecting aberrant succination by immunohistochemistry. Am J Surg Pathol 2014;38: 627–37.

80. Alderson NL, Wang Y, Blatnik M, et al. S-(2-Succinyl)cysteine: a novel chemical modification of tissue proteins by a Krebs cycle intermediate. Arch Biochem Biophys 2006;450:1–8.

81. Buelow B, Cohen J, Nagymanyoki Z, et al. Immunohistochemistry for 2-succinocysteine (2SC) and fumarate hydratase (FH) in cutaneous leiomyomas may aid in identification of patients with HLRCC (Hereditary Leiomyomatosis and Renal Cell Carcinoma Syndrome). Am J Surg Pathol 2016;40: 982–8.

82. Kiuru M, Lehtonen R, Arola J, et al. Few FH mutations in sporadic counterparts of tumor types observed in hereditary leiomyomatosis and renal cell cancer families. Cancer Res 2002;62:4554–7.

83. Ylisaukko-oja SK, Kiuru M, Lehtonen HJ, et al. Analysis of fumarate hydratase mutations in a population-based series of early onset uterine leiomyosarcoma patients. Int J Cancer 2006;119: 283–7.

84. Parker RL, Young RH, Clement PB. Skeletal muscle-like and rhabdoid cells in uterine leiomyomas. Int J Gynecol Pathol 2005;24:319–25.

85. Fornelli A, Pasquinelli G, Eusebi V. Leiomyoma of the uterus showing skeletal muscle differentiation: a case report. Hum Pathol 1999;30:356–9.

86. Blandamura S, Florea G, Chiarelli S, et al. Myometrial leiomyoma with chondroid lipoma-like areas. Histopathology 2005;46:596–8.

87. Kotru M, Gupta R, Aggarwal S, et al. Cartilaginous metaplasia in uterine leiomyoma. Arch Gynecol Obstet 2009;280:671–3.

88. Chander B, Shekhar S. Osseous metaplasia in leiomyoma: a first in a uterine leiomyoma. J Cancer Res Ther 2015;11:661.

89. Clement PB, Young RH. Diffuse leiomyomatosis of the uterus: a report of four cases. Int J Gynecol Pathol 1987;6:322–30.

90. Mulvany NJ, Ostor AG, Ross I. Diffuse leiomyomatosis of the uterus. Histopathology 1995;27:175–9.

91. Baschinsky DY, Isa A, Niemann TH, et al. Diffuse leiomyomatosis of the uterus: a case report with clonality analysis. Hum Pathol 2000;31:1429–32.

92. Roth LM, Reed RJ, Sternberg WH. Cotyledonoid dissecting leiomyoma of the uterus. The Sternberg tumor. Am J Surg Pathol 1996;20:1455–61.

93. Roth LM, Reed RJ. Cotyledonoid leiomyoma of the uterus: report of a case. Int J Gynecol Pathol 2000; 19:272–5.

94. Roth LM, Reed RJ. Dissecting leiomyomas of the uterus other than cotyledonoid dissecting leiomyomas: a report of eight cases. Am J Surg Pathol 1999;23:1032–9.

95. Gurbuz A, Karateke A, Kabaca C, et al. A case of cotyledonoid leiomyoma and review of the literature. Int J Gynecol Cancer 2005;15:1218–21.

96. Smith CC, Gold MA, Wile G, et al. Cotyledonoid dissecting leiomyoma of the uterus: a review of clinical, pathological, and radiological features. Int J Surg Pathol 2012;20:330–41.

97. Fukunaga M, Ushigome S. Dissecting leiomyoma of the uterus with extrauterine extension. Histopathology 1998;32:160–4.

98. Fukunaga M, Suzuki K, Hiruta N. Cotyledonoid dissecting leiomyoma of the uterus: a report of four cases. APMIS 2010;118:331–3.

99. Chawla I, Bhardwaj M, Sareen N, et al. Epithelioid cotyledonoid leiomyoma of uterus. BMJ Case Rep 2014;2014.

100. Soleymani Majd H, Ismail L, Desai SA, et al. Epithelioid cotyledonoid dissecting leiomyoma: a case report and review of the literature. Arch Gynecol Obstet 2011;283:771–4.

101. Blake EA, Cheng G, Post MD, et al. Cotyledonoid dissecting leiomyoma with adipocytic differentiation: a case report. Gynecol Oncol Rep 2015;11: 7–9.

102. Roth LM, Kirker JA, Insull M, et al. Recurrent coty-ledonoid dissecting leiomyoma of the uterus. Int J Gynecol Pathol 2013;32:215–20.

103. Canzonieri V, D'Amore ES, Bartoloni G, et al. Leio-myomatosis with vascular invasion. A unified path-ogenesis regarding leiomyoma with vascular microinvasion, benign metastasizing leiomyoma and intravenous leiomyomatosis. Virchows Arch 1994;425:541–5.

104. Clement PB, Young RH, Scully RE. Intravenous leiomyomatosis of the uterus. A clinicopathological analysis of 16 cases with unusual histologic fea-tures. Am J Surg Pathol 1988;12:932–45.

105. Carr RJ, Hui P, Buza N. Intravenous leiomyomatosis revisited: an experience of 14 cases at a single medical center. Int J Gynecol Pathol 2015;34: 169–76.

106. Du J, Zhao X, Guo D, et al. Intravenous leiomyoma-tosis of the uterus: a clinicopathologic study of 18 cases, with emphasis on early diagnosis and appropriate treatment strategies. Hum Pathol 2011;42:1240–6.

107. Cooper MM, Guillem J, Dalton J, et al. Recurrent intravenous leiomyomatosis with cardiac extension. Ann Thorac Surg 1992;53:139–41.

108. Uchida H, Hattori Y, Nakada K, et al. Successful one-stage radical removal of intravenous leiomyo-matosis extending to the right ventricle. Obstet Gy-necol 2004;103:1068–70.

109. Arinami Y, Kodama S, Kase H, et al. Successful one-stage complete removal of an entire intravenous leiomyomatosis in the heart, vena cava, and uterus. Gynecol Oncol 1997;64:547–50.

110. Norris HJ, Parmley T. Mesenchymal tumors of the uterus. V. Intravenous leiomyomatosis. A clinical and pathologic study of 14 cases. Cancer 1975; 36:2164–78.

111. Brescia RJ, Tazelaar HD, Hobbs J, et al. Intravas-cular lipoleiomyomatosis: a report of two cases. Hum Pathol 1989;20:252–6.

112. Merchant S, Malpica A, Deavers MT, et al. Vessels within vessels in the myometrium. Am J Surg Pathol 2002;26:232–6.

113. Gupta M, Laury AL, Nucci MR, et al. Predictors of adverse outcome in uterine smooth muscle tumours of uncertain malignant potential (STUMP): a clinicopathological analysis of 22 cases with a proposal for the inclusion of addi-tional histological parameters. Histopathology 2018;73:284–98.

114. Kempson RL, Bari W. Uterine sarcomas. Classifica-tion, diagnosis, and prognosis. Hum Pathol 1970;1: 331–49.

115. Soslow RA, Longacre TA. Uterine pathology. Cam-bridge (England): Cambridge University Press; 2012.

116. Devereaux KA, Kunder CA, Longacre TA. ALK-re-arranged tumors are highly enriched in the STUMP subcategory of uterine tumors. Am J Surg Pathol 2019;43(1):64–74.

117. Subbiah V, McMahon C, Patel S, et al. STUMP un"-stumped": anti-tumor response to anaplastic lym-phoma kinase (ALK) inhibitor based targeted therapy in uterine inflammatory myofibroblastic tu-mor with myxoid features harboring DCTN1-ALK fusion. J Hematol Oncol 2015;8:66.

118. Atkins KA, Arronte N, Darus CJ, et al. The Use of p16 in enhancing the histologic classification of uterine smooth muscle tumors. Am J Surg Pathol 2008;32:98–102.

119. Amant F, Moerman P, Vergote I. Report of an un-usual problematic uterine smooth muscle neoplasm, emphasizing the prognostic importance of coagulative tumor cell necrosis. Int J Gynecol Cancer 2005;15:1210–2.

120. Berretta R, Rolla M, Merisio C, et al. Uterine smooth muscle tumor of uncertain malignant potential: a three-case report. Int J Gynecol Cancer 2008;18: 1121–6.

121. Sung CO, Ahn G, Song SY, et al. Atypical leiomyo-mas of the uterus with long-term follow-up after myomectomy with immunohistochemical analysis for p16INK4A, p53, Ki-67, estrogen receptors, and progesterone receptors. Int J Gynecol Pathol 2009;28:529–34.

122. Veras E, Zivanovic O, Jacks L, et al. "Low-grade leiomyosarcoma" and late-recurring smooth mus-cle tumors of the uterus: a heterogenous collection of frequently misdiagnosed tumors associated with an overall favorable prognosis relative to conven-tional uterine leiomyosarcomas. Am J Surg Pathol 2011;35:1626–37.

123. Peters WA 3rd, Howard DR, Andersen WA, et al. Uterine smooth-muscle tumors of uncertain ma-lignant potential. Obstet Gynecol 1994;83: 1015–20.

124. Guntupalli SR, Ramirez PT, Anderson ML, et al. Uterine smooth muscle tumor of uncertain malig-nant potential: a retrospective analysis. Gynecol Oncol 2009;113:324–6.

125. Croce S, Ribeiro A, Brulard C, et al. Uterine smooth muscle tumor analysis by comparative genomic hybridization: a useful diagnostic tool in chal-lenging lesions. Mod Pathol 2015;28:1001–10.

126. Croce S, Ducoulombier A, Ribeiro A, et al. Genome profiling is an efficient tool to avoid the STUMP classification of uterine smooth muscle lesions: a comprehensive array-genomic hybridi-zation analysis of 77 tumors. Mod Pathol 2018; 31:816–28.

127. Abeler VM, Royne O, Thoresen S, et al. Uterine sar-comas in Norway. A histopathological and prog-nostic survey of a total population from 1970 to 2000 including 419 patients. Histopathology 2009;54:355–64.

128. Gadducci A, Landoni F, Sartori E, et al. Uterine leiomyosarcoma: analysis of treatment failures and survival. Gynecol Oncol 1996;62:25–32.

129. Major FJ, Blessing JA, Silverberg SG, et al. Prognostic factors in early-stage uterine sarcoma. A Gynecologic Oncology Group study. Cancer 1993;71:1702–9.

130. Yanai H, Wani Y, Notohara K, et al. Uterine leiomyosarcoma arising in leiomyoma: clinicopathological study of four cases and literature review. Pathol Int 2010;60:506–9.

131. Mittal KR, Chen F, Wei JJ, et al. Molecular and immunohistochemical evidence for the origin of uterine leiomyosarcomas from associated leiomyoma and symplastic leiomyoma-like areas. Mod Pathol 2009;22:1303–11.

132. Lim D, Alvarez T, Nucci MR, et al. Interobserver variability in the interpretation of tumor cell necrosis in uterine leiomyosarcoma. Am J Surg Pathol 2013;37:650–8.

133. Mahler HR, Lindber MR, Quick CM. Predetermined search methods can increase the yield in counting mitotic figures in uterine leiomyosarcomas. Mod Pathol 2012;25:285A.

134. Darby AJ, Papadaki L, Beilby JO. An unusual leiomyosarcoma of the uterus containing osteoclast-like giant cells. Cancer 1975;36:495–504.

135. Marshall RJ, Braye SG, Jones DB. Leiomyosarcoma of the uterus with giant cells resembling osteoclasts. Int J Gynecol Pathol 1986;5:260–8.

136. Leitao MM Jr, Hensley ML, Barakat RR, et al. Immunohistochemical expression of estrogen and progesterone receptors and outcomes in patients with newly diagnosed uterine leiomyosarcoma. Gynecol Oncol 2012;124:558–62.

137. Lee CH, Turbin DA, Sung YC, et al. A panel of antibodies to determine site of origin and malignancy in smooth muscle tumors. Mod Pathol 2009;22:1519–31.

138. Chen L, Yang B. Immunohistochemical analysis of p16, p53, and Ki-67 expression in uterine smooth muscle tumors. Int J Gynecol Pathol 2008;27:326–32.

139. O'Neill CJ, McBride HA, Connolly LE, et al. Uterine leiomyosarcomas are characterized by high p16, p53 and MIB1 expression in comparison with usual leiomyomas, leiomyoma variants and smooth muscle tumours of uncertain malignant potential. Histopathology 2007;50:851–8.

140. Gannon BR, Manduch M, Childs TJ. Differential immunoreactivity of p16 in leiomyosarcomas and leiomyoma variants. Int J Gynecol Pathol 2008;27:68–73.

141. Bodner-Adler B, Bodner K, Czerwenka K, et al. Expression of p16 protein in patients with uterine smooth muscle tumors: an immunohistochemical analysis. Gynecol Oncol 2005;96:62–6.

142. Sah SP, McCluggage WG. DOG1 immunoreactivity in uterine leiomyosarcomas. J Clin Pathol 2013;66:40–3.

143. Wang L, Felix JC, Lee JL, et al. The proto-oncogene c-kit is expressed in leiomyosarcomas of the uterus. Gynecol Oncol 2003;90:402–6.

144. Simpson KW, Albores-Saavedra J. HMB-45 reactivity in conventional uterine leiomyosarcomas. Am J Surg Pathol 2007;31:95–8.

145. Fadare O, Bonvicino A, Martel M, et al. Pleomorphic rhabdomyosarcoma of the uterine corpus: a clinicopathologic study of 4 cases and a review of the literature. Int J Gynecol Pathol 2010;29:122–34.

146. Verma M, Joseph G, McCluggage WG. Uterine composite tumor composed of leiomyosarcoma and embryonal rhabdomyosarcoma with immature cartilage. Int J Gynecol Pathol 2009;28:338–42.

147. Larson B, Silfversward C, Nilsson B, et al. Prognostic factors in uterine leiomyosarcoma. A clinical and histopathological study of 143 cases. The Radiumhemmet series 1936-1981. Acta Oncol 1990;29:185–91.

148. Blom R, Guerrieri C, Stal O, et al. Leiomyosarcoma of the uterus: a clinicopathologic, DNA flow cytometric, p53, and mdm-2 analysis of 49 cases. Gynecol Oncol 1998;68:54–61.

149. Mayerhofer K, Obermair A, Windbichler G, et al. Leiomyosarcoma of the uterus: a clinicopathologic multicenter study of 71 cases. Gynecol Oncol 1999;74:196–201.

150. Nola M, Babic D, Ilic J, et al. Prognostic parameters for survival of patients with malignant mesenchymal tumors of the uterus. Cancer 1996;78:2543–50.

151. Nordal RR, Kristensen GB, Kaern J, et al. The prognostic significance of stage, tumor size, cellular atypia and DNA ploidy in uterine leiomyosarcoma. Acta Oncol 1995;34:797–802.

152. Pautier P, Genestie C, Rey A, et al. Analysis of clinicopathologic prognostic factors for 157 uterine sarcomas and evaluation of a grading score validated for soft tissue sarcoma. Cancer 2000;88:1425–31.

153. Pelmus M, Penault-Llorca F, Guillou L, et al. Prognostic factors in early-stage leiomyosarcoma of the uterus. Int J Gynecol Cancer 2009;19:385–90.

154. Wolfson AH, Wolfson DJ, Sittler SY, et al. A multivariate analysis of clinicopathologic factors for predicting outcome in uterine sarcomas. Gynecol Oncol 1994;52:56–62.

155. Jones MW, Norris HJ. Clinicopathologic study of 28 uterine leiomyosarcomas with metastasis. Int J Gynecol Pathol 1995;14:243–9.

156. Giuntoli RL 2nd, Metzinger DS, DiMarco CS, et al. Retrospective review of 208 patients with leiomyosarcoma of the uterus: prognostic indicators,

surgical management, and adjuvant therapy. Gynecol Oncol 2003;89:460–9.

157. Evans HL, Chawla SP, Simpson C, et al. Smooth muscle neoplasms of the uterus other than ordinary leiomyoma. A study of 46 cases, with emphasis on diagnostic criteria and prognostic factors. Cancer 1988;62:2239–47.

158. D'Angelo E, Espinosa I, Ali R, et al. Uterine leiomyosarcomas: tumor size, mitotic index, and biomarkers Ki67, and Bcl-2 identify two groups with different prognosis. Gynecol Oncol 2011;121: 328–33.

159. Silva EG, Deavers MT, Bodurka DC, et al. Uterine epithelioid leiomyosarcomas with clear cells: reactivity with HMB-45 and the concept of PEComa. Am J Surg Pathol 2004;28:244–9.

160. Levine PH, Mittal K. Rhabdoid epithelioid leiomyosarcoma of the uterine corpus: a case report and literature review. Int J Surg Pathol 2002;10:231–6.

161. Lee FY, Wen MC, Wang J. Epithelioid leiomyosarcoma of the uterus containing sex cord-like elements. Int J Gynecol Pathol 2010;29:67–8.

162. Fadare O. Perivascular epithelioid cell tumor (PEComa) of the uterus: an outcome-based clinicopathologic analysis of 41 reported cases. Adv Anat Pathol 2008;15:63–75.

163. Folpe AL, Mentzel T, Lehr HA, et al. Perivascular epithelioid cell neoplasms of soft tissue and gynecologic origin: a clinicopathologic study of 26 cases and review of the literature. Am J Surg Pathol 2005;29:1558–75.

164. Burch DM, Tavassoli FA. Myxoid leiomyosarcoma of the uterus. Histopathology 2011;59:1144–55.

165. King ME, Dickersin GR, Scully RE. Myxoid leiomyosarcoma of the uterus. A report of six cases. Am J Surg Pathol 1982;6:589–98.

166. Hoang LN, Aneja A, Conlon N, et al. Novel high-grade endometrial stromal sarcoma: a morphologic mimicker of myxoid leiomyosarcoma. Am J Surg Pathol 2017;41:12–24.

167. Marino-Enriquez A, Lauria A, Przybyl J, et al. BCOR internal tandem duplication in high-grade uterine sarcomas. Am J Surg Pathol 2018;42:335–41.

168. Chiang S, Lee CH, Stewart CJR, et al. BCOR is a robust diagnostic immunohistochemical marker of genetically diverse high-grade endometrial stromal sarcoma, including tumors exhibiting variant morphology. Mod Pathol 2017;30: 1251–61.

169. Lee HP, Tseng HH, Hsieh PP, et al. Uterine lipoleiomyosarcoma: report of 2 cases and review of the literature. Int J Gynecol Pathol 2012;31:358–63.

170. Schoolmeester JK, Stamatakos MD, Moyer AM, et al. Pleomorphic liposarcoma arising in a lipoleiomyosarcoma of the uterus: report of a case with genetic profiling by a next generation sequencing panel. Int J Gynecol Pathol 2016;35: 321–6.

171. Rosenblat Y, Rath-Wolfson L, Rabinerson D, et al. Huge uterine tumor in a postmenopausal woman. Arch Pathol Lab Med 2005;129:1189–91.

172. Bapat K, Brustein S. Uterine sarcoma with liposarcomatous differentiation: report of a case and review of the literature. Int J Gynaecol Obstet 1989; 28:71–5.

173. Strinic T, Kuzmic-Prusac I, Eterovic D, et al. Leiomyomatosis peritonealis disseminata in a postmenopausal woman. Arch Gynecol Obstet 2000;264: 97–8.

174. Nguyen GK. Disseminated leiomyomatosis peritonealis: report of a case in a postmenopausal woman. Can J Surg 1993;36:46–8.

175. Bekkers RL, Willemsen WN, Schijf CP, et al. Leiomyomatosis peritonealis disseminata: does malignant transformation occur? A literature review. Gynecol Oncol 1999;75:158–63.

176. Tavassoli FA, Norris HJ. Peritoneal leiomyomatosis (leiomyomatosis peritonealis disseminata): a clinicopathologic study of 20 cases with ultrastructural observations. Int J Gynecol Pathol 1982;1:59–74.

177. Halama N, Grauling-Halama SA, Daboul I. Familial clustering of Leiomyomatosis peritonealis disseminata: an unknown genetic syndrome? BMC Gastroenterol 2005;5:33.

178. Valente PT. Leiomyomatosis peritonealis disseminata. A report of two cases and review of the literature. Arch Pathol Lab Med 1984;108:669–72.

179. Drake A, Dhundee J, Buckley CH, et al. Disseminated leiomyomatosis peritonealis in association with oestrogen secreting ovarian fibrothecoma. BJOG 2001;108:661–4.

180. Willson JR, Peale AR. Multiple peritoneal leiomyomas associated with a granulosa-cell tumor of the ovary. Am J Obstet Gynecol 1952;64:204–8.

181. Quade BJ, McLachlin CM, Soto-Wright V, et al. Disseminated peritoneal leiomyomatosis. Clonality analysis by X chromosome inactivation and cytogenetics of a clinically benign smooth muscle proliferation. Am J Pathol 1997;150:2153–66.

182. Kuo T, London SN, Dinh TV. Endometriosis occurring in leiomyomatosis peritonealis disseminata: ultrastructural study and histogenetic consideration. Am J Surg Pathol 1980;4:197–204.

183. Ma KF, Chow LT. Sex cord-like pattern leiomyomatosis peritonealis disseminata: a hitherto undescribed feature. Histopathology 1992;21:389–91.

184. Gana BM, Byrne J, McCullough J, et al. Leiomyomatosis peritonealis disseminata (LPD) with associated endometriosis: a case report. J R Coll Surg Edinb 1994;39:258–60.

185. Toriyama A, Ishida M, Amano T, et al. Leiomyomatosis peritonealis disseminata coexisting with endometriosis within the same lesions: a case

report with review of the literature. Int J Clin Exp Pathol 2013;6:2949–54.

186. Buttner A, Bassler R, Theele C. Pregnancy-associated ectopic decidua (deciduosis) of the greater omentum. An analysis of 60 biopsies with cases of fibrosing deciduosis and leiomyomatosis peritonealis disseminata. Pathol Res Pract 1993;189:352–9.

187. Ghosh K, Dorigo O, Bristow R, et al. A radical debulking of leiomyomatosis peritonealis disseminata from a colonic obstruction: a case report and review of the literature. J Am Coll Surg 2000;191:212–5.

188. Heinig J, Neff A, Cirkel U, et al. Recurrent leiomyomatosis peritonealis disseminata after hysterectomy and bilateral salpingo-oophorectomy during combined hormone replacement therapy. Eur J Obstet Gynecol Reprod Biol 2003;111:216–8.

189. Hales HA, Peterson CM, Jones KP, et al. Leiomyomatosis peritonealis disseminata treated with a gonadotropin-releasing hormone agonist. A case report. Am J Obstet Gynecol 1992;167:515–6.

190. Lete I, Gonzalez J, Ugarte L, et al. Parasitic leiomyomas: a systematic review. Eur J Obstet Gynecol Reprod Biol 2016;203:250–9.

191. Seidman MA, Oduyebo T, Muto MG, et al. Peritoneal dissemination complicating morcellation of uterine mesenchymal neoplasms. PLoS One 2012;7:e50058.

192. Larrain D, Rabischong B, Khoo CK, et al. "Iatrogenic" parasitic myomas: unusual late complication of laparoscopic morcellation procedures. J Minim Invasive Gynecol 2010;17:719–24.

193. Nezhat C, Kho K. Iatrogenic myomas: new class of myomas? J Minim Invasive Gynecol 2010;17:544–50.

194. Gal AA, Brooks JS, Pietra GG. Leiomyomatous neoplasms of the lung: a clinical, histologic, and immunohistochemical study. Mod Pathol 1989;2:209–16.

195. Fan D, Yi X. Pulmonary benign metastasizing leiomyoma: a case report. Int J Clin Exp Pathol 2014;7:7072–5.

196. Choe YH, Jeon SY, Lee YC, et al. Benign metastasizing leiomyoma presenting as multiple cystic pulmonary nodules: a case report. BMC Womens Health 2017;17:81.

197. Barnas E, Ksiazek M, Ras R, et al. Benign metastasizing leiomyoma: A review of current literature in respect to the time and type of previous gynecological surgery. PLoS One 2017;12:e0175875.

198. Steiner PE. Metastasizing fibroleiomyoma of the uterus: report of a case and review of the literature. Am J Pathol 1939;15:89–110.7.

199. Horstmann JP, Pietra GG, Harman JA, et al. Spontaneous regression of pulmonary leiomyomas during pregnancy. Cancer 1977;39:314–21.

200. Patton KT, Cheng L, Papavero V, et al. Benign metastasizing leiomyoma: clonality, telomere length and clinicopathologic analysis. Mod Pathol 2006;19:130–40.

201. Tietze L, Gunther K, Horbe A, et al. Benign metastasizing leiomyoma: a cytogenetically balanced but clonal disease. Hum Pathol 2000;31:126–8.

202. Nucci MR, Drapkin R, Dal Cin P, et al. Distinctive cytogenetic profile in benign metastasizing leiomyoma: pathogenetic implications. Am J Surg Pathol 2007;31:737–43.

203. Christacos NC, Quade BJ, Dal Cin P, et al. Uterine leiomyomata with deletions of Ip represent a distinct cytogenetic subgroup associated with unusual histologic features. Genes Chromosomes Cancer 2006;45:304–12.

204. Aboualfa K, Calandriello L, Dusmet M, et al. Benign metastasizing leiomyoma presenting as cystic lung disease: a diagnostic pitfall. Histopathology 2011;59:796–9.

205. Fukunaga M. Benign "metastasizing" lipoleiomyoma of the uterus. Int J Gynecol Pathol 2003;22:202–4.

206. Folpe AL, Kwiatkowski DJ. Perivascular epithelioid cell neoplasms: pathology and pathogenesis. Hum Pathol 2010;41:1–15.

207. Tomashefski JF Jr. Benign endobronchial mesenchymal tumors: their relationship to parenchymal pulmonary hamartomas. Am J Surg Pathol 1982;6:531–40.

208. Dekate J, Chetty R. Epstein-Barr virus-associated smooth muscle tumor. Arch Pathol Lab Med 2016;140:718–22.

209. Miller J, Shoni M, Siegert C, et al. Benign metastasizing leiomyomas to the lungs: an institutional case series and a review of the recent literature. Ann Thorac Surg 2016;101:253–8.

210. Ki EY, Hwang SJ, Lee KH, et al. Benign metastasizing leiomyoma of the lung. World J Surg Oncol 2013;11:279.

211. Lewis EI, Chason RJ, DeCherney AH, et al. Novel hormone treatment of benign metastasizing leiomyoma: an analysis of five cases and literature review. Fertil Steril 2013;99:2017–24.

212. Nasu K, Tsuno A, Takai N, et al. A case of benign metastasizing leiomyoma treated by surgical castration followed by an aromatase inhibitor, anastrozole. Arch Gynecol Obstet 2009;279:255–7.

213. Lerwill MF, Sung R, Oliva E, et al. Smooth muscle tumors of the ovary: a clinicopathologic study of 54 cases emphasizing prognostic criteria, histologic variants, and differential diagnosis. Am J Surg Pathol 2004;28:1436–51.

214. Sayeed S, Xing D, Jenkins SM, et al. Criteria for risk stratification of vulvar and vaginal smooth muscle tumors: an evaluation of 71 cases comparing

proposed classification systems. Am J Surg Pathol 2018;42:84–94.

215. Patel V, Xing D, Feely DO, et al. Smooth muscle tumors of the visceral adnexal and uterine ligaments and adnexal connective tissue: a clinicopathologic study of 67 cases. Int J Gynecol Pathol 2019, [Epub ahead of print].

216. Santini D, Ceccarelli C, Leone O, et al. Smooth muscle differentiation in normal human ovaries, ovarian stromal hyperplasia and ovarian granulosa-stromal cells tumors. Mod Pathol 1995; 8:25–30.

217. Doss BJ, Wanek SM, Jacques SM, et al. Ovarian smooth muscle metaplasia: an uncommon and possibly underrecognized entity. Int J Gynecol Pathol 1999;18:58–62.

218. Lastarria D, Sachdev RK, Babury RA, et al. Immunohistochemical analysis for desmin in normal and neoplastic ovarian stromal tissue. Arch Pathol Lab Med 1990;114:502–5.

219. Okamura H, Virutamasen P, Wright KH, et al. Ovarian smooth muscle in the human being, rabbit, and cat. Histochemical and electron microscopic study. Am J Obstet Gynecol 1972;112:183–91.

220. Doss BJ, Wanek SM, Jacques SM, et al. Ovarian leiomyomas: clinicopathologic features in fifteen cases. Int J Gynecol Pathol 1999;18:63–8.

221. Kurai M, Shiozawa T, Noguchi H, et al. Leiomyoma of the ovary presenting with Meigs' syndrome. J Obstet Gynaecol Res 2005;31:257–62.

222. Prayson RA, Hart WR. Primary smooth-muscle tumors of the ovary. A clinicopathologic study of four leiomyomas and two mitotically active leiomyomas. Arch Pathol Lab Med 1992;116:1068–71.

223. Kandalaft PL, Esteban JM. Bilateral massive ovarian leiomyomata in a young woman: a case report with review of the literature. Mod Pathol 1992;5:586–9.

224. Fallahzadeh H, Dockerty MB, Lee RA. Leiomyoma of the ovary: report of five cases and review of the literature. Am J Obstet Gynecol 1972;113: 394–8.

225. Hemalata M, Kusuma V, Sruthi P. Ovarian lipoleiomyoma: a rare benign tumour. J Clin Pathol 2007; 60:939–40.

226. Xing D, Berrebi AA, Liu C, et al. An epithelioid smooth muscle neoplasm mimicking a signet ring cell carcinoma in the ovary. Int J Gynecol Pathol 2018, [Epub ahead of print].

227. Irving JA. Cellular fibromatous neoplasms of the ovary. Surg Pathol Clin 2009;2:731–53.

228. Tiltman AJ, Haffajee Z. Sclerosing stromal tumors, thecomas, and fibromas of the ovary: an immunohistochemical profile. Int J Gynecol Pathol 1999; 18:254–8.

229. Oliva E, Egger JF, Young RH. Primary endometrioid stromal sarcoma of the ovary: a clinicopathologic study of 27 cases with morphologic and behavioral features similar to those of uterine low-grade endometrial stromal sarcoma. Am J Surg Pathol 2014; 38:305–15.

230. Young RH, Prat J, Scully RE. Endometrioid stromal sarcomas of the ovary. A clinicopathologic analysis of 23 cases. Cancer 1984;53:1143–55.

231. Rasmussen CC, Skilling JS, Sorosky JI, et al. Stage IIIC ovarian leiomyosarcoma in a premenopausal woman with multiple recurrences: prolonged survival with surgical therapy. Gynecol Oncol 1997; 66:519–25.

232. Shah A, Finn C, Light A. Leiomyosarcoma of the broad ligament: a case report and literature review. Gynecol Oncol 2003;90:450–2.

233. Bouie SM, Cracchiolo B, Heller D. Epithelioid leiomyosarcoma of the ovary. Gynecol Oncol 2005; 97:697–9.

234. Nogales FF, Ayala A, Ruiz-Avila I, et al. Myxoid leiomyosarcoma of the ovary: analysis of three cases. Hum Pathol 1991;22:1268–73.

235. Fadare O, Ghofrani M, Stamatakos MD, et al. Mesenchymal lesions of the uterine cervix. Pathol Case Rev 2006;11:140–51.

236. Fadare O. Uncommon sarcomas of the uterine cervix: a review of selected entities. Diagn Pathol 2006;1:30.

237. Tiltman AJ. Leiomyomas of the uterine cervix: a study of frequency. Int J Gynecol Pathol 1998;17:231–4.

238. Nichols DH, Hayes LW Jr. Cervical fibroid in pregnancy and delivery. Obstet Gynecol 1953;2:180–2.

239. Abitbol MM, Madison RL. Cervical fibroids complicating pregnancy; report of three cases. Obstet Gynecol 1958;12:397–8.

240. Erian J, El-Toukhy T, Chandakas S, et al. Rapidly enlarging cervical fibroids during pregnancy: a case report. J Obstet Gynaecol 2004; 24:578–9.

241. Pollard RR, Goldberg JM. Prolapsed cervical myoma after uterine artery embolization. A case report. J Reprod Med 2001;46:499–500.

242. Varras M, Hadjilira P, Polyzos D, et al. Clinical considerations and sonographic findings of a large nonpedunculated primary cervical leiomyoma complicated by heavy vaginal haemorrhage: a case report and review of the literature. Clin Exp Obstet Gynecol 2003;30:144–6.

243. Palanichamy G, Authilingom R. Degenerating cervical myoma simulating chronic puerperal inversion and gangrene of uterus - (Report of a case). J Obstet Gynaecol India 1976;26:790–1.

244. Chu CM, Acholonu UC Jr, Chang-Jackson SC, et al. Leiomyoma recurrent at the cervical stump: report of two cases. J Minim Invasive Gynecol 2012;19:131–3.

245. Laskin WB, Fetsch JF, Tavassoli FA. Superficial cervicovaginal myofibroblastoma: fourteen cases

of a distinctive mesenchymal tumor arising from the specialized subepithelial stroma of the lower female genital tract. Hum Pathol 2001;32: 715–25.

246. Abell MR, Ramirez JA. Sarcomas and carcinosarcomas of the uterine cervix. Cancer 1973;31: 1176–92.

247. Kasamatsu T, Shiromizu K, Takahashi M, et al. Leiomyosarcoma of the uterine cervix. Gynecol Oncol 1998;69:169–71.

248. Wright JD, Rosenblum K, Huettner PC, et al. Cervical sarcomas: an analysis of incidence and outcome. Gynecol Oncol 2005;99:348–51.

249. Toyoshima M, Okamura C, Niikura H, et al. Epithelioid leiomyosarcoma of the uterine cervix: a case report and review of the literature. Gynecol Oncol 2005;97:957–60.

250. Gotoh T, Kikuchi Y, Takano M, et al. Epithelioid leiomyosarcoma of the uterine cervix. Gynecol Oncol 2001;82:400–5.

251. Colombat M, Sevestre H, Gontier MF. Epithelioid leiomyosarcoma of the uterine cervix. Report of a case. Ann Pathol 2001;21:48–50, [in French].

252. Fujiwaki R, Yoshida M, Iida K, et al. Epithelioid leiomyosarcoma of the uterine cervix. Acta Obstet Gynecol Scand 1998;77:246–8.

253. Fraga M, Prieto O, Garcia-Caballero T, et al. Myxoid leiomyosarcoma of the uterine cervix. Histopathology 1994;25:381–4.

254. Grayson W, Fourie J, Tiltman AJ. Xanthomatous leiomyosarcoma of the uterine cervix. Int J Gynecol Pathol 1998;17:89–90.

255. Bader LV, Rundle RC. Mesenchymal sarcoma of the cervix uteri: case report. Pathology 1969;1: 251–4.

256. Young RH. Neoplasms of the fallopian tube and broad ligament: a selective survey including historical perspective and emphasising recent developments. Pathology 2007;39:112–24.

257. Honore LH. Parauterine leiomyomas in women: a clinicopathologic study of 22 cases. Eur J Obstet Gynecol Reprod Biol 1981;11:273–9.

258. Brown RS, Marley JL, Cassoni AM. Pseudo-Meigs' syndrome due to broad ligament leiomyoma: a mimic of metastatic ovarian carcinoma. Clin Oncol (R Coll Radiol) 1998;10:198–201.

259. Matthews T, Amanuel B, Tsokos N. Atypical leiomyoma of the broad ligament. Aust N Z J Obstet Gynaecol 2003;43:326–8.

260. Salman MC, Atak Z, Usubutun A, et al. Lipoleiomyoma of broad ligament mimicking ovarian cancer in a postmenopausal patient: case report and literature review. J Gynecol Oncol 2010;21:62–4.

261. Maryanski J, Gulak G, Pawlowski W. Lipoleiomyoma of the broad ligament of the uterus. Int J Gynaecol Obstet 2009;107:257.

262. Clement PB. The pathology of endometriosis: a survey of the many faces of a common disease emphasizing diagnostic pitfalls and unusual and newly appreciated aspects. Adv Anat Pathol 2007;14:241–60.

263. Clement PB. Pathology of endometriosis. Pathol Annu 1990;25(Pt 1):245–95.

264. Wahal SP, Mardi K, Sharma S. "Stump" of broad ligament: a rare entity with review of literature. South Asian J Cancer 2013;2:118.

265. Murialdo R, Usset A, Guido T, et al. Leiomyosarcoma of the broad ligament: a case report and review of literature. Int J Gynecol Cancer 2005;15: 1226–9.

266. Jacoby AF, Fuller AF Jr, Thor AD, et al. Primary leiomyosarcoma of the fallopian tube. Gynecol Oncol 1993;51:404–7.

267. You D, Wang Q, Jiang W, et al. Primary leiomyosarcoma of the fallopian tube: a case report and literature review. Medicine (Baltimore) 2018;97: e0536.

268. Kir G, Eren S, Akoz I, et al. Leiomyosarcoma of the broad ligament arising in a pre-existing pure neurilemmoma-like leiomyoma. Eur J Gynaecol Oncol 2003;24:505–6.

269. Kaba M, Tokmak A, Timur H, et al. A rare case of leiomyosarcoma originating from the left round ligament of the uterus. J Exp Ther Oncol 2016;11: 237–40.

270. Kirkham JC, Nero CJ, Tambouret RH, et al. Leiomyoma and leiomyosarcoma arising from the round ligament of the uterus. J Am Coll Surg 2008;207:452.

271. Clarke BA, Rahimi K, Chetty R. Leiomyosarcoma of the broad ligament with osteoclast-like giant cells and rhabdoid cells. Int J Gynecol Pathol 2010;29: 432–7.

272. Franquemont DW, Frierson HF Jr. Muscle differentiation and clinicopathologic features of gastrointestinal stromal tumors. Am J Surg Pathol 1992;16: 947–54.

273. Sangwan K, Khosla AH, Hazra PC. Leiomyoma of the vagina. Aust N Z J Obstet Gynaecol 1996;36:494–5.

274. Tavassoli FA, Norris HJ. Smooth muscle tumors of the vagina. Obstet Gynecol 1979;53:689–93.

275. Leron E, Stanton SL. Vaginal leiomyoma–an imitator of prolapse. Int Urogynecol J Pelvic Floor Dysfunct 2000;11:196–8.

276. Biankin SA, O'Toole VE, Fung C, et al. Bizarre leiomyoma of the vagina: report of a case. Int J Gynecol Pathol 2000;19:186–7.

277. Vlahos N, Economopoulos K, Skarpidi E, et al. Bizarre leiomyoma of the posterior vaginal fornix. Int J Gynaecol Obstet 2008;102:296–7.

278. Kay S, Schneider V. Reactive spindle cell nodule of the endocervix simulating uterine sarcoma. Int J Gynecol Pathol 1985;4:255–7.

279. Ciaravino G, Kapp DS, Vela AM, et al. Primary leiomyosarcoma of the vagina. A case report and literature review. Int J Gynecol Cancer 2000; 10:340–7.

280. Rastogi BL, Bergman B, Angervall L. Primary leiomyosarcoma of the vagina: a study of five cases. Gynecol Oncol 1984;18:77–86.

281. Peters WA 3rd, Kumar NB, Andersen WA, et al. Primary sarcoma of the adult vagina: a clinicopathologic study. Obstet Gynecol 1985;65: 699–704.

282. Nucci MR, Fletcher CD. Vulvovaginal soft tissue tumours: update and review. Histopathology 2000; 36:97–108.

283. Malkasian GD Jr, Welch JS, Soule EH. Primary leiomyosarcoma of the vagina. Report of 8 cases. Am J Obstet Gynecol 1963;86:730–6.

284. Byrd L, Sikand K, Slade R. Lipoleiomyosarcoma of the vagina. J Obstet Gynaecol 2007;27:334–5.

285. Faber K, Jones MA, Spratt D, et al. Vulvar leiomyomatosis in a patient with esophagogastric leiomyomatosis: review of the syndrome. Gynecol Oncol 1991;41:92–4.

286. Miner JH. Alport syndrome with diffuse leiomyomatosis. When and when not? Am J Pathol 1999;154: 1633–5.

287. Nielsen GP, Rosenberg AE, Koerner FC, et al. Smooth-muscle tumors of the vulva. A clinicopathological study of 25 cases and review of the literature. Am J Surg Pathol 1996;20:779–93.

288. Tavassoli FA, Norris HJ. Smooth muscle tumors of the vulva. Obstet Gynecol 1979;53:213–7.

289. Kim HR, Yi BH, Lee HK, et al. Vulval epithelioid leiomyoma in a pregnant woman. J Obstet Gynaecol 2013;33:210–1.

290. Hopkins-Luna AM, Chambers DC, Goodman MD. Epithelioid leiomyoma of the vulva. J Natl Med Assoc 1999;91:171–3.

291. Steeper TA, Rosai J. Aggressive angiomyxoma of the female pelvis and perineum. Report of nine cases of a distinctive type of gynecologic soft-tissue neoplasm. Am J Surg Pathol 1983;7: 463–75.

292. Nucci MR, Granter SR, Fletcher CD. Cellular angiofibroma: a benign neoplasm distinct from angiomyofibroblastoma and spindle cell lipoma. Am J Surg Pathol 1997;21:636–44.

293. Iwasa Y, Fletcher CD. Cellular angiofibroma: clinicopathologic and immunohistochemical analysis of 51 cases. Am J Surg Pathol 2004; 28:1426–35.

294. Yang EJ, Howitt BE, Fletcher CDM, et al. Solitary fibrous tumour of the female genital tract: a clinicopathological analysis of 25 cases. Histopathology 2018;72:749–59.

295. Gonzalez-Bugatto F, Anon-Requena MJ, Lopez-Guerrero MA, et al. Vulvar leiomyosarcoma in Bartholin's gland area: a case report and literature review. Arch Gynecol Obstet 2009;279:171–4.

296. Mowers EL, Shank JJ, Frisch N, et al. Myxoid leiomyosarcoma of the Bartholin gland. Obstet Gynecol 2014;124:433–5.

297. Nemoto T, Shinoda M, Komatsuzaki K, et al. Myxoid leiomyoma of the vulva mimicking aggressive angiomyxoma. Pathol Int 1994;44:454–9.

298. Di Gilio AR, Cormio G, Resta L, et al. Rapid growth of myxoid leiomyosarcoma of the vulva during pregnancy: a case report. Int J Gynecol Cancer 2004;14:172–5.

299. Tjalma WA, Colpaert CG. Myxoid leiomyosarcoma of the vulva. Gynecol Oncol 2005;96:548–51.

300. Jahanseir K, Xing D, Greipp PT, et al. PDGFB rearrangements in dermatofibrosarcoma protuberans of the vulva: a study of 11 cases including myxoid and fibrosarcomatous variants. Int J Gynecol Pathol 2018;37:537–46.

301. Edelweiss M, Malpica A. Dermatofibrosarcoma protuberans of the vulva: a clinicopathologic and immunohistochemical study of 13 cases. Am J Surg Pathol 2010;34:393–400.

302. Ghorbani RP, Malpica A, Ayala AG. Dermatofibrosarcoma protuberans of the vulva: clinicopathologic and immunohistochemical analysis of four cases, one with fibrosarcomatous change, and review of the literature. Int J Gynecol Pathol 1999;18: 366–73.

Fallopian Tube Neoplasia and Mimics

David L. Kolin, MD, PhD, Marisa R. Nucci, MD*

KEYWORDS

- Fallopian tube • Adenomatoid tumor • Serous tubal intraepithelial carcinoma • Serous neoplasia
- Secretory cell outgrowth • Endometrioid carcinoma

Key Points

- Adenomatoid tumors are the most common benign tumor of the fallopian tube, and display morphology that may overlap with carcinoma

- Serous tubal intraepithelial carcinoma (STIC) is the precursor of many so-called ovarian high-grade serous carcinomas and should be differentiated from histologic mimics

- Metastases to the fallopian tube may be serosal, mural, or mucosal, and mimic primary tubal neoplasia

- Although rare, endometrioid neoplasms of the tube may histologically resemble STIC, sex-cord proliferations, and female adnexal tumors of Wolffian origin (FATWO)

ABSTRACT

This review discusses select fallopian tube entities and their associated mimics. It first focuses on adenomatoid tumors, the most common benign tumor of the fallopian tube. High-grade serous carcinoma and its precursor, serous tubal intraepithelial carcinoma, are then addressed. Finally, attention is turned to endometrioid proliferations of the fallopian tube. A diagnostic approach is provided for these lesions, with an emphasis on differential diagnoses and situations in which a benign lesion may appear malignant, and vice-versa.

ADENOMATOID TUMORS

OVERVIEW

Adenomatoid tumors are the most common benign tumor of the fallopian tube, and are usually solitary and incidentally discovered.[1,2] When multiple, they can be associated with cyclosporine therapy in the setting of renal transplantation.[3] Although the diagnosis is usually straightforward, their varied morphology raises many differential diagnoses. Recent molecular studies have shown that they are defined by mutations in *TRAF7*.[4] However, molecular testing is not routinely used because of their typically easily recognized morphology and distinct immunohistochemical profile.

GROSS FEATURES

Tubal adenomatoid tumors are well-circumscribed, firm masses.[5] They are subserosal, with a grey-white cut surface, and are usually sub-centimeter in size.[1,5]

MICROSCOPIC FEATURES

Adenomatoid tumors can display a wide range of morphologies, including glandular, signet ring, solid, cystic, and angiomatoid (**Fig. 1**); a single tumor often displays more than 1 pattern.[1,5] The tumors are unencapsulated, and unlike those that

---

Disclosure Statement: The authors have no conflicts of interest to disclose.
Division of Women's and Perinatal Pathology, Department of Pathology, Harvard Medical School, Brigham and Women's Hospital, 75 Francis Street, Boston, MA 02115, USA
* Corresponding author.
E-mail address: mnucci@bwh.harvard.edu

Surgical Pathology 12 (2019) 457–479
https://doi.org/10.1016/j.path.2019.01.006
1875-9181/19/© 2019 Elsevier Inc. All rights reserved.

458

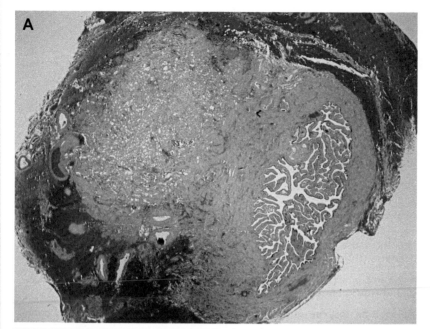

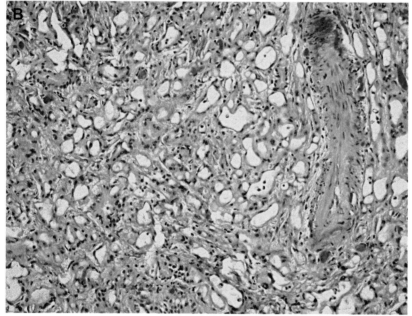

Fig. 1. (*A*) Low-power view of an adenomatoid tumor that forms a mass on the serosal aspect of the fallopian tube. (*B*) Higher magnification shows microcystic spaces lined by mesothelial cells and signet ring morphology.

occur in the uterus, usually well-circumscribed. They are composed of a single layer of flattened mesothelial cells. Atypia is usually absent and mitotic activity should be scarce. Smooth muscle fibers may be admixed with the mesothelial proliferation. Lymphoid aggregates may also be seen (**Fig. 2**).[1] In rare instances, infarcted adenomatoid tumors may show necrosis and raise the possibility of a malignant process.[6] Immunohistochemical staining supports their mesothelial lineage, as they are positive for WT-1, pan-keratin, D2-40, and calretinin (**Fig. 3**).[1,7]

Key features
OF ADENOMATOID TUMOR

1. Most common benign tumor of fallopian tube

2. Well-circumscribed, subserosal nodule

3. Glandular, microcystic, angiomatoid, solid morphologies

4. Immunohistochemistry: positive for mesothelial markers (pan-keratin, WT-1, calretinin)

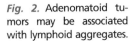

Differential diagnosis
OF ADENOMATOID TUMOR

Metastatic signet ring cell carcinoma

Salpingitis isthmica nodosa

Mesothelioma

Lipoleiomyoma

Lymphangioma

Metastatic Carcinoma

Metastatic carcinoma may involve the fallopian tube and show signet ring morphology, which can mimic an adenomatoid tumor (**Fig. 4**). The most common non-gynecologic malignancies to spread to this site include appendiceal, gastric, colonic, and mammary carcinomas.[8,9] Patients with metastatic lesions usually have a known history of a prior carcinoma, which is helpful in recognizing this potential diagnostic pitfall. In the absence of this history, other features are helpful. For instance, metastases are often multifocal, with an infiltrative growth pattern, which is in contrast to adenomatoid tumors. Immunohistochemistry also can be used to differentiate metastases from an adenomatoid tumor and to confirm a site of origin in difficult cases. Although both adenomatoid tumors and carcinomas are positive for keratins, carcinoma is usually negative for

calretinin and D2-40, and may be positive for site-specific markers (eg, CDX-2 or GATA-3 in gastrointestinal and breast primaries, respectively). Signet ring cell carcinomas also demonstrate intracytoplasmic mucin, whereas adenomatoid tumors do not. D2-40 and calretinin are less helpful if the differential diagnosis includes serous carcinoma of the ovary, as it may display positivity for both of these markers (albeit usually weak and patchy).[10,11]

Salpingitis Isthmica Nodosa

Salpingitis isthmica nodosa may form a nodular mass composed of glands that resemble an adenomatoid tumor (**Fig. 5**). However, the glands are lined by tubal-type epithelium; it is present in the muscular wall of the tube, and it has been likened to a tubal adenomyosis.[12] It is a benign lesion, present in 0.6% to 11% of fallopian tubes, and is associated with ectopic pregnancy.[13]

Malignant Mesothelioma

Malignant mesothelioma, like adenomatoid tumors, is of mesothelial lineage. However, it forms a large, infiltrative mass, with increased cytologic atypia and mitotic activity (**Fig. 6**). In addition to the tubal serosa, other peritoneal surfaces may also be involved. About half of mesotheliomas show loss of BAP1 by immunohistochemistry.[14] Some cases are associated with asbestos exposure.

Fig. 2. Adenomatoid tumors may be associated with lymphoid aggregates.

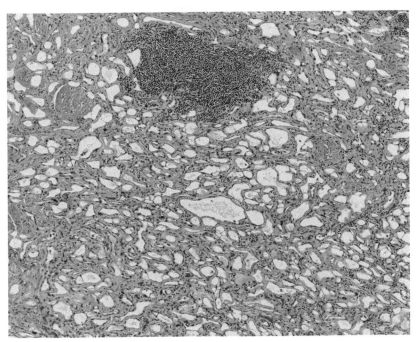

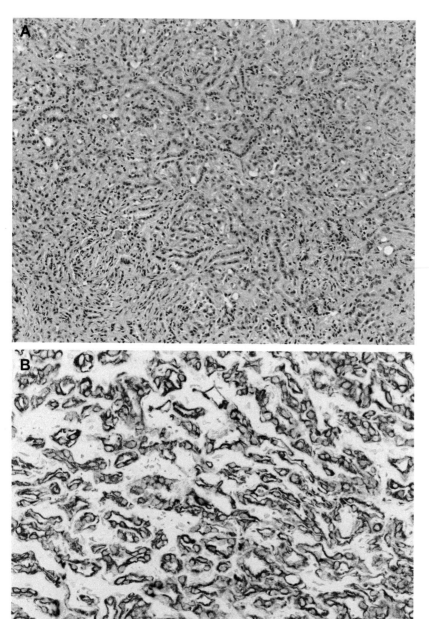

Fig. 3. Adenomatoid tumors may show a glandular architecture (*A*), which mimics a metastatic adenocarcinoma. Like carcinoma, adenomatoid tumors are positive for keratin (*B*). However, they are also positive for calretinin

Lipoleiomyoma

Lipoleiomyoma is a benign tumor usually seen in the myometrium, which is composed of smooth muscle and mature adipocytes, and may resemble the microcystic spaces of an adenomatoid tumor at low power. However, adipocytes are not features of adenomatoid tumors, and immunohistochemistry can confirm the presence of mesothelial-lined spaces rather than true adipocytes in challenging cases.

Lymphangiomas

Lymphangiomas may occur in the fallopian tube. They show cystically dilated lymphatic spaces that resemble the cystic spaces of an adenomatoid tumor. However, the cystic spaces contain

Fig. 3. (*continued*). (*C*), with a low Ki-67 proliferation index (*D*).

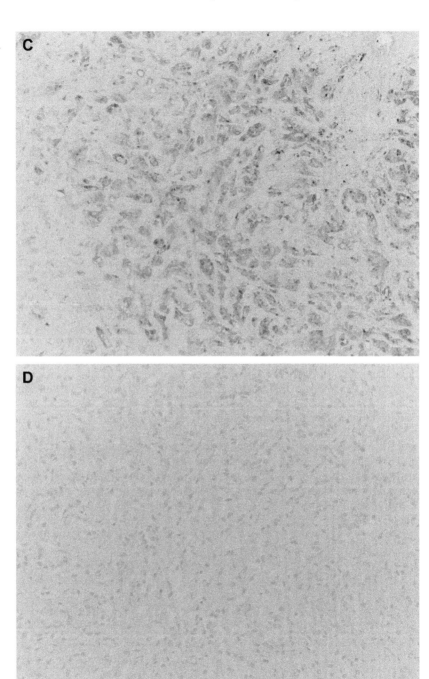

lymphocytes, and they are negative for calretinin. Of note, D2-40 may be positive in both lymphangiomas and adenomatoid tumors.

PROGNOSIS

Adenomatoid tumors are benign, without risk of recurrence.

SEROUS TUBAL INTRAEPITHELIAL CARCINOMA

OVERVIEW

The fallopian tube had been overlooked as a site of origin until relatively recently. Its central role in high-grade serous neoplasia became appreciated

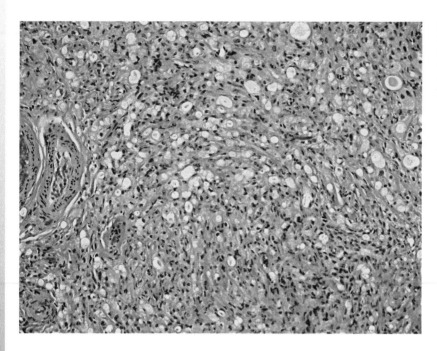

Fig. 4. Metastatic breast carcinoma to the fallopian tube may have a signet ring morphology and mimic an adenomatoid tumor (cf. **Fig. 1B**).

after early tubal precancers and cancers were detected in the fimbria of *BRCA1/2* carriers undergoing prophylactic salpingo-oophorectomies.[15–18] Serous tubal intraepithelial carcinoma (STIC) is now thought to be the precursor of tubal high-grade serous carcinoma (HGSC), and most, if not all, "ovarian" HGSC.[19] The vast majority of STICs are located in the tubal fimbria, although they can occur elsewhere in the tube.[16,20] A STIC is found in about half of HGSC cases,[20,21] and in

5% to 8% of prophylactic salpingectomies.[15,22] In women without either genetic risk factors or HGSC, the incidence of STIC is extremely low (0.1%).[23]

GROSS FEATURES

Serous tubal intraepithelial carcinomas are focal, microscopic lesions that are not grossly visible and therefore require extensive sampling of the

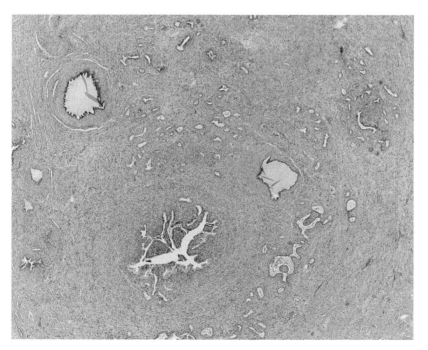

Fig. 5. Salpingitis isthmica nodosa is composed of nodular groups of diverticula-like lumens lined with tubal epithelium.

Fig. 6. Malignant meso-
thelioma forms a large,
infiltrative mass that
may surround the tube.

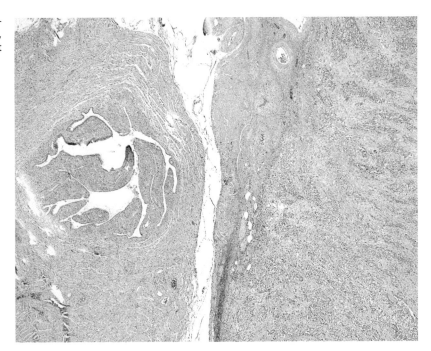

fallopian tube for detection. The sectioning and
extensive examining of the fimbriated end (SEE-
FIM) protocol was developed to carefully examine
the tube in toto, with an emphasis on maximizing
the cross-section of visible fimbria, the location
most likely to harbor a STIC.18

MICROSCOPIC FEATURES

Serous tubal intraepithelial carcinomas are characterized by loss of polarity with stratification,
hyperchromasia, nuclear atypia, prominent
nucleoli, apoptotic bodies, and increased mitotic
activity (**Fig. 7**A). Cilia are usually absent. Both
STIC and HGSC share an immunohistochemical
profile, with a mutant pattern of p53 staining (either
diffuse overexpression, or a null pattern), block
positive staining of p16, and an increased Ki-67
proliferation index (**Fig. 7**B).

Key features
OF SEROUS TUBAL
INTRAEPITHELIAL CARCINOMA

1. Extensive examination of the fallopian tube
   using the SEE-FIM grossing protocol is
   required for prophylactic salpingectomies

2. The precursor lesion for most ovarian high-
   grade serous carcinoma

3. Increased incidence in *BRCA1/2* carriers

4. Characterized by loss of nuclear polarity
   with stratification, nuclear pleomorphism,
   increased nuclear-cytoplasmic ratio, mitotic
   activity, and apoptotic bodies

5. Immunohistochemistry: aberrant p53 staining pattern and increased Ki-67 proliferation
   index

6. Associated with an increased risk of subsequent HGSC, but most clinicians will not
   treat STIC with chemotherapy

DIAGNOSIS AND DIFFERENTIAL DIAGNOSIS

p53 Signatures

p53 signatures are composed of a clonal proliferation of cells with an abnormal pattern of p53 staining (**Fig. 8**). In contrast to STIC, they have
maintained polarity, minimal cytologic atypia, and
a low proliferation index. The clinical significance
of these incidental lesions is not clear and they
are not usually reported as a clinical pathologic
diagnosis.

Serous Tubal Intraepithelial Proliferations or Lesions of Uncertain Significance

Serous tubal intraepithelial proliferations or lesions of uncertain significance may lack ciliated

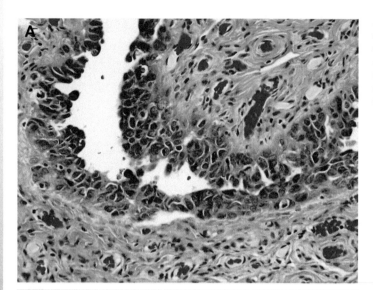

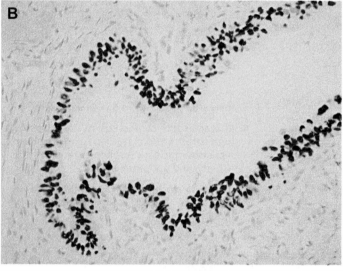

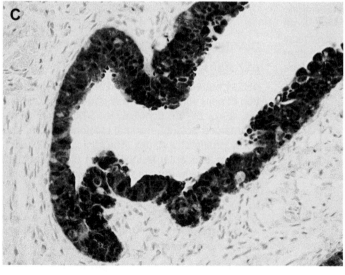

Fig. 7. (*A*) Serous tubal intraepithelial carcinoma (STIC) shows nuclear enlargement, hyperchromasia, loss of polarity, prominent nucleoli, and mitotic activity. (*B*) STICs show a mutant pattern of p53 staining, and (*C*) are diffusely positive for p16.

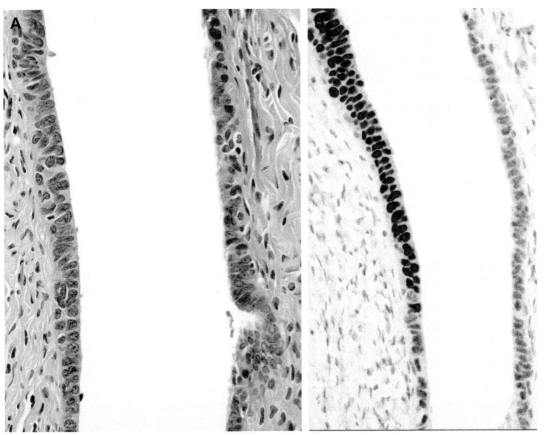

Fig. 8. (*A*) p53 signatures are characterized by an outgrowth of cells with abnormal p53 staining pattern (*B*), but with preserved polarity, minimal cytologic atypia, and a low proliferative index.

differentiation, display an abnormal p53 staining pattern, and show cytologic atypia but have *maintained* polarity.[19] The malignant potential of these lesions is unknown, but is likely less than STIC.[19] Serial sections are recommended to exclude the possibility of an STIC or invasive carcinoma. A recent study has shown a clonal relationship between early serous proliferations, such as p53 signatures and tubal intraepithelial lesions, and metastatic HGSC, even in the absence of an STIC.[24] This finding suggests that these early proliferations may undergo "precursor escape," in that they seed the peritoneum and later develop into HGSC, thereby providing a possible mechanism for the pathogenesis of HGSC in cases without an STIC or involvement of tubal mucosa by HGSC.

High-Grade Serous Carcinoma

High-grade serous carcinoma shares the cytology and immunohistochemical profile of STIC. However, stromal invasion, usually accompanied by mass formation, differentiate it from an STIC.

Metastases

Metastases to the tube are most commonly from the endometrium, ovary, appendix, stomach, colon, and breast,[8,9,25] and may involve any part of the tube, including the fimbria, serosa, muscularis, mucosa, lymphovascular spaces, and tube lumen.[9,25] Of note, some metastases have an intraepithelial growth pattern in the fimbria that may histologically mimic an STIC, and also show a mutant pattern of p53 staining.[8,9,26,27] These STIC mimics may metastasize from gynecologic primaries, including endometrial and endocervical carcinomas, or from distant sites such as colonic, gastric, pancreaticobiliary, and mammary carcinomas.[9,26–29] An appropriate immunohistochemical panel is usually sufficient to differentiate these mucosal metastases from STIC.

Metastases from human papillomavirus-positive endocervical primaries usually stain strongly with p16, such as STIC. However, they have frequent apical mitotic figures, and lack abnormal p53 staining. Human papillomavirus tissue testing can also be performed in difficult cases. Immunohistochemistry for CK7, CK20, CDX2 or SATB2 (colonic), GATA-3 (breast), and SMAD4 (lost in half of metastatic pancreatic adenocarcinomas) can be used, as appropriate, if metastases are considered. PAX8 is useful to confirm Mullerian origin. A history of malignancy is usually available and is the most helpful feature to raise the possibility of a mucosal metastasis.

The metastases may also show bland cytology, occasionally with a deceiving appearance of mucinous metaplasia.[9] p53 immunohistochemistry may be helpful to demonstrate the neoplastic nature of these benign-appearing lesions. STIC and serous carcinoma should not show mucinous differentiation, and a p53 mutant mucinous lesion in the tube should prompt consideration of other entities. True mucinous metaplasia of the fallopian tube can be seen in Peutz-Jeghers syndrome, and this should be considered clinically.[30,31] Positive staining with MUC6 is supportive of gastric differentiation, and can be confirmed with MUC6 immunohistochemistry.

Arias-Stella Effect

Arias-Stella effect can occur in the fallopian tube epithelium of pregnant patients, producing a similar effect to that seen in the endometrium (**Fig. 9**), with stratification and cellular atypia. The clinical setting of pregnancy usually helps to resolve the differential diagnosis, but immunohistochemistry for p53 can be used in challenging cases.

Pseudocarcinomatous Hyperplasia

Pseudocarcinomatous hyperplasia is an inflammatory response of the tubal epithelium that may mimic a neoplastic proliferation (**Fig. 10**). In half of cases, the patients have pelvic inflammatory disease, and it can also be associated with tuberculosis.[32,33] All reported cases have occurred in premenopausal women.[32,34] Clinically and radiographically, it may mimic a primary carcinoma, with tubal distension and increased CA-125.[34] Grossly, the fallopian tube wall may be thickened and distended with pyosalpinx, but there is usually no mass.[32] Microscopically, there is an absence of both severe cytologic atypia and atypical mitotic figures. Immunohistochemistry shows a wild-type p53 pattern of staining, although the Ki-67 proliferation index may be increased. Microscopically, pseudocarcinomatous hyperplasia may show several features concerning for malignancy, including a cribriform, back-to-back glandular, or microcystic sieve-like architecture, apparent infiltration of the tubal wall by glands, and presence of epithelial clusters and/or psammoma bodies in lymphatics.[32] Features inconsistent with pseudocarcinomatous hyperplasia, which should prompt consideration of a

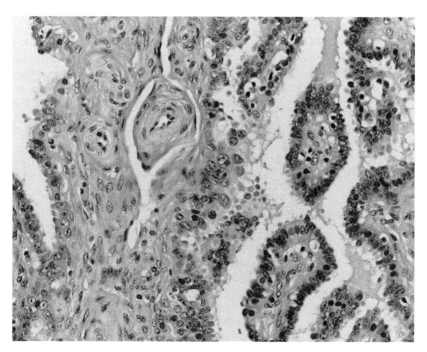

Fig. 9. Arias-Stella effect can cause cytologic atypia that can be morphologically suspicious for a serous tubal intraepithelial lesion.

Fig. 10. (*A*) Pseudocarcinomatous hyperplasia of the tubal epithelium can show complex, cribriform architecture. (*B*) Elsewhere in this tube, there was extensive granulomatous inflammation. Acid-fast bacillus and Gomori methenamine silver stains were negative for microorganisms (not shown).

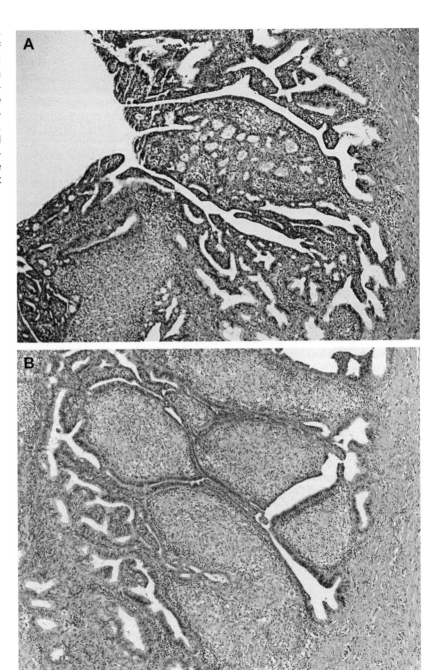

neoplastic process, including a grossly visible mass, post-menopausal age, severe cytologic atypia, and numerous mitotic figures, or any atypical mitoses. HGSC is occasionally associated with brisk inflammatory infiltrate, which can mimic pseudocarcinomatous hyperplasia (**Fig. 11**). A dense inflammatory infiltrate or history of lymphoma should also prompt consideration of a lymphoproliferative disorder. However, when lymphoma involves the tube, it usually consists of nodular aggregates in the tube wall, distinct from the endosalpingeal inflammatory infiltrate in pseudocarcinomatous hyperplasia.

Transitional Metaplasia

Transitional metaplasia of the fallopian tube is common and may be mistaken for STIC with transitional morphology, especially when it occurs in the fimbria of a *BRCA1/2* carrier.[35] In cases in which there is ambiguous morphology, transitional metaplasia shows wild-type p53 staining and a low Ki-67 proliferation index.

PROGNOSIS

Most patients with STIC have an uneventful course with no disease recurrence. However, between 4% and 11% of patients will subsequently develop so-called primary peritoneal serous carcinoma,[22,36,37] suggesting that the tubal lesion seeded the peritoneal cavity before the salpingectomy. After a diagnosis of an isolated STIC, some patients may be observed with pelvic ultrasounds and serum CA-125.[36–38] Germline *BRCA1/2* testing should also be considered. The prognostic significance of pelvic washings in the setting of STIC is unclear.[39]

Pitfalls
In The Diagnosis Of
Serous Intraepithelial
Carcinoma

- Secretory cell outgrowths with conspicuous ciliated (type I) or endometrioid (type II) differentiation look distinct from the surrounding tubal mucosa but lack *TP53* mutations and likely do not carry an increased risk of subsequent neoplasia

- p53 signatures show a clonal appearance and have aberrant p53 immunohistochemistry staining, but have preserved polarity, and minimal cytologic atypia and mitotic activity

- Pseudocarcinomatous epithelial hyperplasia, usually in the setting of pelvic inflammatory disease or other infection (eg, tuberculosis), may show worrisome, complex architecture with mild cytologic abnormalities

- Metastases to the tubal mucosa may histologically mimic an STIC with an intraepithelial growth pattern and show aberrant p53 staining

Differential diagnosis

Differential Diagnosis of Serous Tubal Intraepithelial Carcinoma	Helpful Distinguishing Features
p53 signature	Preserved nuclear polarity, minimal to mild cytologic atypia Low proliferation index
Serous tubal intraepithelial lesion	Abnormal cytomorphology, but insufficient for diagnosis of STIC Preserved polarity
Metastasis	Often serosal or nodular tumor deposits History of previous malignancy or synchronous carcinoma (often endometrial or endocervical)
High-grade serous carcinoma	Mass-forming lesion with stromal invasion Usually disease spread to adjacent structures
Arias-Stella effect	Synchronous intra-uterine or ectopic pregnancy Wild-type p53 pattern
Pseudocarcinomatous hyperplasia	Premenopausal patient, with associated infection Moderate cytologic atypia, no atypical mitotic figures Wild-type p53 pattern
Endometrioid carcinoma	May be associated with endometriosis Columnar/endometrioid cytomorphology Usually wild-type p53 pattern, ± nuclear β-catenin expression
Type I and II secretory cell outgrowths (SCOUTs)	Ciliated (type I) or endometrioid (type II) differentiation Wild-type p53 pattern Preserved polarity and lack of significant cytologic atypia
Transitional metaplasia/Walthard cell rest	Well-circumscribed nests or mucosal lining of transitional cells Absence of mitotic activity and cytologic atypia

Fig. 11. (A–C) High-grade serous carcinoma of the fallopian tube with a brisk inflammatory infiltrate may mimic pseudocarcinomatous hyperplasia.

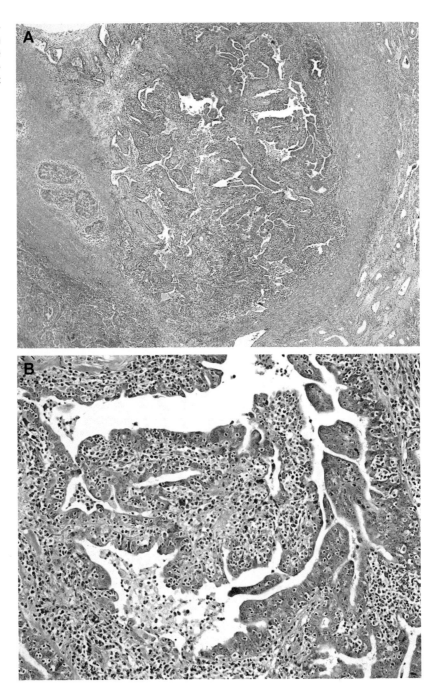

ENDOMETRIOID TUBAL NEOPLASIA

OVERVIEW

Although most primary neoplasias of the fallopian tube are of serous lineage, endometrioid proliferations of the tubal mucosa can occur as well. The spectrum of endometrioid neoplasia includes type II secretory cell outgrowths (SCOUTs), atypical endometrioid proliferations (analogous to hyperplasias of the endometrium), and endometrioid carcinomas.[40] Unlike endometrioid lesions of the ovary and peritoneum, endometrioid proliferations of the tube seem to arise directly from

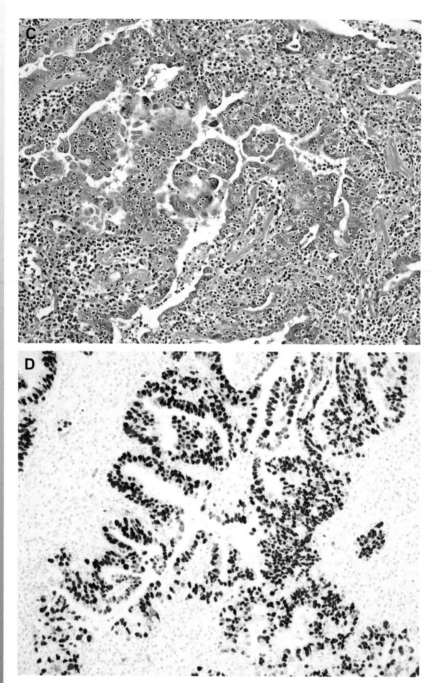

Fig. 11. (continued). (D) p53 staining shows a mutant pattern in HGSC, unlike pseudocarcinomatous hyperplasia.

the tubal epithelium and are not associated with endometriosis.

GROSS FEATURES

Most endometrioid lesions of the tube are microscopic proliferations and are not grossly visible.

Because the SEE-FIM protocol is becoming increasingly common, these lesions are likely to be detected with increasing frequency. Primary endometrioid carcinomas of the tube grossly appear as yellow, friable masses that cause luminal distension.[41] They range in size from 0.4 to 6 cm.[41]

MICROSCOPIC FEATURES

Secretory cell outgrowths are benign epithelial proliferations of the fallopian tube, which are morphologically distinct from the adjacent tubal mucosa. They are subdivided into 2 groups based on their morphology. Type I SCOUTs show ciliated differentiation (Fig. 12), while type II SCOUTs show endometrioid cytomorphology (Fig. 13A). Notably, both have preserved polarity. Although not used routinely in clinical diagnostic practice, type I SCOUTs are positive for FOXJ1, a marker of ciliated differentiation. The conspicuous ciliated differentiation of type I SCOUTs is a helpful feature to differentiate them from an STIC. Type II SCOUTs are composed of a uniform population of columnar cells and are frequently positive (nuclear and cytoplasmic) for β-catenin (Fig. 13B), which is a surrogate for an underlying mutation in CTNNB1. In morphologically ambiguous cases, in which there is concern for STIC, p53 immunostaining can be used. Unlike STIC, type I and II SCOUTs show a wild-type pattern of p53 expression. Atypical endometrioid proliferations of the tube show a distinct population of cells with endometrioid cytomorphology, but which are not diagnostic of adenocarcinoma (Figs. 13C–E).

Primary endometrioid adenocarcinoma of the tube, while rare, shows a morphology similar to that of the endometrium and ovary (Figs. 14A, B). They often show areas of solid growth and small glands that resemble female adnexal tumors of Wolffian origin (FATWO).[41] In contrast to HGSC of the tube, endometrioid tumors usually present at a low stage, do not involve the fimbria, and have a favorable prognosis.[41]

DIAGNOSIS AND DIFFERENTIAL DIAGNOSIS

The differential diagnosis of endometrioid neoplasia in the fallopian tube includes metastatic endometrioid carcinoma, as well as less-common entities that can mimic endometrioid tumors such as microscopic extraovarian sex-cord proliferations, and FATWO. In all cases of endometrioid lesions of the tube, endometrial sampling should be performed to exclude synchronous neoplasia or metastatic disease (Figs. 14C–E). Spread from an ovarian endometrioid tumor should also be excluded. Finally, detached fragments of endometrial carcinoma are often seen intraluminally at the time of hysterectomy. These are artifactually displaced and should not be interpreted as a metastasis or primary lesion of the tube. They do not affect the staging of an endometrial carcinoma.

Female Adnexal Tumors of Probable Wolffian Origin

Female adnexal tumors of probable Wolffian origin are rare tumors that usually occur in the

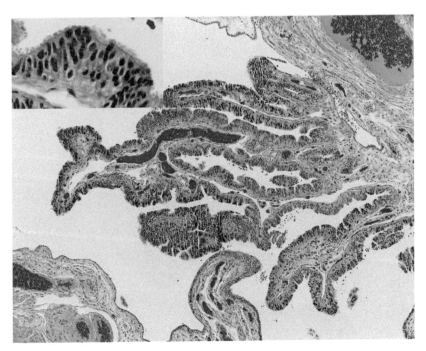

Fig. 12. Type I secretory cell outgrowth (SCOUT) shows a focal proliferation of ciliated cells (inset, high power).

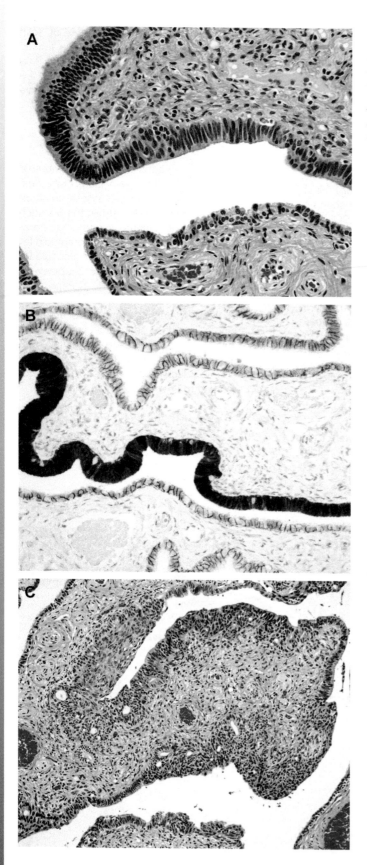

Fig. 13. Type II secretory cell outgrowths (SCOUTs) have endometrioid differentiation (*A*), and may show nuclear β-catenin expression (*B*). The endometrioid proliferations may become more exuberant, analogous to endometrial hyperplasia: (*C*) H&E and (*D*) β-catenin. In some cases, they are multifocal (*E*) highlighted by β-catenin staining.

Fig. 13. (*continued*).

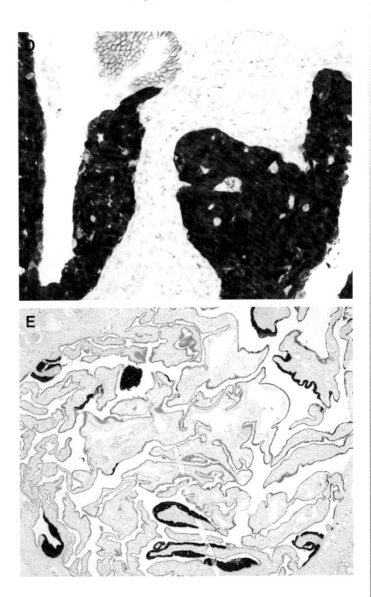

broad ligament and may be adherent to the serosal aspect of the fallopian tube.[42,43] Microscopically, they show a sieve-like architectural pattern, which can mimic endometrioid neoplasia (**Fig. 15**). They can occur over a wide age range (15–87).[43,44] Whereas most cases of FATWO follow a benign course, some may recur or metastasize.[44] Some cases have been shown to express c-kit (CD117), and it has been suggested to treat these patients with imatinib, although KIT mutations have not been identified in FATWO.[45–48]

Microscopic Extraovarian Sex-Cord Proliferations

Microscopic extraovarian sex-cord proliferations may resemble either adult granulosa cell tumors, or sex-cord tumors with annular tubules.[2,49] They are thought to be embryonic rests, and are not associated with a sex-cord stromal tumor in the ovary. Although only a small number of cases have been reported, they seem to be benign.[49] These proliferations are usually composed of small, well-circumscribed nests of round to ovoid cells that may be arranged in follicles or cribriform arrangements (**Fig. 16**). If

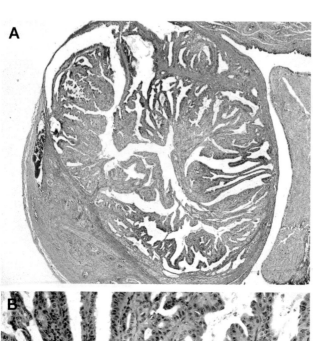

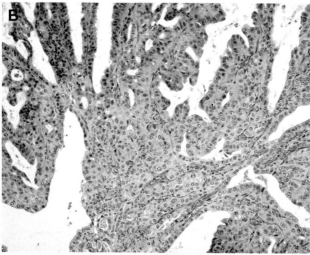

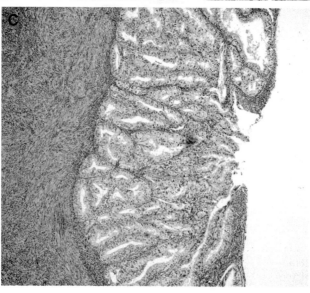

Fig. 14. Primary endometrioid carcinomas of the fallopian tube distend the tube lumen (*A*) and have a morphologic appearance identical to those of the endometrium (higher power) (*B*). The patient in (*A*) and (*B*) also had a synchronous endometrioid tumor of the endometrium (*C*). The pattern of β-catenin immunohistochemical staining was different:

Fig. 14. (*continued*). (*D*) nuclear in the fallopian tube tumor and (*E*) membranous in the endometrial tumor, suggesting that these were synchronous primaries and not clonally related.

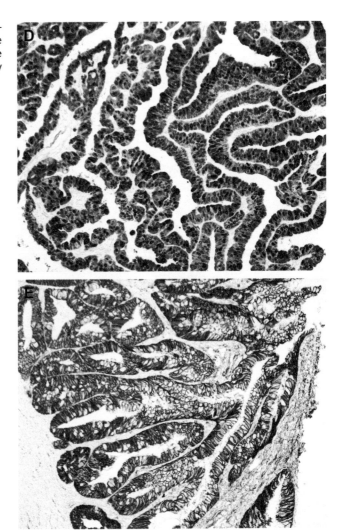

they form tubules or have a cribriform architecture, they may be mistaken for endometrioid neoplasia, especially in the setting of a primary endometrial or ovarian tumor. There should be no to rare mitotic activity and no nuclear pleomorphism. Cytoplasm ranges from scant to moderate, and the nuclei may be grooved. Immunohistochemically, they stain like sexcord cells and are positive for pan-keratin, inhibin, calretinin, WT-1, and SF-1, and are negative for EMA, synaptophysin, and chromogranin.[49] These extraovarian sex-cord proliferations may also be seen in the pelvic peritoneum and appendix. Sex-cord cells can also be seen in a different phenomenon in which granulosa cells are displaced from a developing ovarian follicle and migrate to the fallopian tube.

The granulosa cells may be crushed and mitotically active, mimicking a small cell carcinoma.[50] Of note, heterotopic hilus (Leydig) cells can also be seen in the tube (**Fig. 17**).[51] These incidental lesions are of no clinical significance.

Cautery Artifact

Cautery artifact can mimic endometrioid neoplasia of the tube by causing nuclear enlargement, hyperchromasia, and stratification. The nuclear changes are usually exaggerated compared with the columnar cells seen in endometrioid neoplasia. Further, cautery artifact does not form a mass, and cautery artifact is also usually seen on adjacent stromal tissue.

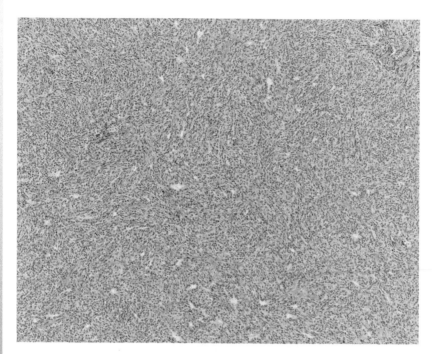

Fig. 15. Female adnexal tumor of probable Wolffian origin (FATWO) usually arises in the broad ligament and may be associated with the fallopian tube.

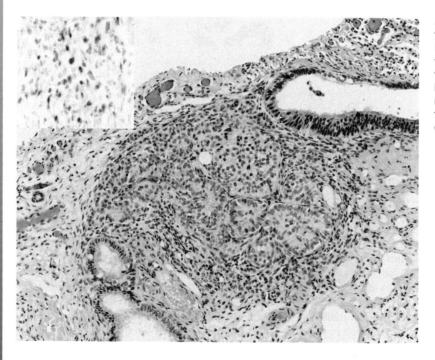

Fig. 16. Microscopic extraovarian sex-cord proliferation involving the fallopian tube. The lesion forms small nests and tubules, and is positive for markers of sex-cord differentiation, such as SF-1 (inset).

Fig. 17. Hilus cell hyperplasia subjacent to the fallopian tube epithelium.

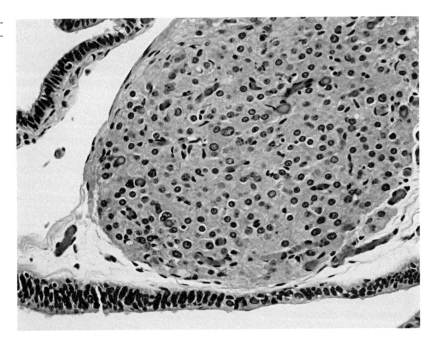

PROGNOSIS

Although there are limited data regarding these lesions, type I and II SCOUTs do not seem to confer an increased risk of subsequent malignancy and are clinically inconsequential.

Atypical endometrioid proliferations of the tube (as illustrated in **Fig. 13C**) may be associated with an increased risk of recurrence. Primary endometrioid carcinomas of the fallopian tube have a stage-dependent prognosis.

△△

Differential diagnosis	
OF ENDOMETRIOID NEOPLASIA OF THE FALLOPIAN TUBE	
Endometrioid Neoplasia versus	**Helpful Distinguishing Features**
Metastasis	Advanced stage endometrioid tumor in endometrium or ovary
Serous neoplasia	Tubal differentiation Psammomatous calcifications Immunohistochemistry: positive for WT-1, with cytoplasmic or membranous β-catenin expression
Cautery artifact	Artifactually elongated columnar cells Adjacent to recognized cautery effect Wild-type p53, low Ki-67, membranous β-catenin
Female adnexal tumor of Wolffian origin (FATWO)	Usually arises from broad ligament, not tubal lumen Low-power "sieve-like" appearance Immunohistochemistry: positive for calretinin
Microscopic extraovarian sex-cord proliferation	Composed of granulosa cells or sex-cord tumor with annular tubules (SCTAT) morphology Immunohistochemistry: positive for sex-cord stromal markers (SF-1, inhibin)

REFERENCES

1. Sangoi AR, McKenney JK, Schwartz EJ, et al. Adenomatoid tumors of the female and male genital tracts: a clinicopathological and immunohistochemical study of 44 cases. Mod Pathol 2009;22(9):1228–35.

2. Crum CP, Nucci MR, Howitt BE, et al. Diagnostic gynecologic and obstetric pathology. 3rd edition. Philadelphia: Elsevier; 2018.

3. Mizutani T, Yamamuro O, Kato N, et al. Renal transplantation-related risk factors for the development of uterine adenomatoid tumors. Gynecol Oncol Rep 2016;17:96–8.

4. Goode B, Joseph NM, Stevers M, et al. Adenomatoid tumors of the male and female genital tract are defined by TRAF7 mutations that drive aberrant NF-kB pathway activation. Mod Pathol 2018;31(4): 660–73.

5. Wachter DL, Wünsch PH, Hartmann A, et al. Adenomatoid tumors of the female and male genital tract. A comparative clinicopathologic and immunohistochemical analysis of 47 cases emphasizing their site-specific morphologic diversity. Virchows Arch 2011;458(5):593–602.

6. Skinnider BF, Young RH. Infarcted adenomatoid tumor: a report of five cases of a facet of a benign neoplasm that may cause diagnostic difficulty. Am J Surg Pathol 2004;28(1):77–83.

7. Schwartz EJ, Longacre TA. Adenomatoid tumors of the female and male genital tracts express WT1. Int J Gynecol Pathol 2004;23(2):123–8.

8. Stewart CJR, Leung YC, Whitehouse A. Fallopian tube metastases of non-gynaecological origin: a series of 20 cases emphasizing patterns of involvement including intra-epithelial spread. Histopathology 2012;60(6B):E106–14.

9. Rabban JT, Vohra P, Zaloudek CJ. Nongynecologic metastases to fallopian tube mucosa. Am J Surg Pathol 2015;39(1):35–51.

10. Takeshima Y, Amatya VJ, Kushitani K, et al. A useful antibody panel for differential diagnosis between peritoneal mesothelioma and ovarian serous carcinoma in Japanese cases. Am J Clin Pathol 2008; 130(5):771–9.

11. Chu AY, Litzky LA, Pasha TL, et al. Utility of D2-40, a novel mesothelial marker, in the diagnosis of malignant mesothelioma. Mod Pathol 2005;18(1):105–10.

12. Wrork DH, Broders AC. Adenomyosis of the fallopian tube. Am J Obstet Gynecol 1942;44(3):412–32.

13. Jenkins CS, Williams SR, Schmidt GE. Salpingitis isthmica nodosa: a review of the literature, discussion of clinical significance, and consideration of patient management. Fertil Steril 1993;60(4):599–607.

14. Andrici J, Jung J, Sheen A, et al. Loss of BAP1 expression is very rare in peritoneal and gynecologic serous adenocarcinomas and can be useful in the differential diagnosis with abdominal mesothelioma. Hum Pathol 2016;51:9–15.

15. Colgan TJ, Murphy J, Cole DE, et al. Occult carcinoma in prophylactic oophorectomy specimens: prevalence and association with BRCA germline mutation status. Am J Surg Pathol 2001;25(10): 1283–9.

16. Medeiros F, Muto MG, Lee Y, et al. The tubal fimbria is a preferred site for early adenocarcinoma in women with familial ovarian cancer syndrome. Am J Surg Pathol 2006;30(2):230–6.

17. Kindelberger DW, Lee Y, Miron A, et al. Intraepithelial carcinoma of the fimbria and pelvic serous carcinoma: evidence for a causal relationship. Am J Surg Pathol 2007;31(2):161–9.

18. Crum CP, Drapkin R, Miron A, et al. The distal fallopian tube: a new model for pelvic serous carcinogenesis. Curr Opin Obstet Gynecol 2007;19(1):3–9.

19. Meserve EEK, Brouwer J, Crum CP. Serous tubal intraepithelial neoplasia: the concept and its application. Mod Pathol 2017;30(5):710–21.

20. Przybycin CG, Kurman RJ, Ronnett BM, et al. Are all pelvic (nonuterine) serous carcinomas of tubal origin? Am J Surg Pathol 2010;34(10):1407–16.

21. Horn L-C, Kafkova S, Leonhardt K, et al. Serous tubal in situ carcinoma (STIC) in primary peritoneal serous carcinomas. Int J Gynecol Pathol 2013; 32(4):339–44.

22. Conner JR, Meserve E, Pizer E, et al. Outcome of unexpected adnexal neoplasia discovered during risk reduction salpingo-oophorectomy in women with germ-line BRCA1 or BRCA2 mutations. Gynecol Oncol 2014;132(2):280–6.

23. Meserve EEK, Mirkovic J, Conner JR, et al. Frequency of "incidental" serous tubal intraepithelial carcinoma (STIC) in women without a history of or genetic risk factor for high-grade serous carcinoma: a six-year study. Gynecol Oncol 2017;146(1):69–73.

24. Soong TR, Howitt BE, Miron A, et al. Evidence for lineage continuity between early serous proliferations (ESPs) in the fallopian tube and disseminated high-grade serous carcinomas. J Pathol 2018; 246(3):344–51.

25. Na K, Kim H-S. Clinicopathological characteristics of fallopian tube metastases from primary endometrial, cervical, and nongynecological malignancies: a single institutional experience. Virchows Arch 2017; 471(3):363–73.

26. Singh R, Cho KR. Serous tubal intraepithelial carcinoma or not? Metastases to fallopian tube mucosa can masquerade as in situ lesions. Arch Pathol Lab Med 2017;141(10):1313–5.

27. Kommoss F, Faruqi A, Gilks CB, et al. Uterine serous carcinomas frequently metastasize to the fallopian tube and can mimic serous tubal intraepithelial carcinoma. Am J Surg Pathol 2017;41(2):161–70.

28. McDaniel AS, Stall JN, Hovelson DH, et al. Next-generation sequencing of tubal intraepithelial carcinomas. JAMA Oncol 2015;1(8):1128.

29. Reyes C, Murali R, Park KJ. Secondary involvement of the adnexa and uterine corpus by carcinomas of the uterine cervix. Int J Gynecol Pathol 2015;34(6):551–63.

30. Kato N, Sugawara M, Maeda K, et al. Pyloric gland metaplasia/differentiation in multiple organ systems in a patient with Peutz-Jeghers syndrome. Pathol Int 2011;61(6):369–72.

31. Seidman JD. Mucinous lesions of the fallopian tube. A report of seven cases. Am J Surg Pathol 1994;18(12):1205–12.

32. Cheung AN, Young RH, Scully RE. Pseudocarcinomatous hyperplasia of the fallopian tube associated with salpingitis. A report of 14 cases. Am J Surg Pathol 1994;18(11):1125–30.

33. Gupta S, Singh P, Bala J, et al. Pseudocarcinomatous hyperplasia of the fallopian tubes which was associated with female genital tract tuberculosis, histologically mimicking tubal adenocarcinoma: a diagnostic challenge. J Clin Diagn Res 2012;6(8):1419–21.

34. Lee NK, Choi KU, Han GJ, et al. Pseudocarcinomatous hyperplasia of the fallopian tube mimicking tubal cancer: a radiological and pathological diagnostic challenge. J Ovarian Res 2016;9(1):79.

35. Rabban JT, Crawford B, Chen L-M, et al. Transitional cell metaplasia of fallopian tube fimbriae: a potential mimic of early tubal carcinoma in risk reduction salpingo-oophorectomies from women with BRCA mutations. Am J Surg Pathol 2009;33(1):111–9.

36. Patrono MG, Iniesta MD, Malpica A, et al. Clinical outcomes in patients with isolated serous tubal intraepithelial carcinoma (STIC): a comprehensive review. Gynecol Oncol 2015;139(3):568–72.

37. Chay WY, McCluggage WG, Lee C-H, et al. Outcomes of incidental fallopian tube high-grade serous carcinoma and serous tubal intraepithelial carcinoma in women at low risk of hereditary breast and ovarian cancer. Int J Gynecol Cancer 2016;26(3):431–6.

38. Weinberger V, Bednarikova M, Cibula D, et al. Serous tubal intraepithelial carcinoma (STIC) – clinical impact and management. Expert Rev Anticancer Ther 2016;16(12):1311–21.

39. Wethington SL, Park KJ, Soslow RA, et al. Clinical outcome of isolated serous tubal intraepithelial carcinomas (STIC). Int J Gynecol Cancer 2013;23(9):1603–11.

40. Brouwer J, Strickland KC, Schmelkin CB, et al. Evidence for a novel endometrioid carcinogenic sequence in the fallopian tube with unique beta-catenin expression. Int J Gynecol Pathol 2019, [Epub ahead of print].

41. Navani SS, Alvarado-Cabrero I, Young RH, et al. Endometrioid carcinoma of the fallopian tube: a clinicopathologic analysis of 26 cases. Gynecol Oncol 1996;63(3):371–8.

42. Kariminejad MH, Scully RE. Female adnexal tumor of probable wolffian origin. A distinctive pathologic entity. Cancer 1973;31(3):671–7.

43. Hong S, Cui J, Li L, et al. Malignant female adnexal tumor of probable Wolffian origin: case report and literature review. Int J Gynecol Pathol 2018;37(4):331–7.

44. Daya D. Malignant female adnexal tumor of probable wolffian origin with review of the literature. Arch Pathol Lab Med 1994;118(3):310–2.

45. Steed H, Oza A, Chapman WB, et al. Female adnexal tumor of probable Wolffian origin: a clinicopathological case report and a possible new treatment. Int J Gynecol Cancer 2004;14(3):546–50.

46. Cossu A, Casula M, Paliogiannis P, et al. Female adnexal tumors of probable Wolffian origin (FATWO): a case series with next-generation sequencing mutation analysis. Int J Gynecol Pathol 2017;36(6):575–81.

47. Mirkovic J, Dong F, Sholl LM, et al. Targeted genomic profiling of female adnexal tumors of probable Wolffian origin (FATWO). Int J Gynecol Pathol 2018. https://doi.org/10.1097/PGP.0000000000000545.

48. Wakayama A, Matsumoto H, Aoyama H, et al. Recurrent female adnexal tumor of probable Wolffian origin treated with debulking surgery, imatinib and paclitaxel/carboplatin combination chemotherapy: a case report. Oncol Lett 2017;13(5):3403–8.

49. McCluggage WG, Stewart CJR, Iacobelli J, et al. Microscopic extraovarian sex cord proliferations: an undescribed phenomenon. Histopathology 2015;66(4):555–64.

50. Vydianath B, Ganesan R, McCluggage WG. Displaced granulosa cells in the fallopian tube mimicking small cell carcinoma. J Clin Pathol 2008;61(12):1323–5.

51. Hirschowitz L, Salmons N, Ganesan R. Ovarian hilus cell heterotopia. Int J Gynecol Pathol 2011;30(1):46–52.

Low-grade Serous Neoplasia of the Female Genital Tract

Ann K. Folkins, MD*, Teri A. Longacre, MD

KEYWORDS

- Low-grade serous carcinoma • Serous borderline tumor • Serous carcinoma

Key points

- Low-grade serous neoplasia of the female gynecologic tract encompasses a spectrum of lesions from serous cystadenoma to serous borderline tumor to low-grade serous carcinoma.
- The defining feature of serous borderline tumors is papillary epithelial proliferation without destructive tissue invasion.
- Low-grade serous carcinoma shows destructive stromal invasion and is associated with decreased overall survival compared with serous borderline tumor.
- Tumor implants in the setting of serous borderline tumor that show destructive tissue invasion should be designated as low-grade serous carcinoma.

ABSTRACT

Low-grade serous neoplasia of the gynecologic tract includes benign (serous cystadenomas), borderline, and malignant lesions (low-grade serous carcinoma). Classification of these lesions relies on rigorous attention to several pathologic features that determine the prognosis and the need for adjuvant therapy. Risk stratification of serous borderline tumor behavior based on histologic findings and criteria for low-grade serous carcinoma are the primary focus of this article, including the redesignation of invasive implants of serous borderline tumor as low-grade serous carcinoma based on the similar survival rates. The molecular underpinnings of these tumors are also discussed, including their potential for prognostication.

OVERVIEW

Low-grade serous neoplasia of the female genital tract encompasses a spectrum of benign, borderline, and malignant lesions that occur predominantly within the ovaries but can also be of fallopian tube or potentially peritoneal origin. Benign serous cystadenomas and cystadenofibromas are common lesions that usually do not pose much diagnostic difficultly. However, low-grade serous carcinomas are uncommon tumors that can be challenging to distinguish from their high-grade counterparts and noninvasive precursor lesions (serous borderline tumors). This article focuses primarily on diagnostic criteria for serous borderline tumors, classification of borderline implants, and diagnostic criteria of invasive low-grade serous carcinoma.

GROSS FEATURES

The gross appearance of low-grade serous neoplasia depends to some extent on whether it is benign, borderline, or malignant, although microscopic examination is required for true stratification of the lesion. Benign serous cystadenomas can be simple cysts and by definition are distinguished from cortical inclusion cysts by a size greater than 1 cm. Benign serous cystadenofibromas show

Disclosure: The authors have no financial relationships to disclose.
Department of Pathology, Stanford University School of Medicine, 300 Pasteur Drive, Stanford, CA 94305, USA
* Corresponding author.
E-mail address: afolkins@stanford.edu

Surgical Pathology 12 (2019) 481–513
https://doi.org/10.1016/j.path.2019.02.006
1875-9181/19/© 2019 Elsevier Inc. All rights reserved.

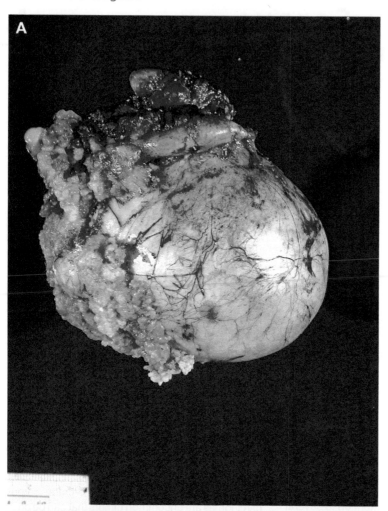

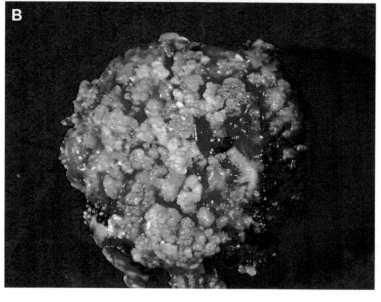

Fig. 1. Serous borderline tumor with smooth external surface (*A*) and prominent papillary projections in internal surface (*B*).

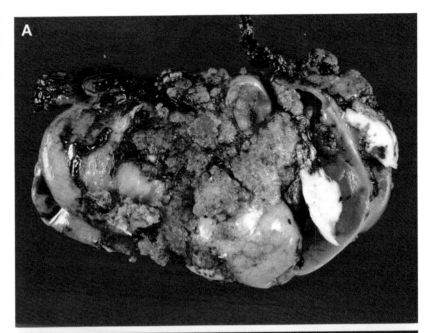

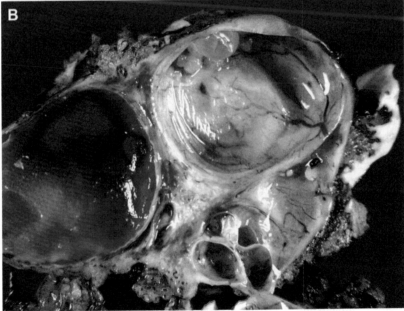

Fig. 2. Serous borderline tumor involving the ovarian surface (*A*) and small papillary excrescences on internal cyst wall (*B*).

cystic components as well as papillary protrusions. As opposed to the papillary excrescences of the borderline and malignant tumors, the papillae in cystadenofibromas tend to be firm. Rarely, benign serous neoplasia shows a completely firm/solid appearance in serous adenofibromas.

Borderline serous tumors show visible papillary excrescences either within cystic spaces of the tumor or on the surface of the ovary/peritoneal implants (Figs. 1 and 2). Invasive low-grade serous carcinoma cannot be reliably distinguished grossly from a borderline tumor, but it usually shows more abundant, fleshy, soft papillary growth. Evaluation of ovaries involved in serous neoplasia should always

involve mention of whether the capsule is ruptured/intact and whether there is surface involvement so that accurate staging can be performed depending on the results of microscopic examination.

MICROSCOPIC FEATURES AND DIAGNOSTIC CRITERIA

SEROUS CYSTADENOMA/ CYSTADENOFIBROMA

Benign serous tumors are defined by a lining of tubal-type epithelium. This epithelium usually consists of a mixture of ciliated and secretory cells

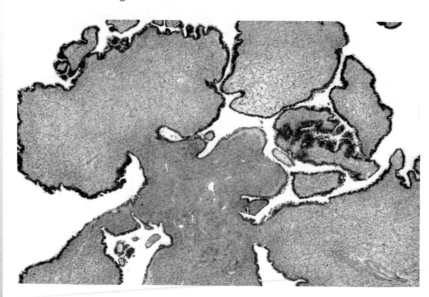

Fig. 3. Serous cystadeno-fibroma. There is no significant epithelial stratification.

similar to that found in the fallopian tube mucosa, but these tumors can also show a bland cuboidal lining in some areas. The appearance of the serous lining varies greatly depending on the amount of fibrous papillary growth in the tumor. Completely cystic tumors show a flat serous lining. However, the serous epithelium can be undulating and irregular in cases with papillary growth (Fig. 3). It is critical to distinguish undulation of the serous epithelium secondary to papillary stromal protrusions from the true epithelial proliferation seen in serous borderline tumors (discussed later). Benign serous lesions can also show glands/crypts adjacent to the lining, which again should not be interpreted as epithelial proliferation.

SEROUS BORDERLINE TUMOR (CONVENTIONAL TYPE)

Serous borderline tumors are defined by serous epithelial growth and stratification in the absence of tissue invasion. In principle, this sounds straightforward; however, defining epithelial proliferation and tissue invasion can both be problematic.

First, epithelial proliferation in conventional serous borderline tumors is characterized by hierarchical branching of the epithelium from the surface of the fibrous papillae (Fig. 4). This pattern needs to be present in greater than 10% of the epithelial surface of the tumor to qualify as a serous borderline tumor; lesions with less than 10% are designated as serous cystadenoma/cystadenofibroma with focal proliferation. This rule is generally applicable, although there are select circumstances that may require modification of this

system. For instance, some tumors show a large cystic component with abundant flat serous lining but there is a discrete nodule of papillary growth with pronouncing epithelial proliferation. Although a strict calculation of the percentage of growth based on the size of the nodule versus the total cyst may not be greater than 10%, the degree of growth in the focal area may be sufficient by itself to quality as a borderline tumor.

Second, although borderline tumors by definition show no tissue invasion, their patterns of growth can be challenging to distinguish from invasion when they expand the ovarian parenchyma. Serous borderline tumors can form expansile masses within the ovary in which there are cystic spaces with papillary intracystic growth. Separating this growth from tissue invasion requires recognition of the subtle patterns of invasion seen in low-grade serous carcinoma, which are discussed in detail later in relation to microscopy.

Cytologically, serous borderline tumors can show similar features to serous cystadenomas or mild atypia, with uniform nuclear enlargement and vesicular chromatin. Mitotic figures should be rare to scattered. Psammomatous calcifications are often present but are not required for the diagnosis and can be seen in any of the spectrum of serous neoplasms. Although mild nuclear enlargement is acceptable for serous borderline tumors, there should not be nuclear pleomorphism or significant mitotic activity. If these features are present, other tumors, such as high-grade serous carcinoma or clear cell carcinoma, should be considered (discussed later in relation to differential diagnosis). Typically, there is an admixture of columnar cells and eosinophilic (pink) cells

Fig. 4. Serous borderline tumor with hierarchical papillary branching (*A*) and epithelial stratification (*B*).

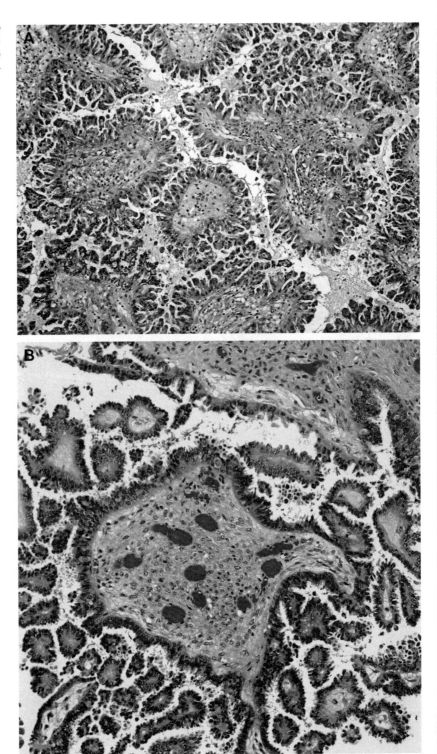

(**Fig.** 5). Rarely, serous borderline tumors can show intraepithelial carcinoma, as discussed next.

SEROUS BORDERLINE TUMOR WITH INTRAEPITHELIAL CARCINOMA

There are rare cases in which a serous borderline tumor shows areas with marked cytologic atypia but no stromal invasion.[1] This tumor should be designated as serous borderline tumor with intraepithelial carcinoma (**Fig.** 6). Liberal sectioning of the tumor in such cases is necessary, because there are often small foci of destructive invasion identified elsewhere. If the cytologic atypia is diffuse or extensive, an alternative diagnosis of a high-grade epithelial malignancy, such as clear cell or serous carcinoma, should be entertained and excluded.

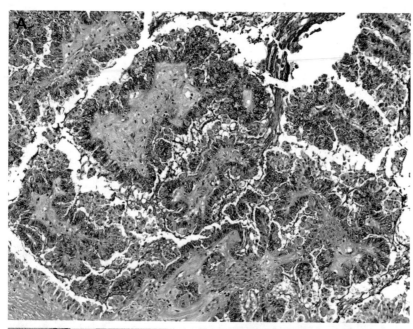

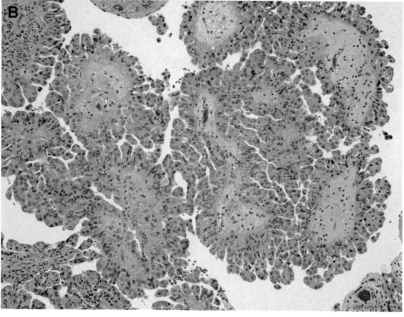

Fig. 5. Serous borderline tumor with hierarchical papillary branching (*A*) and epithelial stratification with eosinophilic and columnar cells (*B*).

Fig. 6. Serous borderline tumor with intracystic solid epithelial proliferation (*A*) and intraepithelial carcinoma (marked cytologic atypia) (*B*).

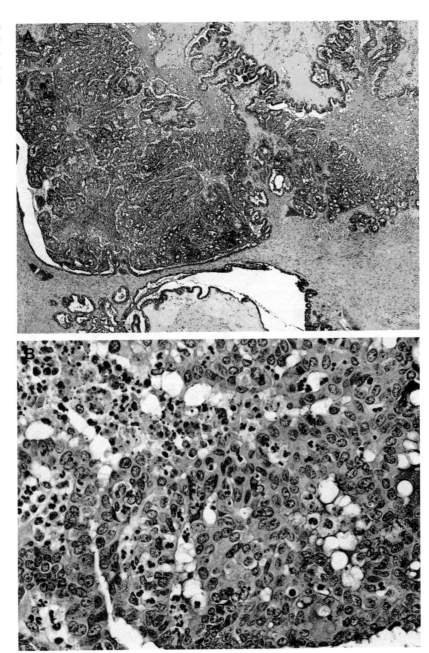

SEROUS BORDERLINE TUMOR, MICROPAPILLARY TYPE

There is a variant of serous borderline tumor termed micropapillary borderline tumor or borderline tumor, micropapillary type, which shows nonhierarchical epithelial proliferation and deserves special mention because of its unique prognostic implications. To qualify as micropapillary growth, the tumor needs to show slender, long papillae with minimal fibrovascular support that are at least 5 times as long as they are wide (**Fig. 7**).[2] This growth pattern needs to be present in a greater than 5-mm area to be designated as micropapillary type.[3] Significant micropapillary growth is present in approximately 5% to 10% of serous borderline tumors.[4] Micropapillary borderline tumors tend to show more exuberant epithelial growth than conventional borderline tumors and often have the appearance of medusa hair. The

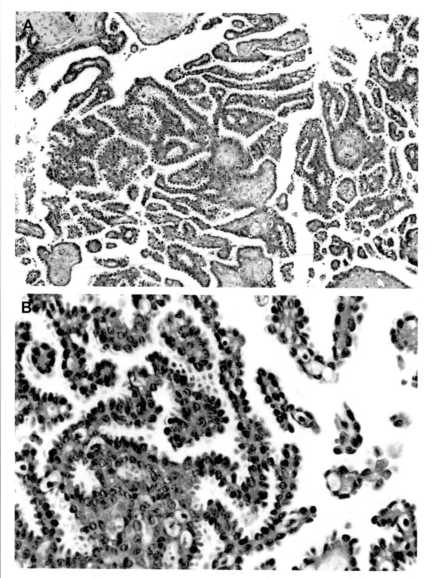

Fig. 7. Serous borderline tumor with a micropapillary pattern. (A) Low-magnification, medusa-head appearance, the area with this change should measure 5 mm in a lineal dimension; (B) higher-magnification, bland cytologic features.

micropapillary growth can also form cribriform spaces, which is also considered in the spectrum of this variant. The micropapillary variant of serous borderline tumor can show a slightly higher degree of cytologic atypia than the conventional variant, although the cells should still lack significant pleomorphism. The cells in the micropapillary variant tend to be uniform and hyperchromatic, sometimes with small nucleoli, and less frequently show a ciliated cell population.

Micropapillary borderline tumors have a higher frequency of bilaterality, surface involvement, and extraovarian implants, which may show invasion.[5] In patients with extraovarian disease, micropapillary tumors are associated with invasive implants (low-grade serous carcinoma) in 50% of cases, whereas the association is only 8% for conventional serous borderline tumors.[6] It is recommended that the extent of micropapillary growth (percentage of the tumor) be reported, although the direct prognostic significance of the proportion is unclear. It should be noted that some pathologists refer to these tumors as noninvasive low-grade serous carcinomas.[3,7]

SOLID EPITHELIAL GROWTH IN SEROUS BORDERLINE TUMOR

Sometimes serous borderline tumors show confluent epithelial growth within cystic spaces that forms almost solid areas (See **Fig. 6**).[8] There is controversy on whether these should qualify as low-grade serous carcinoma in the absence of tissue invasion. These solid proliferations can show similar cytologic features to low-grade serous carcinomas and may represent a form of noninvasive intermediate lesion with potentially higher risk for recurrence and progression. In our practice, we comment on the presence of solid-type epithelial growth and note that this may represent an intermediate lesion between serous borderline tumors and low-grade serous carcinomas.[8] Solid growth can often be seen in the setting of micropapillary borderline tumors, because these tend to have more extensive epithelial proliferation than the conventional types.

IMPLANTS OF SEROUS BORDERLINE TUMOR

The term "implant" specifically describes involvement of peritoneal tissues in the setting of serous borderline tumors; to avoid confusion, this term should not be used to describe involvement of peritoneal tissue by serous carcinoma. About 30% to 47% of patients with serous borderline tumors have extraovarian pelvic and/or abdominal implants.[1,9] Implants were traditionally divided into noninvasive and invasive types based on whether they showed invasion of the underlying tissue. This distinction is the best prognostic indicator in high-stage disease. Noninvasive implants are further subdivided into epithelial and desmoplastic types. Most patients with extraovarian disease at the time of diagnosis have noninvasive implants, with only about 10% to 15% showing invasive extraovarian implants (low-grade serous carcinoma).[10]

Epithelial noninvasive implants show papillary clusters of serous borderline tumor cells on the peritoneal surfaces and in the septa of the omentum (**Fig. 8**). The implants in the omentum tend to be the most difficult to evaluate for "invasion," because the noninvasive implants are allowed to expand the septa but not invade from them. The implants should show well-rounded borders without irregular protrusions of tumor cells into the fat to quality as noninvasive.

Desmoplastic noninvasive implants consist of well-demarcated nodules of desmoplastic and inflamed fibrous tissue with small foci of serous borderline tumor cells in clusters and even as single cells.[10] Within a desmoplastic nodule, the borderline tumor cells look like they are invading the stroma; however, this appearance should be confined to the nodule and not extend into the surrounding native fibroadipose tissue.

Therefore, the desmoplastic implants are described as having a stuck-on appearance adjacent to normal tissue structures. Desmoplastic noninvasive implants usually show predominantly desmoplastic stromal tissue with small amounts of epithelial proliferation. This feature can be helpful in challenging cases, because there tends to be more pronounced epithelial component in invasive implants (low-grade serous carcinoma). Desmoplastic implants on the surface of the ovary that contains a serous borderline tumor are termed autoimplants (**Fig. 9**). Sometimes implants are removed from the surface of the peritoneum without any underlying native tissue. As long as the cytologic features in these implants remain within the spectrum of serous borderline tumors, they can be designated as noninvasive implants based on the current literature.[10]

Because so-called invasive implants behave more like carcinomas than borderline tumors, foci of invasion occurring in implants should be designated as low-grade serous carcinoma and the invasive implant terminology should no longer be used.[1,8,10–14] Invasion, as stated previously, is defined as destructive tissue invasion, because this feature shows independent prognostic significance for overall survival and disease-free survival compared with other features suggested as potential microscopic indicators of invasion, namely micropapillary architecture and cell nests surrounded by clefts.[10] In the omentum, this usually appears as irregular nests of tumor cells in the fat at the edges of the septa (**Fig. 10**). When invasion is encountered in an implant but the ovarian tumor is still a serous borderline tumor, only the invasive implant should be called low-grade serous carcinoma. The comment can then explain that low-grade serous carcinoma can arise at extraovarian sites in the setting of serous borderline ovarian tumors or that there could be an invasive component in the ovaries than was unsampled. In a similar fashion, sometimes only the ovarian tumor shows low-grade serous carcinoma (destructive stroma invasion >5 mm in linear extent) but the extraovarian disease appears to be noninvasive implants of serous borderline tumor. The extraovarian implants should still be considered spread of the serous borderline tumor and not metastatic disease from the low-grade serous carcinoma.

There are rare cases in which it cannot reliably be determined whether an implant is invasive or noninvasive; the term serous borderline tumor implant indeterminate for invasion should be used in these circumstances.

Histologic Features of Extraovarian Serous Epithelial Lesions	
Implant Type	**Diagnostic Features**
Noninvasive Implants[a]	
Epithelial implants	Smooth interface with underlying/surrounding normal tissue. Implant composed of branching papillae, glands with complex papillary infoldings, and single cell and small cell clusters. Mild to moderate atypia. Minimal or no reactive stroma
Desmoplastic implants	Smooth interface with underlying/surrounding normal tissue. Implant composed of branching papillae, simple and complex glands with papillary infoldings, and single cell and small cell clusters. Mild to moderate atypia. Edematous, reactive fasciitislike stroma
Indeterminate implants[b]	Implants with desmoplastic-type stromal response but focal encroachment into underlying or adjacent parenchymal tissue, imparting a subtle irregular interface at low power magnification, or implants with focal micropapillary architecture but no evidence of infiltration into underlying parenchyma (ie, showing a smooth interface) or implants with no evidence of infiltration into underlying parenchyma but with cytologic atypia that exceeds that of the usual implant (ie, moderate atypia, insufficient to warrant a diagnosis of carcinoma)
Invasive implants (low-grade serous carcinoma)[c]	Jagged and irregular interface with underlying/surrounding normal tissue, often entrapping fat lobules in omentum. Typically formed by branching papillae and simple and/or complex glands with papillary and micropapillary infoldings. Abundant epithelial component. Moderate to marked atypia

[a] Implants should be distinguished from endosalpingiosis (which is a benign process and does not warrant upstaging of an accompanying ovarian serous borderline tumor).

[b] Implants with no attached normal tissue (so-called detached implants) are classified as noninvasive (either epithelial or desmoplastic) provided the atypia is moderate at most (eg, no marked carcinomatous cytologic atypia) and the architecture is not overly complex (eg, cribriform or florid micropapillary). When marked cytologic and architectural atypia is present, the implant should probably be classified as invasive or, alternatively, as indeterminate because there is no interface evaluable. Implants in which it is difficult to determine whether the interface is smooth and expansile or focally irregular and infiltrative should also be classified as indeterminate.

[c] Less than 15% of extraovarian implants are invasive (low-grade serous carcinoma).

LYMPH NODE INVOLVEMENT IN SEROUS BORDERLINE TUMORS

Lymph node involvement in serous borderline tumors is a common occurrence and upstages the disease.[15–18] Up to 20% to 30% of serous borderline tumors can show lymph node involvement.[18] Patterns of involvement include intracystic papillary growth, subcapsular sinus aggregates, intraparenchymal deposits, and individual eosinophilic cells (Fig. 11). Lymph node involvement is associated with extraovarian implants, but does not seem to have independent prognostic significance. There is some evidence that confluent aggregates of cells larger than 1 mm have a more aggressive clinical course with decreased disease-free survival and should be considered low-grade serous carcinoma.[18]

The possibility of endosalpingiosis should always be considered when making a diagnosis of serous borderline tumor in a lymph node. Intranodal endosalpingiosis typically forms simple glands or cysts in the subcapsular sinus that are lined by a single layer of bland serous epithelium. Serous borderline tumor in lymph nodes should be morphologically similar to the tumor elsewhere and can show the patterns as mentioned earlier. The presence of bland, simple, serous-lined glands in the lymph nodes should not be automatically classified as serous borderline tumor because it is common to have endosalpingiosis in patients with serous borderline tumors (Fig. 12).

MICROINVASION IN SEROUS BORDERLINE TUMORS

Microinvasion is a distinct pattern of nondestructive stromal invasion measuring less than 5 mm in linear extent. It occurs in approximately 10% to 15% of serous borderline tumors and has a markedly increased incidence in the setting of pregnancy.[19] Microinvasion in serous borderline tumors can show several different morphologic patterns, although the most

Fig. 8. Noninvasive serous borderline implants often show epithelial, desmoplastic, or mixed epithelial and desmoplastic features. There is no significant cytologic atypia and the interface between implant and surrounding tissue is smooth and well delineated (*A–D*).

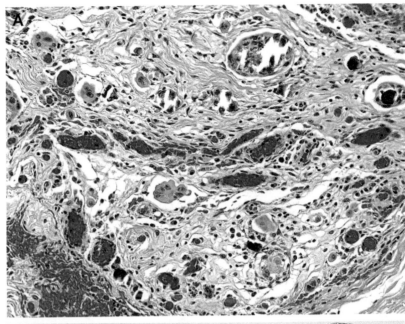

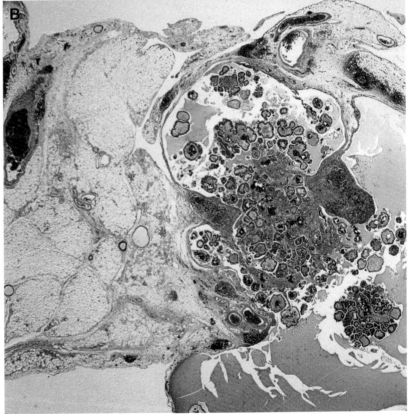

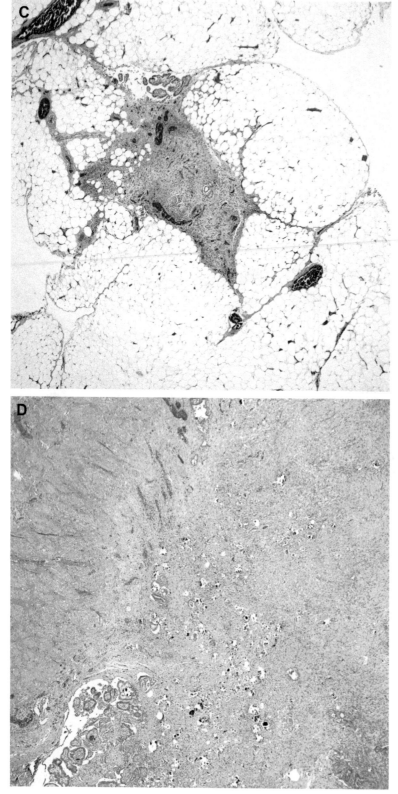

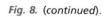

Fig. 8. (continued).

Fig. 9. Noninvasive serous borderline implant on ovary (so-called autoimplant) does not represent invasion.

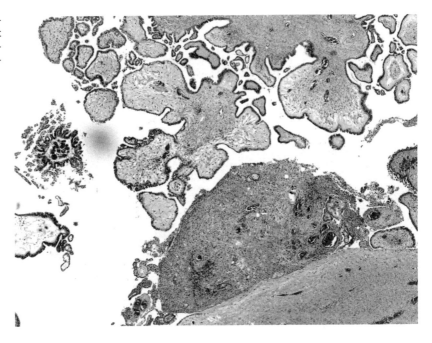

commonly encountered consists of individual cells or clusters of tumor cells with prominent eosinophilic cytoplasm within the stromal stalks. This pattern is referred to as classic stromal microinvasion (**Fig. 13**). Other patterns include simple papillae, cribriform glands, micropapillary structures, and inverted macropapillae (**Fig. 14**). If there are multiple separate foci of microinvasion, they should not be added together to make an aggregate size. Instead, the tumor should be designated as a serous borderline tumor with multifocal microinvasion. Microinvasion is often associated with lymphovascular space invasion (present in up to 60% of cases).[20] If there is an individual area measuring greater than 5 mm, then the tumor should be labeled as low-grade serous carcinoma arising in a serous borderline tumor.

Fig. 10. Invasive implant (low-grade serous carcinoma) in omentum. There is invasion into the surrounding omental fat and a prominent micropapillary epithelial component.

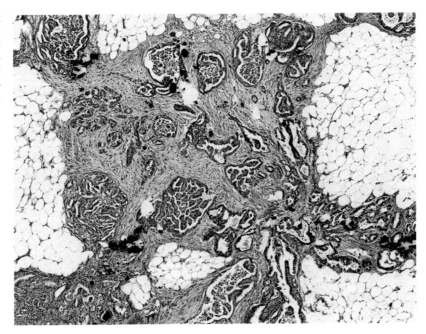

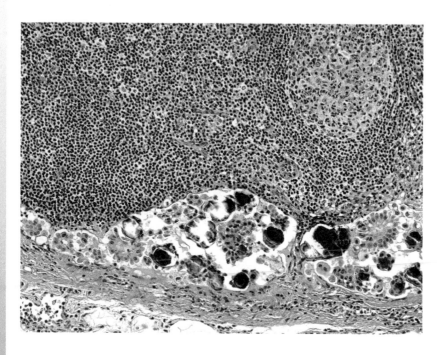

Fig. 11. Lymph node involvement by serous borderline tumor.

Serous borderline tumor with microinvasion should be distinguished from the rare cases of microinvasive low-grade serous carcinoma. Classic stromal microinvasion does not generally show a desmoplastic response in the stroma that would indicate destructive stroma invasion. Rarely, tumors with small foci (<5 mm) of unequivocal destruction stromal invasion are encountered which should be diagnosed as microinvasive low-grade serous carcinoma to indicate the potential for more aggressive behavior than is seen in conventional microinvasion (**Fig. 15**). Small foci of destructive invasion (<5 mm) have been associated with fatal outcomes, providing the rationale for distinguishing small foci of destructive invasion from classic microinvasion.[8]

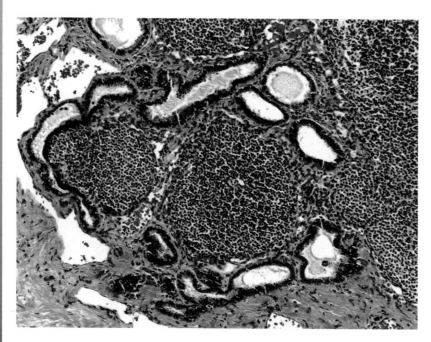

Fig. 12. The presence of bland, simple serous-lined glands in the lymph nodes should not be automatically classified as serous borderline tumor because it is common to have endosalpingiosis in patients with serous borderline tumors.

Special Histologic Features in Serous Borderline Tumors	
Microinvasion	Nondestructive stroma invasion measuring <5mm Classic pattern is individual cells and cell clusters with prominent eosinophilic cytoplasm Other patterns include papillae, cribriform glands, micropapillae, and inverted macropapillae
Intraepithelial carcinoma	Foci of marked cytologic atypia without stromal invasion Liberally sample to exclude invasion Consider the possibility of a high-grade tumor
Solid epithelial growth	Confluent, solid, intraluminal epithelial growth without invasion Could be an intermediate lesion between serous borderline tumor and invasive low-grade serous carcinoma Some groups call this noninvasive low-grade serous carcinoma
Micropapillary growth	Slender, nonbranching papillary or cribriform growth >5 mm to designate as micropapillary variant
Lymph node involvement	Common finding consisting of serous borderline epithelium in nodes Confluent aggregates of tumor cells >1 mm should prompt search for invasive disease and could represent more aggressive disease
Lymphovascular invasion	Commonly present in cases with microinvasion
Implants	Refers to noninvasive implants of serous borderline tumor Can be epithelial or desmoplastic Desmoplastic implants show voluminous fibroinflammatory response with small amounts of serous epithelium Autoimplants are desmoplastic implants on the ovarian surface Destructive tissue invasion should be called low-grade serous carcinoma, not invasive implant

LOW-GRADE SEROUS CARCINOMA

Low-grade serous carcinoma is defined as an invasive serous neoplasm with low-grade cytologic features. The low-grade cytologic features distinguish it from high-grade serous carcinoma, and the invasive growth pattern distinguishes it from serous borderline tumor. Most serous carcinomas are high-grade tumors, with low-grade serous carcinoma accounting for less than 10% of cases.[21] Cytologically, low-grade serous carcinoma is characterized by uniform, round to oval nuclei with evenly distributed chromatin and a low mitotic rate (usually <2–3 per 10 high-power

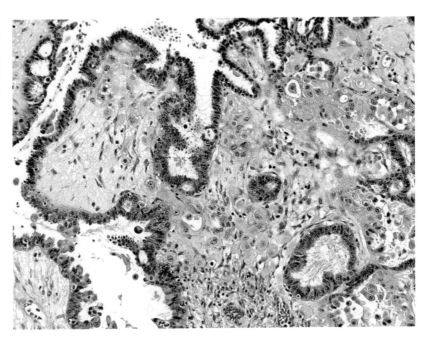

Fig. 13. Stromal microinvasion in serous borderline tumor. Individual cells and cell clusters are present in spaces devoid of epithelial lining within the tumor stroma.

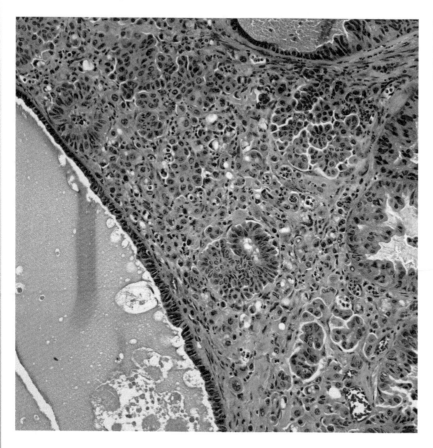

Fig. 14. Extensive stromal microinvasion in this serous borderline tumor shows single cells and small papillae.

fields) (**Fig. 16**).[22] By contrast, high-grade serous carcinoma should show significant nuclear pleomorphism with 3 to 1 variation in the size of nuclei; irregular, coarse chromatin; and increased mitotic activity (>12 mitoses per 10 high-power fields) (see **Fig. 16**). In practice, most cases are easily separable based on the nuclear features and no formal mitotic count is required. However, there are

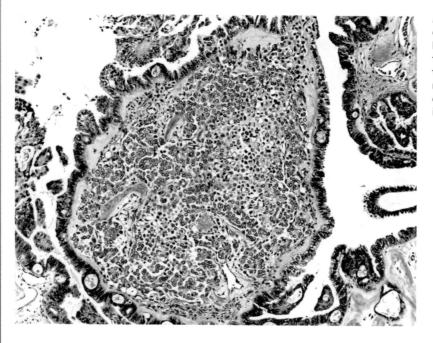

Fig. 15. Microinvasive carcinoma in serous borderline tumor. When this is encountered, additional sampling is recommended in order to ensure a more extensive invasive process.

Fig. 16. Cytologic features of low-grade serous carcinoma (*A*) contrasted with those of high-grade serous carcinoma (*B*). High-grade serous carcinoma shows significant nuclear pleomorphism with 3 to 1 variation in the size of nuclei; irregular, coarse chromatin; and increased mitotic activity (>12 mitoses per 10 high-power fields), whereas low-grade serous carcinoma has more uniform cytology and only occasional mitotic figures.

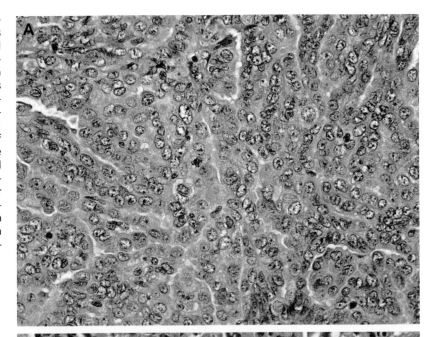

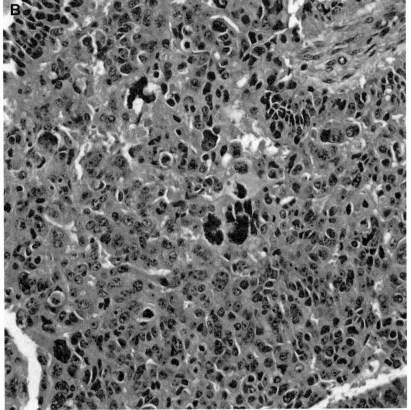

problematic cases that show ambiguous or borderline cytologic features between low-grade and high-grade serous carcinoma. Use of an immunohistochemical stain for p53 can be valuable in these cases, because abnormal expression of p53 (either overexpression in >90% of cells or complete lack of expression) is association with underlying mutations in the

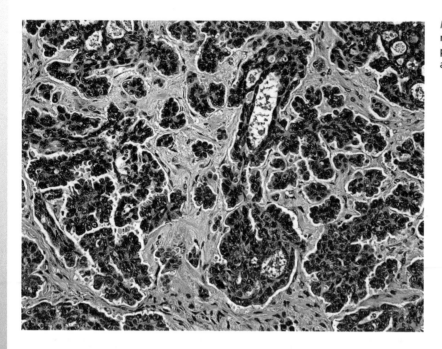

Fig. 17. Low-grade serous carcinoma with complex branching papillary architecture.

TP53. Abnormal expression of p53 would not be expected in a low-grade serous carcinoma, because these tumors generally lack this mutation.

Stromal invasion is the defining characteristic that separates low-grade serous carcinoma from serous borderline tumor, and there are wide variety of invasive patterns that can be encountered (**Figs. 17–19**). Patterns of invasion include micropapillary and/or complex papillary, compact cell nests, inverted macropapillae, cribriform, glandular, solid sheets with slitlike spaces, cystic, and single cells.[8] Again, by definition, these are patterns of destructive stromal invasion, although the stromal response can be subtle to appreciate in some cases. To qualify as low-grade serous carcinoma, the focus of invasion must be at least 5 mm in linear extent; if it is less than 5 mm, it should be designated as microinvasive low-grade serous carcinoma, as mentioned earlier. Cytologically, low-grade serous carcinoma shows slightly more

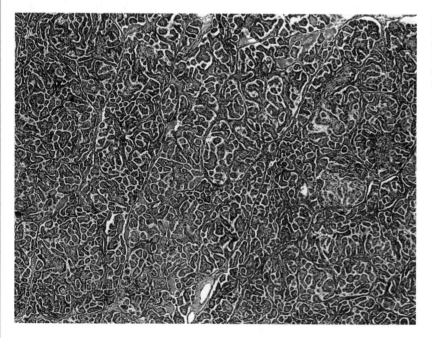

Fig. 18. Low-grade serous carcinoma with complex, back-to-back, branching micropapillary architecture with minimal intervening stroma.

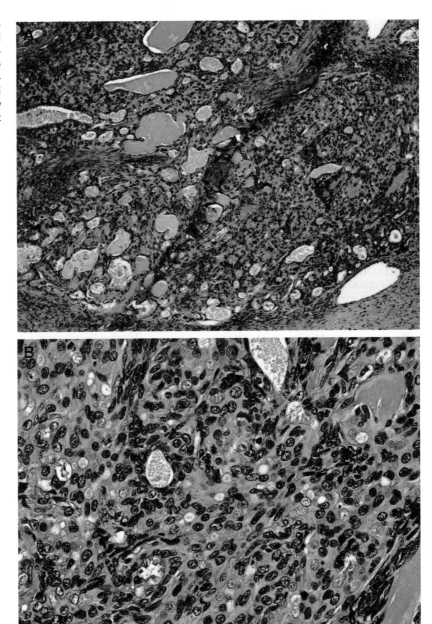

Fig. 19. Low-grade serous carcinoma with solid and micropapillary stromal invasion (*A*). Despite the solid epithelial proliferation, the nuclei are uniform and show only scattered mitotic figures (*B*).

atypia than serous borderline tumor, with higher nuclear to cytoplasmic ratios, nuclear hyperchromasia, and visible nucleoli. The mixture of ciliated and serous cells seen in the borderline tumors is usually absent in low-grade serous carcinoma.

Low-grade serous carcinoma is often associated with background serous borderline tumor, and it is important to independently evaluate individual foci of low-grade serous neoplasms. For example, sections of the ovarian tumor may show straightforward serous borderline tumor but the omental involvement shows destructive invasion consistent with low-grade serous carcinoma. In this case, the diagnosis of low-grade serous carcinoma should be rendered for the omental tumor, but the ovarian tumor should still be designated serous borderline tumor. A comment can explain that this either represents an extraovarian progression of the tumor or spread from an unsampled area of invasion in the ovarian tumors.

SEROUS PSAMMOCARCINOMA

Serous psammocarcinoma, as strictly defined, is rare and is probably a variant of low-grade serous carcinoma in which there are prominent psammomatous calcifications. Serous psammo-carcinoma is composed predominantly of psammomatous calcifications (>75% of the tumor area) with interspersed clusters of tumor cells with a similar appearance to low-grade serous carcinoma (**Fig. 20**).[23] In general, these tumors show primarily peritoneal disease without a clear or dominant ovarian mass. This tumor category is separated from low-grade serous carcinoma by its potentially different prognosis.

Pathologic Key Features
LOW-GRADE SEROUS NEOPLASMS

Serous cystadenoma/ cystadeno-fibroma	Cystic or cystic and solid lesion Bland epithelial lining with mixture of serous and ciliated cells or simple cuboidal cells Minimal epithelial stratification
Serous borderline tumor	Papillary epithelial growth in >10% of the lesion lining Hierarchical epithelial branching in conventional type Slender nonbranching papillary or cribriform growth in micropapillary type Microinvasion defined as nondestructive stromal invasion measuring <5 mm in greatest dimension May involve lymph nodes or form implants in peritoneum
Low-grade serous carcinoma	Characterized by destructive stromal invasion Low-grade cytologic atypia (uniform cells with hyperchromatic chromatin, small nucleoli, and scattered mitotic figures) Normal (patchy) expression of p53 on immunohistochemistry
Serous psammo-carcinoma	Variant of serous carcinoma with >75% of tumor mass composed of psammomatous calcifications Low-grade cytologic atypia similar to low-grade serous carcinoma

---

ANCILLARY STUDIES

There are several immunohistochemical stains that can provide useful adjunct information for making an accurate diagnosis of low-grade serous lesions. Serous lesions, like other müllerian epithelial tumors, reliably express PAX8. WT1 is the best stain to separate low-grade serous neoplasms (positive) from the other ovarian epithelial tumors (negative), but it is also positive in mesothelial lesions. Low-grade serous neoplasia is usually strongly positive for estrogen receptor, with more limited expression of progesterone receptor. P53 should show normal (patchy) nuclear expression (**Fig. 21**).

Molecular techniques are not routinely used for the classification or prognosis of low-grade serous neoplasia; however, it is helpful to understand the current knowledge of molecular alterations, because these may provide more value in the future. Low-grade serous neoplasia is associated with mutations in *BRAF* and *KRAS/NRAS*, as contrasted with the *TP53* mutations typical of high-grade serous carcinoma. *BRAF* mutations are most commonly seen in serous borderline tumors and low-stage, low-grade serous carcinomas.[24–26] Low-grade serous carcinomas and serous borderline tumors that recur as low-grade serous carcinomas more frequently show *KRAS/NRAS* mutations.[27,28] Given these trends, it is possible that molecular alterations could be useful for prognostication and eventually for diagnostic purposes.

DIFFERENTIAL DIAGNOSIS

SEROUS CYSTADENOMA/ CYSTADENOFIBROMA

The primary differential diagnoses for benign serous neoplasms are cortical inclusion cysts, mesothelial cysts, and endometriosis/endometriomas. Cortical inclusion cysts are common benign lesions that are thought to represent inclusion of the ovarian surface epithelium. The epithelium lining these cysts can show a variety of differentiation patterns, including frequent serous (tubal-like) differentiation. Serous cystadenoma are arbitrarily distinguished from inclusion cysts by size greater than 1 cm. Mesothelial (peritoneal) inclusion cysts can occur in the periadnexal tissue and are often associated with adhesions.

Mesothelial cysts are lined by cuboidal cells, which can have a similar appearance to serous epithelium. It is common for mesothelial cysts

Fig. 20. Psammocarcinoma composed predominantly of psammomatous calcifications (>75% of the tumor area) with interspersed clusters of tumor cells with a similar appearance to low-grade serous carcinoma.

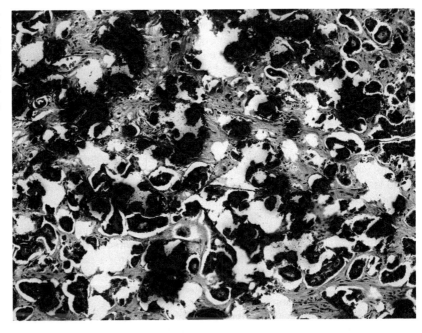

to have squamous metaplasia, which can make the diagnosis more challenging. In general, careful review of a serous cystadenoma shows as least a small area with ciliated cells. If necessary, a limited panel of immunohistochemical stains can be helpful for this differential diagnosis. The authors usually use a panel of PAX-8, MOC-31, and calretinin to make the

Fig. 21. Normal (wild-type) p53 expression in low-grade serous carcinoma.

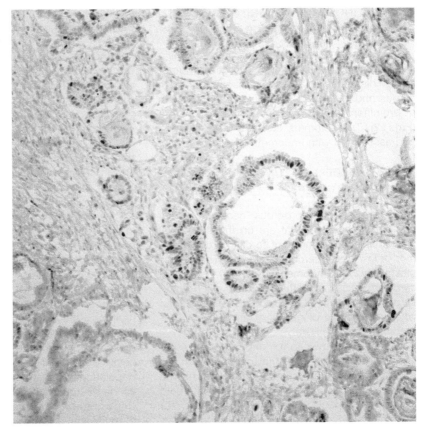

distinction between müllerian epithelium and mesothelial cells. PAX-8 is usually strongly positive in serous epithelium and negative in mesothelial cells. However, mesothelial cells can also be positive for PAX-8, so we additionally rely on MOC-31 as a marker of epithelial differential that it not usually present in mesothelial cells. Calretinin typically highlights mesothelial cells more strongly than serous epithelium.

Serous cystadenomas can show morphologic overlap with ovarian endometriomas, because some lesions show condensation of the ovarian stroma under the serous epithelium that mimics the endometrial-type stroma in endometriomas. Endometriomas can show a variety of metaplasias within the lining cells, including frequent serous differentiation. Most of the time, these 2 entities can be reliably distinguished by evaluation of the stromal cells under the epithelium, the presence of nonserous epithelial differentiation in endometriomas, and the abundance of hemorrhage and reactive change encountered in endometriomas. We have used WT1, because there is strong and diffuse nuclear staining in the lining cells of serous cystadenomas but absent to patchy staining in those of endometriomas.

SEROMUCINOUS BORDERLINE TUMOR AND SEROUS BORDERLINE TUMOR

Seromucinous borderline tumor shows similar architecture features to serous borderline tumor but is distinguished by the presence of both serous and mucinous epithelium, typically with a prominent associated neutrophilic infiltrate (Fig. 22). These tumors are also often bilateral and associated with endometriosis.

SEROUS BORDERLINE TUMOR AND LOW-GRADE SEROUS CARCINOMA

There are several nonserous neoplasms with papillary architecture that are on the differential when making a diagnosis of serous borderline tumor or low-grade serous carcinoma. These neoplasms include endometrioid tumors, clear cell carcinomas, and mesothelial tumors. High-grade serous carcinoma also needs to be excluded when making the diagnosis of any type of low-grade serous neoplasia.

Endometrioid ovarian tumors can show striking papillary architecture that overlaps with the papillary architecture seen in serous borderline tumors (Fig. 23). To recognize an endometrioid tumor with papillary architecture, look for endometrioid-type cytologic features (columnar,

pseudostratified cells with smooth luminal borders), squamous metaplasia, and/or areas with more classic endometrioid architecture (complex glandular growth). It is worth noting that both endometrioid borderline tumors and endometrioid adenocarcinoma can mimic serous borderline tumors. It is important to first decide the line of differentiation (endometrioid vs serous), before deciding on the designation of borderline versus carcinoma, because the criteria for carcinoma are different in the two tumor types. Specifically, to make a diagnosis of serous carcinoma, desmoplastic stromal invasion is needed, whereas low-grade endometrioid carcinomas can show expansile-type growth without desmoplastic stromal invasion. Therefore, a papillary tumor with exuberant epithelial growth showing cribriforming but no destructive invasion of the stroma may be diagnosed as a serous borderline tumor or an endometrioid adenocarcinoma. WT1 is again a useful marker in these cases to confirm serous differentiation (diffuse positive staining) in cases with challenging morphology.

A major pitfall in the diagnosis of serous borderline tumors, especially at the time of intraoperative frozen section, is clear cell carcinoma (Fig. 24). If a clear cell carcinoma shows an exclusive or predominant papillary architectural pattern, cytology is the key to making the correct diagnosis. Serous borderline tumors can show mild nuclear enlargement but should not show the classic cytologic features associated with clear cell carcinoma, which include enlarged, round to angulated nuclei centrally placed in the cells, variably prominent nucleoli, abundant clear to eosinophilic cytoplasm, eosinophilic globules, and hobnailing. Look for other architectural patterns of clear cell carcinoma, such as small papillae with hyalinized cores, tubulocystic growth, and solid areas. Immunohistochemical stains are useful in this differential diagnosis. WT1 and estrogen receptor are usually positive in serous tumors, whereas clear cell tumors are usually negative for these markers but positive for NapsinA.

Mesothelial lesions (multicystic mesothelial cysts, mesothelial proliferations, well-differentiated papillary mesothelioma, and malignant mesothelioma) can sometimes be confused with serous neoplasia. The distribution of disease may be the first clue for a mesothelial process. Mesothelial lesions show a monomorphic population of cells (not mixed ciliated and serous as in serous borderline tumors) (Fig. 25). Compared with the stratification and proliferation of epithelium seen in serous tumors, mesothelial

Fig. 22. Seromucinous borderline ovarian tumor shows hierarchical branching similar to serous borderline tumor (*A*), but contains mixture of serous and mucinous cells with neutrophilic infiltrate (*B*).

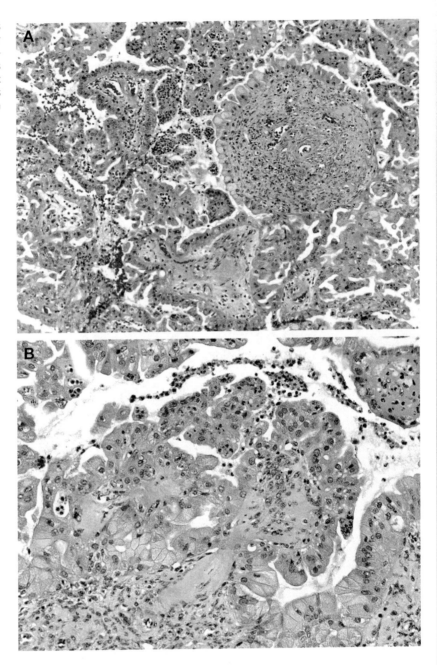

tumors tend to have nonstratified epithelium with well-developed papillary cores (**Fig. 26**). Malignant mesothelial lesions show invasion (like a serous carcinoma) but usually more cytologic atypia. The authors have seen atypical mesothelial proliferations in pelvic peritoneal tissues that form glandlike structures with the appearance of invasive adenocarcinoma, especially at frozen section. A mesothelial-epithelial immunohistochemical panel should be used in difficult cases. An example of a useful panel is calretinin, CK5/6, and D2-40 as mesothelial markers and PAX8, MOC-31, and Ber-EP4 as epithelial markers.

Papillary struma ovarii can mimic serous borderline tumor or low-grade serous carcinoma (**Fig. 27**). The presence of dense colloid material, additional foci of teratoma, and high index

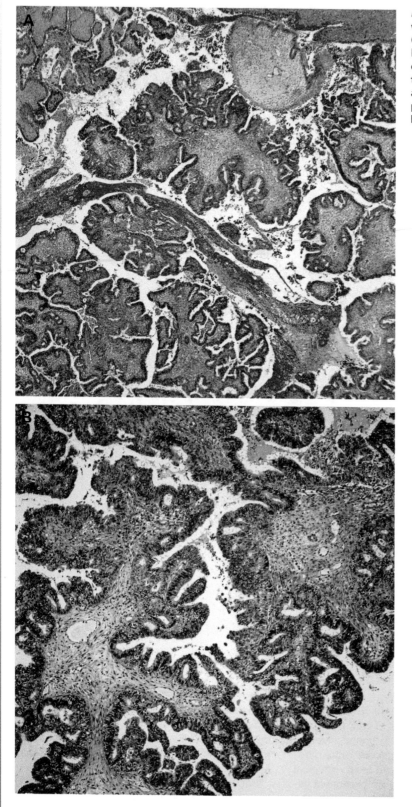

Fig. 23. Endometrioid tumor with papillary architecture (*A*) can mimic serous borderline tumor but can usually be distinguished by presence of taller, columnar cells and absence of the classic eosinophil (pink) cells in serous borderline tumor (*B*).

Fig. 24. Ovarian clear cell carcinoma may show a prominent papillary architecture, mimicking serous borderline tumor, but the characteristic hierarchical branching pattern seen in serous borderline tumor is absent. Also, clear cell carcinoma is typically unilateral and often associated with a background of endometriosis.

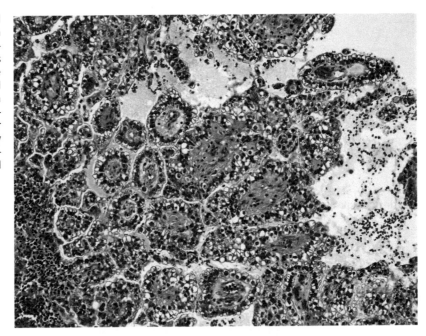

of suspicion prevents misdiagnosis. Struma can be confirmed by positive staining for thyroglobulin.

Both serous borderline tumors and low-grade serous carcinomas show fairly uniform tumor cells, whereas high-grade serous carcinomas show nuclear pleomorphism and increased mitotic activity. The MD Anderson criteria for high-grade serous carcinoma include significant nuclear pleomorphism with 3 to 1 variation in the size of nuclei; irregular, coarse chromatin; and increased mitotic activity (>12 mitoses per 10 high-power fields). Because high-grade serous and low-grade serous lesions usually arise via distinct molecular pathways, most tumors are either pure low grade or pure high grade. However, there are several well-described series of tumors with mixed low-grade and high-grade components or low-grade tumors that progress to high-grade tumors over time, presumably by acquiring mutations in TP53.

IMPLANTS OF SEROUS BORDERLINE TUMOR

Noninvasive implants of serous borderline tumor can show morphologic overlap with endosalpingiosis, psammomatous calcifications, and mesothelial proliferations. Endosalpingiosis refers to the presence of ectopic, benign serous-type epithelial tissue. It is characterized by tubules and cysts lined by bland serous-type

epithelium and can be found anywhere in the peritoneum and even in the lymph nodes. By contrast, implants of serous borderline tumor should show papillary or micropapillary architectural growth (in the case of epithelial implants) or even single cells/clusters of cells (in the case of desmoplastic implants). The term atypical endosalpingiosis is used to refer to lesions that show features of endosalpingiosis with focal papillary growth that are not extensive enough for a diagnosis of a borderline tumor (**Fig. 28**).

Psammomatous calcifications can occur in isolation or in association with serous lesions, including endosalpingiosis, borderline tumors, and carcinomas. When psammomatous calcifications are encountered, judgment about how to classify the lesion (if it is serous) should be made from architectural complexity (simple tubules vs papillary proliferations), presence of invasion (diagnostic of carcinoma), and cytologic features (low grade vs high grade). Serous psammocarcinoma is a specific case in which psammomatous calcifications may predominate and coat peritoneum with only infrequent areas showing papillary clusters of tumor cells. Invasion may be challenging to identify in these cases and relies on liberal sampling.

The spectrum of mesothelial lesions described earlier can also show overlapping morphology with implants of serous borderline tumors. Please see for the earlier discussion.

ΔΔ Differential Diagnosis
OF LOW-GRADE SEROUS NEOPLASIA

Lesion	Helpful Features
Endometriosis/ endometrioma	Distinguish from serous cystadenoma by presence of hemosiderin, endometrial-type stroma, and cuboidal lining cells with eosinophilic cytoplasm WT-1 can be useful
Mesothelial lesions	Distinguish from serous cystadenoma and serous borderline tumor by monomorphic, nonstratified, cuboidal cell population with well-development papillary cores in proliferative lesions Calretinin, CK5/6, D2-40, PAX-8, MOC-31, and Ber-EP4 can be useful
Endosalpingiosis	Distinguish from implants of serous borderline tumor by lack of significant epithelial stratification and papillary architecture
Endometrioid tumors with papillary architecture	Distinguish from serous borderline tumor by more pronounced pseudostratification of columnar-appearing cells, squamous differentiation Look for other areas of classic endometrioid glandular growth
Clear cell carcinoma	Distinguish from serous borderline tumor by enlarged, round, centrally located nuclei with prominent nucleoli, abundant cytoplasm, eosinophilic globules, and hobnailing Look for other patterns of clear cell carcinoma WT-1 and estrogen receptor can be useful
High-grade serous carcinoma	Distinguish from both serous borderline tumor and low-grade serous carcinoma primarily based on cytologic findings of significant nuclear pleomorphism with vesicular chromatin and prominent nucleoli Mitotic figures should be increased (>12 per 10 high-power fields) P53 shows abnormal overexpression (>90% of cells) or complete lack of expression (null)

PROGNOSIS

SEROUS CYSTADENOMA/ CYSTADENOFIBROMA

Serous cystadenomas are benign lesions that require no adjuvant therapy. They do not recur if they are completely excised. When there is focal epithelial proliferation representing less than 10% of the lesion, the prognosis seems to be the same.

SEROUS BORDERLINE TUMOR

Serous borderline tumors have a generally indolent behavior with prolonged periods between disease recurrences or even regression of disease. The stage of the tumor largely determines the overall survival, with greater than 95% survival for low-stage disease (I) versus 65% for high-stage disease (II–IV).[9] In low-stage disease, the presence of bilateral ovarian involvement and ovarian surface involvement is associated with increased risk of progression/recurrence.[13] In the Stanford series, greater than or equal to 5-year overall survival and disease-free survival

were 95% and 78%, respectively.[1] Because the overall survival in the presence of invasive implants is similar to that of low-grade serous carcinoma, it is recommended that these lesions be designated low-grade serous carcinoma. Specifically, a recent study showed that overall survival in the setting of so-called invasive implants was 50% compared with 90% for noninvasive implants and 79% for indeterminate implants.[10]

Classic microinvasion (with or without lymphovascular invasion) and lymph node involvement in serous borderline tumors do not seem to alter the overall prognosis, although careful attention should be paid to excluding more extensive disease in these cases.[18] Microinvasion, even when multifocal, does not change the course of disease; however, pathologists are encouraged to liberally sample the neoplasm in this setting to exclude foci of invasion greater than the 5-mm cutoff or areas of destructive stromal invasion. It is uncommon to encounter cases in which areas of classic stromal microinvasion (nondestructive) exceed the 5 mm cutoff.[19] There are more limited data regarding the behavior of the nonclassic patterns of stromal microinvasion, which may confer a higher risk

Fig. 25. Florid mesothelial hyperplasia may mimic involvement by serous borderline tumor (*A*), but can be recognized by the presence of a more monomorphic pattern of uniform cells, often with intracytoplasmic vacuoles. The reactive nature of the proliferation can be further recognized by the apparent linear arrangement (as opposed to haphazard arrangement) of the cells (*B*).

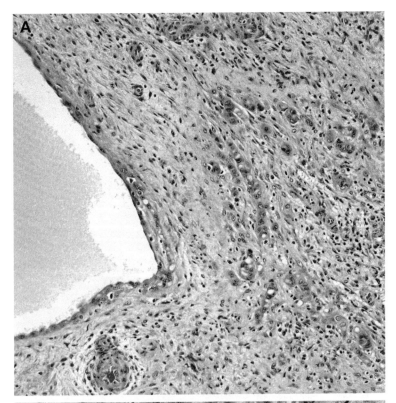

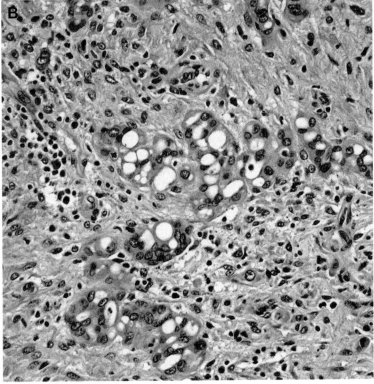

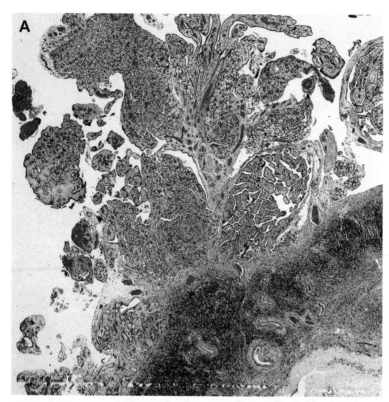

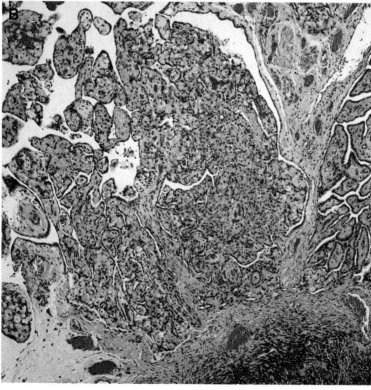

Fig. 26. Papillary mesothelioma shows a monomorphic population of cells (not mixed ciliated and serous as in serous borderline tumors) (*A*). Compared with the stratification and proliferation of epithelium seen in serous tumors, mesothelial tumors tend to have nonstratified epithelium with well-developed papillary cores (*B*).

Fig. 27. Papillary struma ovarii (*A, B*) can mimic serous borderline tumor or low-grade serous carcinoma The presence of dense colloid material, additional foci of teratoma, and high index of suspicion prevent misdiagnosis. Struma can be confirmed by positive staining for thyroglobulin.

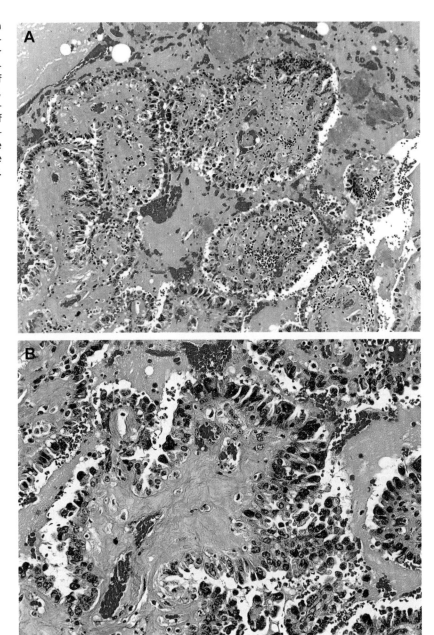

than the classic microinvasion pattern.[19] Lymph node involvement by borderline tumors likewise does not seem to alter the behavior of the disease. There is some evidence that nodular aggregates of tumor cells greater than or equal to 1 mm in lymph nodes should be considered metastatic low-grade serous carcinoma, because these may show more aggressive behavior.[18]

Although most serous borderline tumors recur as borderline tumors, transformation to low-grade serous carcinoma occurs in approximately 7%.[1] Progression to low-grade serous carcinoma can occur over a prolonged period of time, with the risk persistent up to 20 years later.[13,29] Transformation is usually seen in the setting of serous borderline tumors, which are initially high stage; however, it can rarely occur in stage I disease.[13] Occasionally, serous borderline tumors can progress to high-grade serous carcinoma.[13] As expected, transformation to either low-grade or high-grade serous carcinoma is accompanied by an expected

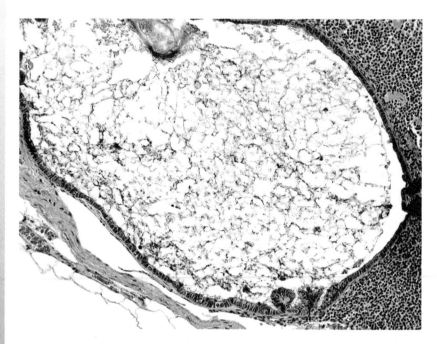

Fig. 28. Atypical endosalpingiosis in this lymph node does not warrant classification as involvement by serous borderline tumor.

decrease in overall survival and increased tempo of recurrences.[13]

Micropapillary serous borderline tumors have a higher propensity for extraovarian disease (implants), including ones with tissue invasion (considered low-grade serous carcinoma). The decreased overall survive in this variant (as opposed to conventional borderline tumors) is probably caused by covariance with the presence of invasive implants.[1,30–32] When making a diagnosis of micropapillary serous borderline tumor, the comment should note that these tumors have a tendency for bilaterality, surface involvement, and implants, which may be invasive. Based on recent population-based data, it is reasonable to conclude that micropapillary tumors have an increased risk of developing serous carcinoma compared with their conventional counterparts.[13]

Given the paucity of data, no clear recommendation has been made as to whether or not women with higher risk ovarian serous borderline tumors (eg, extensive micropapillary or cribriform architecture, microinvasive carcinoma, surface involvement) should undergo an additional formal staging procedure following initial diagnosis, especially for women of reproductive age who wish to maintain fertility. At present, the decision to proceed with formal staging is conducted on an individualized basis and is likely determined by several pathologic and clinical factors.

Fertility-sparing procedures such as cystectomy or unilateral oophorectomy are associated with a higher incidence of recurrent disease compared with bilateral oophorectomy. In most cases, women are instructed to complete childbearing within a short time frame following initial diagnosis because of the high risk of recurrence. Recurrences tend to be seen in the ipsilateral and/or contralateral ovary in patients so treated.

LOW-GRADE SEROUS CARCINOMA

Low-grade serous carcinoma is important to distinguish from high-grade serous carcinoma because it has a unique tempo of disease and is less responsive to standard chemotherapy agents. The mean survival for low-grade serous carcinoma is 90.8 months versus 40.7 months for high-grade serous carcinoma.[33] Transformation from a low-grade serous carcinoma to a high-grade serous carcinoma is rare but has been reported, and mixed high-grade and low-grade tumors are sometimes seen.[34]

Low-grade serous carcinoma shows a more aggressive clinical course than serous borderline tumor with a significant decrease in overall survival. In the Stanford series, 5-year overall survival was 82% and disease-free survival was 47% for low-grade serous carcinoma; similar findings have been reported by other groups.[8,35,36] By contrast, greater than or equal to 5-year overall survival and disease-free survival were 95% and 78%, respectively, for serous borderline tumors.[1] Serous psammocarcinoma has an intermediate behavior between that of low-grade serous carcinoma and serous borderline tumor.[23] Most patients with serous psammocarcinoma present with high-stage disease with minimal ovarian involvement.

Pitfalls

! Because low-grade serous carcinoma is often associated with serous borderline tumor, tumors with increased mitotic figures, increased cytologic atypia, or extensive cribriform and/or micropapillary architecture should be adequately sampling to exclude foci of carcinoma, especially if high stage.

! Stromal microinvasion in serous borderline tumors may be multifocal, simulating low-grade serous carcinoma, but classic stromal microinvasion does not seem to confer a worse prognosis.

! The classification of micropapillary architecture is subjective; in order to achieve greater reproducibility for this diagnosis, a serous tumor should be designated as micropapillary only when the involved papillae are at least 5 times as long as they are wide and they encompass at least 5 mm in continuous linear extent.

! Prominent psammomatous calcifications may be focally present in a variety of peritoneal lesions (eg, usual serous carcinoma, endosalpingiosis, and peritoneal adhesions). Adequate sampling is required to establish the appropriate diagnosis.

! Low-grade serous carcinoma may contain foci of spindle cells, simulating high-grade serous carcinoma, but marked nuclear pleomorphism is absent, and mitotic figures do not exceed 12 figures per 10 high-power fields (and rarely exceed 5–6 figures per 10 high-power fields).

! Areas of tumor infarction may mimic stromal invasion, but they are usually associated with a geographic zone of inflamed and edematous stroma, which may or may not contain disrupted and entrapped epithelial cells.

! Autoimplants (desmoplastic-type implants in the primary ovarian tumor) may mimic stromal invasion, but they are distinguished from stromal invasion by their characteristic position along the tips and lateral borders of papillae and on the ovarian surface and their resemblance to noninvasive desmoplastic extraovarian implants elsewhere.

SUMMARY

Classification of low-grade serous neoplasms remains a challenging area of gynecologic pathology, but recent findings have refined the ability to predict aggressive behavior and changed some of the traditional terminology used for these tumors. Lesions previously termed invasive implants of serous borderline tumor are now designated as low-grade serous carcinoma based on the similar overall survival in these cases to low-grade serous carcinoma. Molecular analysis may also be helpful in the future for prognostication.

REFERENCES

1. Longacre TA, McKenney JK, Tazelaar HD, et al. Ovarian serous tumors of low malignant potential (borderline tumors): outcome-based study of 276 patients with long-term (> or =5-year) follow-up. Am J Surg Pathol 2005;29(6):707–23.

2. Malpica A, Longacre TA. Prognostic indicators in ovarian serous borderline tumours. Pathology 2018;50(2):205–13.

3. Burks RT, Sherman ME, Kurman RJ. Micropapillary serous carcinoma of the ovary. A distinctive low-grade carcinoma related to serous borderline tumors. Am J Surg Pathol 1996;20(11):1319–30.

4. Eichhorn JH, Bell DA, Young RH, et al. Ovarian serous borderline tumors with micropapillary and cribriform patterns: a study of 40 cases and comparison with 44 cases without these patterns. Am J Surg Pathol 1999;23(4):397–409.

5. Bell DA, Longacre TA, Prat J, et al. Serous borderline (low malignant potential, atypical proliferative) ovarian tumors: workshop perspectives. Hum Pathol 2004;35(8):934–48.

6. Hannibal CG, Vang R, Junge J, et al. A nationwide study of serous "borderline" ovarian tumors in Denmark 1978-2002: centralized pathology review and overall survival compared with the general population. Gynecol Oncol 2014;134(2):267–73.

7. Smith Sehdev AE, Sehdev PS, Kurman RJ. Noninvasive and invasive micropapillary (low-grade) serous carcinoma of the ovary: a clinicopathologic analysis of 135 cases. Am J Surg Pathol 2003;27(6):725–36.

8. Ahn G, Folkins AK, McKenney JK, et al. Low-grade Serous carcinoma of the ovary: clinicopathologic analysis of 52 invasive cases and identification of a possible noninvasive intermediate lesion. Am J Surg Pathol 2016;40(9):1165–76.

9. Seidman JD, Kurman RJ. Ovarian serous borderline tumors: a critical review of the literature with emphasis on prognostic indicators. Hum Pathol 2000;31(5):539–57.

10. McKenney JK, Gilks CB, Kalloger S, et al. Classification of extraovarian implants in patients with ovarian serous borderline tumors (tumors of low malignant potential) based on clinical outcome. Am J Surg Pathol 2016;40(9):1155–64.

11. Shvartsman HS, Sun CC, Bodurka DC, et al. Comparison of the clinical behavior of newly diagnosed stages II-IV low-grade serous carcinoma of the ovary with that of serous ovarian tumors of low malignant potential that recur as low-grade serous carcinoma. Gynecol Oncol 2007; 105(3):625–9.

12. Hannibal CG, Vang R, Junge J, et al. A nationwide study of ovarian serous borderline tumors in Denmark 1978-2002. Risk of recurrence, and development of ovarian serous carcinoma. Gynecol Oncol 2017;144(1):174–80.

13. Vang R, Hannibal CG, Junge J, et al. Long-term behavior of serous borderline tumors subdivided into atypical proliferative tumors and noninvasive low-grade carcinomas: a population-based clinicopathologic study of 942 cases. Am J Surg Pathol 2017;41(6):725–37.

14. Karlsen NMS, Karlsen MA, Hogdall E, et al. Relapse and disease specific survival in 1143 Danish women diagnosed with borderline ovarian tumours (BOT). Gynecol Oncol 2016;142(1):50–3.

15. Camatte S, Morice P, Atallah D, et al. Lymph node disorders and prognostic value of nodal involvement in patients treated for a borderline ovarian tumor: an analysis of a series of 42 lymphadenectomies. J Am Coll Surg 2002;195(3):332–8.

16. Djordjevic B, Malpica A. Lymph node involvement in ovarian serous tumors of low malignant potential: a clinicopathologic study of thirty-six cases. Am J Surg Pathol 2010;34(1):1–9.

17. Lesieur B, Kane A, Duvillard P, et al. Prognostic value of lymph node involvement in ovarian serous borderline tumors. Am J Obstet Gynecol 2011; 204(5):438.e1-7.

18. McKenney JK, Balzer BL, Longacre TA. Lymph node involvement in ovarian serous tumors of low malignant potential (borderline tumors): pathology, prognosis, and proposed classification. Am J Surg Pathol 2006;30(5):614–24.

19. McKenney JK, Balzer BL, Longacre TA. Patterns of stromal invasion in ovarian serous tumors of low malignant potential (borderline tumors): a reevaluation of the concept of stromal microinvasion. Am J Surg Pathol 2006;30(10):1209–21.

20. Sangoi AR, McKenney JK, Dadras SS, et al. Lymphatic vascular invasion in ovarian serous tumors of low malignant potential with stromal microinvasion: a case control study. Am J Surg Pathol 2008; 32(2):261–8.

21. Kobel M, Kalloger SE, Huntsman DG, et al. Differences in tumor type in low-stage versus high-stage ovarian carcinomas. Int J Gynecol Pathol 2010; 29(3):203–11.

22. Malpica A, Deavers MT, Lu K, et al. Grading ovarian serous carcinoma using a two-tier system. Am J Surg Pathol 2004;28(4):496–504.

23. Gilks CB, Bell DA, Scully RE. Serous psammocarcinoma of the ovary and peritoneum. Int J Gynecol Pathol 1990;9(2):110–21.

24. Grisham RN, Iyer G, Garg K, et al. BRAF mutation is associated with early stage disease and improved outcome in patients with low-grade serous ovarian cancer. Cancer 2013;119(3):548–54.

25. Wong KK, Tsang YT, Deavers MT, et al. BRAF mutation is rare in advanced-stage low-grade ovarian serous carcinomas. Am J Pathol 2010;177(4): 1611–7.

26. Zeppernick F, Ardighieri L, Hannibal CG, et al. BRAF mutation is associated with a specific cell type with features suggestive of senescence in ovarian serous borderline (atypical proliferative) tumors. Am J Surg Pathol 2014;38(12): 1603–11.

27. Tsang YT, Deavers MT, Sun CC, et al. KRAS (but not BRAF) mutations in ovarian serous borderline tumour are associated with recurrent low-grade serous carcinoma. J Pathol 2013; 231(4):449–56.

28. Emmanuel C, Chiew YE, George J, et al. Genomic classification of serous ovarian cancer with adjacent borderline differentiates RAS pathway and TP53-mutant tumors and identifies NRAS as an oncogenic driver. Clin Cancer Res 2014;20(24): 6618–30.

29. Silva EG, Gershenson DM, Malpica A, et al. The recurrence and the overall survival rates of ovarian serous borderline neoplasms with noninvasive implants is time dependent. Am J Surg Pathol 2006; 30(11):1367–71.

30. Prat J, De Nictolis M. Serous borderline tumors of the ovary: a long-term follow-up study of 137 cases, including 18 with a micropapillary pattern and 20 with microinvasion. Am J Surg Pathol 2002;26(9): 1111–28.

31. Deavers MT, Gershenson DM, Tortolero-Luna G, et al. Micropapillary and cribriform patterns in ovarian serous tumors of low malignant potential: a study of 99 advanced stage cases. Am J Surg Pathol 2002;26(9):1129–41.

32. Slomovitz BM, Caputo TA, Gretz HF 3rd, et al. A comparative analysis of 57 serous borderline tumors with and without a noninvasive micropapillary component. Am J Surg Pathol 2002;26(5): 592–600.

33. Gockley A, Melamed A, Bregar AJ, et al. Outcomes of women with high-grade and low-grade advanced-stage serous epithelial ovarian cancer. Obstet Gynecol 2017;129(3):439–47.

34. Boyd C, McCluggage WG. Low-grade ovarian se-
    rous neoplasms (low-grade serous carcinoma and
    serous borderline tumor) associated with high-
    grade serous carcinoma or undifferentiated carci-
    noma: report of a series of cases of an unusual phe-
    nomenon. Am J Surg Pathol 2012;36(3):368–75.

35. Gershenson DM, Sun CC, Bodurka D, et al. Recur-
    rent low-grade serous ovarian carcinoma is relatively
    chemoresistant. Gynecol Oncol 2009;114(1):48–52.

36. Gershenson DM, Sun CC, Lu KH, et al. Clinical
    behavior of stage II-IV low-grade serous carcinoma
    of the ovary. Obstet Gynecol 2006;108(2):361–8.

Ovarian High-Grade Serous Carcinoma

Assessing Pathology for Site of Origin, Staging and Post-neoadjuvant Chemotherapy Changes

Laura Casey, FRCPath[a], Naveena Singh, MD, FRCPath[b],*

KEYWORDS
- High-grade serous carcinoma • Staging • chemotherapy response score • Primary site
- Serous tubal intraepithelial carcinoma

ABSTRACT

High-grade serous (HGSC) stands apart from the other ovarian cancer histotypes in being the most frequent, in occurring as part of a genetic predisposition in a significant proportion of cases, and in having the poorest clinical outcomes. Although the pathologic diagnosis of HGSC is now made with high accuracy, there remain areas of disagreement regarding viewpoints on tissue site of origin and designation of primary site, with impact on staging in low-stage cases, as well as difficulties in reproducible and clinically relevant reporting of HGSC in specimens taken after neoadjuvant chemotherapy. These areas are discussed in the current article.

OVERVIEW

Over the past 15 years, there have been dramatic changes in our diagnostic approach to ovarian carcinomas. Long considered and treated as a single disease with a common origin in the ovarian surface epithelium, ovarian carcinomas are now known to comprise 5 major clinicopathologically distinct entities[1]: high-grade serous (HGSC), clear cell (CCC), endometrioid (EC), low-grade serous, and mucinous carcinomas. HGSC stands apart from the others in being the most frequent, in occurring in the setting of a genetically inherited cancer risk in approximately one-fifth of all cases, thereby raising the need for reflex referral to genetic counseling services, and in having the poorest clinical outcomes. Despite advances in surgical and nonsurgical treatments, including targeted therapies, survival in HGSC has not improved significantly over the past few decades, underscoring the need for preventive and early detection strategies.

For these reasons, it is vital that the pathologic diagnosis of HGSC and all ovarian cancer subtypes is robust and reproducible. The high reproducibility of ovarian carcinoma histotype diagnosis using current diagnostic criteria has been well demonstrated,[2] both with and without the use of commonly available immunohistochemical markers, with combined WT1 positivity and abnormal p53 expression being highly specific for a diagnosis of HGSC.[3] Although in the past it was common to diagnose "mixed" carcinomas based on combinations of growth patterns, it is now well recognized that most carcinomas thought to be mixtures actually represent HGSC, which can have many different appearances, and that true mixed carcinomas are extremely rare, with most representing combinations of carcinomas occurring in a background of endometriosis, such as mixed EC and CCC.[4]

Although the pathologic diagnosis of HGSC is now made with high accuracy, there remain areas

[a] Department of Pathology, Queen's Hospital, Rom Valley Way, Romford RM7 0AG, UK; [b] Department of Cellular Pathology, Barts Health NHS Trust, The Royal London Hospital, 2nd Floor, 80 Newark Street, London E1 2ES, UK
* Corresponding author.
E-mail address: N.Singh@bartshealth.nhs.uk

Surgical Pathology 12 (2019) 515–528
https://doi.org/10.1016/j.path.2019.01.007
1875-9181/19/Crown Copyright © 2019 Published by Elsevier Inc. All rights reserved.

of disagreement with regard to viewpoints on origin and designation of primary site with impact on staging in low-stage cases, as well as difficulties in reproducible and clinically relevant reporting of HGSC in specimens taken after neoadjuvant chemotherapy (NACT). These areas are the subjects of the current review.

ASSESSING SITE OF ORIGIN

One of the key stipulations of the 2013 International Federation of Gynecology and Obstetrics (FIGO) staging system is that the primary tumor site (fallopian tube, ovary, or peritoneum) should be clearly designated and that, where such assignment is not possible, the term "undesignated" should be used.[5] Unfortunately, FIGO provides no accompanying guidance on the criteria for site assignment, and the World Health Organization (WHO) classification issued in the following year advises only that the site assignment of extraovarian HGSC should be left to the "experience and professional judgment" of the reporting pathologist.[1] Since the publication of these guidelines, however, considerable further evidence on the origin of HGSC has emerged, which should inform current practice in advance of future changes to FIGO/WHO terminology.

The persistent lack of clarity on this issue almost certainly reflects historical and, indeed, ongoing debates as to the true origin of extrauterine HGSC. Early theories centered on the notion that all ovarian carcinomas derived from a common origin (ovarian surface epithelium) and were therefore closely related and frequently admixed.[6] For a number of reasons, this theory was problematic although not least because the ovary is covered by mesothelium whereas the 5 major subtypes of ovarian carcinoma are of Müllerian derivation. Attempts to correct for this led to the idea that ovarian carcinomas arose from cortical inclusion cyst epithelium, itself derived from ovarian surface epithelium but now demonstrating tubal-type cells either through a process of metaplasia or through colonization of a preexisting cyst by cells detached from the fallopian tube.[7] The evidence to support these theories is limited though descriptions of in situ lesions involving the ovarian surface epithelium, and cortical inclusion cyst epithelium do exist in the literature[8,9] and murine experimental models aimed at evoking transformation of ovarian serous epithelium have indeed produced tumors that resemble ovarian carcinoma in humans.[10–12] More recently, there have been reports of serous tubal intraepithelial carcinoma (STIC)-like lesions occurring within benign ciliated epithelium of ovarian serous cystadenofibromas,[13]

as well as evidence that some cases of HGSC without STIC may occur through a process of "precursor escape" as evidenced by HGSC occurring in the presence of clonally identical lesions within the tube that fall short of morphologic criteria of STIC.[14]

A further problem with the search for an ovarian primary is that it is predicated on the notion that tumor volume reflects site of origin, which is to say that if disease is visible in the ovary alone it must, necessarily, have originated in the ovary. Of course, it is now appreciated that the steroid cell stroma of the ovary provides a uniquely fertile environment for transient malignant cells and that tumors of the stomach, colon, appendix, and endocervix may give rise to ovarian metastases that exceed the size of their primary lesion.[15,16] The idea, therefore, that HGSC may arise at an extraovarian site, spread to the ovary and produce a larger tumor focus within that ovary should not be conceptually challenging,[17–19] but the theory of tumor bulk is appealing in its apparent simplicity and forms the basis of the problematic and yet widely used Gynecologic Oncology Group criteria for siting extraovarian serous carcinoma.[1,20]

Another origin model is that of the secondary Müllerian system. The term "Müllerian" is used to describe the structures and epithelia that derive from the embryologic Müllerian ducts; that is, the uterus and fallopian tubes with their serous, endometrial, and endocervical cell linings.[21] In the 1970s, Lauchlan[22] drew a distinction between these, the "primary Müllerian system," and the mesothelium/mesenchyme of the lower abdomen and pelvis, which he believed to be capable of Müllerian differentiation and thus dubbed "the secondary Müllerian system." The theoretic potential of this mesothelium to undergo metaplastic transformation to a Müllerian type epithelium was posited as an explanation for "Müllerianosis," that is, endometriosis, endosalpingiosis, and endocervicosis. It is this theoretic model that gave rise to the concept of "field change" in the HGSC origin debate (whereby the entire peritoneum is subject to a carcinogenic stimulus resulting in multiple coexistent primary sites)[23,24] and, furthermore, to the entity "primary peritoneal carcinoma." Lauchlan[22,23] insisted that, "it has not been seriously suggested…that an ovarian focus of, say, endometriosis acts as a kind of Tinkerbell sprinkling replicas of itself, like stardust, throughout the peritoneum," instead believing that foci of endometriosis might arise synchronously but entirely separately at sites undergoing Müllerian metaplasia. Today, the favored model for the dissemination of endometriosis is that of retrograde menstruation,[25,26] supported by evidence of a clonal relationship between physically distinct endometriotic foci,[27] although, admittedly, the possibility of metaplastic change in this context has not been absolutely excluded. Primary peritoneal carcinoma was first described in 1959[28] and was believed to arise from the totipotential pelvic peritoneum: the "secondary Müllerian system." The concept of primary peritoneal carcinoma persists, as it provides a ready explanation for cases of widely disseminated peritoneal disease in the context of minimal/undetectable ovarian disease[29–31] and it is ostensibly granted credence by reports of its occurrence many years after prophylactic bilateral salpingo-oophorectomy in BRCA mutation carriers.[32–34] However, in most cases, diligent examination of the ovaries and fallopian tubes will reveal foci of disease and recent studies have demonstrated clonal identity in recurrences following HGSC after long intervals,[35,36] and therefore true primary peritoneal carcinoma, if it exists at all, is likely a very rare entity.[37]

Today, the weight of evidence suggests that extrauterine HGSC most frequently arises from the distal, fimbrial end of the fallopian tube and derives from the precursor lesion "serous tubal intraepithelial carcinoma": STIC.[39–42] In 2001, it was reported that prophylactic salpingo-oophorectomy specimens taken from patients with a genetic predisposition to developing ovarian cancer (ie, individuals with BRCA1/2 mutations) contained foci of dysplastic change within the tubal epithelium.[43] This observation led to the development of a detailed sampling system for tubal specimens, the SEE-FIM protocol (Sectioning and Extensively Examining the FIMbriated end of the fallopian tube),[39] and to the validation of a diagnostic algorithm for STIC.[44] The incidence of STIC in prophylactic specimens varies from 1% to 25% in the literature and STIC is now widely accepted as the precursor lesion in hereditary extrauterine HGSC,[45–48] but the transfer of this model to cases of sporadic HGSC continues to be met with caution and skepticism.[49] To demonstrate that STIC is the original lesion in all cases of extrauterine HGSC (ie, both germline and sporadic), 3 key points have been addressed. The first has been to identify the frequency of STIC and small tubal mucosal invasive carcinomas in sporadic cases of HGSC. When the SEE-FIM protocol is properly applied, STIC or invasive tubal mucosal disease is found in up to 60% of cases of sporadic HGSC.[49] Where the disease has progressed to a more advanced stage, it is less likely that a precursor lesion will be identified, as it is frequently subsumed within a larger tumor mass. In a study of 53 cases of chemonaive extrauterine HGSC, SEE-FIM sampling revealed STIC alone in only 9% of specimens (5 of 53), tubal invasive mucosal disease, with or without STIC, in 49% (26 of 53), and incorporation of the fimbrial end into a larger tumor mass (thus preventing identification of a precursor lesion) in 25% (13 of 53).[50] Furthermore, in cases in which early stage or incidental sporadic disease has been examined (ie, where the extent of disease is analogous to that seen in risk-reducing salpingo-oophorectomy specimens), tubal mucosal disease was present in 100% of cases (48 of 48) and STIC was identified in 98% (47 of 48).[51–54] Thus, it has been proven that the incidence of STIC and tubal mucosal invasive carcinoma in both sporadic and germline extrauterine HGSC is comparable and that, in all cases, the fallopian tube is the site of earliest disease. However, these findings do not necessarily counter the "field change" model whereby multiple primary sites of disease are said to arise synchronously in response to a single noxious stimulus and, therefore, the second focus of investigation has been to demonstrate a clonal relationship between STIC and concurrent invasive tumor. In HGSC, mutations in the tumor suppressor TP53 gene have been shown to be both early and ubiquitous,[55] with identical mutations occurring in all samples derived from a single patient (ie, from multiple sites) and in both the in situ (STIC) and invasive foci of disease.[40,56–59] The probability of an identical TP53 mutation occurring simultaneously in multiple distinct primaries is exceedingly low and, therefore, these findings serve (1) to confirm that HGSC arises from a single tumor clone, a clone isolated in even the earliest lesions, and (2) to refute the notion that multiple foci of disease within the peritoneum occur on a background of field change. The timing and direction of metastatic spread remains unresolved and for this reason the third investigative objective has been to confirm that STIC is indeed the definitive primary lesion. Combined data from a series of papers examining a total of 48 cases of incidental HGSC identified unifocal disease on 43 occasions and, in all 43 cases, that single site of disease was the tubal mucosa. Ovarian involvement was identified in 4 of 48 cases and was always associated with tubal mucosal disease, suggesting that this represented secondary extension to the ovary.[51–54] On a different note, it is widely acknowledged that bilateral ovarian involvement by malignancy favors secondary involvement of the organ rather than primary disease. Indeed, colorectal, gastric, pancreato-biliary, breast, and cervical metastases to the ovary are frequently bilateral. In one study, 62% of cases of ovarian HGSC were bilateral, whereas tubal involvement in the same cases was unilateral in 84%.[50] The unilaterality of tubal disease further supports the notion of tubal origin. These are observational findings, but the conclusions reached are bolstered by a variety of sophisticated molecular studies that have sought to establish the developmental relationship between STIC and invasive HGSC. Comparisons of telomere length,[60] mapping of clonal ancestry,[61–63] and modeling of genetic mutational pathways[64] all point to a precursor: carcinoma relationship.

As a result of the ongoing origin debate, and in the absence of a ratified protocol for primary site assignment, there is significant variation in practice among pathologists, and it is possible for a single case to be classified as tubal, ovarian, primary peritoneal, or undesignated (**Fig. 1**). In

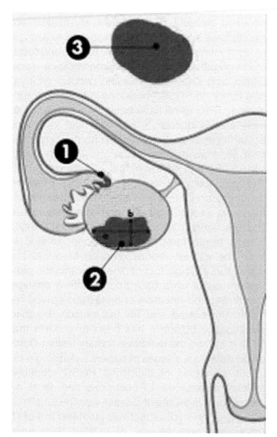

Fig. 1. Potential exists for variation in primary site assignment in HGSC. An example of a case with (1) STIC, (2) a small invasive ovarian HGSC, and (3) large-volume peritoneal disease is illustrated, that could be categorized as *ovarian* (if the pathologist sees the largest dimension (a) and this exceeds 5 mm) or *peritoneal* (if the pathologist sees the smallest dimension (b) and this is less than 5 mm) based on traditional criteria, *tubal* if the newly proposed criteria are accepted,[67] or *undesignated* if it is felt that there remains doubt on site of origin.

2016, an international survey of 173 pathologists and 101 clinicians was conducted.[65] The respondents were asked to assign a primary site to a case of STIC with HGSC in the ovary. Fifty-six percent determined that this was a tubal primary, whereas 44% favored ovarian origin. When asked to stage the same case, 45% of respondents determined that this was stage I disease (presumably because they did not consider STIC in the absence of tubal mucosal invasion sufficient to upstage the tumor), whereas 55% considered this to be stage II (ie, a tubal primary with ovarian metastases). In this same survey, the question was posed, "do you think it is important to assign site of origin for extrauterine HGSC given that most are disseminated at presentation and currently assignment of primary site is of limited or no therapeutic or prognostic significance?" to which 51% of pathologists answered "no," whereas, interestingly, 71% of clinicians answered "yes." Although it is true that neither treatment pathways nor prognostic outcomes will be informed by primary site assignment in widely disseminated disease, this should not discourage efforts toward diagnostic accuracy. Our staging protocols and clinical practice should be rigorously evidence-based and, as such, should reflect the overwhelming weight of data identifying the fallopian tube as the primary site in most cases of extrauterine HGSC. Determination of the true incidence of primary tubal disease will, in turn, indicate the extent to which ovary-conserving therapeutic strategies could be used to reduce the incidence, morbidity, and mortality in HGSC; accurate data collection will aid in comparing outcomes in routine practice and clinical trials; and engendering a greater understanding of extrauterine HGSC will facilitate the development of standardized pathology protocols for specimen dissection and reporting. With this in mind, a uniform approach to site assignment has been recommended by the International Collaboration on Cancer Reporting (ICCR),[66] and a prospective study applying these criteria to 53 cases of chemonaive HGSC produced a high level of interobserver concordance (4 of 4 reviewing pathologists agreed on site assignment in 48 (96%) of 50 cases) with 44 (83%) of 53 cases being designated tubal primaries, 9 (17%) of 53 ovarian, and 0 (0%) of 53 primary peritoneal.[50] The proposed site assignment system is summarized in **Table 1**.[67]

Crucially, it is strongly recommended that the ubiquitous practice of referring to extrauterine HGSC as "ovarian" be discontinued, and that the term "tubo-ovarian HGSC" be used in its stead. In this manner, the disease continues to be clearly distinguishable from both uterine serous carcinoma

Table 1
Criteria for assignment of primary site in tubo-ovarian HGSC

Criteria	Primary Site	Comment
STIC present	Fallopian tube	Regardless of presence and size of ovarian and peritoneal disease
Invasive mucosal carcinoma in tube, with or without STIC	Fallopian tube	Regardless of presence and size of ovarian and peritoneal disease
Fallopian tube partially or entirely incorporated into tubo-ovarian mass	Fallopian tube	Regardless of presence and size of ovarian and peritoneal disease
No STIC or invasive mucosal carcinoma in *either* tube in presence of ovarian mass or microscopic ovarian involvement	Ovary	Both tubes should be clearly visible and examined fully by a standardized SEE-FIM protocol regardless of presence and size of peritoneal disease
Both tubes and both ovaries grossly and microscopically normal (when examined entirely) or involved by benign process in presence of peritoneal HGSC	Primary peritoneal HGSC	As recommended in WHO "blue book" 2014; this diagnosis should be made only in specimens removed at primary surgery before any chemotherapy; see below for samples following chemotherapy
HGSC diagnosed on small sample, peritoneal/omental biopsy or cytology	Tubo-ovarian	Note: this should be supported by clinicopathological findings, including immunohistochemistry to exclude mimics, principally uterine serous carcinoma
Postchemotherapy with residual disease	Tubo-ovarian	Chemotherapy alters disease distribution; this can result in different disease categorization following chemotherapy
Postchemotherapy with no residual disease	Tubo-ovarian	

Abbreviations: HGSC, high-grade serous carcinoma; SEE-FIM, sectioning and extensively examining the fimbria; STIC, serous tubal intraepithelial carcinoma.

From Singh N, Gilks CB, Hirshowitz L, et al. Adopting a uniform approach to site assignment in tubo-ovarian high-grade serous carcinoma: the time has come. Int J Gynecol Pathol 2016;35(3):230–7; with permission.

and ovarian low-grade serous carcinoma, whereas the proper acknowledgment is given to its predominant tubal derivation, as well as to its propensity for rapid spread to the ovary and thereby the traditional and longstanding categorization as an ovarian cancer. Admittedly, this issue has very little if any impact on therapeutic decisions, but its importance derives from the fact that this is a paradigm shift, and for it to gain acceptance among the wider community, the burden of responsibility falls entirely on pathologists.

STAGING

In 2013, the FIGO staging systems for ovarian, tubal, and peritoneal cancers were unified.[5] A comparison of the 2003 and 2013 FIGO staging systems for ovarian carcinoma is provided in **Table 2**. In the 2013 FIGO staging, stage IC has been subdivided to reflect the means by which a risk of spread of tumor cells into the abdominal cavity may arise, namely surgical spill (IC1),

presurgical rupture of the capsule (IC2), or the presence of tumor on the surface of the ovary (also IC2) and the presence of tumor cells in cytologic samples from the peritoneal cavity (IC3). FIGO stage IIC has been eliminated, as the outcome after intrapelvic spread (stage IIA/IIB) is not worsened by the presence of tumor cells in cytologic samples from the peritoneal cavity. Stage III, which addresses spread to the extrapelvic peritoneum and lymph node metastasis, has gained additional nuance such that nodal involvement is assigned a lower substage than previously: stage IIIA, formerly applied to cases of "microscopic metastasis beyond the pelvis," is now separated into IIIA1, positive retroperitoneal lymph nodes, either ≤10 mm (IIIA1[i]) or greater than 10 mm (IIIA1[ii]), and IIIA2, microscopic, extrapelvic peritoneal involvement. "Extrapelvic" is defined as above the pelvic brim. Stages IIIB and IIIC are similar in both iterations of the classification, with the exception of the change in the approach to nodal involvement. The new FIGO staging brings clarity to cases

Table 2
A comparison of the 2003 and 2013 International Federation of Gynecology and Obstetrics staging classifications for ovarian cancer (changed criteria or sub stages are in italics)

	2003		**2013**
STAGE I: Tumor confined to ovaries			
IA	Tumor limited to 1 ovary, capsule intact, no tumor on surface, negative washings/ascites	IA	Tumor limited to 1 ovary, capsule intact, no tumor on surface, negative washings
IB	Tumor involves both ovaries otherwise like IA	IB	Tumor involves both ovaries otherwise like IA
IC	Tumor involves 1 or both ovaries with any of the following: capsule rupture, tumor on surface, positive washings/ascites	*IC Tumor limited to 1 or both ovaries* *IC1* *IC2* *IC3*	*Surgical spill* *Capsule rupture before surgery or tumor on ovarian surface* *Malignant cells in the ascites or peritoneal washings*
STAGE II: Tumor involves 1 or both ovaries with pelvic extension (below the pelvic brim) or primary peritoneal cancer			
IIA	Extension and/or implant on uterus and/or Fallopian tubes	IIA	Extension and/or implant on uterus and/or fallopian tubes
IIB	Extension to other pelvic intraperitoneal tissues	IIB	Extension to other pelvic intraperitoneal tissues
IIC	IIA or IIB with positive washings/ascites		
STAGE III: Tumor involves 1 or both ovaries with cytologically or histologically confirmed spread to the peritoneum outside the pelvis and/or metastasis to the retroperitoneal lymph nodes			
IIIA	Microscopic metastasis beyond the pelvis	*IIIA (Positive retroperitoneal lymph nodes and/or microscopic metastasis beyond the pelvis)* *IIIA1* *IIIA1(i)* *IIIA1(ii)* *IIIA2*	 *Positive retroperitoneal lymph nodes only* *Metastasis ≤10 mm* *Metastasis >10 mm* *Microscopic, extrapelvic (above the brim) peritoneal involvement ± positive retroperitoneal lymph nodes*
IIIB	Macroscopic, extrapelvic, peritoneal metastasis ≤2 cm in greatest dimension	IIIB	*Macroscopic, extrapelvic, peritoneal metastasis ≤2 cm ± positive retroperitoneal lymph nodes. Includes extension to capsule of liver/spleen*
IIIC	Macroscopic, extrapelvic, peritoneal metastasis >2 cm in greatest dimension and/or regional lymph node metastasis	IIIC	*Macroscopic, extrapelvic, peritoneal metastasis >2 cm ± positive retroperitoneal lymph nodes. Includes extension to capsule of liver/spleen*
STAGE IV: Distant metastasis excluding peritoneal metastasis			
IV	Distant metastasis excluding peritoneal metastasis. Includes hepatic parenchymal metastasis	IVA IVB	*Pleural effusion with positive cytology* Hepatic and/or splenic parenchymal metastasis, metastasis to extraabdominal organs (including inguinal lymph nodes and lymph nodes outside of the abdominal cavity)

of tumor extension to the liver and spleen. Where extension is purely capsular, the tumor should be staged as either IIIB (≤2 cm) or IIIC (>2 cm). Parenchymal extension, however, is considered true distant metastasis and designated stage IVB (formerly, simply IV). Stage IVA is a new introduction and is assigned to cases of pleural effusion with positive cytology.

The 2013 FIGO staging is clear and without controversy for the vast majority of HGSC cases, as this disease typically presents at advanced stages. There are, however, 2 specific areas that are controversial when the disease is of low volume, as acknowledged in the staging system,[68] namely:

- What is the appropriate stage designation for a case showing tumor limited to 1 ovary (or a peritoneal site) and STIC?
- Bilateral involvement (stage IB), that is, whether these constitute independent contralateral primary tumors or metastases

For the first question, the FIGO Committee has recommended classification as stage IA ovarian carcinoma with STIC, *unless there is evidence of direct extension from the STIC to the ovary*, in which case, it would be stage IIA carcinoma of the fallopian tube. It is not clear what would be the basis for the evidence of direct extension in such cases. With regard to the second scenario, acknowledged to be relatively uncommon, occurring in only 1% to 5% of stage I cases, it was suggested that the distinction should be based on relative sizes of the 2 masses; a large ovarian tumor associated with a contralateral normal-size ovary exhibiting small and superficial foci of tumor, suggests that the latter are metastatic. It is reported that among stage I tumors with bilateral involvement, one-third have this appearance, but no clear guidance is given.

On the basis of the more recent observational and molecular data discussed previously, it is clear that HGSC originates as fimbrial STIC in the vast majority of cases. A study of 7 cases of bilateral involvement, selected specifically for having had complete staging and only 2 disease sites located on opposite adnexa (bilateral tubal, bilateral ovarian, or one tube and opposite ovary, with no other site of disease) showed that the disease foci at both sites harbored identical *TP53* mutations in all cases, indicating their clonal identity and thereby that these represent combinations of a primary and a metastatic site.[69] The survey referred to previously has demonstrated the lack of uniformity in staging such cases.[65] It is therefore recommended for uniformity and to correctly reflect the underlying disease process, that STIC should be classified as a disease site for staging purposes, and that cases of ovarian HGSC with STIC, and no other disease site, should be staged as IIA. Based on the same reasoning, it is recommended that because bilateral adnexal involvement represents metastasis from one side to the other, such cases should be staged as FIGO stage IIA, similar to those showing tubal with ovarian involvement. This approach has been agreed in the 2018 joint consensus meeting on ovarian cancer management of the European Societies of Gynecologic Oncology and Medical Oncology.[38]

SAMPLING OF THE FALLOPIAN TUBE

Central to all of the previously discussed issues on assigning primary site and staging of low-stage disease is the extent and manner of tubal sampling for histologic examination. The detection of STIC requires meticulous sampling of the fimbrial end of the Fallopian tube and the SEE-FIM protocol has proven accuracy in this regard **(Fig. 2)**.[39] It is

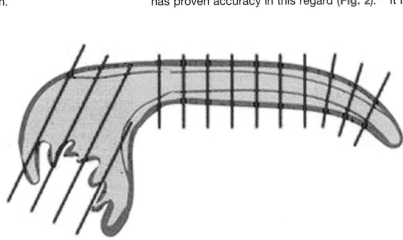

Fig. 2. SEE-FIM protocol for detailed examination of the macroscopically normal fallopian tube in familial and sporadic cases of HGSC. The fimbrial end, comprising the distal 1.5 cm or so, is separated from the rest of the length of the tube and is sliced longitudinally in 4 or more slices. The rest of the tube is sliced in transverse slices. All of the tissue is processed and examined histologically.

important that this protocol is followed in all cases in which this would impact on disease detection/categorization, that is, all risk-reducing salpingo-oophorectomy specimens and all cases of HGSC with macroscopically normal tubes. It is unnecessary to carry this out in all opportunistic salpingectomies except in women at high risk of HGSC, as the yield of clinically relevant disease in such cases is very low.[70] In current practice, a routine sampling section is now often taken from the fimbrial end of the tube rather than the mid portion. The chances of finding STIC increase with the number of levels examined,[71,72] but this should be at the discretion of the pathologist and the clinical relevance. All cases of STIC should be diagnosed using robust morphologic criteria, with the use of adjunct immunohistochemistry for p53 and Ki67 in difficult cases.[44,73] Lesions falling short of a diagnosis of STIC should not be included in the pathology report, or, if included, should be accompanied by a comment on their uncertain significance with regard to clinical management.

PATHOLOGY OF HIGH-GRADE SEROUS CARCINOMA IN THE POST-NEOADJUVANT CHEMOTHERAPY SETTING: MORPHOLOGY AND IMMUNOHISTOCHEMISTRY AFTER CHEMOTHERAPY

The 2 key immunohistochemical markers for tubo-ovarian HGSC are WT1 and p53. Wilms tumor 1 (WT1) is expressed in cells of serous origin. The frequency of WT1 positivity (nuclear staining) in tubo-ovarian HGSC is approximately 97%.[3] p53 is the protein product of the tumor suppressor gene TP53. Mutations in TP53 are early tumorigenetic events in HGSC[56] and, in 95% of cases, the presence of a mutation is reflected in the pattern p53 immunohistochemical staining.[74] In normal tissue, the p53 protein is present in dividing cells and the expression pattern is one of variable nuclear intensity and distribution. The abnormal/mutation-type patterns are as follows: (1) uniform, diffuse, and strong nuclear expression in more than 80% of tumor cell nuclei; (2) complete absence of expression, with the internal control retained; or (3) prominent cytoplasmic expression.[74] The utility of p53 immunohistochemistry is therefore as a surrogate for TP53 mutation status; in addition the pattern may also indicate the nature of the underlying mutation (**Table 3**).[74,75] The strength of combining WT1 and p53 in a diagnostic panel is that nuclear positivity of the former alongside mutant expression of the latter is 99% specific for tubo-ovarian HGSC[3] (though, notably, high-grade uterine serous carcinoma also may show this combination of staining in a minority of cases).[76]

The traditional approach to the treatment of tubo-ovarian HGSC has been surgery followed by adjuvant platinum-based chemotherapy. More recently, however, there has been a shift toward the use of NACT, the aim being to reduce disease volume before surgical intervention.[77,78] NACT has

Table 3
p53 immunohistochemistry (IHC) pattern and interpretation with correlation to TP53 mutation type

Pattern	p53 IHC Interpretation	TP53 Mutation Type	% in HGSC
TP53 mutation absent			
Wild-type	Normal	No mutation	0
TP53 mutation present			
Overexpression	Abnormal	Nonsynonymous (missense); also inframe deletion, splicing	66
Complete absence/null	Abnormal	Indels, stopgains, splicing mutations	25
Cytoplasmic	Abnormal	Indels and stopgains with disruption of the nuclear localization domain	4
Wild-type	Normal[a]	Truncating mutation	5

Abbreviation: HGSC, high-grade serous carcinoma.
[a] Exception from normal: truncating mutations can be associated with a wild-type pattern.
Adapted from Kobel M, Piskorz AM, Lee S, et al. Optimized p53 immunohistochemistry is an accurate predictor of TP53 mutation in ovarian carcinoma. J Pathol Clin Res 2016;2(4): 247–58; and Kobel MM, McCluggage WG, Gilks CB, et al. Interpretation of p53 immunohistochemistry in tubo-ovarian carcinoma: guidelines for reporting interpretation of p53 immunohistochemistry in tubo-ovarian carcinoma: guidelines for reporting. Online resource. 2016. Available at: http://www.thebagp.org/resources, with permission.

been shown to improve rates of optimal debulking, including debulking to no residual disease, and to reduce surgical morbidity and mortality.[79,80] However, it has been shown that exposure to chemotherapeutic agents alters the morphology of ovarian carcinomas, with treated tumors demonstrating enlarged nuclei, a reduced nuclear-cytoplasmic ratio, eosinophilia, bizarre nuclear outlines, and nuclear chromatin smudging/clumping.[81] These changes can confound attempts at histologic tumor typing and, for this reason, it is advised that a pretreatment tissue biopsy be obtained for histotype classification. Although post-treatment hematoxylin-eosin (H&E) diagnosis may be difficult, a recent study has shown that the immunohistochemical expression of p53 and WT1 remain largely concordant before and after chemotherapy, thus underscoring their reliability as diagnostic markers. Paired prechemotherapy and postchemotherapy omental biopsies were stained with p53 (57 pairs) and WT1 (58 pairs). Immunohistochemistry results for p53 were concordant in 55 (96%) of 57 and for WT1 in 56 (97%) of 58 cases. It was, however, noted that there was significant diminution of WT1 staining intensity in the postchemotherapy samples.[82]

ASSESSMENT OF RESPONSE TO NEOADJUVANT CHEMOTHERAPY IN HIGH-GRADE SEROUS CARCINOMA

In 2015, Böhm and colleagues[83] published a scoring system to report the histologic response to NACT in interval debulking specimens. Before this, the question had been addressed by many studies,[84–88] but with each using different criteria and case selection. Although all of these showed that some histologic parameters correlated with outcome, no system was independently validated. As HGSC typically involves multiple sites within the abdomen, Böhm and colleagues[83] aimed to identify which tissue would be the best for reporting chemotherapy changes and whether the morphologic changes in tumor cells, the extent of regressive changes, or the amount of residual tumor would be the most informative. Most important of all, they wanted to see first whether these changes could be reported reproducibly between pathologists using a relatively simple numerical scoring system, and second, whether these would serve to reflect clinical outcomes, namely progression-free survival (PFS) and overall survival (OS), and thereby be worthy of incorporating into routine clinical practice. The chemotherapy response score (CRS) was devised on a test cohort of patients, and its reproducibility and

Table 4
The chemotherapy response score: a summary of criteria

CRS Score	Criteria
CRS 1: No or minimal tumor response	Mainly viable tumor with no or minimal regression-associated fibroinflammatory changes[a] limited to a few foci Note: cases in which it is difficult to decide between regression and tumor-associated desmoplasia or inflammatory cell infiltration
CRS 2: Partial response	Appreciable tumor response amidst viable tumor, both readily identifiable and tumor regularly distributed Note: cases ranging from multifocal or diffuse regression-associated fibroinflammatory changes,[a] with viable tumor in sheets, streaks, or nodules, to extensive regression-associated fibroinflammatory changes[a] with multifocal residual tumor that is easily identifiable
CRS 3: Total or near-total response	No residual tumor OR minimal irregularly scattered tumor foci seen as individual cells, cell groups, or nodules up to 2 mm in maximum size Note: cases showing mainly regression-associated fibroinflammatory changes[a] or, in rare cases, no/very little residual tumor in the complete absence of any inflammatory response; advisable to record whether "no residual tumor" or "microscopic residual tumor present"

Abbreviation: CRS, chemotherapy response score.
[a] Regression-associated fibroinflammatory changes: fibrosis associated with macrophages, including foam cells, mixed inflammatory cells, and psammoma bodies; to distinguish from tumor-related inflammation or desmoplasia.
Adapted from Böhm S, Faruqi A, Said I, et al. Chemotherapy response score: development and validation of a system to quantify histopathologic response to neoadjuvant chemotherapy in tubo-ovarian high-grade serous carcinoma. J Clin Oncol 2015;33(22): 2457–63; Said I, Böhm S, Beasley J, et al. The chemotherapy response score (CRS): interobserver reproducibility in a simple and prognostically relevant system for reporting the histologic response to neoadjuvant chemotherapy in tuboovarian high-grade serous carcinoma. Int J Gynecol Pathol 2017;36(2):172–9; with permission.

prognostic relevance were validated in a completely separate validation cohort, both incorporated in the original report.

Since its publication, the CRS system has been independently validated by multiple studies for its reproducibility[89] and prognostic value[90–93]; separately its correlation with tumor immune response has been demonstrated,[94] with exciting potential for patient selection for immune therapies. The 3-part score is used to assess the routinely processed omental section with the maximum amount of tumor (Table 4). This reliably and reproducibly identifies patients with a total or near-total response to NACT (CRS3), who show significantly better PFS and OS than those with CRS1/CRS2. A recent international collaborative multicentre analysis of pooled individual patient data in more than 900 cases has validated these results, demonstrating CRS to predict outcome independently of age, stage, and debulking status, CRS3 thereby serving as a surrogate for platinum sensitivity and survival. This study has additionally shown CRS3 to correlate with germline *BRCA* mutation status and likelihood of complete surgical resection.[95] What this larger analysis has also demonstrated is that the prognostic difference between CRS1 and CRS2, as currently defined, is not statistically significant; separation of different prognostic categories within this group of patients who show less than a near-total/total response to conventional platinum-based chemotherapy is an area that would benefit from further research. CRS has been incorporated into pathology reporting and clinical guidelines for objective and reproducible reporting,[66,96] with potential to inform therapeutic decision-making as well as being a useful trial end-point. An online training module has been set up to enable pathologists to familiarize and test themselves with the system before incorporating this into their own practice (http://www.bccancer.bc.ca/health-professionals/professional-resources/cancer-management-guidelines/gynecology/ovary-epithelial-carcinoma).[83]

SUMMARY

The diagnosis of HGSC has been shown to be accurate and reproducible using morphologic criteria and immunohistochemistry, but in some areas of disease categorization there remains disagreement. The wider acceptance of the paradigm that most extrauterine HGSC arises in the fallopian tube is dependent on pathologists, as this requires correct handling of the tube as well as uniform categorization of primary site using an evidence-based classification. As the incidence of presentation at low stages increases as a result of opportunistic salpingectomy and through

strategies for earlier detection, it is imperative that such cases are uniformly staged without individual variation. Finally, the objective and reproducible pathologic reporting of treatment response is an urgent need as new treatment protocols emerge.

REFERENCES

1. Kurman RJ, Carcangiu ML, Herrington CS, Young RH, editors. WHO classification of tumors of the female reproductive organs. 4th edition. Lyon (France): International Agency for Research on Cancer (IARC); 2014.
2. Kommoss SG CB, du Bois A, Kommoss F. Ovarian carcinoma diagnosis: the clinical impact of 15 years of change. Br J Cancer 2016;115(8):993–9.
3. Kobel M, Rahimi K, Rambau PF, et al. An immunohistochemical algorithm for ovarian carcinoma typing. Int J Gynecol Pathol 2016;35(5):430–41.
4. Mackenzie R, Talhouk A, Eshragh S, et al. Morphologic and molecular characteristics of mixed epithelial ovarian cancers. Am J Surg Pathol 2015;39(11):1548–57.
5. Prat J, FIGO Committee on Gynecologic Oncology. Staging classification for cancer of the ovary, fallopian tube, and peritoneum. Int J Gynaecol Obstet 2014;124(1):1–5.
6. Auersperg N, Wong AS, Choi KC, et al. Ovarian surface epithelium: biology, endocrinology, and pathology. Endocr Rev 2001;22(2):255–88.
7. Maines-Bandiera S, Woo MM, Borugian M, et al. Oviductal glycoprotein (OVGP1, MUC9): a differentiation-based mucin present in serum of women with ovarian cancer. Int J Gynecol Cancer 2010;20(1):16–22.
8. Scully RE. Early de novo ovarian cancer and cancer developing in benign ovarian lesions. Int J Gynaecol Obstet 1995;49(Suppl):S9–15.
9. Pothuri B, Leitao MM, Levine DA, et al. Genetic analysis of the early natural history of epithelial ovarian carcinoma. PLoS One 2010;5(4):e10358.
10. Orsulic S, Li Y, Soslow RA, et al. Induction of ovarian cancer by defined multiple genetic changes in a mouse model system. Cancer Cell 2002;1(1):53–62.
11. Connolly DC, Bao R, Nikitin AY, et al. Female mice chimeric for expression of the simian virus 40 TAg under control of the MISIIR promoter develop epithelial ovarian cancer. Cancer Res 2003;63(6):1389–97.
12. Flesken-Nikitin A, Choi KC, Eng JP, et al. Induction of carcinogenesis by concurrent inactivation of p53 and Rb1 in the mouse ovarian surface epithelium. Cancer Res 2003;63(13):3459–63.
13. Craig E, Clarke R, Rushton G, et al. Serous tubal intraepithelial carcinoma (STIC)-like lesions arising in

ovarian serous cystadenofibroma: report of 2 cases. Int J Gynecol Pathol 2015;34(6):535–40.

14. Soong TR, Howitt BE, Miron A, et al. Evidence for lineage continuity between early serous proliferations (ESPs) in the Fallopian tube and disseminated high-grade serous carcinomas. J Pathol 2018; 246(3):344–51.

15. Kurman RJ. Origin and molecular pathogenesis of ovarian high-grade serous carcinoma. Ann Oncol 2013;24(Suppl 10):x16–21.

16. Song Z. Ovarian enzymatically active stromal cells can be a promoter of ovarian surface epithelial tumor. Med Hypotheses 2011;77(3):356–8.

17. Holtz F, Hart WR. Krukenberg tumors of the ovary: a clinicopathologic analysis of 27 cases. Cancer 1982;50(11):2438–47.

18. Young RH, Gilks CB, Scully RE. Mucinous tumors of the appendix associated with mucinous tumors of the ovary and pseudomyxoma peritonei. A clinicopathological analysis of 22 cases supporting an origin in the appendix. Am J Surg Pathol 1991; 15(5):415–29.

19. Elishaev E, Gilks CB, Miller D, et al. Synchronous and metachronous endocervical and ovarian neoplasms: evidence supporting interpretation of the ovarian neoplasms as metastatic endocervical adenocarcinomas simulating primary ovarian surface epithelial neoplasms. Am J Surg Pathol 2005;29(3): 281–94.

20. Bloss JD, Liao SY, Buller RE, et al. Extraovarian peritoneal serous papillary carcinoma: a case-control retrospective comparison to papillary adenocarcinoma of the ovary. Gynecol Oncol 1993;50(3): 347–51.

21. Auersperg N. Ovarian surface epithelium as a source of ovarian cancers: unwarranted speculation or evidence-based hypothesis? Gynecol Oncol 2013;130(1):246–51.

22. Lauchlan SC. The secondary Mullerian system. Obstet Gynecol Surv 1972;27(3):133–46.

23. Lauchlan SC. The secondary Mullerian system revisited. Int J Gynecol Pathol 1994;13(1):73–9.

24. Bannatyne P, Russell P. Early adenocarcinoma of the fallopian tubes. A case for multifocal tumorigenesis. Diagn Gynecol Obstet 1981;3(1):49–60.

25. Halme J, Hammond MG, Hulka JF, et al. Retrograde menstruation in healthy women and in patients with endometriosis. Obstet Gynecol 1984; 64(2):151–4.

26. Liu DT, Hitchcock A. Endometriosis: its association with retrograde menstruation, dysmenorrhoea and tubal pathology. Br J Obstet Gynaecol 1986;93(8): 859–62.

27. Anglesio MS, Bashashati A, Wang YK, et al. Multifocal endometriotic lesions associated with cancer are clonal and carry a high mutation burden. J Pathol 2015;236(2):201–9.

28. Swerdlow M. Mesothelioma of the pelvic peritoneum resembling papillary cystadenocarcinoma of the ovary; case report. Am J Obstet Gynecol 1959; 77(1):197–200.

29. Fromm GL, Gershenson DM, Silva EG. Papillary serous carcinoma of the peritoneum. Obstet Gynecol 1990;75(1):89–95.

30. Foyle A, Al-Jabi M, McCaughey WT. Papillary peritoneal tumors in women. Am J Surg Pathol 1981;5(3): 241–9.

31. Dalrymple JC, Bannatyne P, Russell P, et al. Extraovarian peritoneal serous papillary carcinoma. A clinicopathologic study of 31 cases. Cancer 1989;64(1): 110–5.

32. Tobacman JK, Greene MH, Tucker MA, et al. Intraabdominal carcinomatosis after prophylactic oophorectomy in ovarian-cancer-prone families. Lancet 1982;2(8302):795–7.

33. Lynch HT, Bewtra C, Lynch JF. Familial peritoneal ovarian carcinomatosis: a new clinical entity? Med Hypotheses 1986;21(2):171–7.

34. Casey MJ, Synder C, Bewtra C, et al. Intra-abdominal carcinomatosis after prophylactic oophorectomy in women of hereditary breast ovarian cancer syndrome kindreds associated with BRCA1 and BRCA2 mutations. Gynecol Oncol 2005;97(2): 457–67.

35. Castellarin M, Milne K, Zeng T, et al. Clonal evolution of high-grade serous ovarian carcinoma from primary to recurrent disease. J Pathol 2013;229(4):515–24.

36. Anglesio MS, O'Neill CJ, Senz J, et al. Identical TP53 mutations provide evidence that late-recurring tuboovarian high-grade serous carcinomas do not represent new peritoneal primaries. Histopathology 2017; 71(6):1014–7.

37. Seidman JD, Zhao P, Yemelyanova A. "Primary peritoneal" high-grade serous carcinoma is very likely metastatic from serous tubal intraepithelial carcinoma: assessing the new paradigm of ovarian and pelvic serous carcinogenesis and its implications for screening for ovarian cancer. Gynecol Oncol 2011;120(3):470–3.

38. Colombo N, Sessa C, du Bois A, et al. ESMO-ESGO Consensus Recommendations on Ovarian Cancer: Pathology and Molecular Biology, Early and Advanced stages, Borderline Tumours and Recurrent Disease. Annals of Oncology 2019, in press.

39. Medeiros F, Muto MG, Lee Y, et al. The tubal fimbria is a preferred site for early adenocarcinoma in women with familial ovarian cancer syndrome. Am J Surg Pathol 2006;30(2):230–6.

40. Kindelberger DW, Lee Y, Miron A, et al. Intraepithelial carcinoma of the fimbria and pelvic serous carcinoma: evidence for a causal relationship. Am J Surg Pathol 2007;31(2):161–9.

41. Przybycin CG, Kurman RJ, Ronnett BM, et al. Are all pelvic (nonuterine) serous carcinomas of

tubal origin? Am J Surg Pathol 2010;34(10): 1407–16.

42. Lee Y, Miron A, Drapkin R, et al. A candidate precursor to serous carcinoma that originates in the distal fallopian tube. J Pathol 2007;211(1):26–35.

43. Piek JM, van Diest PJ, Zweemer RP, et al. Dysplastic changes in prophylactically removed Fallopian tubes of women predisposed to developing ovarian cancer. J Pathol 2001;195(4):451–6.

44. Visvanathan K, Vang R, Shaw P, et al. Diagnosis of serous tubal intraepithelial carcinoma based on morphologic and immunohistochemical features: a reproducibility study. Am J Surg Pathol 2011; 35(12):1766–75.

45. Gross AL, Kurman RJ, Vang R, et al. Precursor lesions of high-grade serous ovarian carcinoma: morphological and molecular characteristics. J Oncol 2010;2010:126295.

46. Carcangiu ML, Peissel B, Pasini B, et al. Incidental carcinomas in prophylactic specimens in BRCA1 and BRCA2 germ-line mutation carriers, with emphasis on fallopian tube lesions: report of 6 cases and review of the literature. Am J Surg Pathol 2006; 30(10):1222–30.

47. Crum CP, Herfs M, Ning G, et al. Through the glass darkly: intraepithelial neoplasia, top-down differentiation, and the road to ovarian cancer. J Pathol 2013; 231(4):402–12.

48. George SH, Shaw P. BRCA and early events in the development of serous ovarian cancer. Front Oncol 2014;4:5.

49. Chen F, Gaitskell K, Garcia MJ, et al. Serous tubal intraepithelial carcinomas associated with high-grade serous ovarian carcinomas: a systematic review. BJOG 2017;124(6):872–8.

50. Singh N, Gilks CB, Wilkinson N, et al. Assessment of a new system for primary site assignment in high-grade serous carcinoma of the fallopian tube, ovary, and peritoneum. Histopathology 2015;67(3):331–7.

51. Gilks CB, Irving J, Kobel M, et al. Incidental nonuterine high-grade serous carcinomas arise in the fallopian tube in most cases: further evidence for the tubal origin of high-grade serous carcinomas. Am J Surg Pathol 2015;39(3):357–64.

52. Morrison JC, Blanco LZ Jr, Vang R, et al. Incidental serous tubal intraepithelial carcinoma and early invasive serous carcinoma in the nonprophylactic setting: analysis of a case series. Am J Surg Pathol 2015;39(4):442–53.

53. Semmel DR, Folkins AK, Hirsch MS, et al. Intercepting early pelvic serous carcinoma by routine pathological examination of the fimbria. Mod Pathol 2009; 22(8):985–8.

54. Rabban JT, Garg K, Crawford B, et al. Early detection of high-grade tubal serous carcinoma in women at low risk for hereditary breast and ovarian cancer

syndrome by systematic examination of fallopian tubes incidentally removed during benign surgery. Am J Surg Pathol 2014;38(6):729–42.

55. Cole AJ, Dwight T, Gill AJ, et al. Assessing mutant p53 in primary high-grade serous ovarian cancer using immunohistochemistry and massively parallel sequencing. Sci Rep 2016;6:26191.

56. Ahmed AA, Etemadmoghadam D, Temple J, et al. Driver mutations in TP53 are ubiquitous in high grade serous carcinoma of the ovary. J Pathol 2010;221(1):49–56.

57. Kuhn E, Kurman RJ, Vang R, et al. TP53 mutations in serous tubal intraepithelial carcinoma and concurrent pelvic high-grade serous carcinoma–evidence supporting the clonal relationship of the two lesions. J Pathol 2012;226(3):421–6.

58. McDaniel AS, Stall JN, Hovelson DH, et al. Next-generation sequencing of tubal intraepithelial carcinomas. JAMA Oncol 2015;1(8):1128–32.

59. Meserve EE, Strickland KC, Miron A, et al. Evidence of a monoclonal origin for bilateral serous tubal intraepithelial neoplasia. Int J Gynecol Pathol 2018, [Epub ahead of print].

60. Kuhn E, Meeker A, Wang TL, et al. Shortened telomeres in serous tubal intraepithelial carcinoma: an early event in ovarian high-grade serous carcinogenesis. Am J Surg Pathol 2010;34(6):829–36.

61. Bashashati A, Ha G, Tone A, et al. Distinct evolutionary trajectories of primary high-grade serous ovarian cancers revealed through spatial mutational profiling. J Pathol 2013;231(1):21–34.

62. Eckert MA, Pan S, Hernandez KM, et al. Genomics of ovarian cancer progression reveals diverse metastatic trajectories including intraepithelial metastasis to the fallopian tube. Cancer Discov 2016;6(12): 1342–51.

63. Labidi-Galy SI, Papp E, Hallberg D, et al. High grade serous ovarian carcinomas originate in the fallopian tube. Nat Commun 2017;8(1):1093.

64. Kuhn E, Wang TL, Doberstein K, et al. CCNE1 amplification and centrosome number abnormality in serous tubal intraepithelial carcinoma: further evidence supporting its role as a precursor of ovarian high-grade serous carcinoma. Mod Pathol 2016;29(10):1254–61.

65. McCluggage WG, Hirschowitz L, Gilks CB, et al. The fallopian tube origin and primary site assignment in extrauterine high-grade serous carcinoma: findings of a survey of pathologists and clinicians. Int J Gynecol Pathol 2017;36(3):230–9.

66. McCluggage WG, Judge MJ, Clarke BA, et al. Data set for reporting of ovary, fallopian tube and primary peritoneal carcinoma: recommendations from the International Collaboration on Cancer Reporting (ICCR). Mod Pathol 2015;28(8):1101–22.

67. Singh N, Gilks CB, Hirshowitz L, et al. Adopting a uniform approach to site assignment in tubo-

ovarian high-grade serous carcinoma: the time has come. Int J Gynecol Pathol 2016;35(3):230–7.

68. Prat J. Ovarian, fallopian tube and peritoneal cancer staging: rationale and explanation of new FIGO staging 2013. Best Pract Res Clin Obstet Gynaecol 2015;29(6):858–69.

69. Singh N, Faruqi A, Kommoss F, et al. Extrauterine high-grade serous carcinomas with bilateral adnexal involvement as the only two disease sites are clonal based on tp53 sequencing results: implications for biology, classification, and staging. Mod Pathol 2018;31(4):652–9.

70. Meserve EEK, Mirkovic J, Conner JR, et al. Frequency of "incidental" serous tubal intraepithelial carcinoma (STIC) in women without a history of or genetic risk factor for high-grade serous carcinoma: a six-year study. Gynecol Oncol 2017; 146(1):69–73.

71. Mahe E, Tang S, Deb P, et al. Do deeper sections increase the frequency of detection of serous tubal intraepithelial carcinoma (STIC) in the "sectioning and extensively examining the FIMbriated end" (SEE-FIM) protocol? Int J Gynecol Pathol 2013;32(4): 353–7.

72. Singh N, Benson JL, Gan C, et al. Disease distribution in low-stage tubo-ovarian high-grade serous carcinoma (HGSC): implications for assigning primary site and FIGO stage. Int J Gynecol Pathol 2018;37(4):324–30.

73. Carlson JW, Jarboe EA, Kindelberger D, et al. Serous tubal intraepithelial carcinoma: diagnostic reproducibility and its implications. Int J Gynecol Pathol 2010;29(4):310–4.

74. Kobel M, Piskorz AM, Lee S, et al. Optimized p53 immunohistochemistry is an accurate predictor of TP53 mutation in ovarian carcinoma. J Pathol Clin Res 2016;2(4):247–58.

75. Kobel MM, McCluggage WG, Gilks CB, et al. Interpretation of p53 immunohistochemistry in tubo-ovarian carcinoma: guidelines for reporting interpretation of p53 immunohistochemistry in tubo-ovarian carcinoma: guidelines for reporting. Online resource. 2016. Available at: http://www.thebagp. org/resources. Accessed August 31, 2018.

76. Chen W, Husain A, Nelson GS, et al. Immunohistochemical profiling of endometrial serous carcinoma. Int J Gynecol Pathol 2017;36(2):128–39.

77. Ledermann JA, Raja FA, Fotopoulou C, et al. Newly diagnosed and relapsed epithelial ovarian carcinoma: ESMO Clinical Practice Guidelines for diagnosis, treatment and follow-up. Ann Oncol 2013; 24(Suppl 6):vi24–32.

78. Vergote I, Trope CG, Amant F, et al. Neoadjuvant chemotherapy or primary surgery in stage IIIC or IV ovarian cancer. N Engl J Med 2010;363(10):943–53.

79. Gill SE, McGree ME, Weaver AL, et al. Optimizing the treatment of ovarian cancer: neoadjuvant

chemotherapy and interval debulking versus primary debulking surgery for epithelial ovarian cancers likely to have suboptimal resection. Gynecol Oncol 2017;144(2):266–73.

80. Kehoe S, Hook J, Nankivell M, et al. Primary chemotherapy versus primary surgery for newly diagnosed advanced ovarian cancer (CHORUS): an open-label, randomised, controlled, non-inferiority trial. Lancet 2015;386(9990):249–57.

81. McCluggage WG, Lyness RW, Atkinson RJ, et al. Morphological effects of chemotherapy on ovarian carcinoma. J Clin Pathol 2002;55(1):27–31.

82. Casey L, Kobel M, Ganesan R, et al. A comparison of p53 and WT1 immunohistochemical expression patterns in tubo-ovarian high-grade serous carcinoma before and after neoadjuvant chemotherapy. Histopathology 2017;71(5):736–42.

83. Böhm S, Faruqi A, Said I, et al. Chemotherapy response score: development and validation of a system to quantify histopathologic response to neoadjuvant chemotherapy in tubo-ovarian high-grade serous carcinoma. J Clin Oncol 2015;33(22): 2457–63.

84. Sassen S, Schmalfeldt B, Avril N, et al. Histopathologic assessment of tumor regression after neoadjuvant chemotherapy in advanced-stage ovarian cancer. Hum Pathol 2007;38(6):926–34.

85. Le T, Williams K, Senterman M, et al. Histopathologic assessment of chemotherapy effects in epithelial ovarian cancer patients treated with neoadjuvant chemotherapy and delayed primary surgical debulking. Gynecol Oncol 2007;106(1): 160–3.

86. Le T, Williams K, Senterman M, et al. Omental chemotherapy effects as a prognostic factor in ovarian cancer patients treated with neoadjuvant chemotherapy and delayed primary surgical debulking. Ann Surg Oncol 2007;14(9):2649–53.

87. Muraji M, Sudo T, Iwasaki S, et al. Histopathology predicts clinical outcome in advanced epithelial ovarian cancer patients treated with neoadjuvant chemotherapy and debulking surgery. Gynecol Oncol 2013;131(3):531–4.

88. Petrillo M, Zannoni GF, Tortorella L, et al. Prognostic role and predictors of complete pathologic response to neoadjuvant chemotherapy in primary unresectable ovarian cancer. Am J Obstet Gynecol 2014; 211(6):632 e1–8.

89. Said I, Bohm S, Beasley J, et al. The chemotherapy response score (CRS): interobserver reproducibility in a simple and prognostically relevant system for reporting the histologic response to neoadjuvant chemotherapy in tuboovarian high-grade serous carcinoma. Int J Gynecol Pathol 2017;36(2):172–9.

90. Coghlan E, Meniawy TM, Munro A, et al. Prognostic role of histological tumor regression in patients

receiving neoadjuvant chemotherapy for high-grade serous tubo-ovarian carcinoma. Int J Gynecol Cancer 2017;27(4):708–13.

91. Singh P, Kaushal V, Rai B, et al. The chemotherapy response score is a useful histological predictor of prognosis in high-grade serous carcinoma. Histopathology 2018;72(4):619–25.

92. Ditzel HM, Strickland KC, Meserve EE, et al. Assessment of a chemotherapy response score (CRS) system for tubo-ovarian high-grade serous carcinoma (HGSC). Int J Gynecol Pathol 2018, [Epub ahead of print].

93. Lee JY, Chung YS, Na K, et al. External validation of chemotherapy response score system for histopathological assessment of tumor regression after neoadjuvant chemotherapy in tubo-ovarian high-grade serous carcinoma. J Gynecol Oncol 2017;28(6):e73.

94. Bohm S, Montfort A, Pearce OM, et al. Neoadjuvant chemotherapy modulates the immune microenvironment in metastases of tubo-ovarian high-grade serous carcinoma. Clin Cancer Res 2016;22(12): 3025–36.

95. Cohen P, Böhm S, Powell A, et al. Pathological chemotherapy response score predicts survival in patients with advanced ovarian cancer receiving neoadjuvant chemotherapy: an individual patient meta-analysis. Int J Gynecol Cancer 2018; 28(supp2):14.

96. Movahedi-Lankarani S, Krishnamurti U, Bell DA, et al. Protocol for the Examination of Specimens From Patients With Primary Tumors of the Ovary, Fallopian Tube, or Peritoneum. College of American Pathologists. Protocol Posting Date: August 2018. Version: OvaryFallopian 1.1.0.0. Accessed February 27, 2019.

Pathology of Endometrioid and Clear Cell Carcinoma of the Ovary

Oluwole Fadare, MD[a,*], Vinita Parkash, MD[b]

KEYWORDS

- Ovary • Endometrioid carcinoma • Clear cell carcinoma • Endometriosis • Borderline tumor
- Adenofibroma • ARID1A

Key points

- Endometrioid adenocarcinoma and clear cell carcinoma are two histotypes of ovarian carcinoma that are related by their shared association with endometriosis and, accordingly, a possibly shared histogenesis and pathogenesis.

- Both tumors tend to present at an early stage, especially when associated with endometriosis. They also show an association with Lynch syndrome, often accompanied by synchronous endometrial carcinoma.

- Both tumors show multiple histologic patterns and therefore have a wide range of differential diagnoses, including a variety of epithelial, sex cord stromal, and germ cell tumors.

- Morphology and differential expression of immunohistochemical markers aids in distinguishing these tumors from each other and from other potential mimics.

ABSTRACT

This review is an appraisal of the current state of knowledge of 2 enigmatic histotypes of ovarian carcinoma: endometrioid and clear cell carcinoma. Both show an association endometriosis and the hereditary nonpolyposis colorectal cancer (Lynch) syndrome, and both typically present at an early stage. Pathologic and immunohistochemical features that distinguish these tumors from high-grade serous carcinomas, each other, and other potential mimics are discussed, as are staging, grading, and molecular pathogenesis.

OVERVIEW

Dr John A. Sampson,[1] an Albany gynecologist, is generally credited with the seminal description of endometrioid carcinoma of the ovary (OEC). In his expansive 1925 report, he described several examples of endometrial carcinoma of the ovary that were frequently associated with endometriosis, and that closely resembled the most common carcinoma of the uterine corpus, now recognized as endometrioid carcinoma of the endometrium.[1] Additional cases of OEC were described primarily in isolated case reports or small case series for the next few decades,[2] which was likely a function of the stringent criteria for malignant transformation of endometriosis that were originally outlined by Sampson.[1] However, reports from Thompson[2] in 1957 and Long and Taylor[3] in 1964 firmly established that endometriosis may undergo malignant transformation and that such tumors represent a significant subset of ovarian carcinomas. The tumor that is currently classified as clear cell carcinoma of the ovary (CCC) was most likely originally

---

Disclosures: None.
[a] Department of Pathology, University of California San Diego, San Diego, CA, USA; [b] Department of Pathology, Yale School of Medicine, 20 York Street, EP2-607, New Haven, CT 06510, USA
* Corresponding author. Department of Pathology, Anatomic Pathology Division, University of California San Diego Health, 9300 Campus Point Drive, Suite 1-200, MC 7723, La Jolla, CA 92037.
E-mail address: oluwole.fadare@gmail.com

Surgical Pathology 12 (2019) 529–564
https://doi.org/10.1016/j.path.2019.01.009
1875-9181/19/© 2019 Elsevier Inc. All rights reserved.

described in 1899 by Peham[4] as "hypernephroma of the ovary," based on the striking similarity of the reported case to clear cell renal cell carcinoma. Saphir and Lackner[5] described 2 additional cases in 1944 and applied the term adenocarcinoma with clear cells. In 1939, Dr Walter Schiller[6] described and proposed the name mesonephroma ovarii for a group of ovarian tumors that showed glomeruluslike bodies and microcysts into which small papillae project. Numerous cases were subsequently reported that most likely represent a heterogeneous mix of histotypes by currently applicable diagnostic criteria, mostly as mesonephric carcinoma, mesonephroma, or mesonephric clear cell carcinoma.[7–10] In 1959, Dr Gunter Teilum[11] noted that at least a subset of the cases previously classified by as mesonephroma ovarii resembled extraembryonic (yolk sac–allantoic) structures of the rat's placenta, and as such are better classified as tumors of endodermal sinus derivation. That proposal quickly gained acceptance and helped to establish yolk sac tumor of the ovary as a definitive clinicopathologic entity.[12] For the other subset of mesonephric ovarii (ie, tumors other than yolk sac tumor), Scully and Barlow[13] noted in 1960 that "evidence of mesonephric origin or direction of differentiation" is inconclusive, and that the "term *mesonephroma* is unwarranted for almost all the neoplasms to which it has been applied."[13] Scully and Barlow's[13] seminal report was also significant as the first to (1) detail a strong association between endometriosis and CCC, (2) note their frequent admixture with EEC, and (3) introduce the term CCC for these tumors.[13] In 1973, CCC was included in the World Health Organization (WHO) classification of ovarian tumors,[14] a reflection of the strong consensus that had emerged that CCC is a tumor of mullerian derivation with distinctive clinicopathologic features. This article details the pathologic attributes of OEC and CCC, with an emphasis on diagnostic aspects.

ASSOCIATION WITH ENDOMETRIOSIS

Endometriosis (the existence of morphologically normal endometrial tissues outside of the uterine corpus) is a common disease that affects up to 10% of reproductive-aged women. In the narrower population of patients with ovarian cancer, the prevalence of endometriosis has varied by geographic region, but has reportedly been between 3% and 15%.[15–19] In one meta-analysis of 15 studies that described more than 2500 patients, the prevalence of endometriosis in ovarian

carcinoma was strongly histotype dependent: 3.3% in serous carcinoma, 3.0% in mucinous carcinoma, 39.2% in CCC, and 21.2% in OEC.[20] Although these figures are highly dependent on how the ovarian cancer/endometriosis association is defined, approximately similar findings were found in another analysis wherein this association was simply defined as endometriosis in the same adnexal organ that is harboring a carcinoma.[21] The frequency of endometriosis-associated OEC is much higher than endometriosis-associated CCC in Western countries compared with Japan and nearby countries, reflecting the differences in prevalence of these histotypes in these two regions of the world.[20] Regarding the risk of malignancy in patients with endometriosis, Brinton and colleagues[22] performed a cohort study of 20,686 women with a hospital discharge diagnosis of endometriosis and who had substantial follow-up. The overall ovarian cancer risk was found to be increased (relative risk, 1.92; 95% confidence interval [CI], 1.3–2.8).[22] Similarly, in a pooled analysis of 35 studies that included more than 400,000 patients, Kim and colleagues[23] found that endometriosis increased ovarian cancer risk in case-control or 2-arm cohort studies (relative risk, 1.265; 95% CI, 1.214–1.318) as well as single-arm cohort studies (standard incidence ratio, 1.797; 95% CI, 1.276–2.531). Nevertheless, the raw prevalence of ovarian carcinoma in patients with ovarian or pelvic endometriosis is estimated to only be between 0.7% and 2.5%.[21,24,25] In comparisons with their counterparts that are unassociated with endometriosis, endometriosis-associated ovarian carcinomas are more likely to be diagnosed in younger patients and to be early stage, and, as such, have a better prognosis on univariate analyses.[23,26–34] However, the apparently improved prognosis is likely a function of the comparative earlier stage at detection of endometriosis-associated carcinomas; this advantage disappears on adjusting for stage in most,[23,26–34] but not all,[35,36] studies.

The diagnostic criteria for endometriosis are well established and are reviewed in detail elsewhere.[37] The term atypical endometriosis has been applied to endometriotic cysts that are lined by atypical epithelium, although what constitute atypia has varied in different studies.[38,39] The spectrum of potential changes includes focal glandular crowding, tufting, nuclear stratification or disorganization, and sporadic pleomorphism. In one study, atypical foci were identified in 1.7% of ovarian endometriosis cases and in 61% of endometriosis cases that were associated with an ovarian carcinoma.[39] Foci of atypical endometriosis may be observed in direct morphologic contiguity with their associated carcinomas.[38,39] Metaplasias of various types are frequently present in both atypical and nonatypical endometriosis.[40] Cases that show cytologically demarcated glandular crowding or other architectural epithelial abnormalities are likely analogous to atypical hyperplasia of the endometrium, and should be classified as such. Cases that show minimal architectural complexity but are defined primary by cytologic atypia are substantially more common. It is unclear whether these foci represent degenerative nuclear changes, cystic degeneration of the associated carcinoma, lepidic growth of the associated carcinoma, or a precancerous precursor lesion. Evidence that may support a precancerous, precursor lesion include (1) the rare cases of patients with atypical endometriosis that subsequently went on to develop endometrioid carcinoma[39]; (2) the high frequency with which atypical endometriosis is associated with a malignancy[39,41]; (3) the frequently observed morphologic contiguity between atypical endometriosis and their associated carcinoma[38,39]; (4) the demonstration of a progressively increasing mutational load between nonatypical endometriosis, atypical endometriosis, and associated carcinoma[42]; and (5) cases with shared molecular events between atypical endometriosis and their associated carcinomas, including PTEN, ERCC1, PIK3CA, PPP2R1A, and ARID1A mutations, and upregulation of HNF-1β.[42,43] Endometriosis foci that are associated with a carcinoma show a high mutational burden, including, in some cases, a nearly total complement of driver somatic mutations that are present in the concurrent carcinoma. This mutational burden is present irrespective of whether atypia is present or whether the endometriotic focus is near or distant from the carcinoma.[44–46] These alterations are generally absent in eutopic endometrium, suggesting that the process of neoplastic transition begins with endometriosis. In addition, the insides of endometriotic cysts are thought to be a hypoxic microenvironment rich in potentially mutagenic iron-induced reactive oxygen species, inflammatory cytokines, and chemokines.[47] When this environment is superimposed on already-mutated epithelia, the development of a morphologically recognizable, immediate cancer precursor lesion is possible. Nevertheless, whether an isolated diagnosis of atypical endometriosis warrants any directed treatments, or even increased surveillance, is unclear at present time.

HISTOGENESIS AND MOLECULAR PATHOGENESIS

As previously noted, OEC and CCC, two clinicopathologically distinct neoplasms, are both associated with endometriosis and can often be observed in direct morphologic contiguity with endometriotic epithelium, from which they presumably originated. It has been postulated that both tumors are primarily derived from progenitor cells in endometriotic endometrium that differentiate toward secretory cell lineage (OEC) or ciliated cell lineage (CCC) depending on their specific microenvironment.[48] The epithelial compartment in endometriosis shows clonally dominant somatic passenger mutations relative to stroma and is accordingly a likely point of carcinogenesis.[45,49] There is significant overlap in the molecular events that have been identified in OEC and CCC, although the frequencies differ[50–65] and are briefly discussed later for each histotype. The most commonly recurring events in CCC involve mutations of the ARID1A gene and dysregulation of the phosphatidylinositol 3-kinase (PI3K)/AKT/mammalian target of rapamycin (mTOR) pathway, the latter most commonly manifested as mutation of the PIK3CA gene. The protein product of the ARID1A gene is BAF250a, a component of the human mating-type switch (SWI) and nutrient switch (SNF) complex, which is involved in ATP-dependent chromatin remodeling. ARID1A mutations have been reported to be present in 47% to 57% of CCC,[51,66] manifested at the protein level as loss of expression of the BAF-250a. These mutations are present in morphologically typical as well as atypical endometriosis associated with carcinoma, which suggests that they occur early in carinogenesis.[51,52,59,67–69] Indeed, loss of BAF-250a expression in CCC has been reported to be significantly associated with the presence of adjacent endometriosis.[67] PIK3CA mutations are present in 30% to 50% of CCC.[56,65] ARID1A mutations frequently co-occur with other mutations, including PIK3CA, leading to an activation of the phosphatidylinositol 3-kinase (PI3K)/AKT pathway and promoting carcinogenesis in a possibly synergistic manner. Other mutations in the PI3K pathway and the SWI/SNF complex have been reported, including ARID1B (10%), PIK3R1 (7%–8%), MET (37%), AKT2 (14%), SMARCA4 (5%), and SMARCD3,[58,61,70,71] which together show the significance of pathways that pertain to cytoskeletal organization, chromatin remodeling, cell proliferation, DNA repair, and cell cycle regulation in ovarian clear cell carcinogenesis. However, in general, whole-exome sequencing of CCC has shown them to show complex mutational profiles that significantly exceed just the primary (PI3K/AKT/mTOR and chromatin remodeling) pathways.[70–75] Other genes that have been found to be mutated or to show significant copy number alterations in subsets of CCC include *CTNNB1*, *CSMD3*, *LPHN3*, *LRP1B*, *TP53*, *NTRK1*, *MYC*, *GNAS*, *TET2*, *TSC1*, *BRCA2*, *SMAD4*, *BRAF*, *BCL1B*, *ERBB2*, *PDGFRB*, *PGR*, *KRAS*, *ETS1*, *MLH1*, *PRKDC*, *AMER1*, *ARID2*, *BCL11A*, *CREBBP*, *EXT1*, *FANCD2*, *MSH6*, *NF1*, *NOTCH1*, *NUMA1*, *PDE4-DIP*, *PPP2R1A*, *MLL3*, *RNF213*, and *SYNE1*.[42,71,73,75] Chromosomal regions that have been found to show recurrent copy number alterations include 17q, 8q.24.3, and 20q.13.2-20q.13.33 (amplifications) and 13q12.11-13q14.3, 17p13.2-17p13.1, 19p13.2-19p13.1, 9q, and 18q (deletions).[71,76] Numerical variations at chromosome 20q13.2 are significant because this region harbors the *ZNF217* gene, amplifications of which have been associated with poor prognosis and whose expression may be a pharmacotherapeutic target.[77–79] Gene microarray analyses have identified a 66-gene CCC signature that distinguished CCC from non-CCC samples, and that included genes such as *HNF-1β*, *cyclin-dependent kinase inhibitor 1A (p21)*, *HIF-1a*, *IL-6*, and *STAT3*, as well as other genes that reflect the oxidative, hypoxic, and inflammatory microenvironment that characterizes the endometriotic cyst in which many CCCs originate.[80] Expression profiling has highlighted that inflammation-related genes are differentially expressed in cohorts of endometriosis, CCC, and OEC,[81] and examination of gene signatures has also shown that OEC with concurrent endometriosis shows inflammation-related molecular signatures that are distinct from EEC without concurrent endometriosis, both of which highlight the significance of inflammatory dysregulation in malignant transformation in endometriotic cysts.[81,82] It has been postulated that HNF1β, possibly induced by the hypoxic and stressful environment within an endometriotic cyst, modulates the intracellular metabolism of endometriotic epithelium to enhance aerobic glycolysis, which in turn facilitates the survival, and eventually malignant transformation, of these cells in such a microenvironment.[83,84] Ultimately, although the process of clear cell carcinogenesis is

unclear at the present time, there is enough information to indicate that it is a complex and possibly unique interplay of genetic/epigenetic alterations and immune factors that are induced or directly influenced by their specific microenvironments.

Even less is known about endometrioid carcinogenesis. The principal molecular alterations in OEC are outlined in **Table 1**. These alterations include mutations in the Wnt, PI3K, and mitogen-activated protein kinase (MAPK) pathways, *POLE* exonuclease domain mutations, the SWI/SNF complex, and microsatellite instability or DNA mismatch repair deficiency.[85–90] Overall, the most common alterations include mutations in *CTNNB1* (31%–53.3%), *PIK3CA* (15%–40%), *ARID1A* (30%), and *PPP2R1A* (7%–16.6%).[66,85–90] Largely, these events are similar to those that have been reported for the more common endometrial endometrioid carcinoma. Similar to their endometrial counterparts, OECs seem to be classifiable into molecular subgroups that correlate with survival.[84] Parra-Herran and colleagues[91] classified 72 cases of OEC using a surrogate The Cancer Genome Atlas–like classifier into 4 subgroups, namely *POLE*-mutated/ultramutated (10%), DNA mismatch repair (MMR) deficient (8%), p53 abnormal (24%), and p53 wild type (58%). This molecular classification was reportedly associated with disease-free survival independent of tumor grade and stage.[84]

Both OEC and CCC are associated with Lynch syndrome,[87,91–96] an autosomal dominant syndrome that primarily derives from a germline mutation in DNA MMR mechanisms, which increases the risk of carcinogenesis in various organs. It is been estimated that patients with Lynch syndrome have a 10% lifetime risk of developing OEC or CCC.[92] Loss of expression of the DNA MMR proteins MSH2, MSH6, PMS2, and/or MLH1 have been identified in 6% to 13% of CCCs[65,95] and 3.8 to 12.5% of OECs.[86–89,91,92] DNA MMR-deficient OECs show a concurrent endometrioid carcinoma of the uterus, mostly low grade and early stage, in 57% to 71% of cases.[92,95] Similarly, for DNA MMR-deficient CCCs, at least 28% show a concurrent carcinoma elsewhere, although the data are less robust.[93,95] DNA MMR-deficient CCCs have been reported to show significantly more stromal inflammation that MMR-proficient controls, and they have also been reported to occur in younger patients[95]; such associations have not been clearly demonstrable for DNA MMR-deficient OECs.[92] In 1 meta-analysis on Lynch syndrome–associated ovarian cancer, the mean

Table 1
Frequencies of selected mutations in clear cell carcinoma of the ovary and endometrioid carcinoma of the ovary

Molecular Aberration	CCC Frequency (%)	OEC Frequency (%)	References
ARID1A mutation	47–57	30	51,66,85
PIK3CA mutation	30–60	15–40	42,56,57,85,86
PPP2R1A mutation	7	7–16.6	53,66,85
KRAS mutation	5–14	12–33.3	52,54,62,85,86
BRAF V600 mutation	0–1	NI	52,60,62
DNA MMR deficiency or MSI H	6–13	3.8–12.5	65,86–89,91,92,94
PTEN mutation	5	NI	52,55
CDKN2A/2B deletion	9	NI	56
NRAS mutation	0	NI	62
TP53 mutation	15–53	6.6–24	52,57,63,85,91
BRCA1/2 mutation	6	NI	50
TERT promoter mutation	16	NI	64
AKT2 amplification	14	NI	58
MET amplification	37	NI	58,61
CTNNB1 mutation	3	31–53.3	52,85,86
POLE exonuclease domain mutation	NI	4.5–10	90,91

Abbreviations: ARID1A, AT rich interactive domain 1A; *BRCA*, breast cancer; *CDKN*, cyclin-dependent kinase inhibitor; NI, no information; *PIK3CA*, phosphatidylinositol-45-bisphosphate 3-kinase catalytic subunit alpha; *PPP2R1A*, protein phosphatase 2 regulatory subunits 1A; *PTEN*, phosphatase and tensin homolog *KRAS*, Kirsten Rat Sarcoma; *TERT*, Telomerase reverse transcriptase; MSI H, microsatellite instability high; *BRAF*, B-Raf Proto-Oncogene; *TP53*, Tumor protein 53; *CTNNB1*, Catenin Beta 1; *NRAS*, neuroblastoma RAS viral oncogene homolog; *AKT2*, AKT Serine/Threonine Kinase 2; *POLE*, Polymerase epsilon; *MET*, mesenchymal-epithelial transition factor; *CDKN*, Cyclin Dependent Kinase Inhibitor.

patient age at diagnosis was 45.3 years (range, 19–82 years). The most frequent mutations were *MSH2* (47%) and *MLH1* (38%), and 65% were diagnosed at an early stage.[96] Some authorities, including the Austrian Association of Gynecologic Oncology, recommend the routine screening of all CCC and OEC for DNA MMR expression.[97,98]

ENDOMETRIOID CARCINOMA

GENERAL FEATURES

When classified using WHO 2014 criteria and current diagnostic approaches,[99] OECs represent 13% to 15.8% of all ovarian cancers.[100,101] It is estimated that grades I and II cancers represent 84% to 95% of all endometrioid carcinomas, with grade III cancers representing the remaining 5% to 16% of cases.[87,102,103] In one series, the patients ranged from 31 to 85 years (median, 53 years) and 42% were 50 years of age or younger.[87] It is estimated that 18%–71% of OECs in Western countries are associated with endometriosis in 1 or both ovaries or elsewhere in the pelvis.[20,87] Cancer antigen 125 (CA-125) level at presentation varies

widely but is most commonly modestly increased.[103] A family history of OEC in a first-degree relative, or any ovarian cancer, has been associated with an increased risk of OEC, with relative risks that range from 2.81 to 3.81.[104] Between 11% and 30% of patients diagnosed with OEC also have a concurrent endometrioid carcinoma in the uterus.[87,105–107]

GROSS FEATURES

The average tumor size for OEC is larger than 10 cm.[103] The external surface is often smooth. The gross appearance of a tumor's cut surface is a direct reflection of its composition. For tumors that originated from endometriotic cysts, cut surfaces show 1 or more sessile polypoid masses protruding into the lumen of a hemorrhagic cyst. Other cases show small papillary masses lining the wall of a cyst that is not overtly hemorrhagic. Cases that have a significant adenofibromatous background may be entirely solid with a tan-red cut surface and foci of hemorrhage and necrosis. Other cases are purely solid with a fleshy cut surface and are devoid of an adenofibromatous background.

MORPHOLOGIC FEATURES

OECs show broad morphologic similarities to their endometrial counterparts. Most grade 1 tumors are composed of architecturally confluent (back to back or cribriform) glands or papillae that are lined by columnar cells with mildly pleomorphic, variably stratified nuclei[87,103] (**Fig.** 1A), and 99% of cases show a mitotic index of less than 12 mitotic figures per 10 high-power microscopic fields (HPF).[103] Most cases show a confluent pattern of invasion, but a subset show destructive invasion whereby single glands or cells infiltrate in a haphazard pattern in fibrous stroma.[108] From

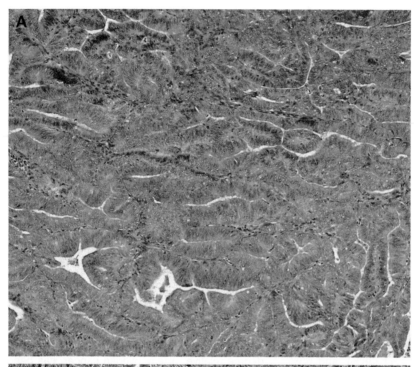

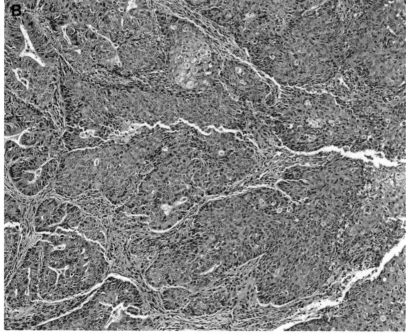

Fig. 1. (*A*, *B*): Endometrioid carcinoma, prototypical morphology for low grade (*A*) and high grade (*B*) (H&E, original magnification x20).

58% to 63% show squamous differentiation (**Fig. 2**), mostly in the form in intraglandular squamous morules.[87,103] Squamous differentiation may also be present in nonmorular forms, or may be configured as spindle cells.[109] Rarely, the squamous elements are overtly malignant.[110] Clear cell changes are present in 32% of cases of all grades.[87] Most take the form of glycogenated alterations in foci of squamous differentiation (**Fig. 3A**), or classic secretory change (**Fig. 3B**), the latter characterized by organized columnar epithelium with supranuclear and/or subnuclear cytoplasmic clearing. Various other forms of nonspecific clear cell change include less organized iterations of secretory change (**Fig. 3C**), dropletlike vacuolization (**Fig. 4**), solid clear cells (**Fig. 5**), glands and papillae lined by cuboidal cells with clear cytoplasm, and diffuse water-clear cytoplasmic clearing often associated with small nuclei.[111] The tubulocystic and small papillary patterns, hobnail nuclei, and sporadic atypia that characterize many CCCs are typically absent. Twenty-four percent of OECs show mucinous differentiation, typically as small segments of cells with intracytoplasmic mucin (**Fig. 6**) in an otherwise cytoarchitecturally typical tumor.[87] Other morphologic variations include significant cytoplasmic oxyphilia[112] (**Fig. 7**), nonspecific spindle cells admixed with typical glandular areas[87] (**Fig. 8**), extensive ciliated cell change OECs[113] (**Fig. 9**), broad hierarchical papillation (usually in a background of an endometrioid borderline tumor) mimicking serous borderline tumor[114] (**Fig. 10**), corded and hyalinized patterns, and small nonvillous papillae (**Fig. 11**). One variant that is deserving of specific mention is that with a sex cord stromal–type pattern,[115–117] which is observed in 13% of cases.[87] These tumors show features that may cause them to be misinterpreted as granulosa cell tumors (small acinar tubules in solid background), Sertoli cell/Sertoli-Leydig cell tumor (hollow, solid, winding, elongated tubular structures), or both (those described earlier in addition to stromal luteinization or spindled stroma)[115–117] (**Fig. 12**). Grade III OECs by definition show a predominant solid architecture. Most cases show greater than 80% solid architecture. The solid areas may show a solid, trabecular, vaguely nested appearance (**Fig. 1B**). The cells are cohesive, imparting an appearance that is reminiscent of squamous cell carcinoma. Mitotic activity may vary, with approximately half of cases showing greater than or equal to 12 or more mitotic figures per 10 HPF, and the other half showing less active mitotic activity. Pleomorphism is similarly variable, with half of cases being atypical but monomorphic, and the other half showing focal or diffuse pleomorphism.[103] Squamous cells are absent in most cases.[103] Nonsolid components show conventional endometrioid carcinoma morphology, albeit with poorly formed glands.

IMMUNOPHENOTYPIC FEATURES

In a large recent study,[103] grade 1 OEC showed the following immunophenotypes: PAX8 positive

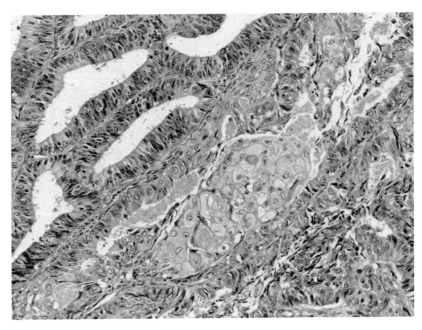

Fig. 2. Endometrioid carcinoma with squamous differentiation (H&E, original magnification x40).

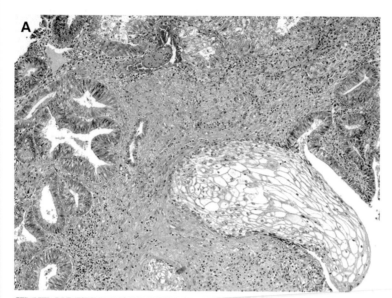

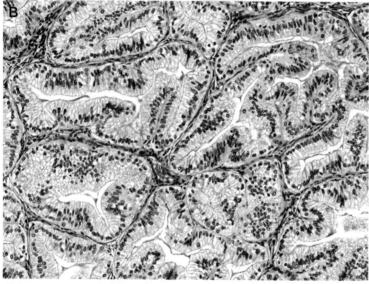

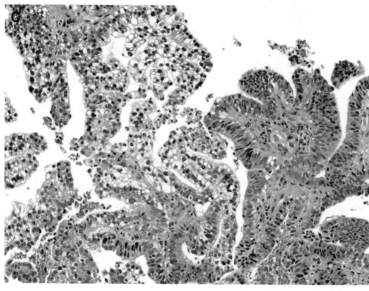

Fig. 3. Endometrioid carcinoma with clear cell change, including glycogenated squamous epithelium (*A*), classic secretory change (*B*), and less organized iterations of secretory change (*C*) (H&E, original magnification [*A,C*] x20; [*B*] x40).

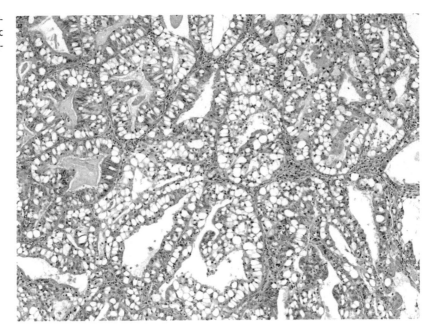

Fig. 4. Endometrioid carcinoma with nonspecific vacuolization (H&E, original magnification x20).

(78%), WT1 positive (7.1%), p53 aberrant (5.6%), DNA MMR deficient (8.8%), p16-block positive (3.2%), ARID1A loss (77%), vimentin diffuse positive (67.2%), PTEN retained (54.8%), estrogen receptor (ER) positive (93%), progesterone receptor (PR) positive (93.6%). Comparable immunophenotypes for grade 3 tumors were as follows: PAX8 positive (63%), WT1 positive (10.3%), p53 aberrant (30%), DNA MMR deficient (23.3%), p16-block positive (16.7%), BAF-250a loss (60%), vimentin diffuse positive (40%), PTEN retained (53.3%), ER positive (76.7%), PR positive (80%).[103] HNF1β, Napsin A, and α-methylacyl–coenzyme A racemase are expressed in 37%, 5.3%, and 0% of OECs, respectively[118]

Fig. 5. Endometrioid carcinoma, grade III, with solid clear cells (H&E, original magnification x20).

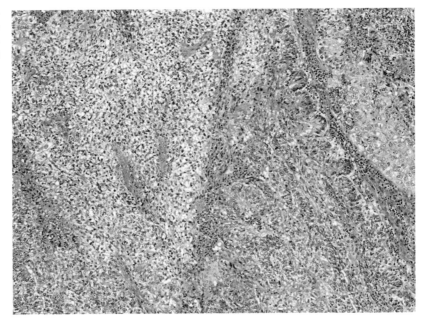

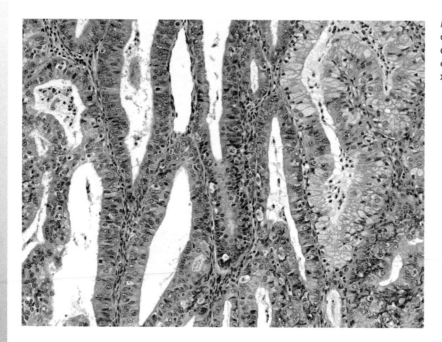

Fig. 6. Endometrioid carcinoma with mucinous differentiation (H&E, original magnification x40).

GRADING AND GRADE DISTRIBUTION

For OEC, the WHO classification recommends the same International Federation of Gynecology and Obstetrics (FIGO) grading that is applicable for endometrioid carcinomas of the uterus.[99] This grading scheme is based on the percentage of nonsquamous solid components in a tumor (≤5% solid, grade 1%; 6%–50%, grade 2; >50%, grade 3), with severe nuclear atypia exceeding 50% of tumoral volume causing a 1-step upgrade.[99] The FIGO grade distribution in 2 recent analyses that included 283 tumors were as follows: grade 1, 67.8%; grade 2, 17.7%; grade 3, 14.5%.[87,103] FIGO grading has been found be significantly correlated with disease-free, disease-specific, and overall survival on univariate analyses for all tumors,[105,119] but not between grade 3 and grade 2 tumors, which raises the possibility of combining grades 2 and 3 tumors into a

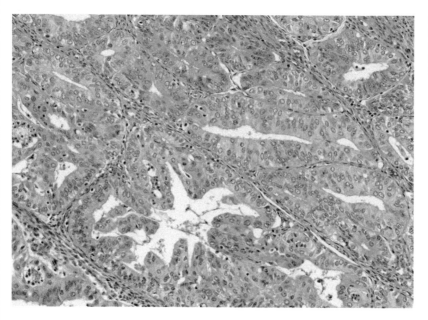

Fig. 7. Endometrioid carcinoma with prominently oxyphilic cytoplasm (H&E, original magnification x40).

Fig. 8. (*A, B*) Endometrioid carcinoma with spindle cells. Note the spindle and glandular cells seamlessly intertwine and are composed of cytologically identical cells (H&E, original magnification [*A*] x20; [*B*] x40).

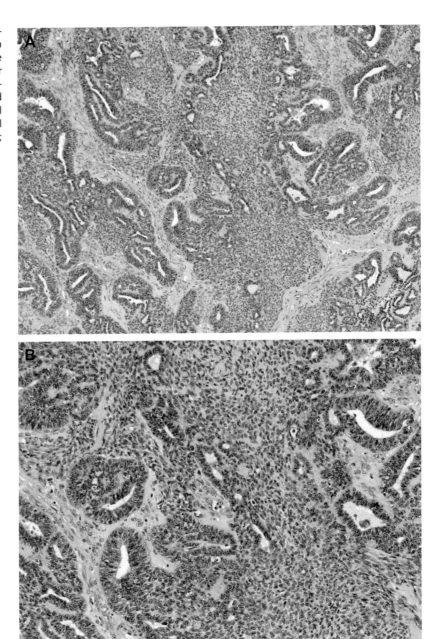

single grade.[103] The Silverberg grading system,[120] which stratifies based on architectural grade, nuclear grade, and mitotic count, is concordant with the FIGO system in about 75% of cases, but the former may be a better predictor of survival than the FIGO system.[119]

STAGE DISTRIBUTION AND PROGNOSIS

The FIGO stage distribution at presentation in 1 analysis of 104 cases was as follows: 72% stage I, 11% stage II, 14% stage III, and 3% stage IV. Within the stage I group, 59% were IA, 4% stage IB, and 37% stage IC.[87] In another recent analysis, the distribution was different: 50% stage I, 36.4% stage II, 12.3% stage III, and 1% stage IV.[103] Stage has been shown to be a significant prognostic factor in OEC, even in population-based analyses without central pathologic review.[121,122] The 5-year cause-specific survival in one such analysis was 82% overall, and was 95%, 84%, 59%, and 29% for stages I, II, III, and IV respectively.[121]

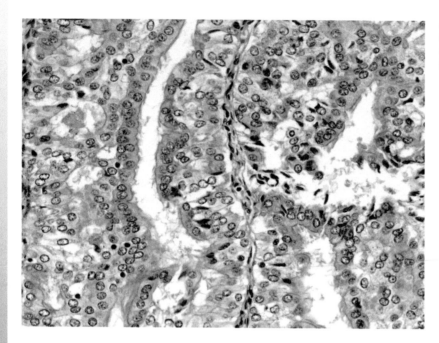

Fig. 9. Endometrioid carcinoma with ciliated cell change (H&E, original magnification x40).

Data from the Surveillance, Epidemiology, and End Results (SEER) program indicate that the 1-year, 5-year, and 10-year overall survival for localized OEC are 96.9%, 87.1%, and 72.5% respectively.[122] In addition to stage, other reported prognostic factors in OEC include ER and PR expression as positive prognostic factors,[123] and lymphovascular invasion, p16-block positivity, BAF250a loss, nuclear beta-catenin expression, and aberrant p53 expression as negative prognostic factors.[119,124–126]

DIFFERENTIAL DIAGNOSIS

Endometrioid Carcinoma of the Ovary Versus Endometrioid Adenofibroma or Borderline Tumor

A background endometrioid adenofibroma is identifiable in at least 14% of cases[87] and a background borderline tumor in about 5%. Approximately 50% of the latter are seen in a background of the former. These areas show either single tubular, variably

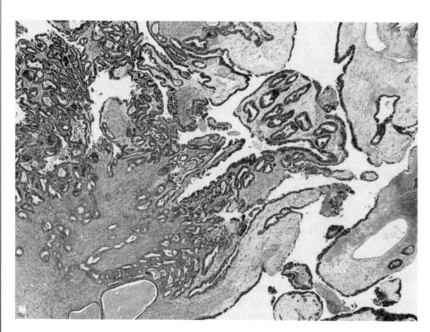

Fig. 10. An endometrioid borderline tumor with foci of confluent microinvasion. Note broad papillary formations mimicking a serous borderline tumor (H&E, original magnification x20).

Fig. 11. Endometrioid carcinoma with small nonvillous papillae (H&E, original magnification x40).

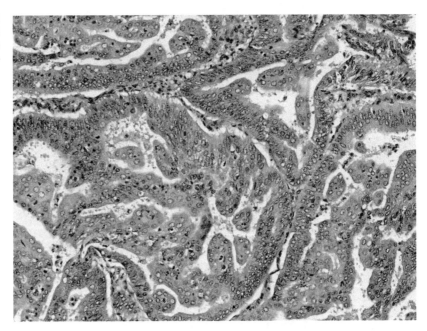

cystic glands lined by proliferative endometrium-type epithelium in a fibromatous background (adenofibroma) or variably atypical, crowded, back-to-back or cribriform glands akin to atypical hyperplasia in a densely fibrous stroma, occasionally in a papillary pattern (borderline tumor)[127,128] (**Fig. 13**). The presence of either supports a histotype assignment as endometrioid.[87,127,128] Adenofibromas do not show glandular crowding or invasion and are rarely the source of diagnostic difficulty. Endometrioid borderline tumors may show small foci of confluent or infiltrative microinvasion (<5 mm); these cases should be classified as endometrioid borderline tumor with microinvasion. Squamous morules are commonly present in endometrioid borderline tumors and should not be mistaken for foci of solid or confluent growth (see **Fig. 10**). Squamous morules are positive for CDX2 and SATB2 and show diminished expression of ER and PR, immunophenotypes that may be diagnostically useful in their distinction from foci of solid growth. When strictly defined, endometrioid borderline tumors are clinically benign.[127–129] A diagnosis of OEC in the aforementioned backgrounds requires the presence of confluent or destructive stromal invasion that exceeds 5 mm in at least 1 focus.

Grade II or III Endometrioid Carcinoma of the Ovary Versus Dedifferentiated Endometrioid Carcinoma

A subset of OECs (<1% of in our experience) show foci of dedifferentiation, characterized by the presence of typically demarcated foci of undifferentiated carcinoma (solid sheets of monomorphic, dyshesive round cells with high nucleocytoplasmic ratios, rhabdoid or epithelioid cells, necrosis, and abundant mitotic figures). These clinically aggressive dedifferentiated endometrioid carcinomas frequently show loss of expression of SWI/SNF proteins, such as SMARCA4 (BRG1), SMARCA2 (BRM), and SMARCB1 (INI1), and are thought to arise, at least in part, because of aberrations in SWI/SNF-mediated transcriptional regulation.[130,131] The morphologic overlap between differentiated endometrioid and grade III endometrioid carcinoma stems from the fact that both may show endometrioid glands and large areas of solid growth. This distinction is of clinical significance because dedifferentiated endometrioid carcinomas are likely much more clinically aggressive. No single feature is absolutely discriminatory, but features favoring grade III OEC include large nested and ribbon patterns in the solid areas, cells that appear cohesive, foci of squamous differentiation, foci of adenofibroma or endometriosis, and retained/diffuse expression of pancytokeratins, SWI/SNF proteins, and PAX8 in the solid areas.

Grade III Endometrioid Carcinoma of the Ovary Versus High-grade Serous Carcinoma

This distinction should be made because of potentially different implications for genetic counseling, treatment, and prognosis. Many high-grade serous carcinomas (HGSCs) were

542

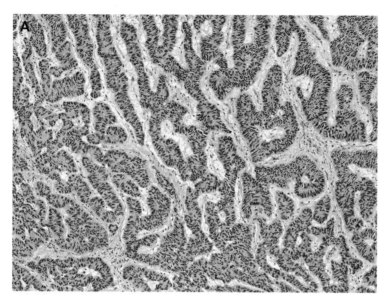

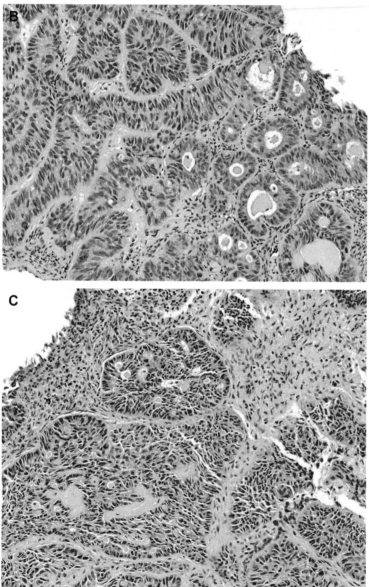

Fig. 12. Endometrioid carcinoma with sex cord stromal type patterns resembling Sertoli cell tumor (sertoliform endometrioid carcinoma) (*A*, *B*) and adult granulosa cell tumor, microfollicular type (*C*) (H&E, original magnification [*A,C*] x20; [*B*] x40).

Fig. 13. Endometrioid borderline tumor, characterized by crowded, endometrioid-type glands in a fibrous background (*A*). Squamous morules are commonly present (*B*) (H&E, original magnification [*A*] x20; [*B*] x40).

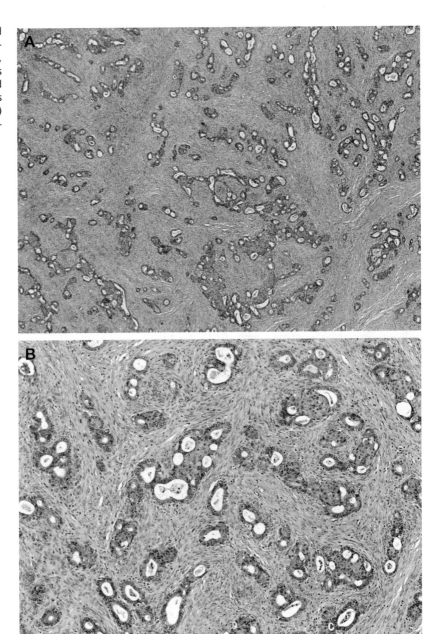

historically classified as grade III OEC.[102] At the morphologic level, these two tumors may overlap because both may show glandular and solid architecture and nuclear anaplasia, and because a significant subset of HGSCs shows the so-called SET features (solid, pseudoendometrioid, and transitional cell carcinoma–like morphology).[102,132] Eighty percent of OECs (of all grades) show at least 1 of the confirmatory endometrioid features: (1) squamous metaplasia,

(2) endometriosis, (3) adenofibromatous background, and (4) borderline endometrioid or mixed mullerian component,[102] although these features tend to be uncommon in grade III OEC.[102] Nevertheless, they are diagnostically useful if present. Features favoring grade III OEC include (1) presence of foci of classic endometrioid carcinoma morphology, (2) absence of classic serous carcinoma morphology, and (3) a WT1-negative/p53–wild-type staining pattern.

Grade I or II Endometrioid Carcinoma of the Ovary with Clear Cells Versus Clear Cell Carcinoma of the Ovary or Mixed Clear Cell Carcinoma of the Ovary/Endometrioid Carcinoma of the Ovary

Clear cell change in endometrioid carcinoma may be related to glycogenated squamous epithelium, secretory change, or may be a nonspecific alteration related to cytoplasmic accumulation of lipid, glycogen, or other unknown substances[87,111] (see **Figs. 2–5**). OEC with clear cell change typically lacks the tubulocystic and small papillary patterns that characterize CCC. The presence of classic glands of EEC (lined by columnar, pseudostratified cells), areas of squamous or mucinous differentiation, or an adenofibromatous background all favor OEC. Glands and papillae of CCC tend to be lined not by columnar epithelium but by low cuboidal, hobnail, flat, or polygonal cells with minimal stratification. OEC and CCC also show a distinctly different immunophenotype, with CCC being negative for ER and PR and highly positive for Napsin A and HNF1β, and OEC showing the opposite phenotype.[118,133] OEC is occasionally admixed with CCC.[13] CCC/OEC represent approximately 56.5% of all mixed cell carcinomas of the ovary, and as such are the most common combination.[133–135] Nevertheless, clear cells in a case of OEC are much more likely represent one of the aforementioned iterations of clear cell change in OEC than a true small CCC component. For any putative focus of CCC, the morphologic and immunophenotypic changes, if viewed in isolation, must be diagnostic.

Grade I or II Endometrioid Carcinoma of the Ovary with Spindle Cells Versus Carcinosarcoma

Spindle cell change is an uncommon finding in OEC.[109] Conventional low-grade glands merge with the spindle cell areas almost imperceptibly, with both components being composed of cells with identical cytologic features, including typically minimal pleomorphism (see **Fig. 8**). Glands and spindle cells are usually in the same region without any distinct demarcations. The spindle cells may be mitotically active, depending on the mitotic index of the glandular components. Both express keratins, EMA, and ER/PR diffusely.[109] In many cases, spindle cell change is most likely a manifestation of squamous differentiation, because the spindle cells can be observed to merge with more conventional foci of squamous differentiation. Carcinosarcomas usually show overt anaplasia in the epithelial and mesenchymal elements, and do not typically show the aforementioned epithelial-to-stromal morphologic transitions. Compared with OEC with spindle cells, carcinosarcomas are much more likely to be at an advanced stage; to show a p53-aberrant, ER/PR-negative phenotype; and to be devoid of squamous elements, adenofibromatous areas, or endometriosis.

Endometrioid Carcinoma of the Ovary with Sex Cord Stromal–Type Patterns Versus Sex Cord Stromal Tumors

Some OECs may mimic AGCT by virtue of comprising benign small acinar tubules in a solid background[136] (see **Fig. 12C**), or may mimic Sertoli cell/Sertoli-Leydig cell tumor by being composed of hollow, solid, or elongated tubular structures[115–117] (see **Fig. 12A, B**). These cases may also show stromal luteinization or spindled stroma.[115–117] Although there is some overlap, patients with OEC with these patterns have an age range that is substantially older than their counterparts with Sertoli cell or Sertoli/Leydig tumors, and rarely have any androgenic or estrogenic clinical manifestations.[117] At the morphologic level, they may show at least focal endometrioid features, including large endometrioid glands, squamous differentiation, luminal mucin accumulation, and adenofibromatous areas, although it is uncommon for a single case to have more than 1 of these features. For OEC that is solid with microacinar areas mimicking adult granulosa cell tumor, more conventional areas of OEC or other endometrioid features are typically present. Immunohistochemistry allows definitive classification in almost all cases. OEC with sex cord stromal–type patterns are mostly diffusely positive for cytokeratin (CK) 7, epithelial membrane antigen, ER, and PR, and are negative for inhibin, calretinin, and SF-1, whereas Sertoli cell tumors, Sertoli-Leydig cell tumors, and AGCT show the opposite phenotype.[115,137–139] OEC with sex cord stromal–type patterns should be distinguished from the extremely rare cases of true OEC-AGCT collision tumors wherein the components are discrete and each shows diagnostic morphologic and immunophenotypic features.[140]

Endometrioid Carcinoma of the Ovary with Metastatic Adenocarcinoma from Extragenital Sites

Some metastatic adenocarcinomas have a distinctly endometrioid appearance in the ovary, including poorly discernible intracytoplasmic mucin[141,142] and extensive cystic change (Fig. 14); these are the most commonly metastases from the gastrointestinal tract. Accurate classification requires a careful integration of all available data, including clinical, macroscopic, microscopic, and immunophenotypic findings. Clinical features favoring metastases include a clinical history of an extragenital malignancy, or advanced stage/diffuse intraperitoneal disease. Gross features that favor metastases include bilaterality, surface tumor nodules, and/or small tumor size. Microscopic features that favor metastases include a nodular growth pattern, morphologic heterogeneity between nodules, extensive lymphovascular invasion, ovarian surface tumor or mucin, a garland pattern of necrosis in glands, the absence of endometrioid features (squamous differentiation, adenofibromatous areas, endometriosis), extensive destructive pattern of invasion, hilar involvement, signet rings, and single-cell pattern of invasion.[141,142] Immunohistochemistry becomes more diagnostically useful the less cytoplasmic mucin a case shows. Expression of CK7, ER, PR, and PAX8 is expected in a gland-forming OEC. Other markers, such as CDX2, CK20, SATB2, SMAD4, and TTF1, may also have diagnostic utility, depending on the potential sites of origin of the tumor. However, there is significant overlap because endometrioid carcinoma may express any and all of these markers.

Endometrioid Carcinoma of the Ovary Versus Glandular Yolk Sac Tumor

OEC may be mistaken for the glandular/pseudoendometrioid variant of yolk sac tumor (YST).

In the seminal series,[143] patients with glandular YSTs ranged in age from 11 to 34 years (mean, 22 years) and all had increased serum alpha fetoprotein (AFP) levels. In their most prototypical form, columnar glands show hyperchromatic nuclei with subnuclear/supranuclear cytoplasmic clearing and easily discernible mitotic figures. However, cytoplasmic clearing need not be present. Other patterns of YST are frequently present concurrently, including reticular, polyvesicular-vitelline, and hepatoid patterns. Minor teratomatous foci (epidermislike squamous epithelium and cartilage) can also be present, albeit less frequently.[143] Most YSTs are immunoreactive for SALL4, Glypican 3, and AFP; show patchy or absent CK7 and EMA expression; and are negative for ER, PR, and PAX8. Most OECs show the opposite immunophenotype.[144–146] The combination of an older age at presentation, normal AFP levels, presence of endometrioid morphologic features (including adenofibromatous areas, endometriosis and morular areas), absence of other YST-like morphologic patterns, and the aforementioned immunophenotypes should facilitate their distinction from glandular YST. Some ovarian carcinomas have areas that are morphologically and immunophenotypically indistinguishable from YST and OEC is the histotype wherein this phenomenon is most frequently observed.[147,148] These cases are recognized using the same morphologic and immunohistochemical approaches outlined earlier, which should highlight the different phenotypes of the constituent areas. In older adults, YSTs are clinically aggressive if an underlying somatic-type epithelial malignancy is pathologically demonstrable.[149] As such, they should be distinguished from pure OEC.

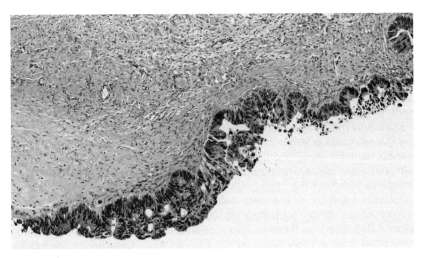

Fig. 14. Metastatic colorectal carcinoma, showing extensive cystic change in the metastatic mass (H&E, original magnification x40).

Endometrioid carcinoma of the ovary versus metastatic endometrioid carcinoma from the uterus

Between 11% and 30% of patients diagnosed with OEC are also found to have a concurrent endometrioid carcinoma in the uterus.[87,105–107] The question of whether, in a given case, the ovarian tumor is metastatic from the uterus, the uterus tumor is metastatic from the ovary, or both represent independent primary tumors has been the subject of significant discussion that has only recently been reviewed.[150] A significant body of literature has accumulated that indicates these tumors are typically low grade and confined to the uterine corpus and ovary, and that, despite being clonally related, behave much more indolently than would be expected from a single advanced-stage cancer at either site.[150,151] Some features allow pathologists to favor one site or the other as the primary site, but there is often uncertainty, and the pathology report should reflect this uncertainty when it is present. When an OEC is concurrently present with an endometrial carcinoma of similar morphology, features that would favor an ovarian primary and endometrial metastases include single endometrial mass with unusually rounded peritumoral borders; absence of atypical and/or nonatypical endometrial hyperplasia; no more than superficial myometrial invasion; the presence of a unilateral ovarian mass greater than 10 cm; and ovarian mass with associated endometriosis, adenofibromatous, or endometrioid borderline areas. Features that would favor an endometrial primary and ovarian metastases include deep myometrial invasion by a large endometrial mass, extensive lymphovascular invasion in the uterus, presence of atypical and/or nonatypical hyperplasia in the endometrium, significant involvement of the ovarian hilum and hilar vessels, small bilateral ovarian masses or nodules with surface involvement, involvement of extrauterine sites other than the ovaries, absence of endometriosis, and adenofibromatous or endometrioid borderline areas in the ovary. Independent primaries essentially become the default interpretation if the tumor cannot be clearly assigned based on these features. In most cases that are classified as independent primaries, the tumors at each site show features that mostly favor that site being a primary: the ovarian mass is larger than 10 cm; unilateral; without surface involvement or multinodularity; with endometriosis, adenofibromatous, or borderline areas; whereas the uterine tumor is variably myoinvasive and shows precursor lesions. As previously noted, these guidelines do not always allow a definitive classification, and a given case may show contradictory features. Of note, DNA MMR-deficient OECs show a concurrent endometrioid carcinoma of the uterus in 57% to 71% of cases, which is significantly more frequently than DNA MMR-proficient OECs.[87,92,95] In addition, more patients with synchronous ovarian and uterine endometrioid carcinomas show MLH1/PMS2 deficiency and *PTEN* aberrations compared with OEC unassociated with a uterine cancer.[152] These findings may highlight the necessity for DNA MMR or MSI testing in patients with such synchronous tumors, but they also suggest that a shared pattern of DNA MMR deficiency between the ovarian and uterine tumors may not necessarily be informative regarding primary site assignment.

CLEAR CELL CARCINOMA

GENERAL FEATURES

CCCs represent 6.8% to 8.7% of all ovarian cancers in Western countries[100,101] and 20% to 25% of ovarian cancers in Japan.[153] Clear cell carcinomas are associated with background ovarian endometriosis and/or more broadly in the pelvis in 22% to 47% and 67% to 68% of cases respectively.[154–156] In one series, the patients ranged in age from 19 to 82 years (mean, 53.1 years).[154] Patients frequently present with a sizable pelvic mass and mild to moderate increase in serum CA-125 levels (usually $\leq$200 U/mL).[157] Patients with CCC have a higher rate of venous thromboembolic events than their counterparts with other histotypes.[158–160] Among the histotypes of epithelial ovarian cancer, CCC has the highest association with paraneoplastic hypercalcemia.[161] A family history of ovarian cancer in a first-degree relative has been associated with an increased risk of CCC.[104] CCC also has a significant association with Lynch syndrome, as previously discussed.

GROSS FEATURES

In one series, the tumors ranged in size from 0.8 to 35 cm (mean, 13.0 cm), with surface involvement by tumor being present in 11%.[154] Tumoral cut surfaces were solid and cystic in 63%, cystic in 21%, and solid in 15%.[154] In another series, these cut surface appearances were equally distributed.[162]

MORPHOLOGIC FEATURES

The diagnostic hallmarks of CCC are their traditional architectural patterns: tubulocystic, papillary, and solid. Most cases show more than a single pattern. The papillary pattern is most frequently present, occurring in 70% of tumors, followed by the tubulocystic (65%) and papillary patterns (51%).[154] A purely solid pattern is generally not seen, although tumors with near-total papillary or tubulocystic patterns may be present.[133,154] The papillary architecture varies, and ranges from small rounded papillae in which a fibrous/hyalinized, myxoid, seemingly fluid-filled, or nonspecifically edematous stroma is surrounded by tumor cells, micropapillary tufts, or broad papillae mimicking serous borderline tumor[163] (Figs. 15 and 16). The tubulocystic pattern ranges from large ectatic cysts to small, round, nonspecific glandular structures (Fig. 17). The solid component ranges from nested clusters to diffuse sheets interspersed by other patterns. It is uncommon for any single slide to be composed entirely of solid areas. Papillae and tubulocystic units are lined by clear cells, eosinophilic/oxyphilic cells, flat cells with minimal cytoplasm, or hobnail cells, typically in various combinations (see Figs. 15–17; Fig. 18). Greater than 90% of cases show

Fig. 15. Papillary pattern of clear cell carcinoma, including papillae with hyalinized (*A*, *B*), nonspecifically fibroblastic

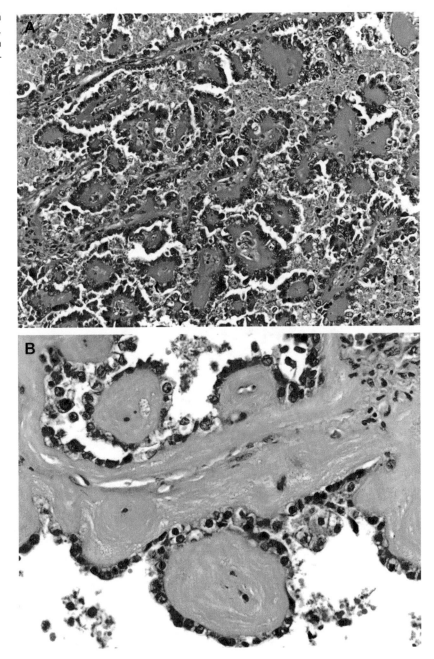

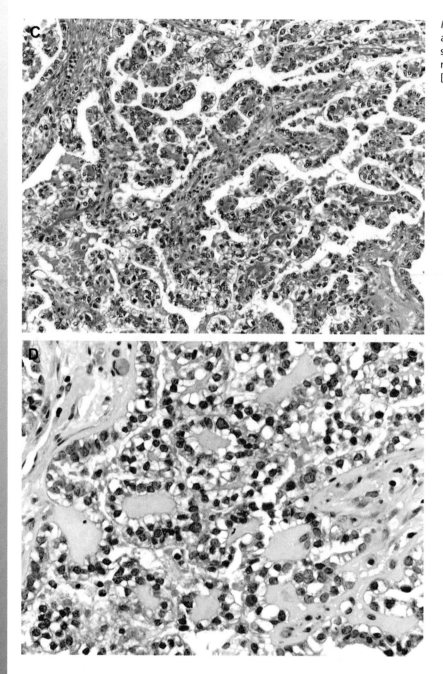

Fig. 15. (*continued*). (*C*), and myxoid/edematous stroma (*D*) (H&E, original magnification [*A,C*] x20; [*B,D*] x40).

at least focal clear cells and most cases also show hobnail cells.[133,154,162] The cells with clear and/or eosinophilic cytoplasm are typically low cuboidal rather than columnar and are mostly less than 1 to 2 cells thick.[133] However, some cases show abundant intraglandular cellular sloughing that may superficially mimic the budding of high-grade serous carcinoma. A rare group are predominantly composed of eosinophilic/oxyphilic cells, but these cases maintain the typical architecture of CCC, at least focally.[164] Pleomorphism may vary significantly, with about 20% being cytologically bland, 40% showing moderate pleomorphism with foci of anaplasia, and 40% showing easily identifiable severely pleomorphic cells. It would be unusual for a true CCC to show continuous severe pleomorphism.[154] The mitotic index of CCC is typically low but may vary significantly

Fig. 16. Clear cell carcinoma with broad papillary structures mimicking serous borderline tumor (H&E, original magnification x20).

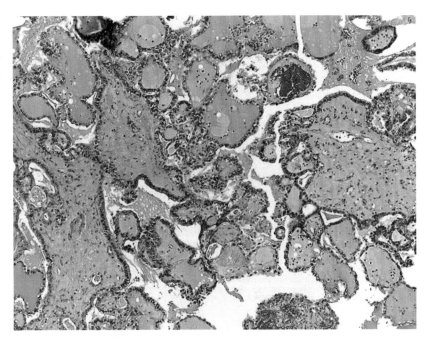

between cases and even between different areas of a single case. In one series, mitotic figure counts ranged from 0 to 13 (mean, 3–4 per 10 HPF).[133] Seventy-three percent show fewer than 6 mitoses per 10 HPFs.[154] Features that may be identified in significant subsets include hyaline globules, psammomatous bodies, and nuclear pseudoinclusions.[154] The stroma is unremarkable in most cases, but significant proportions are notably hyalinized, edematous, or both, whereas others show significant inflammation, most commonly a stromal lymphoplasmacytic infiltrate.[133,154,162] An adenofibromatous component is present in 11% to 33% of cases.[154,165,166] These areas frequently resemble a clear cell adenofibroma or a clear cell borderline tumor.[165–172]

IMMUNOPHENOTYPIC FEATURES

The typical immunophenotype for CCC is HNF1β, Napsin A, CK7, PAX8, and AMACR positive; ER-alpha, WT-1, and PR are typically negative; ER-beta is expressed in 39% of cases; and p53 is aberrant in approximately 25%. p16 is block positive in about 20%.[118,133,173–175] Among the CCC-related markers (HNF1β, Napsin A, and AMACR), HNF1β is highly sensitive but is suboptimally specific if used by itself; AMACR is specific but is not ideally sensitive. Napsin A is specific and shows intermediate sensitivity.[118] These markers are best used as part of the panel depending on the differential diagnostic consideration for a given case.

GRADING AND GRADE DISTRIBUTION

The FIGO grading scheme has not proved to be significantly associated with survival in CCC, and neither has the Silverberg system.[120,176] A grading scheme for CCC was proposed by Yamamoto and colleagues[177] in 2012: group A if greater than or equal to 90% of a tumor showed well-differentiated tubulocystic and/or papillary architecture; group C if greater than or equal to 10% of the tumor was composed of solid masses or individual infiltrating tumor cells with no or little glandular/papillary formation; group B if tumoral features did not fit either group.[177] The grade distribution using this system was 29%, 50%, and 21% for groups A, B, and C, respectively.[177] The investigators found group A to show significantly better outcomes than group C in both early-stage and late-stage cases.[177] However, Bennett and colleagues[154] found no significant correlation between outcomes and specific cytoarchitectural features, and the investigators argued against assigning a histologic grade for these tumors. The authors consider CCC to be a high-grade tumor by definition in the sense that there is insufficient evidence to assert that there is a better-performing, low-grade subset.

STAGE DISTRIBUTION AND PROGNOSIS

Most CCCs present at an early stage. The FIGO stage distribution at presentation in one analysis of 100 cases was as follows: 71% stage I, 4%

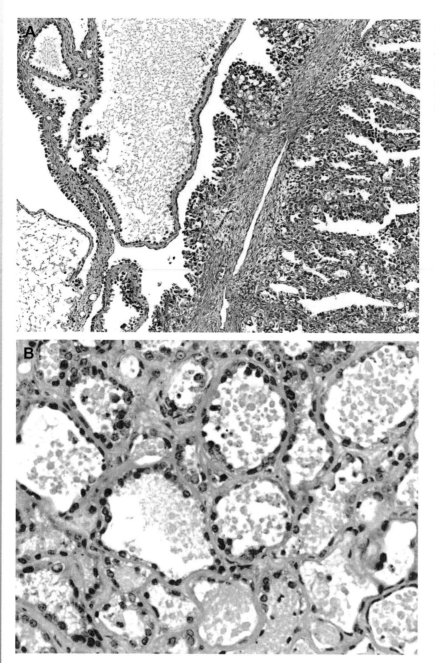

Fig. 17. Clear cell carcinoma, tubulocystic pattern. Tubulocystic patterns range from widely ectatic ducts (*A*), variably confluent smaller cysts (*B–D*), all lined by hobnail (*A*), flat

stage II, 17% stage III, and 8% stage IV.[154] Within the stage I group in another analysis, 54.6% were stage IA, 28.2% were stage IC because of tumor rupture only, and 17.3% were stage IC because of surface involvement and/or positive cytology of ascites or washings.[178] Stage has been shown in numerous analyses to be the most important prognostic factor in CCC.[154,157] The 5-year cause-specific survival in one population-based analysis was 66% overall, and was 85%, 71%, 35%, and 16% for stages I, II, III, and IV respectively.[121] Data from the SEER program indicate that the 1-year, 5-year, and 10-year overall survival for localized CCC are 96.6%, 81.7%, and 71.3% respectively.[122] Comparative figures for advanced-stage disease are 63.3%, 22.3%, and 15.5% respectively.[122] Substaging for stage

Fig. 17. (continued). (D), or low cuboidal cells with eosinophilic to clear cytoplasm *(B, C)* (H&E, original magnification *[A,C]* x20; *[B,D]* x40).

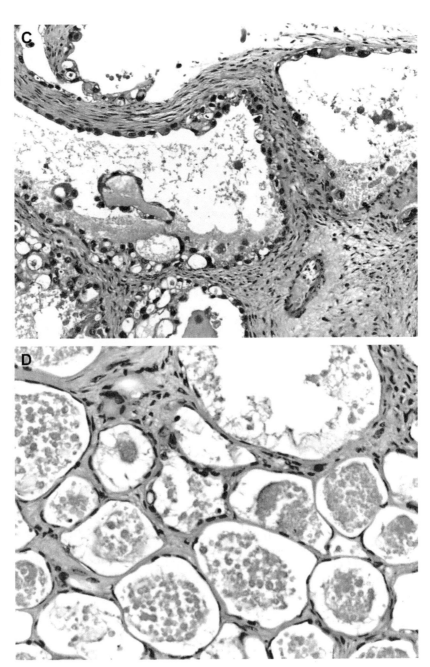

I also has significance, with most, but not all, studies identifying stage IC disease other than surgical spills (ie, stage IC1) to be associated with significantly worse outcomes compared with stage IA.[157,178–180] Numerous other prognostic factors have been proffered in addition to stage.[58,77,79,124,126,181–191] A nonexhaustive selection of reportedly negative prognostic factors includes lymphovascular invasion[192]; block p16 expression[124]; lack of BAF250a expression, beta-catenin nuclear expression, p53-aberrant staining pattern[126]; expression of IMP3,[181] fibroblast growth factor receptor 2,[185] chromobox homolog 7 (CBX7),[186] Emi1,[187] CXCR4,[188] HOXA10,[189] Glypican 3,[190] and Rsf-1 (HBXAP)[191]); *Met* amplification[58]; *CCNE1* copy number gain[182]; *MDM2* amplification (in *TP53*-wild type cases);[183] and a variety of somatic

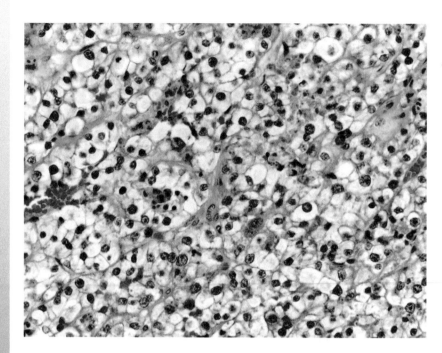

Fig. 18. Clear cell carcinoma, solid pattern (H&E, original magnification x40).

copy number variations, including at chr20q13.2, which harbors the *ZNF217* gene.[77,79,184] *PIK3CA* mutations have been found to be a positive prognostic factor.[193] There are conflicting data on the prognostic significance of an adenofibromatous component[170–172] or background endometriosis[23,26–34]

DIFFERENTIAL DIAGNOSIS

Numerous neoplasms that involve the ovary may potentially show clear cells or hobnail cells, and accordingly are potentially in the differential diagnosis of CCC. These neoplasms include primary and secondary tumors of epithelial, neural/neuroepithelial, melanocytic, and mesenchymal differentiation.[194] Discussed later are a few scenarios wherein CCC may be a diagnostic consideration. It is emphasized that there are other tumors that may bear some superficial resemblance to CCC that are not discussed here because of space considerations, including steroid cell tumor or dysgerminoma mimicking solid pattern CCC; serous borderline tumor mimicking papillary CCC or vice versa; and juvenile granulosa cell tumors, lipidized Sertoli cell tumor, or metastatic tumors mimicking solid or tubulocystic CCC. These scenarios can usually be resolved by careful assessment of clinical factors, including patient age, and consideration of whether a tumor adheres to the known morphologic and immunophenotypic profile of CCC.

Clear Cell Carcinoma of the Ovary Versus High-grade Serous Carcinoma with Clear Cells

Making the distinction between HGSC and CCC is potentially of clinical significance, because these histotypes have different implications for genetic counseling, and because of differences between them in chemoresponsiveness, stage distribution, and possibly prognosis. HGSCs may show clear cells, which occasionally may be diffuse,[195–197] as shown in **Fig. 19**A. This clear cell change may be particularly accentuated after neoadjuvant chemotherapy (**Fig. 19**B). In contrast, CCCs may show foci of significant pleomorphism (**Fig. 20**) as well as small serous carcinoma–like micropapillae.[154] However, such foci are usually minor in CCC, with most areas showing the more characteristic morphology and low mitotic indices. Similarly, HGSCs with clear cells are otherwise cytoarchitecturally typical for HGSC in most cases, and are devoid of tubulocystic architecture or CCC-like small rounded papillae. Although true mixed HGSC/CCC exists,[134] almost all HGSCs that appear to have a CCC component are just HGSC with nonspecific clear cell change.[195] Immunohistochemistry, using a panel that includes WT1, ER, Napsin A, and HNF-1β, should resolve most difficult cases.[174,196,197]

Clear Cell Carcinoma of the Ovary Versus Yolk Sac Tumor

Points of pathologic overlap between CCC and YST, two tumors that are clinically managed

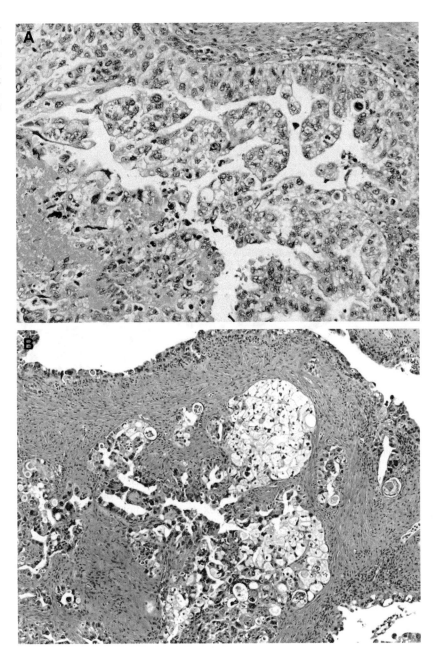

Fig. 19. High-grade serous carcinoma with clear cell change, with (*B*) and without (*A*) associated neoadjuvant chemotherapy (H&E, original magnification x20).

differently, include clear cells, solid architecture, papillae lined by a monolayer of cells, hyaline globules, and expression of HNF-1β (**Fig. 21**). Compared with CCC, patients with YST are substantially younger and have increased serum AFP levels. Pathologically, YSTs have higher tumoral mitotic indices, may have Schiller-Duval bodies, are devoid of background endometriosis or adenofibromatous areas, and may show other histologic patterns of YST, such as the reticular, microcystic, glandular, parietal, or hepatoid changes, which are absent in CCC. Most YSTs are immunoreactive for SALL4, Glypican 3, and AFP; show patchy or absent CK7 and EMA expression; and are negative for ER, PR, and PAX8. Most CCCs show the opposite phenotype.[145,146,174] Seventeen percent of YSTs may show focal or patchy expression of Napsin A, and 17% of CCCs may similarly show focal expression of Glypican 3, but this contrasts

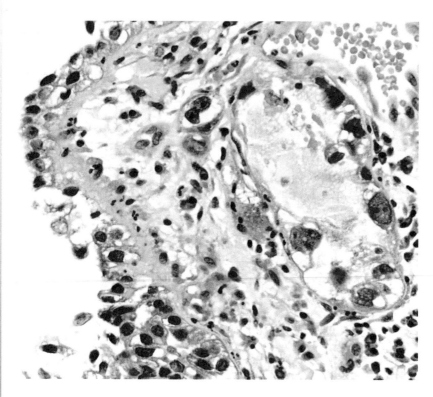

Fig. 20. Foci of severe pleomorphism in clear cell carcinoma. Such foci are typically sporadic and noncontinuous (H&E, original magnification x40).

with the diffuse expression of these markers that is typically seen in the differential consideration.[146,174] In older patients, YSTs may be mixed with (and presumably arising from) epithelial tumors, including CCC, and the immunophenotypes in these cases tend to be more complex. In one study, CK7, EMA, and Glypican 3 were frequently expressed in both components, Napsin A and PAX8 were expressed only in CCC, and SALL4 and AFP were positive in the glandular YST component but negative in the CCC component.[198]

Clear Cell Carcinoma of the Ovary Versus Clear Cell Adenofibroma and Clear Cell Borderline Tumor

An adenofibromatous component is present in 11% to 33% of CCC cases,[154,165,166] and they often show shared patterns of allelic loss that imply an evolutionary relationship.[168,169] However, these foci may also be identified in isolation as a mass lesion wherein they are classified as clear cell adenofibroma or clear cell borderline tumor.[170–172] Both are seen in patients of the same age range (35–65 years; mean, 52 years) who present with a mostly unilateral firm mass, occasionally with areas of endometriosis in the ipsilateral adnexa or elsewhere in the pelvis. Both are

clinically benign when strictly defined. Clear cell adenofibromas by definition show scattered glandular structures lined by HNF-1β/Napsin A–positive, monomorphic flat or low cuboidal cells with clear to eosinophilic cytoplasm in a densely fibrous background. Clear cell adenofibromas are extraordinarily rare, because some degree of cytologic atypia can almost always be found, and the presence of atypia by definition classifies an otherwise typical clear cell adenofibroma as a clear cell borderline tumor (**Fig. 22**). In our experience, the diagnosis of a clear cell adenofibroma unassociated with a carcinoma is exceedingly rare. Clear cell borderline tumors may show destructive or confluent microinvasion of less than 5 mm (clear cell adenofibroma with microinvasion) or show localized foci of intraepithelial severe atypia distinct from background glands (clear cell borderline tumor with intraepithelial carcinoma). Clear cell adenofibromas and borderline tumors should be extensively sampled to rule out an obviously invasive CCC. However, even for cases that appear to be clear cell borderline tumor, the possibility that the entire tumor represents a tubulocystic CCC with fibrous background should be carefully considered. The glands and cysts of tubulocystic CCC are not uniformly scattered but show a greater degree of confluence than would typically be observed in a borderline tumor. Any

Fig. 21. (*A*, *B*) Yolk sac tumor may mimic clear cell carcinoma (H&E, original magnification [*A*] x20; [*B*] x40).

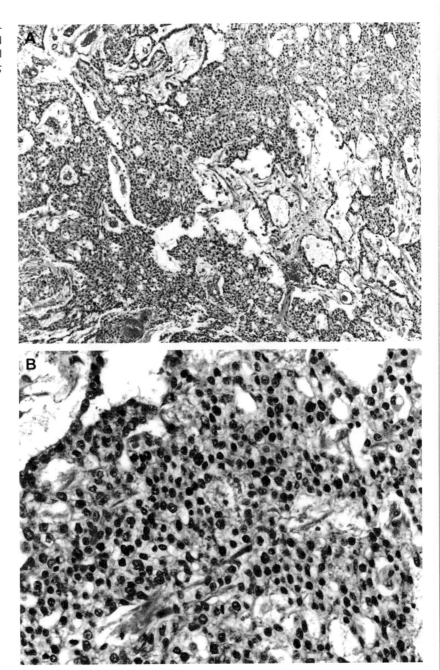

solid or papillary growth is incompatible with a borderline tumor. Similarly, glands throughout the tumor showing severe atypia suggest the entire mass is malignant. It has been suggested that cystic endometriosis and clear cell adenofibromatous lesions represent 2 different and distinct pathways to clear cell carcinogenesis, and that these pathways may result in differences in patient outcomes, but the published data are not entirely congruent.[165–169]

Clear Cell Carcinoma of the Ovary Versus Metastatic Clear Cell Renal Cell Carcinoma

Metastatic clear cell renal cell carcinoma (CCRCC) to the ovary is uncommon, but the adnexa is the most common site of metastatic CCRCC involving the gynecologic tract.[199] Clinically, metastatic CCRCC to the ovary is usually diagnosed as a recurrence in patients with a prior diagnosis of CCRCC.[199] Therefore, knowledge about this

556

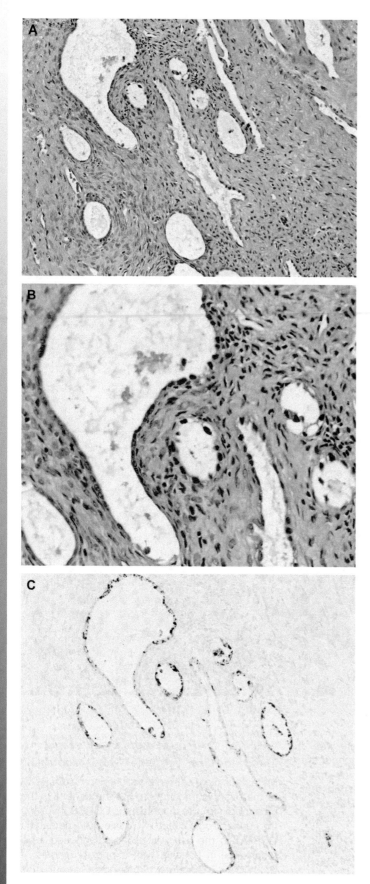

Fig. 22. Clear cell borderline tumors are characterized by scattered glands lined by Napsin A–positive (*C*) (Immunohisto-chemistry, original magnification x20), cytologically atypical epithelium in a fibromatous stroma (*A*). Even the mild atypia (*B*) depicted is incompatible with a diagnosis of clear cell adenofi-broma (H&E, original magnification [*A*] x20; [*B*] x40).

Fig. 23. Metastatic clear cell renal cell carcinoma to the ovary. Note the nested pattern and the interalveolar vascularity (H&E, original magnification x40).

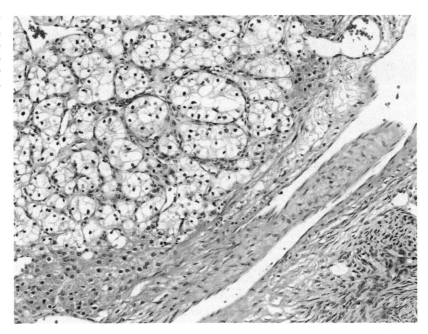

clinical history is essential, especially during intraoperative pathologic assessments. Metastatic CCRCC in the ovary is most frequently unilateral, with a small size (mean, 3.7 cm), and is typically devoid of ovarian surface nodules.[199] As such, its gross appearance is not immediately suggestive of metastases.[199] Microscopically, metastatic CCRCC shows the distinctive nested alveolar pattern with interalveolar stromal vascularity and cells with mostly clear cytoplasm (**Fig. 23**). Solid areas in CCC are frequently nested, but the nests are much larger, and stromal vascularity is not characteristic. In addition, solid patterns in CCC are usually admixed with other patterns and are rarely predominant. In contrast, tubulocystic patterns, small rounded papillae, and hobnail cells are not seen in metastatic CCRCC. By immunohistochemistry, both express PAX8 and HNF1β; CA-IX, CD10, and renal cell carcinoma antigen are more frequently expressed in CCRCC than CCC, whereas Napsin A, CK7, and p504S showed the opposite pattern.

REFERENCES

1. Sampson JA. Endometrial carcinoma of the ovary arising in endometrial tissue in that organ. Arch Surg 1925;10:1–72.
2. Thompson JD. Primary ovarian adenoacanthoma; its relationship to endometriosis. Obstet Gynecol 1957;9:403–16.
3. Long ME, Taylor HC Jr. Endometrioid carcinoma of the ovary. Am J Obstet Gynecol 1964;90:936–50.
4. Peham H. Aus accessorischen nebennierenanlagenentstandene. Ovarial tumoren. Monatsschr F Geburtsh U Gynak 1899;10:685–94.
5. Saphir O, Lackner JE. Adenocarcinoma with clear cells (hypernephroid) of the ovary. Surg Gynec Obstet 1944;79:539.
6. Schiller W. Mesonephroma ovarii. Am J Cancer 1939;35:1–21.
7. Novak ER, Woodruff JD. Mesonephroma of the ovary; thirty-five cases from the Ovarian Tumor Registry of the American Gynecological Society. Am J Obstet Gynecol 1959;77:632–44.
8. Parker TM, Dockerty MB, Randall LM. Mesonephric clear cell carcinoma of the ovary: a clinical and pathologic study. Am J Obstet Gynecol 1960;80:417–25.
9. Kay S, Hoge RH. Mesonephric carcinomas of the ovary. Surg Gynecol Obstet 1958;107:84–94.
10. Bowles HE, Tilden IL. Mesonephric carcinoma of the ovary; report of a case. Obstet Gynecol 1957; 9:64–70.
11. Teilum G. Endodermal sinus tumors of the ovary and testis. Comparative morphogenesis of the so-called mesonephroma ovarii (Schiller) and extra-embryonic (yolk sac-allantoic) structures of the rat's placenta. Cancer 1959;12:1092–105.
12. Young RH. The yolk sac tumor: reflections on a remarkable neoplasm and two of the many intrigued by it–Gunnar Teilum and Aleksander Talerman–and the bond it formed between them. Int J Surg Pathol 2014;22:677–87.
13. Scully RE, Barlow JF. "Mesonephroma" of ovary. Tumor of Müllerian nature related to the endometrioid carcinoma. Cancer 1967;20:1405–17.

14. Serov SF, Scully RE, Sobin LH. Histologic typing of ovarian tumours in international histological classification of tumours, vol. 9. Geneva (Switzerland): World Health Organization; 1973. p. 51–3.

15. Machado-Linde F, Sánchez-Ferrer ML, Cascales P, et al. Prevalence of endometriosis in epithelial ovarian cancer. Analysis of the associated clinical features and study on molecular mechanisms involved in the possible causality. Eur J Gynaecol Oncol 2015;36:21–4.

16. Jimbo H, Yoshikawa H, Onda T, et al. Prevalence of ovarian endometriosis in epithelial ovarian cancer. Int J Gynaecol Obstet 1997;59:245–50.

17. Dzatic-Smiljkovic O, Vasiljevic M, Djukic M, et al. Frequency of ovarian endometriosis in epithelial ovarian cancer patients. Clin Exp Obstet Gynecol 2011;38:394–8.

18. Boyraz G, Selcuk I, Yazıcıoğlu A, et al. Ovarian carcinoma associated with endometriosis. Eur J Obstet Gynecol Reprod Biol 2013;170:211–3.

19. Wang S, Qiu L, Lang JH, et al. Clinical analysis of ovarian epithelial carcinoma with coexisting pelvic endometriosis. Am J Obstet Gynecol 2013;208:413.e1-5.

20. Yoshikawa H, Jimbo H, Okada S, et al. Prevalence of endometriosis in ovarian cancer. Gynecol Obstet Invest 2000;50(Suppl 1):11–7.

21. Van Gorp T, Amant F, Neven P, et al. Endometriosis and the development of malignant tumours of the pelvis. A review of literature. Best Pract Res Clin Obstet Gynaecol 2004;18:349–71.

22. Brinton LA, Gridley G, Persson I, et al. Cancer risk after a hospital discharge diagnosis of endometriosis. Am J Obstet Gynecol 1997;176:572–9.

23. Kim HS, Kim TH, Chung HH, et al. Risk and prognosis of ovarian cancer in women with endometriosis: a meta-analysis. Br J Cancer 2014;110:1878–90.

24. Matalliotakis M, Matalliotaki C, Goulielmos GN, et al. Association between ovarian cancer and advanced endometriosis. Oncol Lett 2018;15:7689–92.

25. Nishida M, Watanabe K, Sato N, et al. Malignant transformation of ovarian endometriosis. Gynecol Obstet Invest 2000;50(Suppl 1):18–25.

26. Dinkelspiel HE, Matrai C, Pauk S, et al. Does the presence of endometriosis affect prognosis of ovarian cancer? Cancer Invest 2016;34:148–54.

27. Wang S, Qiu L, Lang JH, et al. Prognostic analysis of endometrioid epithelial ovarian cancer with or without endometriosis: a 12-year cohort study of Chinese patients. Am J Obstet Gynecol 2013;209:241.e1-9.

28. Cuff J, Longacre TA. Endometriosis does not confer improved prognosis in ovarian carcinoma of uniform cell type. Am J Surg Pathol 2012;36:688–95.

29. Bounous VE, Ferrero A, Fuso L, et al. Endometriosis-associated ovarian cancer: a distinct clinical entity? Anticancer Res 2016;36:3445–9.

30. Erzen M, Rakar S, Klancnik B, et al. Endometriosis-associated ovarian carcinoma (EAOC): an entity distinct from other ovarian carcinomas as suggested by a nested case-control study. Gynecol Oncol 2001;83:100–8.

31. Kumar S, Munkarah A, Arabi H, et al. Prognostic analysis of ovarian cancer associated with endometriosis. Am J Obstet Gynecol 2011;204:63.e1-7.

32. Barreta A, Sarian L, Ferracini AC, et al. Endometriosis-associated ovarian cancer: population characteristics and prognosis. Int J Gynecol Cancer 2018;28:1251–7.

33. Ye S, Yang J, You Y, et al. Comparative study of ovarian clear cell carcinoma with and without endometriosis in People's Republic of China. Fertil Steril 2014;102:1656–62.

34. Komiyama S, Aoki D, Tominaga E, et al. Prognosis of Japanese patients with ovarian clear cell carcinoma associated with pelvic endometriosis: clinicopathologic evaluation. Gynecol Oncol 1999;72:342–6.

35. Schnack TH, Høgdall E, Thomsen LN, et al. Demographic, clinical, and prognostic factors of ovarian clear cell adenocarcinomas according to endometriosis status. Int J Gynecol Cancer 2017;27:1804–12.

36. Park JY, Kim DY, Suh DS, et al. Significance of ovarian endometriosis on the prognosis of ovarian clear cell carcinoma. Int J Gynecol Cancer 2018;28:11–8.

37. Clement PB. The pathology of endometriosis: a survey of the many faces of a common disease emphasizing diagnostic pitfalls and unusual and newly appreciated aspects. Adv Anat Pathol 2007;14:241–60.

38. LaGrenade A, Silverberg SG. Ovarian tumors associated with atypical endometriosis. Hum Pathol 1988;19:1080–4.

39. Fukunaga M, Nomura K, Ishikawa E, et al. Ovarian atypical endometriosis: its close association with malignant epithelial tumours. Histopathology 1997;30:249–55.

40. Fukunaga M, Ushigome S. Epithelial metaplastic changes in ovarian endometriosis. Mod Pathol 1998;11:784–8.

41. Stamp JP, Gilks CB, Wesseling M, et al. BAF250a expression in atypical endometriosis and endometriosis-associated ovarian cancer. Int J Gynecol Cancer 2016;26:825–32.

42. Er TK, Su YF, Wu CC, et al. Targeted next-generation sequencing for molecular diagnosis of endometriosis-associated ovarian cancer. J Mol Med (Berl) 2016;94:835–47.

43. Gadducci A, Lanfredini N, Tana R. Novel insights on the malignant transformation of endometriosis into ovarian carcinoma. Gynecol Endocrinol 2014;30:612–7.

44. Anglesio MS, Bashashati A, Wang YK, et al. Multifocal endometriotic lesions associated with cancer are clonal and carry a high mutation burden. J Pathol 2015;236:201–9.

45. Anglesio MS, Papadopoulos N, Ayhan A, et al. Cancer-associated mutations in endometriosis without cancer. N Engl J Med 2017;376:1835–48.

46. Zou Y, Zhou JY, Guo JB, et al. The presence of KRAS, PPP2R1A and ARID1A mutations in 101 Chinese samples with ovarian endometriosis. Mutat Res 2018;809:1–5.

47. Wendel JRH, Wang X, Hawkins SM. The endometriotic tumor microenvironment in ovarian cancer. Cancers (Basel) 2018;10(8), [pii:E261].

48. Cochrane DR, Tessier-Cloutier B, Lawrence KM, et al. Clear cell and endometrioid carcinomas: are their differences attributable to distinct cells of origin? J Pathol 2017;243:26–36.

49. Noë M, Ayhan A, Wang TL, et al. Independent development of endometrial epithelium and stroma within the same endometriosis. J Pathol 2018;245:265–9.

50. Alsop K, Fereday S, Meldrum C, et al. BRCA mutation frequency and patterns of treatment response in BRCA mutation-positive women with ovarian cancer: a report from the Australian Ovarian Cancer Study Group. J Clin Oncol 2012;30:2654–63.

51. Wiegand KC, Shah SP, Al-Agha OM, et al. ARID1A mutations in endometriosis-associated ovarian carcinomas. N Engl J Med 2010;363:1532–43.

52. Kuo KT, Mao TL, Jones S, et al. Frequent activating mutations of PIK3CA in ovarian clear cell carcinoma. Am J Pathol 2009;174:1597–601.

53. McConechy MK, Anglesio MS, Kalloger SE, et al. Subtype-specific mutation of PPP2R1A in endometrial and ovarian carcinomas. J Pathol 2011;223:567–73.

54. Mayr D, Hirschmann A, Löhrs U, et al. KRAS and BRAF mutations in ovarian tumors: a comprehensive study of invasive carcinomas, borderline tumors and extraovarian implants. Gynecol Oncol 2006;103:883–7.

55. Sato N, Tsunoda H, Nishida M, et al. Loss of heterozygosity on 10q23.3 and mutation of the tumor suppressor gene PTEN in benign endometrial cyst of the ovary: possible sequence progression from benign endometrial cyst to endometrioid carcinoma and clear cell carcinoma of the ovary. Cancer Res 2000;60:7052–6.

56. Kuo KT, Mao TL, Chen X, et al. DNA copy numbers profiles in affinity-purified ovarian clear cell carcinoma. Clin Cancer Res 2010;16:1997–2008.

57. Friedlander ML, Russell K, Millis S, et al. Molecular profiling of clear cell ovarian cancers: identifying potential treatment targets for clinical trials. Int J Gynecol Cancer 2016;26:648–54.

58. Yamashita Y, Akatsuka S, Shinjo K, et al. Met is the most frequently amplified gene in endometriosis-associated ovarian clear cell adenocarcinoma and correlates with worsened prognosis. PLoS One 2013;8:e57724.

59. Yamamoto S, Tsuda H, Takano M, et al. Loss of ARID1A protein expression occurs as an early event in ovarian clear-cell carcinoma development and frequently coexists with PIK3CA mutations. Mod Pathol 2012;25:615–24.

60. Zannoni GF, Improta G, Pettinato A, et al. Molecular status of PI3KCA, KRAS and BRAF in ovarian clear cell carcinoma: an analysis of 63 patients. J Clin Pathol 2016;69:1088–92.

61. Yamamoto S, Tsuda H, Miyai K, et al. Accumulative copy number increase of MET drives tumor development and histological progression in a subset of ovarian clear-cell adenocarcinomas. Mod Pathol 2012;25:122–30.

62. Zannoni GF, Improta G, Chiarello G, et al. Mutational status of KRAS, NRAS, and BRAF in primary clear cell ovarian carcinoma. Virchows Arch 2014;465:193–8.

63. Rechsteiner M, Zimmermann AK, Wild PJ, et al. TP53 mutations are common in all subtypes of epithelial ovarian cancer and occur concomitantly with KRAS mutations in the mucinous type. Exp Mol Pathol 2013;95:235–41.

64. Wu RC, Ayhan A, Maeda D, et al. Frequent somatic mutations of the telomerase reverse transcriptase promoter in ovarian clear cell carcinoma but not in other major types of gynaecological malignancy. J Pathol 2014;232:473–81.

65. Willis BC, Sloan EA, Atkins KA, et al. Mismatch repair status and PD-L1 expression in clear cell carcinomas of the ovary and endometrium. Mod Pathol 2017;30:1622–32.

66. Jones S, Wang TL, Shih IeM, et al. Frequent mutations of chromatin remodeling gene ARID1A in ovarian clear cell carcinoma. Science 2010;330(6001):228–31.

67. Yamamoto S, Tsuda H, Takano M, et al. PIK3CA mutations and loss of ARID1A protein expression are early events in the development of cystic ovarian clear cell adenocarcinoma. Virchows Arch 2012;460:77–87.

68. Samartzis EP, Noske A, Dedes KJ, et al. ARID1A mutations and PI3K/AKT pathway alterations in endometriosis and endometriosis-associated ovarian carcinomas. Int J Mol Sci 2013;14:18824–49.

69. Chene G, Ouellet V, Rahimi K, et al. The ARID1A pathway in ovarian clear cell and endometrioid carcinoma, contiguous endometriosis, and benign endometriosis. Int J Gynaecol Obstet 2015;130:27–30.

70. Itamochi H, Oishi T, Oumi N, et al. Whole-genome sequencing revealed novel prognostic biomarkers and promising targets for therapy of ovarian clear cell carcinoma. Br J Cancer 2017;117:717–24.

71. Murakami R, Matsumura N, Brown JB, et al. Exome sequencing landscape analysis in ovarian clear cell carcinoma shed light on key chromosomal regions and mutation gene networks. Am J Pathol 2017;187:2246–58.

72. Oda K, Hamanishi J, Matsuo K, et al. Genomics to immunotherapy of ovarian clear cell carcinoma: unique opportunities for management. Gynecol Oncol 2018. https://doi.org/10.1016/j.ygyno.2018.09.001.

73. Kim SI, Lee JW, Lee M, et al. Genomic landscape of ovarian clear cell carcinoma via whole exome sequencing. Gynecol Oncol 2018;148:375–82.

74. Shibuya Y, Tokunaga H, Saito S, et al. Identification of somatic genetic alterations in ovarian clear cell carcinoma with next generation sequencing. Genes Chromosomes Cancer 2018;57:51–60.

75. Maru Y, Tanaka N, Ohira M, et al. Identification of novel mutations in Japanese ovarian clear cell carcinoma patients using optimized targeted NGS for clinical diagnosis. Gynecol Oncol 2017;144:377–83.

76. Abou-Taleb H, Yamaguchi K, Matsumura N, et al. Comprehensive assessment of the expression of the SWI/SNF complex defines two distinct prognostic subtypes of ovarian clear cell carcinoma. Oncotarget 2016;7:54758–70.

77. Rahman MT, Nakayama K, Rahman M, et al. Gene amplification of ZNF217 located at chr20q13.2 is associated with lymph node metastasis in ovarian clear cell carcinoma. Anticancer Res 2012;32:3091–5.

78. Rahman MT, Nakayama K, Rahman M, et al. Prognostic and therapeutic impact of the chromosome 20q13.2 ZNF217 locus amplification in ovarian clear cell carcinoma. Cancer 2012;118:2846–57.

79. Huang HN, Huang WC, Lin CH, et al. Chromosome 20q13.2 ZNF217 locus amplification correlates with decreased E-cadherin expression in ovarian clear cell carcinoma with PI3K-Akt pathway alterations. Hum Pathol 2014;45:2318–25.

80. Yamaguchi K, Mandai M, Oura T, et al. Identification of an ovarian clear cell carcinoma gene signature that reflects inherent disease biology and the carcinogenic processes. Oncogene 2010;29:1741–52.

81. Chang CM, Wang ML, Lu KH, et al. Integrating the dysregulated inflammasome-based molecular functionome in the malignant transformation of endometriosis-associated ovarian carcinoma. Oncotarget 2017;9:3704–26.

82. Zhang C, Wang X, Anaya Y, et al. Distinct molecular pathways in ovarian endometrioid adenocarcinoma with concurrent endometriosis. Int J Cancer 2018. https://doi.org/10.1002/ijc.31768.

83. Okamoto T, Mandai M, Matsumura N, et al. Hepatocyte nuclear factor-1β (HNF-1β) promotes glucose uptake and glycolytic activity in ovarian clear cell carcinoma. Mol Carcinog 2015;54:35–49.

84. Amano Y, Mandai M, Yamaguchi K, et al. Metabolic alterations caused by HNF1β expression in ovarian clear cell carcinoma contribute to cell survival. Oncotarget 2015;6(28):26002–17.

85. McConechy MK, Ding J, Senz J, et al. Ovarian and endometrial endometrioid carcinomas have distinct CTNNB1 and PTEN mutation profiles. Mod Pathol 2014;27:128–34.

86. Huang HN, Lin MC, Tseng LH, et al. Ovarian and endometrial endometrioid adenocarcinomas have distinct profiles of microsatellite instability, PTEN expression, and ARID1A expression. Histopathology 2015;66:517–28.

87. Bennett JA, Pesci A, Morales-Oyarvide V, et al. Incidence of mismatch repair protein deficiency and associated clinicopathologic features in a cohort of 104 ovarian endometrioid carcinomas. Am J Surg Pathol 2018. https://doi.org/10.1097/PAS.0000000000001165.

88. Rambau PF, Duggan MA, Ghatage P, et al. Significant frequency of MSH2/MSH6 abnormality in ovarian endometrioid carcinoma supports histotype-specific Lynch syndrome screening in ovarian carcinomas. Histopathology 2016;69:288–97.

89. Gras E, Catasus L, Argüelles R, et al. Microsatellite instability, MLH-1 promoter hypermethylation, and frameshift mutations at coding mononucleotide repeat microsatellites in ovarian tumors. Cancer 2001;92(11):2829–36.

90. Hoang LN, McConechy MK, Köbel M, et al. Polymerase epsilon exonuclease domain mutations in ovarian endometrioid carcinoma. Int J Gynecol Cancer 2015;25:1187–93.

91. Parra-Herran C, Lerner-Ellis J, Xu B, et al. Molecular-based classification algorithm for endometrial carcinoma categorizes ovarian endometrioid carcinoma into prognostically significant groups. Mod Pathol 2017;30(12):1748–59.

92. Nakonechny QB, Gilks CB. Ovarian cancer in hereditary cancer susceptibility syndromes. Surg Pathol Clin 2016;9:189–99.

93. Aysal A, Karnezis A, Medhi I, et al. Ovarian endometrioid adenocarcinoma: incidence and clinical significance of the morphologic and immunohistochemical markers of mismatch repair protein defects and tumor microsatellite instability. Am J Surg Pathol 2012;36:163–72.

94. Vierkoetter KR, Ayabe AR, VanDrunen M, et al. Lynch syndrome in patients with clear cell and endometrioid cancers of the ovary. Gynecol Oncol 2014;135:81–4.

95. Bennett JA, Morales-Oyarvide V, Campbell S, et al. Mismatch repair protein expression in clear cell carcinoma of the ovary: incidence and

morphologic associations in 109 cases. Am J Surg Pathol 2016;40:656–63.

96. Helder-Woolderink JM, Blok EA, Vasen HF, et al. Ovarian cancer in Lynch syndrome; a systematic review. Eur J Cancer 2016;55:65–73.

97. Zeimet AG, Mori H, Petru E, et al. AGO Austria recommendation on screening and diagnosis of Lynch syndrome (LS). Arch Gynecol Obstet 2017; 296:123–7.

98. Chui MH, Gilks CB, Cooper K, et al. Identifying Lynch syndrome in patients with ovarian carcinoma: the significance of tumor subtype. Adv Anat Pathol 2013;20(6):378–86.

99. Kurman RJ, Cancangiu ML, Herrington CS, et al. WHO classification of tumours of female reproductive organs. Lyon (France): IARC; 2014.

100. Peres LC, Cushing-Haugen KL, Anglesio M, et al. Histotype classification of ovarian carcinoma: a comparison of approaches. Gynecol Oncol 2018; 151:53–60.

101. Barnard ME, Pyden A, Rice MS, et al. Inter-pathologist and pathology report agreement for ovarian tumor characteristics in the Nurses' Health Studies. Gynecol Oncol 2018;150:521–6.

102. Lim D, Murali R, Murray MP, et al. Morphological and immunohistochemical reevaluation of tumors initially diagnosed as ovarian endometrioid carcinoma with emphasis on high-grade tumors. Am J Surg Pathol 2016;40:302–12.

103. Assem H, Rambau PF, Lee S, et al. High-grade endometrioid carcinoma of the ovary: a clinicopathologic study of 30 cases. Am J Surg Pathol 2018;42: 534–44.

104. Zheng G, Yu H, Kanerva A, et al. Familial risks of ovarian cancer by age at diagnosis, proband type and histology. PLoS One 2018;13(10): e0205000.

105. Grosso G, Raspagliesi F, Baiocchi G, et al. Endometrioid carcinoma of the ovary: a retrospective analysis of 106 cases. Tumori 1998;84:552–7.

106. Tidy J, Mason WP. Endometrioid carcinoma of the ovary: a retrospective study. Br J Obstet Gynaecol 1988;95:1165–9.

107. Storey DJ, Rush R, Stewart M, et al. Endometrioid epithelial ovarian cancer: 20 years of prospectively collected data from a single center. Cancer 2008; 112:2211–20.

108. Chen S, Leitao MM, Tornos C, et al. Invasion patterns in stage I endometrioid and mucinous ovarian carcinomas: a clinicopathologic analysis emphasizing favorable outcomes in carcinomas without destructive stromal invasion and the occasional malignant course of carcinomas with limited destructive stromal invasion. Mod Pathol 2005;18: 903–11.

109. Tornos C, Silva EG, Ordonez NG, et al. Endometrioid carcinoma of the ovary with a prominent spindle-cell component, a source of diagnostic confusion. A report of 14 cases. Am J Surg Pathol 1995;19(12):1343–53.

110. Terada T. Adenosquamous carcinoma of the ovary arising from endometriosis: two case reports. Cases J 2009;2:6661.

111. Silva EG, Young RH. Endometrioid neoplasms with clear cells: a report of 21 cases in which the alteration is not of typical secretory type. Am J Surg Pathol 2007;31:1203–8.

112. Pitman MB, Young RH, Clement PB, et al. Endometrioid carcinoma of the ovary and endometrium, oxyphilic cell type: a report of nine cases. Int J Gynecol Pathol 1994;13:290–301.

113. Eichhorn JH, Scully RE. Endometrioid ciliated-cell tumors of the ovary: a report of five cases. Int J Gynecol Pathol 1996;15:248–56.

114. Mansor S, McCluggage WG. Endometrioid adenocarcinoma of the ovary mimicking serous borderline tumor: report of a series of cases. Int J Gynecol Pathol 2014;33(5):470–6.

115. Ordi J, Schammel DP, Rasekh L, et al. Sertoliform endometrioid carcinomas of the ovary: a clinicopathologic and immunohistochemical study of 13 cases. Mod Pathol 1999;12:933–40.

116. Roth LM, Liban E, Czernobilsky B. Ovarian endometrioid tumors mimicking Sertoli and Sertoli-Leydig cell tumors: Sertoliform variant of endometrioid carcinoma. Cancer 1982;50(7):1322–31.

117. Young RH, Prat J, Scully RE. Ovarian endometrioid carcinomas resembling sex cord-stromal tumors. A clinicopathological analysis of 13 cases. Am J Surg Pathol 1982;6(6):513–22.

118. Fadare O, Zhao C, Khabele D, et al. Comparative analysis of Napsin A, alpha-methylacyl-coenzyme A racemase (AMACR, P504S), and hepatocyte nuclear factor 1 beta as diagnostic markers of ovarian clear cell carcinoma: an immunohistochemical study of 279 ovarian tumours. Pathology 2015;47: 105–11.

119. Parra-Herran C, Bassiouny D, Vicus D, et al. FIGO versus Silverberg grading systems in ovarian endometrioid carcinoma: a comparative prognostic analysis. Am J Surg Pathol 2018. https://doi.org/ 10.1097/PAS.0000000000001160.

120. Silverberg SG. Histopathologic grading of ovarian carcinoma: a review and proposal. Int J Gynecol Pathol 2000;19:7–15.

121. Torre LA, Trabert B, DeSantis CE, et al. Ovarian cancer statistics, 2018. CA Cancer J Clin 2018; 68:284–96.

122. Peres LC, Cushing-Haugen KL, Köbel M, et al. Invasive epithelial ovarian cancer survival by histotype and disease stage. J Natl Cancer Inst 2018. https://doi.org/10.1093/jnci/djy071.

123. Rambau P, Kelemen LE, Steed H, et al. Association of hormone receptor expression with survival in

ovarian endometrioid carcinoma: biological validation and clinical implications. Int J Mol Sci 2017; 18(3), [pii:E515].

124. Rambau PF, Vierkant RA, Intermaggio MP, et al. Association of p16 expression with prognosis varies across ovarian carcinoma histotypes: an Ovarian Tumor Tissue Analysis consortium study. J Pathol Clin Res 2018. https://doi.org/10.1002/cjp2.109.

125. Okuda T, Otsuka J, Sekizawa A, et al. p53 mutations and overexpression affect prognosis of ovarian endometrioid cancer but not clear cell cancer. Gynecol Oncol 2003;88:318–25.

126. Heckl M, Schmoeckel E, Hertlein L, et al. The ARID1A, p53 and ß-catenin statuses are strong prognosticators in clear cell and endometrioid carcinoma of the ovary and the endometrium. PLoS One 2018;13(2):e0192881.

127. Bell KA, Kurman RJ. A clinicopathologic analysis of atypical proliferative (borderline) tumors and well-differentiated endometrioid adenocarcinomas of the ovary. Am J Surg Pathol 2000;24:1465–79.

128. Roth LM, Emerson RE, Ulbright TM. Ovarian endometrioid tumors of low malignant potential: a clinicopathologic study of 30 cases with comparison to well-differentiated endometrioid adenocarcinoma. Am J Surg Pathol 2003;27:1253–9.

129. Bell DA, Scully RE. Atypical and borderline endometrioid adenofibromas of the ovary. A report of 27 cases. Am J Surg Pathol 1985;9:205–14.

130. Ramalingam P, Croce S, McCluggage WG. Loss of expression of SMARCA4 (BRG1), SMARCA2 (BRM) and SMARCB1 (INI1) in undifferentiated carcinoma of the endometrium is not uncommon and is not always associated with rhabdoid morphology. Histopathology 2017;70:359–66.

131. Coatham M, Li X, Karnezis AN, et al. Concurrent ARID1A and ARID1B inactivation in endometrial and ovarian dedifferentiated carcinomas. Mod Pathol 2016;29:1586–93.

132. Soslow RA, Han G, Park KJ, et al. Morphologic patterns associated with BRCA1 and BRCA2 genotype in ovarian carcinoma. Mod Pathol 2012;25: 625–36.

133. DeLair D, Oliva E, Köbel M, et al. Morphologic spectrum of immunohistochemically characterized clear cell carcinoma of the ovary: a study of 155 cases. Am J Surg Pathol 2011;35:36–44.

134. Mackenzie R, Talhouk A, Eshragh S, et al. Morphologic and molecular characteristics of mixed epithelial ovarian cancers. Am J Surg Pathol 2015;39:1548–57.

135. Ye S, You Y, Yang J, et al. Comparison of pure and mixed-type clear cell carcinoma of the ovary: a clinicopathological analysis of 341 Chinese patients. Int J Gynecol Cancer 2014;24:1590–6.

136. Fujibayashi M, Aiba M, Iizuka E, et al. Granulosa cell tumor-like variant of endometrioid carcinoma

of the ovary exhibiting nuclear clearing with biotin activity: a subtype showing close macroscopic, cytologic, and histologic similarity to adult granulosa cell tumor. Arch Pathol Lab Med 2005;129: 1288–94.

137. Zhao C, Bratthauer GL, Barner R, et al. Comparative analysis of alternative and traditional immunohistochemical markers for the distinction of ovarian Sertoli cell tumor from endometrioid tumors and carcinoid tumor: a study of 160 cases. Am J Surg Pathol 2007;31:255–66.

138. Zhao C, Barner R, Vinh TN, et al. SF-1 is a diagnostically useful immunohistochemical marker and comparable to other sex cord-stromal tumor markers for the differential diagnosis of ovarian Sertoli cell tumor. Int J Gynecol Pathol 2008;27: 507–14.

139. Zhao C, Vinh TN, McManus K, et al. Identification of the most sensitive and robust immunohistochemical markers in different categories of ovarian sex cord-stromal tumors. Am J Surg Pathol 2009;33: 354–66.

140. Schoolmeester JK, Keeney GL. Collision tumor of the ovary: adult granulosa cell tumor and endometrioid carcinoma. Int J Gynecol Pathol 2012;31: 538–40.

141. Judson K, McCormick C, Vang R, et al. Women with undiagnosed colorectal adenocarcinomas presenting with ovarian metastases: clinicopathologic features and comparison with women having known colorectal adenocarcinomas and ovarian involvement. Int J Gynecol Pathol 2008; 27:182–90.

142. Lee KR, Young RH. The distinction between primary and metastatic mucinous carcinomas of the ovary: gross and histologic findings in 50 cases. Am J Surg Pathol 2003;27:281–92.

143. Clement PB, Young RH, Scully RE. Endometrioid-like variant of ovarian yolk sac tumor. A clinicopathological analysis of eight cases. Am J Surg Pathol 1987;11:767–78.

144. Ramalingam P, Malpica A, Silva EG, et al. The use of cytokeratin 7 and EMA in differentiating ovarian yolk sac tumors from endometrioid and clear cell carcinomas. Am J Surg Pathol 2004;28:1499–505.

145. Cao D, Guo S, Allan RW, et al. SALL4 is a novel sensitive and specific marker of ovarian primitive germ cell tumors and is particularly useful in distinguishing yolk sac tumor from clear cell carcinoma. Am J Surg Pathol 2009;33:894–904.

146. Esheba GE, Pate LL, Longacre TA. Oncofetal protein glypican-3 distinguishes yolk sac tumor from clear cell carcinoma of the ovary. Am J Surg Pathol 2008;32:600–7.

147. Rutgers JL, Young RH, Scully RE. Ovarian yolk sac tumor arising from an endometrioid carcinoma. Hum Pathol 1987;18:1296–9.

148. Nogales FF, Bergeron C, Carvia RE, et al. Ovarian endometrioid tumors with yolk sac tumor component, an unusual form of ovarian neoplasm. Analysis of six cases. Am J Surg Pathol 1996;20(9): 1056–66.

149. Roth LM, Talerman A, Levy T, et al. Ovarian yolk sac tumors in older women arising from epithelial ovarian tumors or with no detectable epithelial component. Int J Gynecol Pathol 2011;30:442–51.

150. Gilks CB, Kommoss F. Synchronous tumours of the female reproductive tract. Pathology 2018;50: 214–21.

151. Anglesio MS, Wang YK, Maassen M, et al. Synchronous endometrial and ovarian carcinomas: evidence of clonality. J Natl Cancer Inst 2016;108: djv428.

152. Kelemen LE, Rambau PF, Koziak JM, et al. Synchronous endometrial and ovarian carcinomas: predictors of risk and associations with survival and tumor expression profiles. Cancer Causes Control 2017;28:447–57.

153. Ushijima K. Current status of gynecologic cancer in Japan. J Gynecol Oncol 2009;20:67–71.

154. Bennett JA, Dong F, Young RH, et al. Clear cell carcinoma of the ovary: evaluation of prognostic parameters based on a clinicopathological analysis of 100 cases. Histopathology 2015;66:808–15.

155. Crozier MA, Copeland LJ, Silva EG, et al. Clear cell carcinoma of the ovary: a study of 59 cases. Gynecol Oncol 1989;35:199–203.

156. Brescia RJ, Dubin N, Demopoulos RI. Endometrioid and clear cell carcinoma of the ovary. Factors affecting survival. Int J Gynecol Pathol 1989;8: 132–8.

157. Tang H, Liu Y, Wang X, et al. Clear cell carcinoma of the ovary: clinicopathologic features and outcomes in a Chinese cohort. Medicine (Baltimore) 2018;97(21):e10881.

158. Matsuura Y, Robertson G, Marsden DE, et al. Thromboembolic complications in patients with clear cell carcinoma of the ovary. Gynecol Oncol 2007;104:406–10.

159. Fadare O. Clear cell carcinomas of the gynecologic tract and thromboembolic events: what do we know so far? Womens Health (Lond) 2014;10: 479–81.

160. Duska LR, Garrett L, Henretta M, et al. When 'never-events' occur despite adherence to clinical guidelines: the case of venous thromboembolism in clear cell cancer of the ovary compared with other epithelial histologic subtypes. Gynecol Oncol 2010;116:374–7.

161. Savvari P, Peitsidis P, Alevizaki M, et al. Paraneoplastic humorally mediated hypercalcemia induced by parathyroid hormone-related protein in gynecologic malignancies: a systematic review. Onkologie 2009;32(8–9):517–23.

162. Doshi N, Tobon H. Primary clear cell carcinoma of the ovary. An analysis of 15 cases with review of the literature. Cancer 1977;39:2658–64.

163. Sangoi AR, Soslow RA, Teng NN, et al. Ovarian clear cell carcinoma with papillary features: a potential mimic of serous tumor of low malignant potential. Am J Surg Pathol 2008;32:269–74.

164. Young RH, Scully RE. Oxyphilic clear cell carcinoma of the ovary. A report of nine cases. Am J Surg Pathol 1987;11:661–7.

165. Zhao C, Wu LS, Barner R. Pathogenesis of ovarian clear cell adenofibroma, atypical proliferative (borderline) tumor, and carcinoma: clinicopathologic features of tumors with endometriosis or adenofibromatous components support two related pathways of tumor development. J Cancer 2011; 2:94–106.

166. Yamamoto S, Tsuda H, Yoshikawa T, et al. Clear cell adenocarcinoma associated with clear cell adenofibromatous components: a subgroup of ovarian clear cell adenocarcinoma with distinct clinicopathologic characteristics. Am J Surg Pathol 2007;31: 999–1006.

167. Veras E, Mao TL, Ayhan A, et al. Cystic and adenofibromatous clear cell carcinomas of the ovary: distinctive tumors that differ in their pathogenesis and behavior: a clinicopathologic analysis of 122 cases. Am J Surg Pathol 2009;33:844–53.

168. Yamamoto S, Tsuda H, Takano M, et al. Clear-cell adenofibroma can be a clonal precursor for clear-cell adenocarcinoma of the ovary: a possible alternative ovarian clear-cell carcinogenic pathway. J Pathol 2008;216:103–10.

169. Yamamoto S, Tsuda H, Suzuki K, et al. An allelotype analysis indicating the presence of two distinct ovarian clear-cell carcinogenic pathways: endometriosis-associated pathway vs. clear-cell adenofibroma-associated pathway. Virchows Arch 2009;455:261–70.

170. Bell DA, Scully RE. Benign and borderline clear cell adenofibromas of the ovary. Cancer 1985;56: 2922–31.

171. Roth LM, Langley FA, Fox H, et al. Ovarian clear cell adenofibromatous tumors. Benign, of low malignant potential, and associated with invasive clear cell carcinoma. Cancer 1984;53:1156–63.

172. Gu WY, Zhang LL, Zhang H, et al. Ovarian clear cell borderline tumour: a clinicopathologic analysis. Zhonghua Bing Li Xue Za Zhi 2018;47:622–6.

173. Fujimura M, Hidaka T, Kataoka K, et al. Absence of estrogen receptor-alpha expression in human ovarian clear cell adenocarcinoma compared with ovarian serous, endometrioid, and mucinous adenocarcinoma. Am J Surg Pathol 2001;25: 667–72.

174. Rekhi B, Deodhar KK, Menon S, et al. Napsin A and WT 1 are useful immunohistochemical markers for

differentiating clear cell carcinoma ovary from high-grade serous carcinoma. APMIS 2018;126:45–55.

175. Kandalaft PL, Gown AM, Isacson C. The lung-restricted marker napsin A is highly expressed in clear cell carcinomas of the ovary. Am J Clin Pathol 2014;142:830–6.

176. Montag AG, Jenison EL, Griffiths CT, et al. Ovarian clear cell carcinoma. A clinicopathologic analysis of 44 cases. Int J Gynecol Pathol 1989;8:85–96.

177. Yamamoto S, Tsuda H, Shimazaki H, et al. Histological grading of ovarian clear cell adenocarcinoma: proposal for a simple and reproducible grouping system based on tumor growth architecture. Int J Gynecol Pathol 2012;31:116–24.

178. Shu CA, Zhou Q, Jotwani AR, et al. Ovarian clear cell carcinoma, outcomes by stage: the MSK experience. Gynecol Oncol 2015;139:236–41.

179. Hoskins PJ, Le N, Gilks B, et al. Low-stage ovarian clear cell carcinoma: population-based outcomes in British Columbia, Canada, with evidence for a survival benefit as a result of irradiation. J Clin Oncol 2012;30:1656–62.

180. Higashi M, Kajiyama H, Shibata K, et al. Survival impact of capsule rupture in stage I clear cell carcinoma of the ovary in comparison with other histological types. Gynecol Oncol 2011;123:474–8.

181. Köbel M, Xu H, Bourne PA, et al. IGF2BP3 (IMP3) expression is a marker of unfavorable prognosis in ovarian carcinoma of clear cell subtype. Mod Pathol 2009;22:469–75.

182. Ayhan A, Kuhn E, Wu RC, et al. CCNE1 copy-number gain and overexpression identify ovarian clear cell carcinoma with a poor prognosis. Mod Pathol 2017;30:297–303.

183. Makii C, Oda K, Ikeda Y, et al. MDM2 is a potential therapeutic target and prognostic factor for ovarian clear cell carcinomas with wild type TP53. Oncotarget 2016;7:75328–38.

184. Morikawa A, Hayashi T, Kobayashi M, et al. Somatic copy number alterations have prognostic impact in patients with ovarian clear cell carcinoma. Oncol Rep 2018;40:309–18.

185. Itamochi H, Oumi N, Oishi T, et al. Fibroblast growth factor receptor 2 is associated with poor overall survival in clear cell carcinoma of the ovary and may be a novel therapeutic approach. Int J Gynecol Cancer 2015;25:570–6.

186. Shinjo K, Yamashita Y, Yamamoto E, et al. Expression of chromobox homolog 7 (CBX7) is associated with poor prognosis in ovarian clear cell adenocarcinoma via TRAIL-induced apoptotic pathway regulation. Int J Cancer 2014;135:308–18.

187. Min KW, Park MH, Hong SR, et al. Clear cell carcinomas of the ovary: a multi-institutional study of 129 cases in Korea with prognostic significance of Emi1 and Galectin-3. Int J Gynecol Pathol 2013;32:3–14.

188. Sekiya R, Kajiyama H, Sakai K, et al. Expression of CXCR4 indicates poor prognosis in patients with clear cell carcinoma of the ovary. Hum Pathol 2012;43:904–10.

189. Li B, Jin H, Yu Y, et al. HOXA10 is overexpressed in human ovarian clear cell adenocarcinoma and correlates with poor survival. Int J Gynecol Cancer 2009;19(8):1347–52.

190. Maeda D, Ota S, Takazawa Y, et al. Glypican-3 expression in clear cell adenocarcinoma of the ovary. Mod Pathol 2009;22:824–32.

191. Maeda D, Chen X, Guan B, et al. Rsf-1 (HBXAP) expression is associated with advanced stage and lymph node metastasis in ovarian clear cell carcinoma. Int J Gynecol Pathol 2011;30:30–5.

192. Matsuo K, Yoshino K, Hasegawa K, et al. Survival outcome of stage I ovarian clear cell carcinoma with lympho-vascular space invasion. Gynecol Oncol 2015;136:198–204.

193. Rahman M, Nakayama K, Rahman MT, et al. Clinicopathologic and biological analysis of PIK3CA mutation in ovarian clear cell carcinoma. Hum Pathol 2012;43:2197–206.

194. Young RH, Scully RE. Differential diagnosis of ovarian tumors based primarily on their patterns and cell types. Semin Diagn Pathol 2001;18:161–235.

195. Han G, Gilks CB, Leung S, et al. Mixed ovarian epithelial carcinomas with clear cell and serous components are variants of high-grade serous carcinoma: an interobserver correlative and immunohistochemical study of 32 cases. Am J Surg Pathol 2008;32:955–64.

196. DeLair D, Han G, Irving JA, et al. HNF-1β in ovarian carcinomas with serous and clear cell change. Int J Gynecol Pathol 2013;32:541–6.

197. Köbel M, Kalloger SE, Carrick J, et al. A limited panel of immunomarkers can reliably distinguish between clear cell and high-grade serous carcinoma of the ovary. Am J Surg Pathol 2009;33:14–21.

198. Nogales FF, Prat J, Schuldt M, et al. Germ cell tumour growth patterns originating from clear cell carcinomas of the ovary and endometrium: a comparative immunohistochemical study favouring their origin from somatic stem cells. Histopathology 2018;72:634–47.

199. Fadare O, Desouki MM, Gwin K, et al. Clear cell renal cell carcinoma metastatic to the gynecologic tract: a clinicopathologic analysis of 17 cases. Int J Gynecol Pathol 2018;37:525–35.

Mucinous Ovarian Tumors

Anne M. Mills, MD*, Elisheva D. Shanes, MD

KEYWORDS

- Ovarian mucinous tumors • Mucinous adenocarcinoma • Mucinous borderline tumor
- Mucinous cystadenoma

Key Points

- Ovarian mucinous tumors may show intestinal-type or, less commonly, endocervical-type morphology. Differentiating primary cases from gastrointestinal and endocervical metastases can therefore be challenging.

- Ovarian mucinous tumors range from benign cystadenomas to mucinous borderline tumors to frank adenocarcinomas. Each of these patterns may be mimicked by metastasis.

- Cystadenomas have no more than focal epithelial proliferation (<10%). Borderline tumors show more widespread epithelial proliferation and may exhibit intraepithelial carcinoma or even focal microinvasion.

- Concomitant findings often associated with primary ovarian mucinous tumors include Brenner tumors, teratomas, and sarcoma-like mural nodules.

- When confined to the ovary, all types of mucinous ovarian tumor have an good prognosis, however advanced stage adenocarcinomas have a very poor outcome.

ABSTRACT

Ovarian mucinous tumors range from benign cystadenomas to borderline tumors to frankly malignant adenocarcinomas, and may display either intestinal-type morphology or, less frequently, endocervical-type differentiation. The latter category has been the subject of recent controversy owing to its morphologic overlap with so-called "seromucinous" ovarian tumors, a group that shares more molecular features with endometrioid tumors than it does with either serous or mucinous ovarian neoplasias. Endocervical-type differentiation in ovarian mucinous tumors may also represent an endocervical metastasis. Distinction of primary ovarian mucinous tumors from gastrointestinal metastases can be difficult, as the morphology of intestinal-type ovarian mucinous primaries sometimes differs only subtly if at all from gastrointestinal metastases.

INTRODUCTORY PARAGRAPH

Ovarian mucinous tumors account for 15% of all primary ovarian tumors and present a variety of diagnostic challenges. First, they display a broad spectrum of appearances and behaviors ranging from benign cystadenomas to borderline tumors to frankly malignant adenocarcinomas. Appropriate classification can be particularly vexing because the recommended criteria have shifted over recent decades. Overdiagnosis of mucinous borderline tumors, for instance, was once common, and many cases that would have previously been assigned this distinction are now classified as cystadenomas. Second, primary ovarian tumors may display either intestinal-type morphology or, less frequently, endocervical-type differentiation. The latter category has been the subject of recent controversy owing to its morphologic overlap with so-called

---

Disclosure Statement: The authors have no relevant disclosures to report.
Department of Pathology, University of Virginia, PO Box 800214, 1215 Lee Street, Charlottesville, VA 22908, USA
* Corresponding author.
E-mail address: amm7r@virginia.edu

Surgical Pathology 12 (2019) 565–585
https://doi.org/10.1016/j.path.2019.01.008
1875-9181/19/© 2019 Elsevier Inc. All rights reserved.

"seromucinous" ovarian tumors, a group that shares more molecular features with endometrioid tumors than it does with either serous or mucinous neoplasias. Endocervical-type differentiation also presents challenges when the differential diagnosis includes an endocervical metastasis. Distinction from gastrointestinal metastases can be similarly difficult, as the morphology of intestinal-type ovarian mucinous primaries sometimes differs only subtly from gastrointestinal metastases. This morphologic overlap has led to contamination of the literature on this topic, with erroneous inclusion of extraovarian metastases in investigations on primary tumors. As a result, the aggressive potential of both borderline and malignant mucinous ovarian tumors has potentially been overestimated in some series.

GROSS FEATURES

Primary mucinous tumors of the ovary are typically unilateral and have a mean size of ~10 cm. Some tumors grow quite large, exceeding 30 cm. The tumor surface is usually smooth, even in malignant cases. On cross-section they are typically cystic and multiloculated with locules containing viscous fluid, although occasional benign tumors present as simple unilocular cysts. Unlike serous borderline tumors, mucinous borderline tumors tend to lack grossly prominent velvety excrescences. Solid areas may be appreciated in all mucinous tumor types because of varying contributions of fibrous stroma, and occasionally malignant tumors are almost entirely solid. The heterogeneous nature of mucinous tumors necessitates extensive sampling at the time of frozen section and for permanent microscopic examination, with 2 sections per centimeter of greatest tumor dimension representing a standard suggestion.[1–3] At the time of frozen section, 2 to 4 sections is reasonable. Solid areas or excrescences on the inner cyst wall are most likely to contain malignant foci and should be preferentially sampled.

Primary mucinous ovarian tumors are sometimes associated with teratomas; in this scenario, one may find corresponding gross features including hair, sebaceous material, and teeth.[4] The presence of these teratomatous components therefore does not exclude the possibility of a coexistent mucinous neoplasm, including potentially a mucinous carcinoma, and thus cystic or mucinous-appearing areas associated with teratomas should be sampled thoroughly, in the same manner as mucinous tumors not associated with teratoma.

MICROSCOPIC FEATURES

BENIGN (CYSTADENOMAS, CYSTADENOFIBROMAS)

Mucinous cystadenomas are composed of thin-walled cysts lined by a single layer of mucinous columnar cells with basally oriented nuclei (**Fig. 1**). The associated stroma is typically fibrous and, when abundant, merits classification of the tumor as mucinous cystadenofibroma. Stromal luteinization can often be appreciated (**Fig. 2**).

Small papillary formations can be seen, and when present, are typically characterized by stromal protrusions lined by a single layer of cells. Epithelial proliferation, stratification, and branching papillae should be rare (<10%) if present at all (**Fig. 3**). Tumors with less than 10% epithelial proliferation can be classified as "mucinous cystadenoma/cystadenofibroma with focal proliferation" with a comment that clarifies that the features are not sufficient for a diagnosis of borderline tumor.

BORDERLINE: MUCINOUS BORDERLINE TUMORS

Mucinous borderline tumors, also known as mucinous tumors of low malignant potential or atypical proliferative mucinous tumors, consist of variably-sized cysts with at least 10% of the total tumor area demonstrating epithelial stratification with small papillae or tufts.[2,5–7] Often, the lining cells show some degree of maturation from the base to the surface. Importantly, the tumors often show heterogeneity with cystadenoma-like areas admixed with more classical borderline architecture (**Fig. 4**). The constituent cells most often show intestinal-type morphology, although gastric-type cells may be present. The background stroma ranges from fibrous to edematous to collagenous, and stromal luteinization may be seen. A subset of tumors demonstrate acellular mucin pools within the stroma, and granulomatous responses to ruptured glands and extracellular mucin may present.[3,6] Associated necrosis may be prominent and is not associated with increased risk of malignancy.

Mucinous borderline tumors can show foci of intraepithelial carcinoma, which are defined by the presence of overtly malignant cytologic features (hyperchromasia, prominent nucleoli, and a significantly increased mitotic count) confined to the epithelium[2,5–7] (**Fig. 5**). Although these proliferations are typically associated with some focal cribriform architecture, the presence of such architecture in the absence of atypia does not

Fig. 1. Mucinous cystadenoma. These tumors are composed of thin-walled cysts with a fibrous stroma (*A*) lined by a single layer of mucinous columnar cells with basally oriented nuclei (*B*).

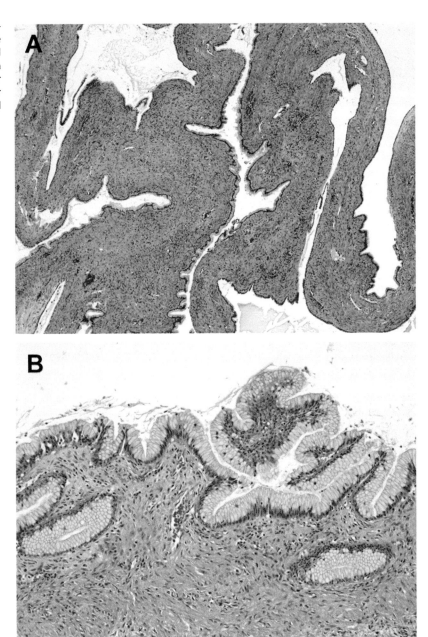

warrant an intraepithelial carcinoma diagnosis (**Fig. 6**). Gland cribriforming should be only focal and should not result in confluent, expansile growth, as that is consistent with a form of "true" invasion. The presence of intraepithelial carcinoma should be included in the diagnostic line ("mucinous borderline tumor with intraepithelial carcinoma").

Foci of stromal microinvasion are also permitted within the diagnostic umbrella of mucinous borderline tumors, provided those foci measure less than 5 mm in greatest dimension.[2,5–7]

Microinvasion is defined as isolated tumor cells in clear lacunae; irregular glands embedded in reactive stroma; small foci of cribriform growth; or nests of cells associated with extracellular mucin.[2,7,8] Some authors suggest that the presence of microinvasion warrants a bottom-line diagnosis of "borderline tumor with microinvasion," or "borderline tumor with microinvasive carcinoma," with the former term reserved for cytologically low-grade cases and the latter applying to cases with more marked cytologic atypia.[8–10]

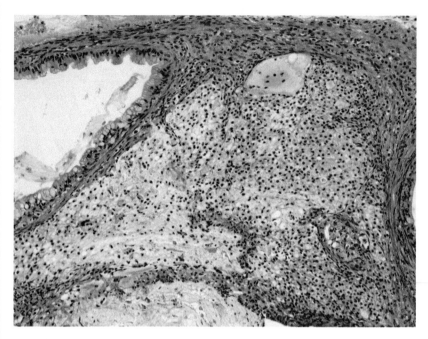

Fig. 2. Stromal luteinization in the wall of a mucinous cystadenoma.

MALIGNANT (MUCINOUS ADENOCARCINOMAS)

The vast majority of primary mucinous adenocarcinomas exhibit a morphologic spectrum that includes admixed benign, borderline, and malignant morphologies[1,5,8] (**Fig. 7**). The malignant areas are cytologically atypical with brisk mitotic activity (**Fig. 8**). Invasion is most often expansile and characterized by confluent glandular growth with pushing borders, which is admittedly a subjective determination. Infiltrative growth with destructive invasion by jagged glands embedded in desmoplastic stroma is less common, and when present should raise concern for metastasis (particularly in the setting of bilaterality).

ASSOCIATED FINDINGS (TERATOMAS, BRENNER TUMORS, AND MURAL NODULES)

Mucinous ovarian tumors are affiliated with mature cystic teratomas with some frequency, and may therefore be juxtaposed with the various

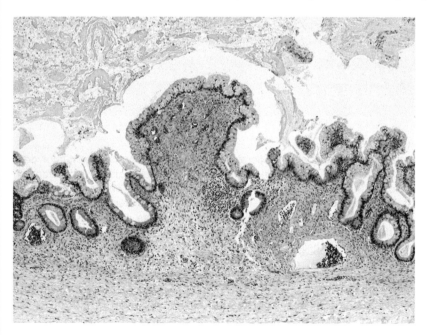

Fig. 3. Mucinous cystadenoma with small papillary formations composed of stromal protrusions lined by a single layer of mucinous cells. Note the absence of epithelial proliferation, stratification, or branching papillae.

Fig. 4. Mucinous border-line tumor. (*A*) The wall of this cystic tumor demonstrates one side with a simple lining as seen in a cystadenoma (bottom of cyst wall), whereas the opposite side demonstrates epithelial stratification with small papillae (*A*) (top of cyst wall) and (*B*) higher magnification.

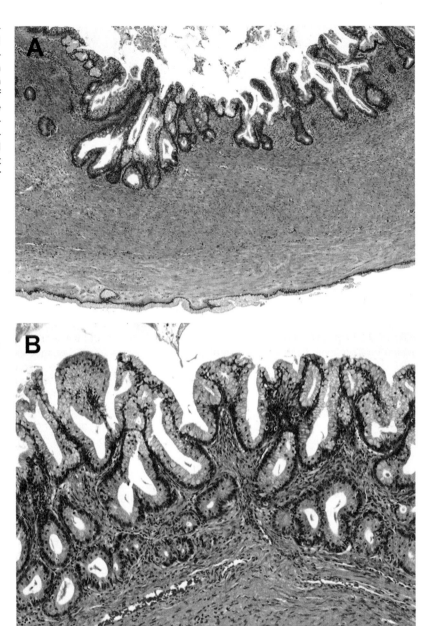

well-developed elements that can be found in teratomas (eg, squamous epithelium, sebaceous units, adipose, cartilage, thyroid tissue), as well as with neoplasms that derive from teratomas, such as carcinoid tumors (**Fig. 9**). There is some evidence that at least a subset of intestinal-type mucinous tumors ultimately derive from teratomas, and that the glandular pattern is either monophasic or has simply overgrown the other teratomatous elements.[4,11,12]

In addition to occurring in tandem with teratomas, ovarian mucinous tumors are often associated with Brenner tumors[13] (see **Fig. 9**). The solid

stroma of the Brenner component may provoke concern for malignancy grossly, but microscopic review reveals reassuringly banal nests of transitional-type epithelium embedded in fibrous stroma.

Mural nodules can also be seen in association with ovarian mucinous neoplasms and come in 3 types: sarcoma-like mural nodules, anaplastic carcinoma, and sarcomatous nodules. Sarcoma-like mural nodules are well-circumscribed, reactive proliferations of atypical spindled cells associated with inflammation and, often, areas of hemorrhage (**Fig. 10**). Bizarre and osteoclast-like multinucleated

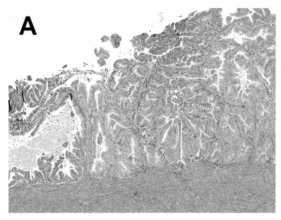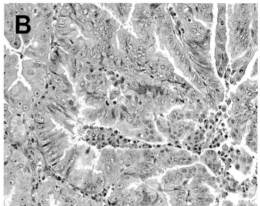

Fig. 5. Mucinous borderline tumor with intraepithelial carcinoma. This tumor exhibits architectural complexity together with malignant nuclear features (prominent nucleoli, mitoses), all confined to the epithelium. Note that to be classified as intraepithelial carcinoma, this growth pattern must be focal and not result in confluent, expansile growth, which would merit designation as invasive carcinoma. In this instance, the proliferation was limited to this field (A: low power; B: high-power highlighting cytologic atypia.).

cells are common, and mitoses may be abundant. Despite their eye-catching appearance, these are benign proliferations. Critically, cytokeratin is typically entirely absent or at most very focal.[14]

Pathologic key features

Mucinous cystadenomas/cystadenofibromas:
- Simple lining
- Cytologically bland
- Less than 10% epithelial proliferation
- Variable contributions of fibrous stroma

Mucinous borderline tumors:
- Greater than 10% epithelial proliferation with stratification and tufting
- May demonstrate focal intraepithelial carcinoma
- May demonstrate microinvasion (<5 mm)
- Often admixed with cystadenoma-like areas

Mucinous adenocarcinomas:
- Glandular complexity, atypical cytology, and brisk mitotic activity
- Expansile growth with confluent glands and pushing borders
- Infiltrative invasion less common
- Often mixed with areas of benign and borderline morphology

Anaplastic carcinomas and sarcomatous nodules, in contrast, are malignant proliferations associated with adenocarcinomas which lack the inflammation and circumscription that typifies their benign mimic. Anaplastic carcinomas demonstrate pleomorphic cytology but are strongly keratin positive. Sarcomatous nodules may be keratin negative but demonstrate rhabdoid to fibrosarcomatous morphology.

DIFFERENTIAL DIAGNOSIS

DISTINCTION FROM OTHER OVARIAN TUMORS

Mucinous differentiation can be seen in a variety of primary ovarian histotypes. Endometrioid ovarian carcinomas, for example, may demonstrate mucinous metaplasia as is often observed in endometrial endometrioid carcinomas. In such cases, the mucinous features are typically endocervical type and admixed with conventional endometrioid morphology. Squamous metaplasia is a common concomitant finding and is useful in securing the endometrioid histotype classification. Also in the differential is the relatively recently described category of seromucinous ovarian tumors. This controversial group is characterized by admixed endocervical-type mucinous, serous, endometrioid, and squamous morphologies[15–17] (**Fig. 11**). Some authors have argued that the seromucinous terminology is a misnomer as they are really more akin to endometrioid and clear cell carcinomas based on their association with endometriosis and frequent *ARID1A* mutations.[17] The term "mixed Müllerian tumor" has therefore been proposed as a more biologically appropriate

Fig. 6. This mucinous borderline tumor has foci of cribriform growth, but no associated cytologic atypia. The focal architecture alone does not warrant a diagnosis of intraepithelial carcinoma. (A: low-power; B: high power of cribriform area).

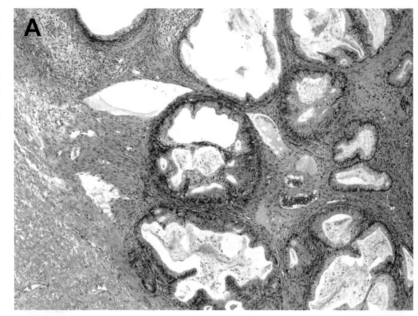

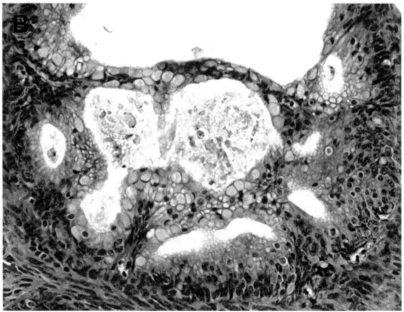

descriptor of this entity, but runs the risk of generating confusion with carcinosarcomas.[17] For the purposes of this differential, the presence of multiple admixed histotypes essentially excludes a conventional mucinous ovarian primary. Although it can been argued based on immunohistochemical and molecular evidence that even mucinous tumors showing pure endocervical-type differentiation are better lumped with their seromucinous sisters rather than grouped with intestinal-type mucinous primaries,[18] this distinction has not yet permeated formal classification systems.[5]

DISTINCTION FROM METASTASES

One of the chief diagnostic challenges in ovarian mucinous neoplasia is the exclusion of metastasis. Gastrointestinal metastases of gastric, appendiceal, intestinal, and pancreatobiliary origin may all mimic primary ovarian mucinous tumors.[19–22] The classic Krukenberg tumor, defined as a poorly differentiated carcinoma with greater than 10% signet ring component, rarely presents difficulties as this morphology is associated with metastasis in the vast majority of instances[23] (**Fig. 12**). More

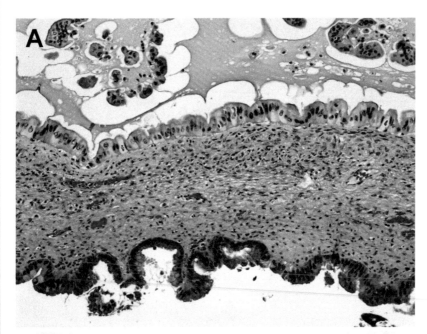

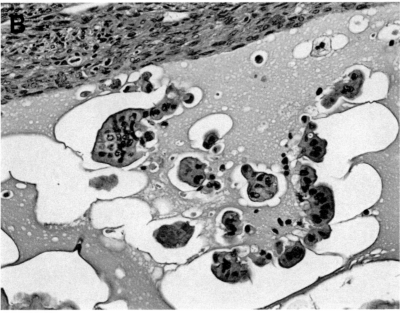

Fig. 7. Mucinous adeno-carcinoma of the ovary. This tumor had features of cystadenoma (single layer of bland mucinous epithelium, *A*, top of cyst wall), borderline tumor (proliferative epithelium with tufts, *A*, bottom of cyst wall), as well as a frankly malignant component that included free-floating malignant cells within intracystic mucin (*B*).

challenging, however, are tumors with classical intestinal or pancreatobiliary-type features as these can closely imitate ovarian primaries (**Fig. 13**). Metastases from colorectal sites are particularly problematic when the primary has not yet been identified, as these individuals often present at a younger age with an elevated serum CA125 and no symptoms referable to the bowel.[24] Pancreatic metastases may similarly masquerade as ovarian primaries owing to frequent unilaterality and histology that recapitulates benign, borderline, and/or

malignant ovarian mucinous tumors.[20,21] Ovarian involvement by appendiceal tumors may also run the histologic gamut from benign to malignant mucinous morphology.[19]

Less commonly, the endocervix represents the nidus of origin for ovarian mucinous tumors.[9] Both human papillomavirus (HPV)-associated and HPV-unassociated endocervical primaries can occasionally spread to the ovary, and can display both conventional endocervical-type differentiation as well as intestinal-type morphology (**Fig. 14**). Most

Fig. 8. Mucinous adeno-carcinoma. This prolifera-tion demonstrates architectural complexity with a broad-based, push-ing border (*A*), which is the most common pattern of invasion for primary ovarian adeno-carcinomas. Higher po-wer (*B*) reveals marked cytologic atypia and crib-riform growth.

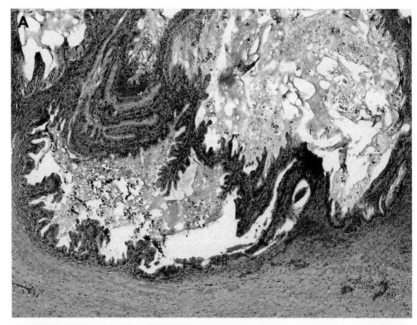

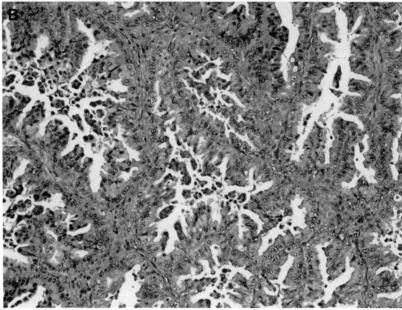

ovarian metastases from endocervical primaries demonstrate borderline-like growth characterized by confluent glandular and villogulandular patterns with limited to absent infiltration.[9] In some in-stances, the prior cervical pathology reveals only adenocarcinoma in situ with no evidence of inva-sion[9,25,26] Whether adenocarcinoma in situ truly bears the capacity for ovarian spread remains somewhat controversial, although retrograde spread represents a putative mechanism of involvement even in the absence of true invasion.

Clinically speaking, it is important to consider endo-cervical derivation in women with a history of endo-cervical neoplasia, even if those lesions were classified as in situ. In addition, if an ovarian mucinous tumor displays prominent features seen in HPV-associated cervical adenocarcinoma, such as apical mitoses and conspicuous apoptotic bodies, consideration should be given for metas-tasis from the endocervix; this diagnostic consider-ation is easily resolved with immunohistochemistry (p16) and/or in situ hybridization for HPV.

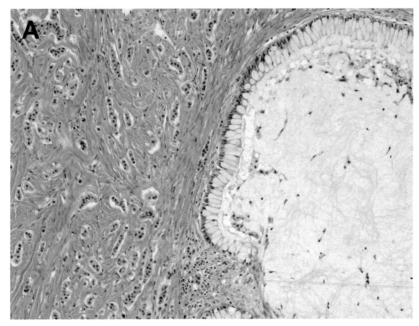

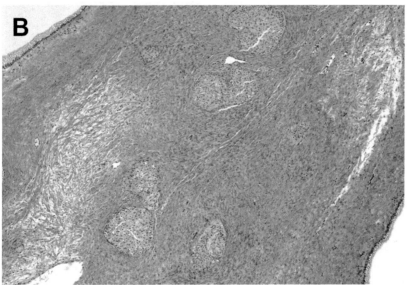

Fig. 9. Ovarian tumors with concomitant pathology. (*A*) Mucinous cystadenoma associated with a carcinoid tumor deriving from a mature cystic teratoma. (*B*) Mucinous cystadenoma associated with a Brenner tumor.

Whether the differential diagnosis includes gastrointestinal or endocervical primaries, the features favoring metastasis include bilaterality, microscopic epithelial surface involvement, and infiltrative stromal growth[27] (**Fig. 15**). Less-sensitive but more specific are nodular growth, ovarian hilar involvement, signet ring cells, single-cell invasion, vascular invasion, and microscopic surface mucin (see **Fig. 15**). Pseudomyxoma peritoneii is also more often associated with extraovarian sites of origin (most often appendiceal) rather than ovarian primaries.[28] In contrast, expansive growth type of invasion, unilateral tumors with size greater than 10 cm, and a smooth external surface usually suggest ovarian origin.[27] Associated Brenner tumors, teratomatous components, and/or sarcoma-like mural nodules also argue against metastasis. Features that have proven unhelpful in differentiating between primaries and metastases include the nature of the cyst contents, stromal mucin, hemorrhage, an intestinal-type appearance (including goblet cells), and tumor grade[27] (**Fig. 16**).

Differential diagnosis I
DISTINCTION FROM OTHER OVARIAN TUMORS

Tumor Characteristics	Ovarian Mucinous Tumors	Ovarian Endometrioid Tumors	Ovarian Seromucinous Tumors
Mucinous morphology	Intestinal-type > endocervical-type	Endocervical-type only	Endocervical-type only
Other associated tumor histologies	Brenner tumor; mature teratomas; sarcoma-like mural nodules	Endometrioid morphology; squamous metaplasia	Serous features, endometrioid, and squamous morphology
Endometriosis association	No	Yes	Yes
Immunohistochemistry	Intestinal-type ER-PR-negative; endocervical-type variable	Often ER/PR-positive	Often ER/PR-positive
Molecular	• *KRAS, CDKN2A* mutations common • *TP53* mutations seen in 50% of adenocarcinomas • Subset (10%–15%) of adenocarcinomas show HER2 amplification • No association with *PTEN* mutations or MMRd	• *ARID1A* and *CTNNB1* mutations common • *PTEN* mutations seen in 10%–20% • Subset (~10%) show MMRd	*ARID1A* mutations common

Abbreviations: ER, estrogen receptor; MMRd, mismatch repair deficiency; PR, progesterone receptor.

ΔΔ	Differential diagnosis II DISTINCTION FROM METASTASIS	
	Ovarian Mucinous Primary	**Metastasis**
Laterality	Unilateral >>> Bilateral	Bilateral > Unilateral
Size	Often >10 cm	Rarely >10 cm
Growth pattern	Usually expansile	Usually infiltrative, may show nodular growth and/or single-cell invasion
Lymphovascular invasion	Usually absent	Often present
Surface involvement	Usually absent	Often present; may also see acellular surface mucin
Hilar involvement	Usually absent	Often present
Associated ovarian findings	May see associated teratomas, Brenner tumors, and/or sarcoma-like mural nodules	Associated ovarian pathology typically absent
Associated extraovarian findings	• Only rarely associated with pseudomyxoma peritoneii • Other extraovarian findings typically absent	• May have known or suspected gastrointestinal or endocervical neoplasia by clinical history, imaging, and/or intraoperative findings • Pseudomyxoma peritoneii in a subset of cases, particularly with appendiceal primaries
Immunohistochemistry/ancillary studies	• SATB2 usually negative • PAX8 may be positive (but not always) • CK7 often diffuse but may be patchy or absent in intestinal-type • CK20 and CDX2 may be positive in intestinal-type • ER may be positive, particularly in endocervical-type • HPV-negative	• SATB2 usually positive in gastrointestinal metastasis • PAX8 usually negative • ER usually negative • CK7 usually negative in lower GI metastases but may be diffuse in endocervical and upper GI metastases • HPV-positive and p16-positive in endocervical metastases *when primary is HPV-associated*

Abbreviation: GI, gastrointestinal.

DIAGNOSIS

The diagnosis of ovarian mucinous tumors relies most heavily on tumor morphology and clinical correlation. In particular, the classification of ovarian primaries into benign, borderline, and malignant categories is exclusively based on histologic impressions derived from well-sampled tumors (**Fig. 17**). In challenging cases, a return to the specimen for additional sampling can be invaluable, and supersedes the potential of any ancillary study for informing the diagnosis.

Although of essentially no utility in the classification of primary tumors into benign, borderline, or malignant, ancillary studies can play an important role when the differential diagnosis is ovarian primary versus metastasis. It is worth emphasizing that such studies should be used as supplements to a clear understanding of the clinical scenario, and that any concern for a metastasis should

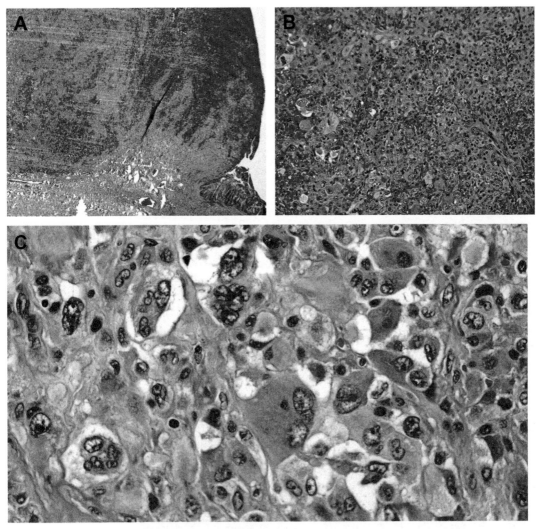

Fig. 10. Sarcoma-like mural nodule in the wall of a benign mucinous tumor. This well-circumscribed nodule (*A*) is associated with hemorrhage and is composed of reactive cells including epithelioid and spindled cells (*B*), as well as bizarre osteoclast-like multinucleated cells (*C*). (*Courtesy of* Dr Kriztina Hanley, Emory University Department of Pathology, Atlanta, GA.)

prompt an inquiry into the history and imaging findings, a conversation with the clinical team regarding other potential primary sites, and any appropriate intraoperative assessment such as running the bowel and consideration for appendectomy.

IMMUNOHISTOCHEMISTRY

Immunohistochemical stains have been used to varying effect to differentiate between primary ovarian tumors and metastases. CK7 often shows diffuse expression in primary ovarian tumors, endocervical metastases, and upper gastrointestinal metastases, but is typically limited or absent in

tumors of lower gastrointestinal origin, whereas CK20 and CDX2 classically show the inverse pattern of expression.[29,30] In practice, however, the expression profiles of all three of these markers can show tremendous overlap across individual tumors.

The relatively new immunomarker SATB2, which was first identified through mining of the Human Protein Atlas expression database, has proven much more useful for the work-up of possible gastrointestinal metastasis as its expression is extremely uncommon among ovarian primaries but typical of gastrointestinal tumors of both lower and upper origin,[31,32] (**Fig. 18**). The transcription factor PAX8, in contrast, is expressed

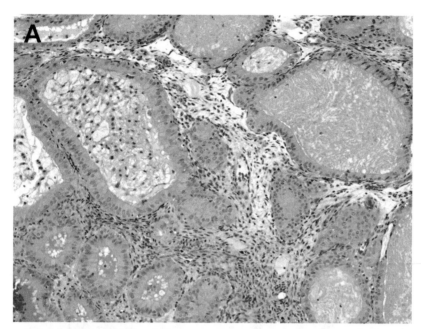

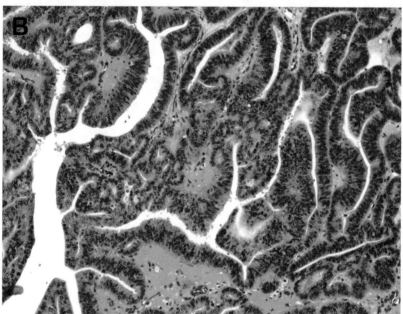

Fig. 11. Seromucinous borderline tumor demonstrating a mix of morphologies, including endocervical-type mucinous (*A*) and endometrioid (*B*) differentiation. The presence of admixed histotypes excludes a diagnosis of conventional mucinous ovarian primary.

by a significant number of ovarian mucinous primaries but is uncommon among metastatic gastric, colorectal, and pancreatobiliary tumors.[31] Estrogen receptor is also highly specific for ovarian origin but has extremely limited sensitivity.[31] Notably, even the specificity of this marker cannot be expected to be entirely perfect as gastric cancers may occasionally express estrogen receptor.[33] To this end generally a panel of immunohistochemical markers is most helpful.

IN SITU HYBRIDIZATION

Human papillomavirus RNA in situ hybridization can be invaluable in the work-up of ovarian mucinous tumors with a differential that includes involvement by HPV-associated endocervical neoplasia, as shared strong HPV positivity is expected in both the ovarian mass and endocervical primary when the former represents a metastasis (see **Fig. 14**).[9,25,26] It is important to emphasize, however, that such ancillary testing

Fig. 12. Krukenberg tumors. Krukenberg tumors may demonstrate abundant extracellular mucin (*A*) or may be predominantly solid (*B*). This poorly differentiated signet ring morphology is not typical of ovarian mucinous primary adenocarcinomas and almost always represents a metastasis.

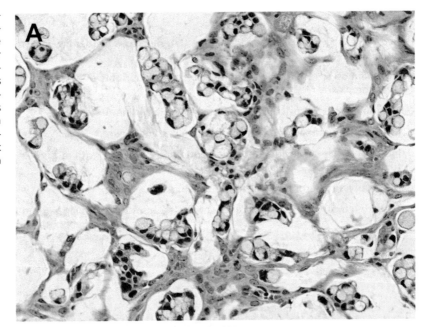

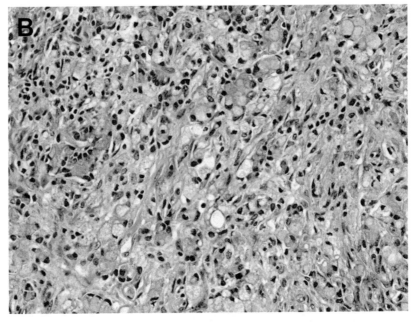

fails to narrow the differential for rare cases wherein an endocervical tumor is HPV unassociated.

MOLECULAR

Molecular studies do not currently play a significant role in ovarian mucinous tumor diagnosis, but may prove useful for prognostication and directing targeted therapy in the future. *KRAS* mutations are identified in most ovarian mucinous tumors and are thought to represent a key early event in neoplastic progression.[34] The *CDKN2A* gene, which encodes the p16 tumor suppressor protein, is also commonly mutated in borderline tumors and adenocarcinomas.[35–37] Roughly half of malignant cases will also show mutations involving *TP53*.[37] Finally, a subset (15%–20%) of ovarian mucinous adenocarcinomas will demonstrate HER2 overexpression and/or amplification, suggesting a possible role for targeted therapy in some cases.[38,39]

Pitfalls

! Overclassifying a mucinous cystadenoma as a mucinous borderline tumor based on focal epithelial projections.

! Overdiagnosing a mucinous borderline tumor as a mucinous adenocarcinoma based on focal architectural complexity.

! Missing invasion associated with a mucinous borderline tumor.

! Misinterpreting a sarcoma-like mural nodule as malignant.

! Inappropriately classifying an ovarian endometrioid tumor with mucinous metaplasia as a mucinous tumor.

! Misclassifying a seromucinous tumor as a mucinous tumor.

! Mistaking a gastrointestinal or endocervical metastasis as an ovarian primary (and vice versa).

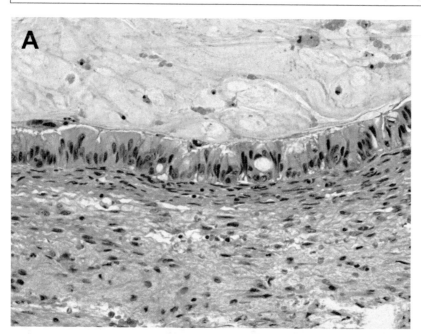

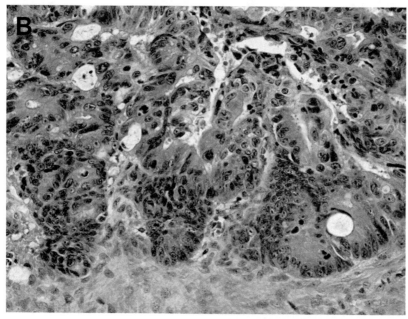

Fig. 13. Gastrointestinal metastasis with a spectrum of morphologies. Like primary ovarian mucinous tumors, metastases may demonstrate a histologic spectrum ranging from cytologically bland, cystadenoma-like areas (*A*) to frankly malignant morphologies (*B*).

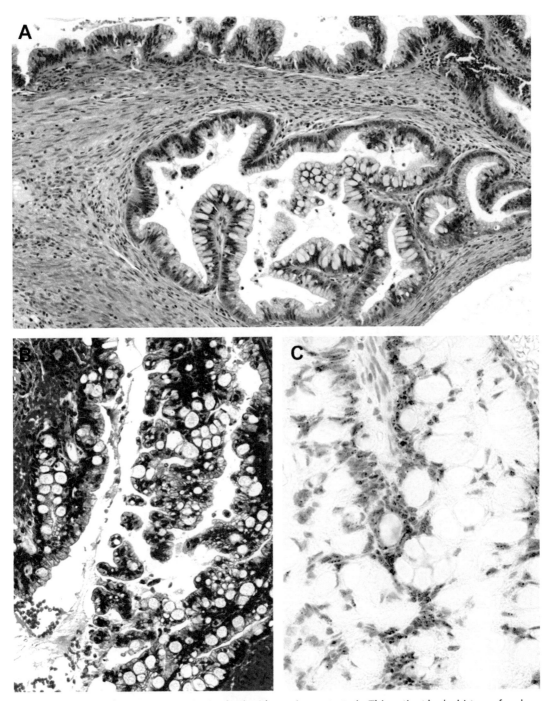

Fig. 14. Endocervical adenocarcinoma in situ (AIS) with ovarian metastasis. This patient had a history of endocervical AIS (*A*) and presented with bilateral ovarian mucinous tumors (*B*). Both the endocervical AIS and the ovarian tumor demonstrated prominent intestinal-type differentiation. Human papillomavirus DNA PCR on both specimens revealed high-risk HPV, type 18, in the cervix and the ovary, and HPV RNA in situ hybridization was positive in the ovarian tumors. (*C*).

PROGNOSIS

Mucinous cystadenomas and cystadenofibromas are benign neoplasms that are managed by complete surgical resection. Mucinous borderline tumors have an excellent survival rate (5 years >95%) when the tumor is confined to the ovary at presentation.[1,7,10] In contrast to serous

582

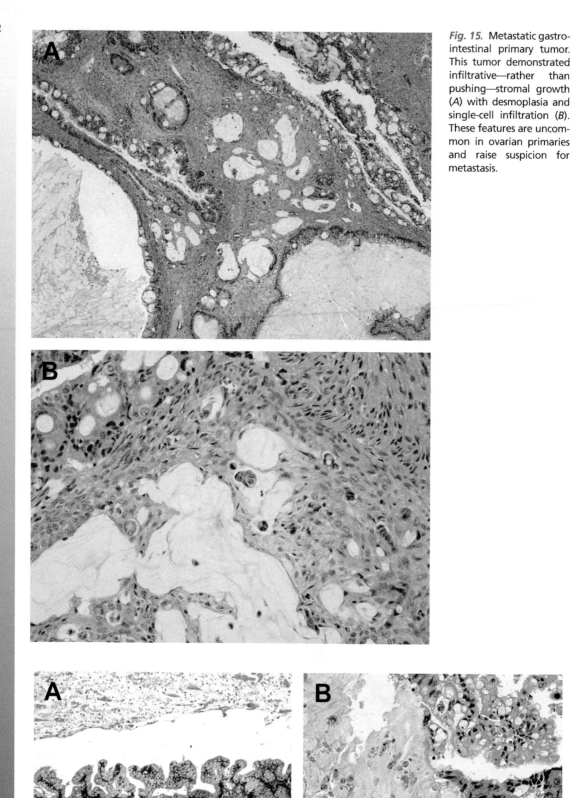

Fig. 15. Metastatic gastro-intestinal primary tumor. This tumor demonstrated infiltrative—rather than pushing—stromal growth (*A*) with desmoplasia and single-cell infiltration (*B*). These features are uncommon in ovarian primaries and raise suspicion for metastasis.

Fig. 16. Ovarian mucinous tumors with associated necrosis. Necrosis can be seen in association with ovarian primaries (*A*) and in metastases, particularly tumors of colorectal origin (*B*). Thus, whereas necrosis is often discussed as a feature supporting extraovarian origin, it should not be considered specific.

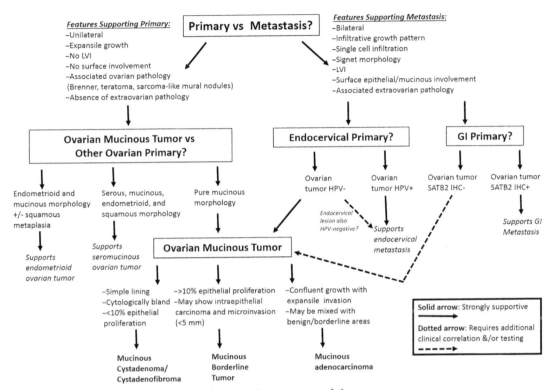

Fig. 17. Diagnostic algorithm for approaching mucinous tumors of the ovary.

borderline tumors, mucinous borderline tumors are not associated with peritoneal or omental studding.[40] Historically, some literature has reported very poor outcome for advanced-stage borderline tumors; however, subsequent reviews revealed that many of these studies were contaminated with both gastrointestinal metastases and primary tumors with frank invasion that ought to have been classified as adenocarcinomas.[7,41,42]

Stage I mucinous ovarian adenocarcinomas also have a good prognosis and the majority can be cured with resection.[43] Interestingly, foci of anaplastic carcinoma are actually associated with a favorable prognosis provided the tumor is confined to the ovary.[44] The outlook is less bright, however, for advanced-stage tumors. Although bona fide advanced-stage primary adenocarcinomas are rare (indeed, in 1 series by Zaino and

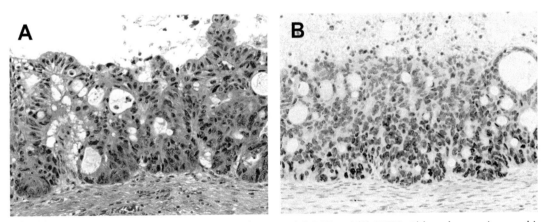

Fig. 18. SATB2 in a gastrointestinal metastasis to the ovary (A) H&E and (B) SATB2. Although many immunohistochemical markers have proven unhelpful for clarifying the site-of-origin for ovarian mucinous tumors, SATB2 has proven relatively sensitive and specific for gastrointestinal metastases.

colleagues[45] almost two-thirds of cases were reclassified as metastases on review), when they do occur they demonstrate a dismal prognosis, with an overall survival that is considerably lower than for advanced-stage serous carcinomas (~14 months versus 42 months in the series by Zaino and colleagues).[45] This poor outcome is thought to reflect not only an inherently aggressive tumor biology, but also resistance to currently available chemotherapeutic approaches.

REFERENCES

1. Chaitin BA, Gershenson DM, Evans HL. Mucinous tumors of the ovary. A clinicopathologic study of 70 cases. Cancer 1985;55(9):1958–62.
2. Silverberg SG, Bell DA, Kurman RJ, et al. Borderline ovarian tumors: key points and workshop summary. Hum Pathol 2004;35(8):910–7.
3. Rodriguez IM, Prat J. Mucinous tumors of the ovary: a clinicopathologic analysis of 75 borderline tumors (of intestinal type) and carcinomas. Am J Surg Pathol 2002;26(2):139–52.
4. Vang R, Gown AM, Zhao C, et al. Ovarian mucinous tumors associated with mature cystic teratomas: morphologic and immunohistochemical analysis identifies a subset of potential teratomatous origin that shares features of lower gastrointestinal tract mucinous tumors more commonly encountered as secondary tumors in the ovary. Am J Surg Pathol 2007;31(6):854–69.
5. Kurman RJ, International Agency for Research on Cancer, World Health Organization. WHO classification of tumours of female reproductive organs. 4th edition. Lyon (France): International Agency for Research on Cancer; 2014. p. 307.
6. Lee KR, Scully RE. Mucinous tumors of the ovary: a clinicopathologic study of 196 borderline tumors (of intestinal type) and carcinomas, including an evaluation of 11 cases with 'pseudomyxoma peritonei'. Am J Surg Pathol 2000;24(11):1447–64.
7. Riopel MA, Ronnett BM, Kurman RJ. Evaluation of diagnostic criteria and behavior of ovarian intestinal-type mucinous tumors: atypical proliferative (borderline) tumors and intraepithelial, microinvasive, invasive, and metastatic carcinomas. Am J Surg Pathol 1999;23(6):617–35.
8. Hoerl HD, Hart WR. Primary ovarian mucinous cystadenocarcinomas: a clinicopathologic study of 49 cases with long-term follow-up. Am J Surg Pathol 1998;22(12):1449–62.
9. Ronnett BM, Yemelyanova AV, Vang R, et al. Endocervical adenocarcinomas with ovarian metastases: analysis of 29 cases with emphasis on minimally invasive cervical tumors and the ability of the metastases to simulate primary ovarian neoplasms. Am J Surg Pathol 2008;32(12):1835–53.
10. Khunamornpong S, Russell P, Dalrymple JC. Proliferating (LMP) mucinous tumors of the ovaries with microinvasion: morphologic assessment of 13 cases. Int J Gynecol Pathol 1999;18(3):238–46.
11. Fujii K, Yamashita Y, Yamamoto T, et al. Ovarian mucinous tumors arising from mature cystic teratomas–a molecular genetic approach for understanding the cellular origin. Hum Pathol 2014;45(4):717–24.
12. Elias KM, Tsantoulis P, Tille JC, et al. Primordial germ cells as a potential shared cell of origin for mucinous cystic neoplasms of the pancreas and mucinous ovarian tumors. J Pathol 2018. https://doi.org/10.1002/path.5161.
13. Seidman JD, Khedmati F. Exploring the histogenesis of ovarian mucinous and transitional cell (Brenner) neoplasms and their relationship with Walthard cell nests: a study of 120 tumors. Arch Pathol Lab Med 2008;132(11):1753–60.
14. Bague S, Rodriguez IM, Prat J. Sarcoma-like mural nodules in mucinous cystic tumors of the ovary revisited: a clinicopathologic analysis of 10 additional cases. Am J Surg Pathol 2002;26(11):1467–76.
15. Taylor J, McCluggage WG. Ovarian seromucinous carcinoma: report of a series of a newly categorized and uncommon neoplasm. Am J Surg Pathol 2015;39(7):983–92.
16. Shappell HW, Riopel MA, Smith Sehdev AE, et al. Diagnostic criteria and behavior of ovarian seromucinous (endocervical-type mucinous and mixed cell-type) tumors: atypical proliferative (borderline) tumors, intraepithelial, microinvasive, and invasive carcinomas. Am J Surg Pathol 2002;26(12):1529–41.
17. Kurman RJ, Shih I. Seromucinous tumors of the ovary. what's in a name? Int J Gynecol Pathol 2016;35(1):78–81.
18. Vang R, Gown AM, Barry TS, et al. Immunohistochemistry for estrogen and progesterone receptors in the distinction of primary and metastatic mucinous tumors in the ovary: an analysis of 124 cases. Mod Pathol 2006;19(1):97–105.
19. Moore L, Gajjar K, Jimenez-Linan M, et al. Prevalence of appendiceal lesions in appendicectomies performed during surgery for mucinous ovarian tumors: a retrospective study. Int J Gynecol Cancer 2016;26(8):1386–9.
20. Young RH. From Krukenberg to today: the ever present problems posed by metastatic tumors in the ovary: part I. Historical perspective, general principles, mucinous tumors including the Krukenberg tumor. Adv Anat Pathol 2006;13(5):205–27.
21. Young RH. From Krukenberg to today: the ever present problems posed by metastatic tumors in the ovary. Part II. Adv Anat Pathol 2007;14(3):149–77.
22. Hristov AC, Young RH, Vang R, et al. Ovarian metastases of appendiceal tumors with goblet cell

carcinoidlike and signet ring cell patterns: a report of 30 cases. Am J Surg Pathol 2007;31(10):1502–11.

23. Kiyokawa T, Young RH, Scully RE. Krukenberg tumors of the ovary: a clinicopathologic analysis of 120 cases with emphasis on their variable pathologic manifestations. Am J Surg Pathol 2006;30(3): 277–99.

24. Judson K, McCormick C, Vang R, et al. Women with undiagnosed colorectal adenocarcinomas presenting with ovarian metastases: clinicopathologic features and comparison with women having known colorectal adenocarcinomas and ovarian involvement. Int J Gynecol Pathol 2008;27(2):182–90.

25. Chang MC, Nevadunsky NS, Viswanathan AN, et al. Endocervical adenocarcinoma in situ with ovarian metastases: a unique variant with potential for long-term survival. Int J Gynecol Pathol 2010;29(1): 88–92.

26. Shah AA, Mills AM, Nichols AR, et al. The pap smear caught it!: harmonizing the findings of an abnormal pap smear and a right ovarian mass. Diagn Cytopathol 2015;43(12):1039–41.

27. Lee KR, Young RH. The distinction between primary and metastatic mucinous carcinomas of the ovary: gross and histologic findings in 50 cases. Am J Surg Pathol 2003;27(3):281–92.

28. Prayson RA, Hart WR, Petras RE. Pseudomyxoma peritonei. A clinicopathologic study of 19 cases with emphasis on site of origin and nature of associated ovarian tumors. Am J Surg Pathol 1994;18(6): 591–603.

29. Vang R, Gown AM, Barry TS, et al. Cytokeratins 7 and 20 in primary and secondary mucinous tumors of the ovary: analysis of coordinate immunohistochemical expression profiles and staining distribution in 179 cases. Am J Surg Pathol 2006;30(9):1130–9.

30. Vang R, Gown AM, Wu LS, et al. Immunohistochemical expression of CDX2 in primary ovarian mucinous tumors and metastatic mucinous carcinomas involving the ovary: comparison with CK20 and correlation with coordinate expression of CK7. Mod Pathol 2006;19(11):1421–8.

31. Strickland S, Wasserman JK, Giassi A, et al. Immunohistochemistry in the diagnosis of mucinous neoplasms involving the ovary: the added value of SATB2 and biomarker discovery through protein expression database mining. Int J Gynecol Pathol 2016;35(3):191–208.

32. Schmoeckel E, Kirchner T, Mayr D. SATB2 is a supportive marker for the differentiation of a primary mucinous tumor of the ovary and an ovarian metastasis of a low-grade appendiceal mucinous neoplasm (LAMN): a series of seven cases. Pathol Res Pract 2018;214(3):426–30.

33. Tang W, Liu R, Yan Y, et al. Expression of estrogen receptors and androgen receptor and their clinical significance in gastric cancer. Oncotarget 2017; 8(25):40765–77.

34. Lee YJ, Lee MY, Ruan A, et al. Multipoint Kras oncogene mutations potentially indicate mucinous carcinoma on the entire spectrum of mucinous ovarian neoplasms. Oncotarget 2016;7(50):82097–103.

35. Bowden NA, Smyth M, Jaaback K, et al. Genetic changes correlate with histopathology in a benign, borderline and malignant mucinous ovarian tumour. J Obstet Gynaecol 2016;36(1):119–21.

36. Mackenzie R, Kommoss S, Winterhoff BJ, et al. Targeted deep sequencing of mucinous ovarian tumors reveals multiple overlapping RAS-pathway activating mutations in borderline and cancerous neoplasms. BMC Cancer 2015;15. https://doi.org/10. 1186/s12885-015-1421-8.

37. Ryland GL, Hunter SM, Doyle MA, et al. Mutational landscape of mucinous ovarian carcinoma and its neoplastic precursors. Genome Med 2015;7(1). https://doi.org/10.1186/s13073-015-0210-y.

38. McAlpine JN, Wiegand KC, Vang R, et al. HER2 overexpression and amplification is present in a subset of ovarian mucinous carcinomas and can be targeted with trastuzumab therapy. BMC Cancer 2009;9. https://doi.org/10.1186/1471-2407-9-433.

39. Mohammed RAA, Makboul R, Elsers DAH, et al. Pattern of HER-2 gene amplification and protein expression in benign, borderline, and malignant ovarian serous and mucinous neoplasms. Int J Gynecol Pathol 2017;36(1):50–7.

40. De Decker K, Speth S, Ter Brugge HG, et al. Staging procedures in patients with mucinous borderline tumors of the ovary do not reveal peritoneal or omental disease. Gynecol Oncol 2017;144(2):285–9.

41. Guerrieri C, Hogberg T, Wingren S, et al. Mucinous borderline and malignant tumors of the ovary. A clinicopathologic and DNA ploidy study of 92 cases. Cancer 1994;74(8):2329–40.

42. Kaern J, Trope CG, Abeler VM. A retrospective study of 370 borderline tumors of the ovary treated at the Norwegian radium hospital from 1970 to 1982. A review of clinicopathologic features and treatment modalities. Cancer 1993;71(5):1810–20.

43. Schiavone MB, Herzog TJ, Lewin SN, et al. Natural history and outcome of mucinous carcinoma of the ovary. Am J Obstet Gynecol 2011;205(5):480.e1-8.

44. Provenza C, Young RH, Prat J. Anaplastic carcinoma in mucinous ovarian tumors: a clinicopathologic study of 34 cases emphasizing the crucial impact of stage on prognosis, their histologic spectrum, and overlap with sarcomalike mural nodules. Am J Surg Pathol 2008;32(3):383–9.

45. Zaino RJ, Brady MF, Lele SM, et al. Advanced stage mucinous adenocarcinoma of the ovary is both rare and highly lethal: a gynecologic oncology group study. Cancer 2011;117(3):554–62.

Practical Review of Ovarian Sex Cord–Stromal Tumors

Krisztina Z. Hanley, MD[a],*, Marina B. Mosunjac, MD[b]

KEYWORDS

- Sex cord–stromal tumor • Immunohistochemistry • DICER1 syndrome • Histomorphology

ABSTRACT

Ovarian sex cord–stromal tumors are uncommon tumors and clinically differ from epithelial tumors. They occur across a wide age range and patients often present with hormone-related symptoms. Most are associated with an indolent clinical course. Sex cord–stromal tumors are classified into 3 main categories: pure stromal tumors, pure sex cord tumors, and mixed sex cord–stromal tumors. The rarity, overlapping histomorphology and immunoprofile of various sex cord–stromal tumors often contributes to diagnostic difficulties. This article describes the various types of ovarian sex cord–stromal tumors and includes practical approaches to differential diagnoses and updates in classification.

OVERVIEW

Sex cord–stromal tumors (SCSTs) of the ovary are uncommon nonepithelial tumors that encompass a heterogeneous group of neoplasms with variable clinical presentation, morphologic features, behavior, and prognosis. Benign stromal tumors represent 0.5% to 3.7% of all benign ovarian tumors. SCSTs are the fifth most common ovarian malignancy and account for approximately 5% to 8% of all ovarian malignancies, with a yearly incidence rate of 2.1 per 1 million women.[1] Most cases are indolent and slow growing, but some are aggressive and have a fatal clinical course. The morphologic appearance may be highly variable within 1 tumor type, and there is morphologic and immunohistochemical (IHC) overlap between different SCST types, as well as fluctuations in nomenclature, which contributes to the diagnostic challenges these tumors pose.[2] SCST nomenclature is intimidating. Even for the most enthusiastic fan of histology and embryology, it is challenging to picture and immediately place the sex cord cells in one of the defined morphologic and embryologic categories.

To date, the true origin of gonadal sex cords is still controversial. Although some investigators support their derivations from coelomic epithelium, others favor an origin from mesenchyme. More recently, the possibility of mesonephric derivation of the sex cord was proposed.[2] Sex cords, also called primitive sex cords or gonadal cords, are structures that develop from the embryologic gonadal ridges. After sexual differentiation, sex cords in boys become testis cords, which helps to develop and nourish Sertoli cells and are precursors to the rete testis. In girls sex cords become cortical cords, also called secondary cords. After further development they give rise to cells surrounding the oocyte and forming the granulosa cells of the follicle.[3]

Ovarian stroma is highly vascular and may contain a variety of cells in addition to ordinary spindle-shaped connective tissue, such as Leydig cells, luteinized stromal cells, decidual cells, smooth muscle cells, and neuroendocrine cells. Ovarian stroma differs from typical connective tissue in that it is highly cellular, appears whorled or storiform, and may acquire endocrine function. Theca cells are the stromal cells associated with ovarian follicles that play an essential role in fertility

[a] Department of Pathology, Emory University Hospital, Rm H-187, 1364 Clifton Road, Northeast, Atlanta, GA 30322, USA; [b] Department of Pathology, Grady Memorial Hospital, 80 Jesse Hill Jr Dr SE, Atlanta, GA 38303, USA

* Corresponding author.

E-mail address: khanley@emory.edu

Surgical Pathology 12 (2019) 587–620
https://doi.org/10.1016/j.path.2019.02.005
1875-9181/19/© 2019 Elsevier Inc. All rights reserved.

surgpath.theclinics.com

by producing the androgen substrate required for ovarian estrogen biosynthesis.[3]

The most recent World Health Organization (WHO) classification divides SCSTs according to the cell of origin into 3 major groups (**Box 1**): pure stromal tumors that originate from ovarian stromal cells, pure sex cord tumors that originate from sex cord, and mixed tumors that have origins from both sex cord and stromal cells.[4] Two new pure stromal tumors are now recognized by the 2014 WHO classification of tumors of the female reproductive system: microcystic stromal tumor and luteinized thecoma associated with sclerosing peritonitis.

Gynandroblastoma is entirely excluded from the new classification.

Box 1
World Health Organization classification scheme for ovarian sex cord–stromal tumors, 2014.

Pure stromal tumors
Fibroma

Cellular fibroma

Thecoma

Luteinized thecoma associated with sclerosing peritonitis

Fibrosarcoma

Sclerosing stromal tumor

Signet ring stromal tumor

Microcystic stromal tumor

Leydig cell tumor

Steroid cell tumor

Steroid cell tumor, malignant

Pure sex cord tumors

Adult granulosa cell tumor

Juvenile granulosa cell tumor

Sertoli cell tumor

Sex cord tumor with annular tubules

Mixed sex cord–stromal tumors

Sertoli-Leydig cell tumor

  Well differentiated

  Moderately differentiated

    With heterologous elements

  Poorly differentiated

    With heterologous elements

  Retiform

    With heterologous elements

Sex cord–stromal tumors, NOS

Abbreviation: NOS, not otherwise specified.

From Burandt E, Young RH. Thecoma of the ovary: a report of 70 cases emphasizing aspects of its histopathology different from those often portrayed and its differential diagnosis. Am J Surg Pathol 2014;38(8):1023–32; with permission.

CLINICAL PRESENTATION, GROSS AND MICROSCOPIC MORPHOLOGY OF SEX CORD–STROMAL TUMORS

PURE STROMAL TUMORS: CLINICAL PRESENTATION

Pure stromal tumors of the ovary are uncommon; however, fibroma and thecoma account for almost 90% of all SCSTs, and fibromas are by far the most common spindle cell tumors of the ovary (**Table 1**).[1]

In general, women with pure stromal tumors present with similar symptoms as women with ovarian epithelial neoplasms, which is abdominal or pelvic pain with the discovery of adnexal mass on imaging or physical examination. In addition, various age-specific clinical symptoms caused by hormone secretion (estrogens or androgens) may be observed, such as precocious puberty in children, abnormal uterine bleeding, or postmenopausal bleeding.[4–6]

In addition, fibroma can be associated with Meigs syndrome or basal cell nevus (Gorlin) syndrome. The more well-known Meigs syndrome is found in only 1% to 2% of patients and is defined as presence of pleural effusion and ascites that resolves after tumor excision.[7] Patients with Meigs syndrome may present with increased cancer antigen (CA) 125 and mimic symptoms of ovarian carcinoma.[8,9] When ovarian fibroma is associated with basal cell nevus syndrome it usually occurs in younger women, and it is almost always bilateral, multiple, and calcified.[10,11]

Luteinized thecoma with sclerosing peritonitis often presents with abdominal pain, ascites, and bowel obstruction caused by the diffuse sclerosing peritoneal process.[12]

Treatment of the most of the tumors in this category is conservative excisional surgery with excellent prognosis, with a few exceptions. The exceptions are ovarian fibrosarcoma, which portends a poor prognosis, and malignant steroid cell tumors, which are treated with debulking surgery and staging followed by chemotherapy and radiation.[13]

Table 1
Clinical presentation of pure stromal tumors

	Age (y)	Presentation	Associated Syndrome	Treatment Prognosis
Fibroma	>30 Average 48	Abdominal pain Ascites Pleural effusion (Meigs syndrome) No hormonal manifestations	Gorlin syndrome Meigs syndrome	Oophorectomy Excellent
Cellular fibroma	Same as fibroma	Same as fibroma	Same as fibroma	Same as fibroma
Thecoma	Postmenopausal Mean 60	Estrogenic presentation Uterine bleeding	None	Same as fibroma
Fibrosarcoma	Postmenopausal women Average 58	None or abdominal pain and ascites	None	Poor
Sclerosing stromal tumor	Young patients <30	Abdominal pain Ascites Estrogenic and androgenic symptoms rare Most are nonfunctioning	None	Same as fibroma
Signet ring stromal tumor	Reproductive age Average 36	Abdominal pain Ascites Nonfunctioning	None	Same as fibroma
Microcystic stromal tumor	Wide age range (26–63) Average 45	Abdominal pain Pelvic mass Rare hormonal manifestations	None	Same as fibroma
Leydig cell tumor	Wide range (32–82)	Androgen symptoms in 80%	None	Same as fibroma
Steroid cell tumor	Wide age range Average 43	Androgen symptoms 50% Estrogen 10%	Rarely Cushing syndrome	Salpingo-oophorectomy
Steroid cell tumor, malignant	Same as benign steroid tumors	Same as benign steroid tumors	None	Salpingo-oophorectomy and hysterectomy

Data from IARC. WHO Classification of Tumours of the Female Reproductive Organs. Geneva (Switzerland): World Health Organization; 2014.

PURE STROMAL TUMORS: GROSS, MICROSCOPIC, AND IMMUNOHISTOCHEMICAL FEATURES

Fibroma, Cellular Fibroma, and Fibrosarcoma

Ovarian fibromas are the most commonly encountered stromal tumors, and their cytologically bland interlacing or storiform fascicles rarely pose a diagnostic challenge (Fig. 1, Table 2). Diagnostic dilemmas occur if the tumor shows increased cellularity, mitotic activity, or cytologic atypia. Increased cellularity in the absence of cytologic atypia and without increased mitotic activity warrants a diagnosis of cellular fibroma. Mitotic activity greater than 4 per 10 high-power fields (HPF) with at least focally increased cellularity, without significant atypia, is considered a variant of fibroma and is designated as mitotically active cellular fibroma (Fig. 2). Mitotic activity in cellular fibromas lacking cytologic atypia is not associated with adverse prognosis. Nevertheless, occasionally local recurrences have been reported caused by incomplete resection and/or associated tumor rupture or surface adhesions.[14] Fibrosarcomas are diffusely hypercellular, with brisk mitotic activity and striking cytologic atypia (Fig. 3). They are not only extremely rare but also carry dismal prognosis, therefore this diagnosis should be made with caution and perhaps with help from consultant pathologist specialized in gynecologic pathology.[13]

Fibromas, cellular fibromas, and fibrosarcomas are uncommonly inhibin positive but often show positive staining for calretinin and splicing factor 1 (SF-1), and weak to moderate Wilms tumor 1 (WT-1) staining.[15,16]

Key Points
FIBROMA, CELLULAR FIBROMA, FIBROSARCOMA

Cellular fibroma	Increased mitotic activity Increased cellularity Lack of cytologic atypia
Fibrosarcoma	Exceedingly rare Increased mitotic activity Increased cellularity Striking cytologic atypia

△△ Differential Diagnosis

AGCT vs fibroma	Reticulin stain, inhibin immunohistochemistry and presence of FOXL 2 mutation distinguishes spindled cell and diffuse variant of AGCT from fibroma. In fibroma, reticulin stains fibers around individual cells, whereas in AGCT it stains bundles or nests of cells
	AGCT tend to be strongly inhibin positive, whereas fibromas are typically negative or weak/focal, but occasionally show more significant inhibin staining

Abbreviation: AGCT, adult granulosa cell tumor.

Signet Ring Stromal Tumor

Signet ring cell stromal tumors are exceedingly rare and are associated with a benign clinical course. Signet ring stromal tumors resemble cellular fibromas but also show dispersed signet ring–like cells that contain no lipid or mucin[17] (Fig. 4). Although these tumors are rare, they need to be distinguished from Krukenberg tumors, which contain intracytoplasmic mucin and represent bilateral ovarian metastasis from a gastrointestinal primary site, which is associated with a poor clinical outcome.[18]

Pitfall
SIGNET RING STROMAL TUMOR

! Krukenberg tumor should always be considered before making a diagnosis of signet ring cell stromal tumor.

Thecoma

Thecoma are rare, estrogen-producing tumors often described as tumors composed of cells with eosinophilic cytoplasm resembling theca cells (Fig. 5). The largest retrospective series, of 70 ovarian thecomas, was described recently,[4] in which the most common morphologic feature was a diffuse or nodular growth of cells with readily appreciable clear cells and indistinct cell borders imparting a syncytial growth appearance. Nuclear

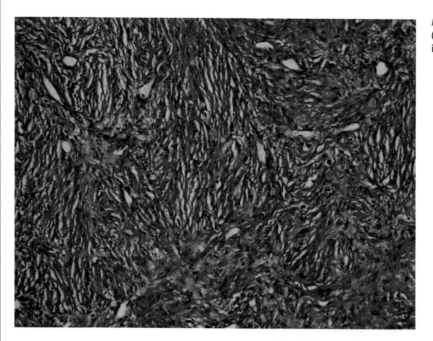

Fig. 1. Ovarian fibroma (hematoxylin-eosin, original magnification ×100).

Table 2
Gross, microscopic, immunohistochemical, and molecular profile of pure stromal tumors

	Macroscopic Features	Laterality	Microscopic Features	IHC	Molecular	DD
Fibroma	Well circumscribed White-tan-gray Firm Solid Calcifications and hemorrhage common Average 6 cm	Unilateral Bilateral in Gorlin syndrome	Storiform and fascicular spindle proliferation Variable cellularity Up to 3 mitoses/10 HPF No or minimal atypia Background of edema, collagen deposition, or calcifications May contain foci with sex cord elements	Positive: WT1 FOXL2 Vimentin SF-1 Negative: CD10 Variable: Inhibin	Trisomy 12	Thecoma Sclerosing Stromal tumor Edema Fibromatosis Spindled (diffuse) AGCT Leiomyoma
Cellular fibroma	White-yellow Fleshy Lager than fibroma Average size 12 cm	Unilateral	Same as fibroma with striking cellularity Mild to moderate atypia	Same as fibroma	Same as fibroma	Same as fibroma
Thecoma	Solid Lobulated Yellow Average size 7 cm	Unilateral	Vacuolated spindled cells with ill-defined pale cytoplasm Collagen depositions and hyaline plaques No atypia and mitosis May contained sex cord elements	Positive Calretinin Inhibin WT1 CD56 ER/PR CD10 FOXL2 Characteristic reticulin pattern	FOXL2 Trisomy 12	Fibroma Thecoma with sclerosing peritonitis Sclerosing stromal tumor Granulosa cell
Luteinized thecoma	Similar to thecoma Edematous with cystic change if associated with sclerosing peritonitis	Bilateral if associated with sclerosing peritonitis	Features of Thecoma + lutein cells in clusters or single If associated with sclerosing peritonitis Mitosis and edema are prominent	Same as thecoma	FOXL2 Trisomy 12	Steroid cell tumors Pregnancy luteoma Sclerosing stromal tumor Edema Cellular fibroma

(continued on next page)

Table 2
(continued)

	Macroscopic Features	Laterality	Microscopic Features	IHC	Molecular	DD
Fibrosarcoma	Fleshy lobulated surface Hemorrhage and necrosis	Unilateral	Densely cellular Spindle shaped Herringbone or storiform pattern Atypia and pleomorphism 4–25 mitoses per 10 HPF	Positive: Vimentin Variable: Inhibin Calretinin	None	Cellular fibroma
Sclerosing stromal tumor	Lobulated tan-yellow Average 10 cm	Unilateral	Spindle-shaped cells admixes with rounded and vacuolated cell Distinct network of thin blood vessels reminiscent of SFT Low-power, lobular appearance with hypercellular and hypocellular zones	Positive Inhibin Calretinin CD34 FOXL2 ER, PR CD10 Negative Keratin EMA	None	Fibroma Thecoma Metastatic signet ring cell
Signet ring stromal tumor	Solid and cystic Lobulated Yellow-tan Necrosis and hemorrhage	Unilateral	Background of cellular fibroma with variable numbers of cells with signet ring features Signet ring cells are with no atypia and vacuoles are empty with no mucin, lipid or glycogen	Positive Keratin SMA Negative Mucicarmine PAS Oil red O EMA Desmin S100 Inhibin Calretinin Variable Vimentin Reticulin	None	Krukenberg Thecoma Granulosa cell tumor with signet ring stromal cells

Microcystic stromal tumor	Mixed pattern of solid and cystic, rarely only solid or only cystic appearance	Unilateral	Composed of 3 major components: 1. Microcystic 2. Solid cellular zones 3. Collagenous stroma Basophilic or clear cyst contents Collagenous bands Bland cytology Bizarre nuclei up to 60% No mitosis Abundant pale to granular cytoplasm Intracytoplasmic vacuoles	Positive: Vimentin Beta-catenin Negative: EMA Variable: Cytokeratin Inhibin Calretinin	Beta-catenin (CTNNB1) gene mutation (exon 3)	Juvenile granulosa cell tumor Yolk sac tumor Struma ovarii Solid pseudopapillary tumor
Leydig cell tumor	Lobulated solid Yellow-orange to red-brown even black	Unilateral	Nonencapsulated, lobular sheets and nests of uniform polygonal cells with eosinophilic to vacuolated cytoplasm Rectangular, hexagonal crystals (Reinke) are necessary for diagnosis Lipochrome pigment often present Mitoses rare	Positive Vimentin Inhibin Calretinin Melan-A CD99 Negative Oil red O	None	Stromal luteoma Pregnancy luteoma Luteinized thecoma Sertoli-Leydig cell tumors

(continued on next page)

Table 2
(continued)

	Macroscopic Features	Laterality	Microscopic Features	IHC	Molecular	DD
Steroid cell tumor	Well circumscribed, solid yellow to orange/brown to black Average size 8 cm	Unilateral	Sheets, nests, cords of polygonal cells with granular eosinophilic cytoplasm or vacuolated lipid-rich cytoplasm Distinct nuclear and cytoplasmic borders No atypia <2 mitoses/10 HPF	Positive Vimentin Inhibin Calretinin Melan-A CD99 Variable AE1/3 Cam 5.2 HMB45 S100	None	Stromal luteoma Pregnancy luteoma Luteinized thecoma Malignant melanoma Granulosa cell tumor
Steroid cell tumor, malignant	Yellow-orange/brown with cystic degeneration hemorrhage and necrosis	Unilateral	Same as benign steroid tumor with moderate to severe atypia, >2 mitoses/10 HPF	Same as benign steroid tumor	None	Same as benign steroid tumor

Abbreviations: AE1/3, pankeratin; AGCT, adult granulosa cell tumor; Cam 5.2, pankeratin; CTNNB1, catenin beta 1; DD, differential diagnosis; EMA, epithelial membrane antigen; ER, estrogen receptor; FOXL2, forkhead box L2; HMB45, human melanoma black 45; HPF, high-power field; IHC, immunohistochemistry; PAS, periodic acid–Schiff; PR, progesterone receptor; SF-1, splicing factor 1; SFT, solitary fibrous tumor; SMA, smooth muscle actin; WT-1, Wilms tumor 1.

Fig. 2. (*A*) Cellular fibroma (hematoxylin-eosin, original magnification ×400). (*B*) Mitotically active fibroma (hematoxylin-eosin, original magnification ×200).

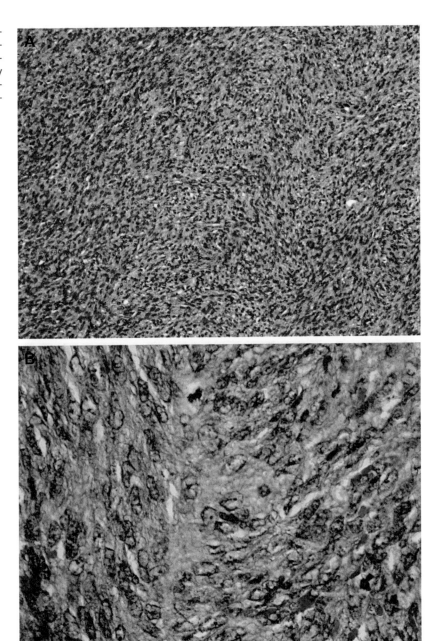

atypia is generally absent and mitotic activity is low. In 41% of cases, there were isolated foci of fibroma. Tumors showing both fibroma and thecoma components should be classified as either thecoma or fibroma according to the prevailing morphologic pattern, although it is noted that the diagnosis of fibrothecoma is not harmful to the patient because both fibroma and thecoma are indolent tumors. Vacuoles presumed to be lipid filled were observed in one-third of the tumors; however, lipid oil red O stain was positive in only 1 of 70 cases, suggesting that these are not lipid-rich vacuoles.

Luteinized Thecoma Associated with Sclerosing Peritonitis

Diagnostic Pitfalls
! Mitotic activity is often brisk in luteinized thecoma.

! Vacuoles may be seen in thecomas; however, lipid stain is typically negative.

Luteinized thecoma refers to a specific type of thecoma tumor that occurs in patients with

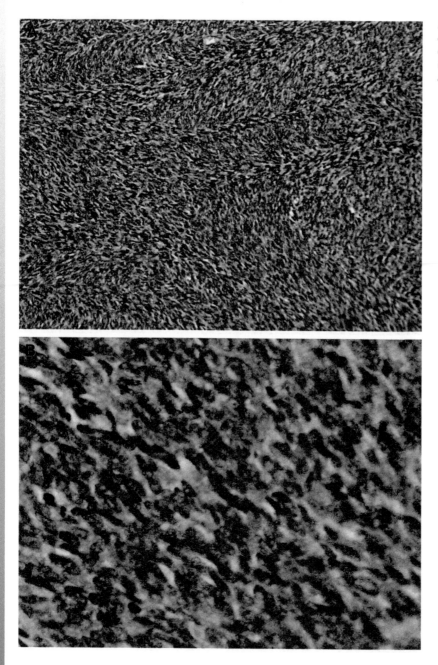

Fig. 3. (*A, B*) Primary ovarian fibrosarcoma (hematoxylin-eosin, original magnification ×100 and ×400).

sclerosing peritonitis. On histology, luteinized thecoma contains clusters of eosinophilic luteinized cells.[19] Mitotic activity can be brisk in these tumors and rarely nuclear atypia are present.[20] Stromal tumors with luteinized cells may present with androgenic manifestations, and therefore their presence should be mentioned to correlate with clinical presentation.

Sclerosing Stromal Tumor

Sclerosing stromal tumor was first described in 1973 as a distinct stromal tumor based on its gross and microscopic characteristics. They usually present in young patients and their characteristic lobular pattern of hypocellular and hypercellular areas with vascular pattern reminiscent of hemangiopericytoma on low-power

Fig. 4. Signet ring stromal tumor of the ovary (hematoxylin-eosin, original magnification ×200).

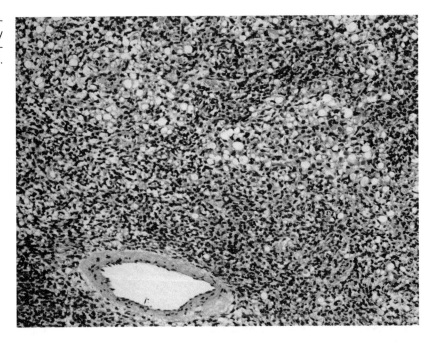

view[21,22] is the most important diagnostic clue. This tumor is composed of lutein epithelioid cells with eosinophilic or clear cytoplasm admixed with spindle cells (**Fig. 6**). If this tumor occurs in a pregnant patient it may be misinterpreted as steroid cell tumor or rarely a Krukenberg tumor because the luteinized cells tend to increase in number and in size, and acquire abundant vacuolated cytoplasm.[23] Rarely it contains minor sex cord–stromal elements represented by small tubules and cords.[24] Immunohistochemistry has a limited role in distinguishing sclerosing stromal

Fig. 5. Ovarian thecoma (hematoxylin-eosin, original magnification ×200).

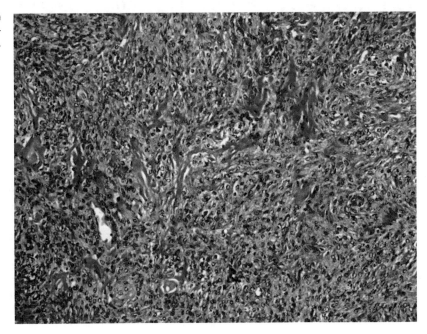

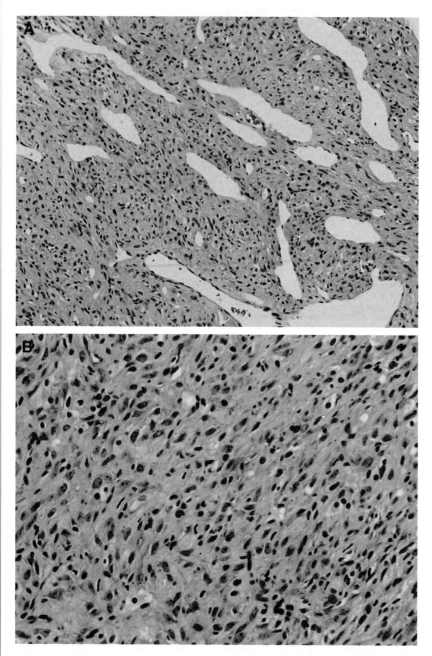

Fig. 6. (*A, B*) Sclerosing stromal tumor (hematoxylin-eosin, original magnification ×100 and ×200).

tumor from steroid cell tumor. Calretinin, inhibin, and Melan-A tend to show diffuse and stronger staining in steroid cell tumors, compared with focal positivity in sclerosing stromal tumors. CD56 and FOXL2 tend to be positive in both tumors.[25] Androgen manifestation and rarely hirsutism have been reported in pregnant patients diagnosed with sclerosing stromal tumor.[23] These symptoms usually resolve following delivery.

Microcystic Stromal Tumor

Microcystic stromal tumor is an exceedingly rare and recently[26] described ovarian stromal tumor. Fewer than 30 cases have been reported in the literature so far. The hallmark of this tumor is a mixture of microcystic and solid areas and collagenous bands. This tumor has overlapping histologic features with primary solid pseudopapillary neoplasm of the ovary, the ovarian counterpart of the same tumor in the pancreas. However, solid and pseudopapillary tumor of the ovary does not express any of the sex cord markers, such as inhibin, calretinin, or SF-1, and often shows positivity for neuroendocrine markers.[27]

Diagnostic Pitfalls

! Branching vascular pattern reminiscent of hemangiopericytoma is the major hallmark of sclerosing stromal tumor that differentiates it from fibroma, thecoma, or Krukenberg tumor.

! Microcystic stromal tumor can be distinguished from solid and pseudopapillary tumor of ovary by positive staining for inhibin, calretinin, and SF-1.

! Microcystic pattern of yolk sac tumor can look very similar to microcystic stromal tumor. Presence of Schiller-Duval bodies, brisk mitotic activity, and SAL-like 4 (SALL-4) positivity can distinguish the two.

Steroid Cell Tumors, Including Leydig Cell Tumor

These tumors are rare subtypes of SCST that usually occur in postmenopausal women and are often associated with symptoms related to hormone production.[28] Grossly they present as unilateral solid ovarian tumors golden yellow to brown in color.

Leydig cell tumors are often testosterone producing and occur in the hilus (hilus cell tumor) or in the stroma.[25,29] The classic histologic features include a nested growth of eosinophilic tumor cells with abundant granular or vacuolated cytoplasm (Fig. 7A). Nuclei are central and have a small prominent nucleolus. Reinke crystals (Fig. 7B), a diagnostic finding of these tumors, are eosinophilic rod-shaped crystalloids in the cytoplasm.[25] They are more likely to be found in the tumors arising in the ovarian stroma. In the absence of Reinke crystals, if the tumor shows classic histologic findings, the diagnosis can still be made, because the crystals may only be seen by electron microscopy. Other common histologic findings include bizarre cytologic atypia, acellular eosinophilic areas between the cellular areas, and fibrinoid necrosis of the vessels.[28]

Steroid cell tumors not otherwise specified (NOS) are those steroid cell tumors that cannot be classified as Leydig cell tumors, because of lack of Reinke crystals, or because of their location.[28,30] They produce androgens or estrogens, but other hormones such as progesterone or cortisol secretion have been reported.[31] Grossly

they have similar appearance to Leydig cell tumors, but tend to be larger, and may contain hemorrhage, necrosis, or cystic degeneration.[30] Microscopically the tumor cells show solid growth or small aggregates, and cytologically show distinct cell borders, abundant eosinophilic granular or lipid-rich clear and vacuolated cytoplasm (Fig. 8). Cytologic atypia is usually minimal and mitotic activity is low, less than 2 per 10 HPF.[30] Extraovarian disease at the time of presentation, large size (>7 cm), increased mitotic index (>2 per 10 HPF), necrosis, and significant cytologic atypia are reported to correlate with malignant clinical behavior.[30]

Diagnostic Pitfalls

! Steroid tumor of pregnancy (pregnancy luteoma) is often bilateral, multifocal and presents in pregnant patients. Morphologically they are indistinguishable from steroid cell tumors (Fig. 9).

! Lipid-rich Sertoli cell tumor usually has other more characteristic areas with Sertoli cell differentiation.

! Metastatic renal cell carcinoma has a glycogen-rich cytoplasm and eccentric nuclei. CD10 is positive in both tumors; however, additional more specific immunomarkers can readily distinguish the two tumors.

! Some Leydig cell tumors show bizarre cytologic atypia with no prognostic significance.

! Presence of cytologic atypia, extraovarian disease, large size, and increased mitotic activity correlate with clinical behavior in steroid tumors (NOS) of the ovary.

! Leydig cell tumors and steroid cell tumors may contain lipochrome pigment and are Melan-A positive. Cytologic atypia can be present in both, which may raise the concern for malignant melanoma.

PURE SEX CORD TUMORS

GRANULOSA CELL TUMORS (ADULT AND JUVENILE)

The adult granulosa cell tumor (AGCT) occurs in middle-aged women (peak mid-50s) and the most common endocrine manifestation of AGCT is hyperestrogenism resulting in abnormal uterine bleeding (Table 3). Low-power features in these two variants are different, because the adult form typically has microfollicles or solid patterns with fairly uniform angulated or oval cells, with scant

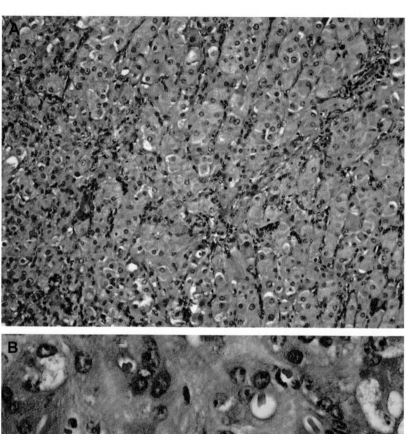

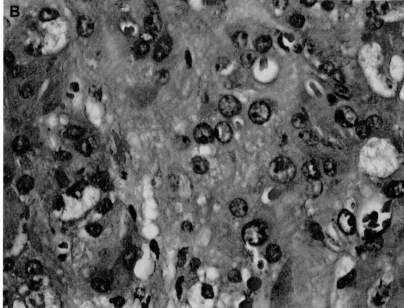

Fig. 7. (*A, B*) Leydig cell tumor with Reinke crystals (hematoxylin-eosin, original magnification ×200 and ×400).

cytoplasm and pale bland nuclei with nuclear grooves[28] (**Fig. 10**). Grooves and Call-Exner bodies (**Fig. 11**), the characteristic and well-known findings of adult AGCT, are not seen in juvenile granulosa cell tumor (JGCT). The absence of Call-Exner bodies should not preclude the diagnosis of AGCT, because they are often absent.[32] Severe cytologic atypia and increased mitotic activity are occasionally seen in AGCT.

Approximately 2% of AGCT tumors show extensive luteinization, in which the tumor cells show abundant eosinophilic cytoplasm and prominent nucleoli (**Fig. 12**). In a small subset of tumors there is significant nuclear pleomorphism, including multinucleated cells and bizarre cytologic atypia,[33] but these areas are often focal, whereas the remainder of the tumor shows characteristic histologic features. Mitotic rate of AGCT is variable;

Fig. 8. (*A, B*) Steroid cell tumor (hematoxylin-eosin, original magnification ×100 and ×100).

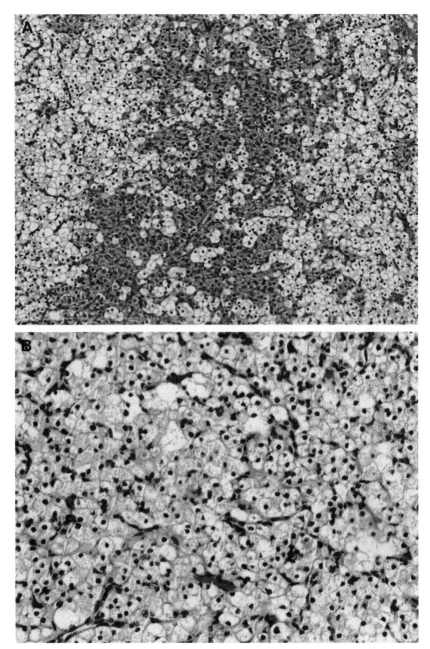

however, if atypical forms are noted, the diagnosis of granulosa cell tumor should be reconsidered. The molecular hallmark of AGCT is a somatic missense point mutation in codon 134 (C402G) of the FOXL2 gene, which is thought to be the driver mutation of these tumors but is not exclusive to AGCT.[34] The same mutation has been reported in a small subset of thecomas and Sertoli-Leydig cell tumors (SLCTs) as well. Not surprisingly, FOXL2 immunohistochemistry is now also used

in the diagnostic work-up of sex cord–stromal tumors and is expressed in most AGCTs and JGCTs. Although it is a sensitive and specific marker for sex cord–stromal tumors, its expression does not correlate with the presence of FOXL2 mutation.[35] In addition, because it is expressed in a large variety of sex cord–stromal tumors, it has limited utility in further subclassifying these tumors. The presence of Sertoli cells can be ignored as long as they comprise less than 10% of the tumor,

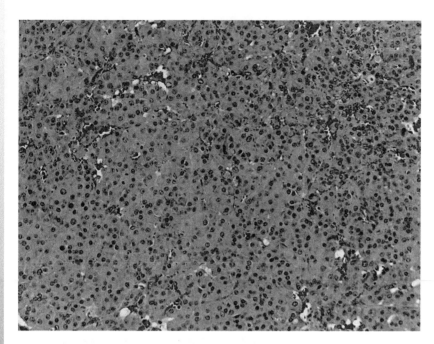

Fig. 9. Pregnancy luteoma (hematoxylin-eosin, original magnification ×200).

otherwise the diagnosis of gynandroblastoma may be considered. Gynandroblastoma is no longer listed in the 2014 WHO classification of tumors of the female reproductive organs. A recent study has revealed the presence of *DICER1* hot-spot mutations in moderately or poorly differentiated SLCT components and JGCT components of these mixed sex cord–stromal tumors.[36] Other hallmark mutations of granulosa cell tumors (FOXL2 and AKT1) have not been found in gynandroblastomas, suggesting that the pathogenesis of these tumors in the setting of mixed germ cell tumors is different from those seen in the pure variants. Of note, both the female and male components of these sex cord–stromal tumors show strong IHC staining for FOXL2, further pointing out its limited value in distinguishing various subtypes of sex cord–stromal tumors.

JGCT occurs in children and young adults, and, if it occurs in prepubertal children, patients often present with isosexual pseudoprecocity. On histology, JGCT shows myxoid or edematous stroma and macrofollicular pattern (follicles are irregular and contain eosinophilic or basophilic secretions) (**Fig. 13**), and the cells have abundant and often vacuolated or eosinophilic cytoplasm and darker chromatin.[32,37] Call-Exner bodies are absent. Rarely JGCT shows cystic architecture lined by friable papillary tumor fronds or solid nodular growth pattern. Findings of more classic foci of JGCT and identifying the characteristic cytologic features of these tumors are often helpful and may require additional sampling. In

contrast with AGCT, FOXL2 mutations are not seen in JGCT. The 2 most common mutations in JGCT are activating mutations of alpha subunit of G protein at position 201,[38] which are seen in up to 30% of JGCTs, and in-frame tandem duplication of point mutations of exon 3 of AKT-1.[39,40]

△△ Differential Diagnosis
ADULT GRANULOSA CELL TUMOR

- Small cell carcinoma hypercalcemic type, characterized by folliclelike pattern, small hyperchromatic cells, and high mitotic index, may have overlapping features with both AGCT and JGCT. Very high mitotic index, small hyperchromatic tumor cells, and increased serum calcium levels are helpful in distinguishing these two tumors. In addition, small cell carcinoma of hypercalcemic type often presents with extraovarian disease.

- Fibroma, fibrothecoma, endometrial stromal sarcoma: diffuse pattern of AGCT appears similar. Reticulin stain and immunostains (CD10, smooth muscle actin) are helpful in the diagnostic work-up of these morphologically similar tumors.

- Unilocular cystic AGCT can look identical to large follicle cyst, but the latter is often luteinized and occurs during pregnancy (**Fig. 14**).

- Well-differentiated endometrioid adenocarcinoma may show sex cord–like areas, such as microfollicular, trabecular, or insular patterns (Fig. 15). Identification of more characteristic patterns for each tumor and difference in cytologic features is helpful when distinguishing these two tumors.

- Misinterpretation of Call-Exner bodies: acini of carcinoid tumors and tubules of sex cord tumor with annular tubules (SCTAT) may resemble Call-Exner bodies, but the center of carcinoid acini contains eosinophilic secretions (sometimes calcified), surrounded by hyperchromatic tumor cells with coarse chromatin. Tubules containing hyaline deposits in SCTAT are larger than Call-Exner bodies and hyaline-type basement membrane deposits are present throughout the tumor (Fig. 16).

△△ **Differential Diagnosis**
JUVENILE GRANULOSA CELL TUMOR

- JGCT may be misinterpreted as yolk sac tumor. However, macrofollicles are not a feature of yolk sac tumors, and often, with additional sampling, more characteristic patterns for each tumor with the aid of IHC stains make the diagnosis easier.

- The tubulocystic pattern of clear cell carcinoma may be confused with JGCT tumor, but clear cell carcinoma rarely occurs in the same age group as JGCT.

- Metastatic breast carcinoma (especially lobular type) and melanoma can also be confused with granulosa cell tumor; however, IHC stains can easily sort out these diagnostic dilemmas.

The most important prognostic feature for granulosa cell tumors is the pathologic stage, because stage I tumors have significantly better 10-year survival (>85%) compared with stage II or higher (<50%).[28] Late recurrences are common, often decades after the initial diagnosis. Other histologic parameters that may have prognostic implications, including tumor size more than 5 cm, cytologic atypia, sarcomatoid foci,[41] mitotic index,[42] and GATA4 or Her2[43] expression, have been investigated with inconclusive results. Cytologic atypia and mitotic activity (even the presence of atypical forms) has no impact on prognosis in JGCT.[37]

SERTOLI CELL TUMORS

These rare tumors occur at any age and may present with endocrine symptoms, including estrogen, androgen, and even renin production.[44] Association with Peutz-Jeghers syndrome (PJS) has been reported.[45] The histologic hallmark of these tumors is closely packed tubules, without or containing only very rare Leydig cells in the stroma. Tubules can be hollow or solid, composed of tumor cells with abundant eosinophilic or vacuolated cytoplasm (Fig. 17). Areas of cords and solid growth may be seen. A variant, so-called lipid-rich Sertoli cell tumor, is characterized by tumor cells with abundant clear cytoplasm. Marked cytologic atypia and increased mitotic index (>5 per 10 HPF) have been reported to carry adverse prognosis.[46] Most tumors are stage I and carry good prognosis.[28]

△△ **Differential Diagnosis**

- In poorly differentiated SLCTs Leydig cells become sparse and can be overlooked.

- Endometrioid carcinoma may have areas of tubular growth pattern; however, presence of more characteristic endometrioid histology and foci of squamous differentiation are helpful findings. In addition, IHC stains that are positive in endometrioid carcinoma, such as epithelial membrane antigen, can aid the diagnosis.

- Female adnexal tumor of probable wolffian origin often presents with various histologic patterns, and areas of tubular growth may be mistaken for Sertoli cell tumor. These tumors most commonly arise in the broad ligament and are positive for GATA3.

- Carcinoid tumors with rosettes and solid nested growth may mimic Sertoli cell tumors on low power, but the neuroendocrine chromatin pattern and different immunoprofile help distinguishing these two tumors.

- Sertoli cell tumors rarely show alveolar pattern, which on low power may resemble dysgerminoma.

SEX CORD–STROMAL TUMOR WITH ANNULAR TUBULES

Clinical presentation depends on whether they occur in a sporadic setting or in association with PJS.[47] In the latter they are often small, incidental, and bilateral, whereas sporadic tumors are large,

Table 3
Gross, microscopic, immunohistochemical and molecular features of pure sex cord tumors

	Gross	Microscopic Features	IHC	Molecular Features
AGCT	Unilateral ~10 cm Solid and cystic Yellow, soft, hemorrhagic	Cords, trabeculae, ribbons, nests, microfollicles (Call-Exner bodies), macrofollicles, diffuse pattern Oval pale nuclei with groves, mitotic index variable, rarely marked atypia	Positive: Inhibin, calretinin, FOXL2, SF-1, WT-1, CD56 Negative: CK7, EMA Variable: AE1/3, Cam 5.2, CD99, desmin, SMA, S100	Mutation of FOXL-2 gene in 90% Trisomy 12, 14 Monosomy 16
JGCT	Unilateral ~12 cm, solid and cystic, yellow and hemorrhagic	Variable size and shape follicles with secretions. Abundant eosinophilic cytoplasm, round nuclei without groves, mitotic index high, significant atypia present 10%–15%	Positive: inhibin, calretinin, SF-1, WT-1, CD56, CD99 Negative: EMA Variable: FOXL2, Cam 5.2	Trisomy 12 FOXL2 mutation is absent. Activating mutation of alpha subunit of G protein (30%) In-frame tandem duplication of AKT1
SCT	Unilateral, ~8 cm, solid tan-yellow, rarely necrosis and hemorrhage	Tubular, trabecular, diffuse, alveolar, pseudopapillary, retiform, spindled. Lipid-rich or eosinophilic cytoplasm, round nuclei	Positive: SF-1, WT-1, AE1/3, inhibin, calretinin, CD99. Negative: EMA Variable: SMA, S100	—
SCTAT	In PJ syndrome: multiple, microscopic, bilateral Sporadic: >3 cm, yellow, solid, cystic, unilateral	Nests of simple or complex annular tubules without lumens, antipodal arrangement of nuclei, fibrous stroma, hyaline material around tubules, calcifications common More complex growth patterns in sporadic forms	Positive: SF-1, FOXL2, inhibin, calretinin, WT-1, CD56 Negative: EMA Variable: AE1/3	Germline mutation of STK11 in 19p13.3 in PJ syndrome

Abbreviations: JGCT, juvenile granulosa cell tumor; PJ, Peutz-Jeghers; SCT, sertoli cell tumor; SCTAT, sex cord tumor with annular tubules.

Fig. 10. (*A, B*) Adult granulosa cell tumor (hematoxylin-eosin, original magnification ×100).

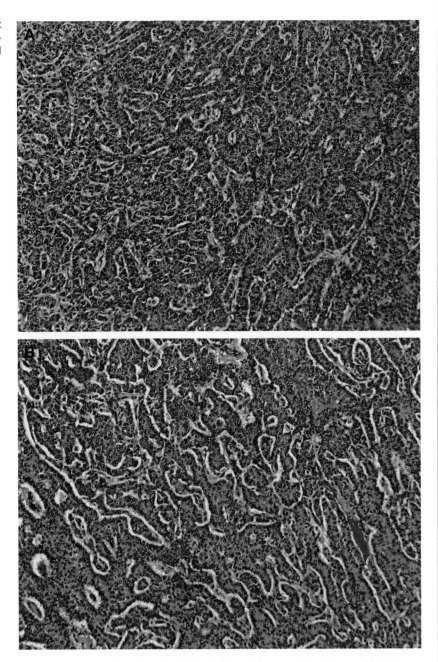

often palpable, and unilateral. Estrogen production is more common in sporadic tumors; rare progesterone secretion has been reported.[48] These tumors have a characteristic histologic appearance, which includes a dominant pattern of simple or complex tubules, containing eosinophilic basement membrane material (hyaline bodies) (**Fig. 18**). The nuclei of the tumor cells are oriented peripherally from the hyaline center (**Fig. 19**). Sporadic tumors tend to show more complex growth patterns,[47] in which tubules are round, well demarcated, and composed of several interconnecting smaller tubules, solid and cystic foci, and acellular patches of eosinophilic hyaline material may be seen (**Fig. 20**). Cytologic atypia and mitotic figures are uncommon. Calcification is often seen in those arising in association with PJS.[47] In the background, rare foci of other common sex cord tumors may be seen (granulosa cell tumor or SLCT). Although sex cord–stromal tumor with

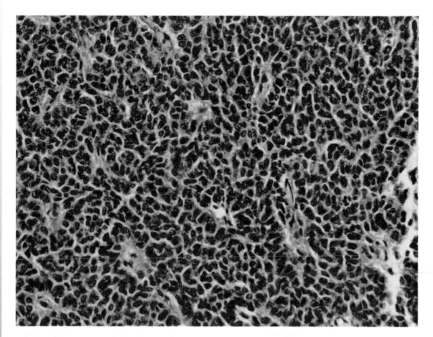

Fig. 11. Adult granulosa cell tumor with Call-Exner bodies (hematoxylin-eosin, original magnification ×200).

annular tubules (SCTAT) occurring in the setting of PJS has a typically benign clinical course, a small subset of sporadic SCTAT behaves in a malignant fashion and can metastasize to regional lymph nodes.[49]

MIXED SEX CORD–STROMAL TUMORS

SERTOLI-LEYDIG CELL TUMORS

SLCTs occur in young women, usually 30 years of age or younger (**Tables 4** and **5**). The retiform

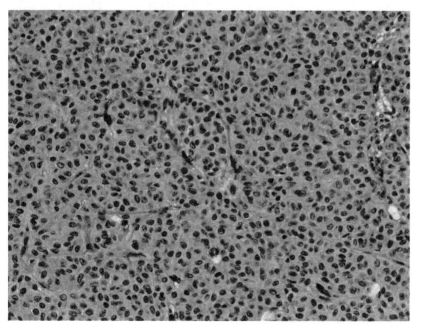

Fig. 12. Luteinized adult granulosa cell tumor (hematoxylin-eosin, original magnification ×100).

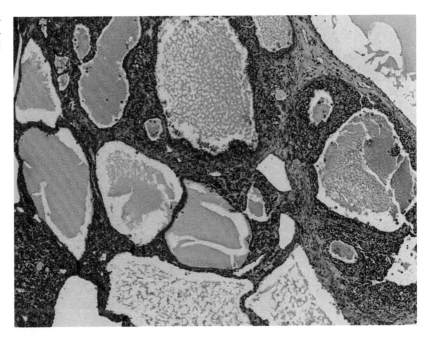

Fig. 13. Juvenile granulosa cell tumor (hematoxylin-eosin, original magnification ×100).

variant and those arising in the setting of germline mutations of the *DICER1* gene tend to occur in even younger patients,[50] whereas well-differentiated SLCTs generally occur a decade later. Virilization may be seen in 40% to 60% of young women, mainly in the setting of moderately and poorly differentiated SLCT forms.[51] Grossly, SLCT are often solid, lobulated, tan to yellow masses. Cystic components may be seen in the retiform variant, or in those with heterologous elements, whereas hemorrhage and necrosis are features of poorly differentiated SLCT. SLCTs are subdivided based on the degree of differentiation and growth patterns of the Sertoli cell component.[28] Well-formed tubules and readily identifiable Leydig cells are characteristic of well-differentiated SLCT, whereas tubules are absent in poorly differentiated SLCT and Leydig cells are very rare. Heterologous elements (ectodermal and mesodermal) can be seen in both moderately and poorly differentiated types, in up to 20% of cases.[32,52] The most common form is the presence of mucinous epithelium (**Fig. 21**), which can show a spectrum of cytologic atypia from benign to borderline to frank carcinoma. Rhabdomyosarcomatous (**Fig. 22**) and chondroid differentiation,[53] carcinoid tumors, and even hepatocytes (benign to atypical) have been reported.[47] Stage and degree of differentiation are the most important prognostic factors. Presence of a retiform component and mesenchymal heterologous

elements have been associated with adverse prognosis.[52] Extraovarian spread at the time of diagnosis is seen in 2% to 3% of patients[28]

Well-differentiated SLCT: Sertoli cells form tubules, and lack cytologic atypia or mitosis. Sertoli cells are columnar have abundant pale or eosinophilic cytoplasm and basally located nuclei. Leydig cells are in the stroma in clusters of single. The 2 distinct cell types are easy to identify (**Fig. 23**).

Moderately differentiated SLCT: this is the most common type. These tumors show lobular architecture and are cellular. Sertoli cells are usually arranged in nests, lobules, alveolar spaces, and rare tubules. Folliclelike spaces may be seen with eosinophilic secretion. Sertoli cells are immature appearing, hyperchromatic, and have high nuclear to cytoplasmic ratio (**Fig. 24**). Bizarre nuclear atypia may be seen and mitotic activity is around 5 per 10 HPF.[32] Leydig cells are dispersed in clusters or single at the periphery of the tumor. They may be hard to identify, which can make the identification of 2 cell types challenging. Background stroma is often edematous.

Poorly differentiated SLCT: these tumors have a solid growth of poorly differentiated cells with high mitotic rate. Foci resembling various differentiations from epithelial to mesenchymal and even germ cell tumors may be seen.[53] The initial impression on low-power and medium-power views is often that of a sarcoma (**Fig. 25A**) and, unless more characteristic Sertoli cell elements are seen

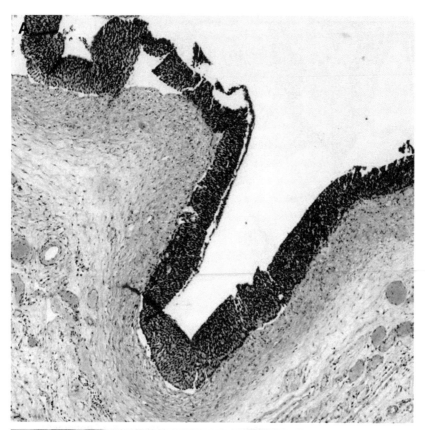

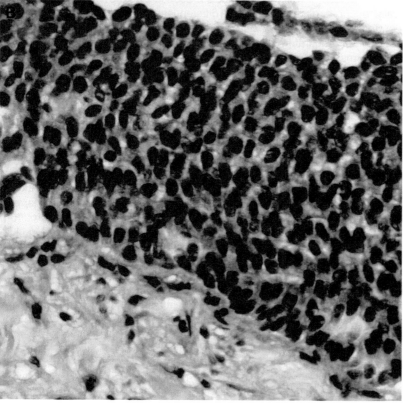

Fig. 14. (*A*, *B*) Cystic granulosa cell tumor (hematoxylin-eosin, original magnification ×100 and ×200).

Fig. 15. Primary ovarian endometrioid carcinoma, well differentiated with sex cord–like areas (hematoxylin-eosin, original magnification ×40).

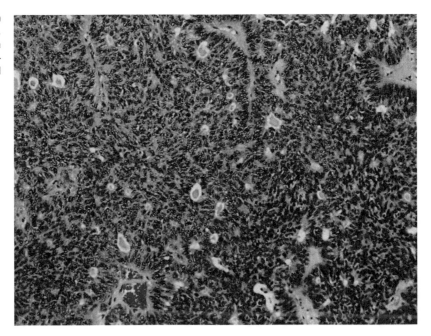

(Fig. 25B), the diagnosis can be difficult. Increased serum alpha fetoprotein (AFP) levels may be encountered.[48] Leydig cells are often difficult to identify.

Retiform variant of SLCT: the characteristic pattern of slitlike spaces, clefts, and papillae, resembling rete testis, lined by cuboidal to columnar cells is found in 15% of moderately and poorly differentiated forms of SLCT.[49] Eosinophilic secretion and florid papillary proliferations of the epithelium may be seen in the lumens. Stroma is commonly hyalinized.

Somatic *DICER1* mutation has been linked to moderately or poorly differentiated subtypes of Sertoli-Leydig tumors in about 60% of cases.[55,56] Germline *DICER1* mutations have been identified in families with pleuropulmonary blastoma, cystic nephroma, multinodular goiter, and SCST and is also associated with increased risk of multiple rare and unusual tumors.[57] Neither *DICER1* nor *FOXL2* mutations were detected in microcystic stromal tumors.[58]

The use of standard IHC panel for SCST in addition to *FOXL2* mutation analysis can help narrow

---

Diagnostic Pitfalls: Sertoli-Leydig Cell Tumor

- Endometrioid carcinoma: well-differentiated SLCT can mimic endometrioid carcinoma.

- Krukenberg tumor: tubular pattern of SLCT with mucinous differentiation may resemble metastasis from gastrointestinal primary site, because those can also present with tubules and the often expected signet ring cells may not be the predominant pattern. Low-power lobular appearance of metastasis and luteinized stromal cells nearby can also be misleading histologic findings.

- Serous neoplasm: florid papillary proliferation in the retiform variant may mimic serous papillary tumors and presence of heterologous elements may resemble carcinosarcoma. However, they occur in different age groups.

- Germ cell tumors, especially yolk sac tumors: poorly differentiated SLCTs may have areas that resemble microcystic or reticular patterns of yolk sac tumor. Focal AFP staining is common in SLCT, which further complicates differentiating it from yolk sac tumor. SLCT arising in a pregnant patient often shows significant stromal and intercellular edema, which also resembles yolk sac tumor. Characteristic histologic foci of SLCT (may require further sampling) often help in the diagnosis.

- Retiform variant of SLCT: less often androgenic, increased serum AFP level may be seen, often large and cystic masses.[54] Overall, their presentation is not classic for SLCT.

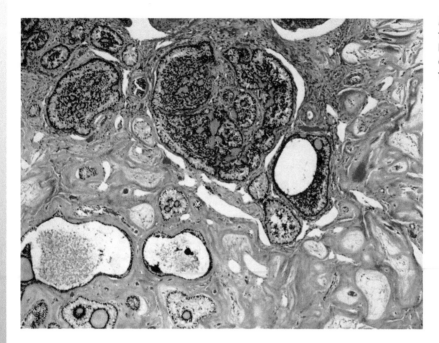

Fig. 16. Sex cord–stromal tumor with annular tubules (hematoxylin-eosin, original magnification ×40).

the differential diagnosis in difficult cases. Testing for *DICER1* mutation can be used in diagnosis of moderately and poorly differentiated Sertoli-Leydig tumors, particularly if the tumor occurs in young patients, because it is more likely to occur in association with an underlying *DICER1* syndrome.

A better understanding of underlying molecular and genetic pathogenesis can help further improve on tumor classification, prognosis, and treatment.

INTRAOPERATIVE EVALUATION OF SEX CORD–STROMAL TUMORS

It is essential to be familiar with ovarian SCST types, including frequency and age at which they occur, common clinical and gross presentations,

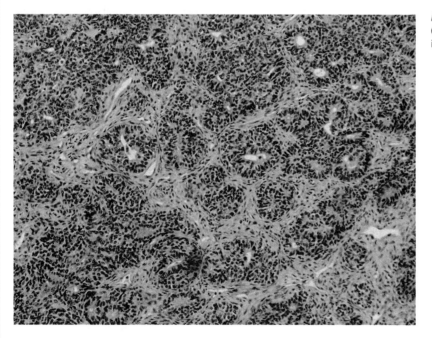

Fig. 17. Sertoli cell tumor (hematoxylin-eosin, original magnification ×100).

Fig. 18. Sex cord-stromal tumor with annual tubules (hematoxylin-eosin, original magnification, 40×)

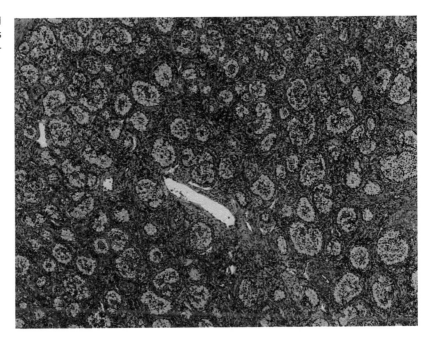

and histologic characteristics, to accurately diagnose them during intraoperative consultation. The sensitivity and specificity of frozen section diagnosis for ovarian tumors overall is high, especially in malignant surface epithelial tumors, which represent more than 80% of ovarian malignancies.[59] The most common SCSTs in young adults include JGCT and SLCTs. Although they are less common, they represent 20% to 30% of primary ovarian malignancies in women 30 years of age or younger.[52] SCST are rarely bilateral, with the exception of fibromas. Gross presentation of SCST varies from solid to solid and cystic masses. Fibromas and sclerosing stromal tumors often present as solid, firm, tan tumors (Fig. 26). Thecomas are typically yellow, whereas fibrothecoma may vary in the amount of yellow coloration related to the amount of thecomatous component

Fig. 19. Sex cord–stromal tumor with annular tubules (hematoxylin-eosin, original magnification ×100).

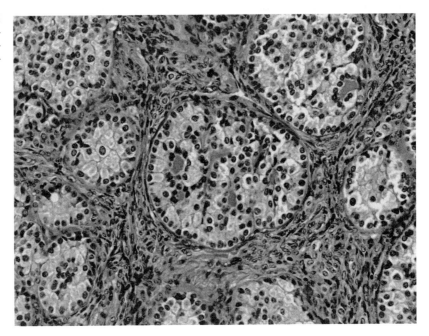

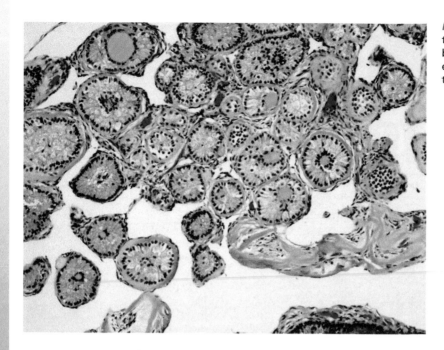

Fig. 20. Sex cord–stromal tumor with annular tubules (hematoxylin-eosin, original magnification ×200).

(**Fig. 27**). Granulosa cell tumors and SLCTs commonly present as solid and cystic tumors; the solid areas are soft to fleshy and tan or yellow and may be associated with necrosis and hemorrhage. Golden yellow to orange appearance in an ovarian tumor may indicate a steroid-producing neoplasm, such as steroid cell tumor or a well-differentiated SLCT. Nevertheless, frozen section in the intraoperative evaluation of sex cord–stromal tumors has significant limitations. Sex cord–like differentiation can be seen in endometrioid carcinomas, endometrial stromal tumors, and adenosarcoma, among others, which may result in misclassification as a granulosa cell tumor.[60] Large, mitotically active fibromas can be challenging to distinguish from fibrosarcoma, although the latter is exceedingly rare. Granulosa cell tumors may be entirely cystic and misclassified as a functional ovarian cyst or follicular cyst. Intestinal epithelium in an SLCT, although often a helpful diagnostic clue, can also pose a challenge and be interpreted as metastasis, a component of a mature teratoma, or primary mucinous neoplasm.[61]

Table 4
Clinical characteristics and prognosis of mixed sex cord–stromal tumors

	Incidence (%)	Age	Presentation	Associated Syndrome	Prognosis
SLCT	<0.5	Wide age range, mean 25 y, younger in DICER1 syndrome	Virilization in 40%–60% patients Rarely estrogenic effects 2%–3% extraovarian involvement	DICER1 syndrome in moderately and poorly differentiated forms	Grade dependent, adverse prognosis in retiform, moderately or poorly differentiated types are malignant in 10%
SCST NOS	—	Reproductive age, often during pregnancy	Often hormonal manifestations	—	Good if confined to ovary, 92% 5-y survival

Table 5
Gross, microscopic, immunohistochemical, and molecular characteristics of mixed sex cord–stromal tumors

	Gross	Microscopic Features	IHC	Molecular Features
SLCT	Unilateral, large (up to 35 cm), average 15 cm; solid, cystic (retiform variant), yellow fleshy, necrosis and hemorrhage common (PD variant)	WD: Sertoli cells in tubules, Leydig cells in clusters or cords MD: Sertoli cells in nests and tubules with cytologic atypia, increased mitosis mixed with Leydig cells, heterologous elements PD: lack of tubular differentiation, increased mitosis, primitive gonadal stroma, decreased Leydig cells, heterologous elements Retiform variant: Slitlike spaces, papillary and multicystic	Positive: vimentin, inhibin, calretinin, keratin, Sertoli cells stain for SF-1, WT-1, CD56, DICER1 Variable: FOXL2	DICER1 gene mutations in 60% in MD and PD variants
SCST NOS	—	Variable and not characteristic of any specific SCST, often stromal edema, luteinization	—	—

Abbreviations: MD, moderately differentiated; PD, poorly differentiated; WD, well differentiated.

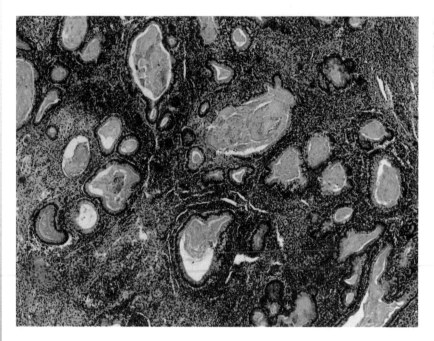

Fig.   21. Sertoli-Leydig cell tumor with heterologous (mucinous epithelium) differentiation (hematoxylin-eosin, original magnification ×40).

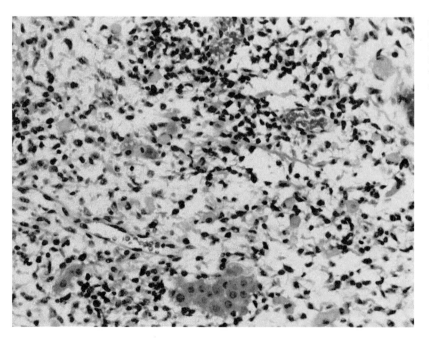

Fig.   22. Sertoli-Leydig cell tumor poorly differentiated with rhabdomyoblastic differentiation (hematoxylin-eosin, original magnification ×400).

Fig. 23. Sertoli-Leydig cell tumor, well differentiated (hematoxylin-eosin, original magnification ×100).

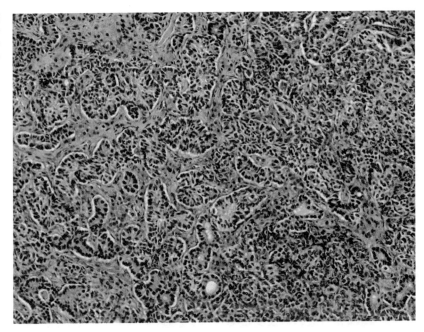

Fig. 24. Sertoli-Leydig cell tumor, moderately differentiated (hematoxylin-eosin, original magnification ×100).

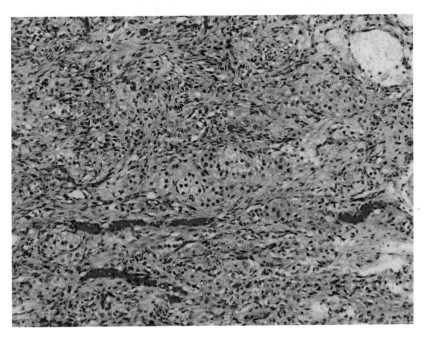

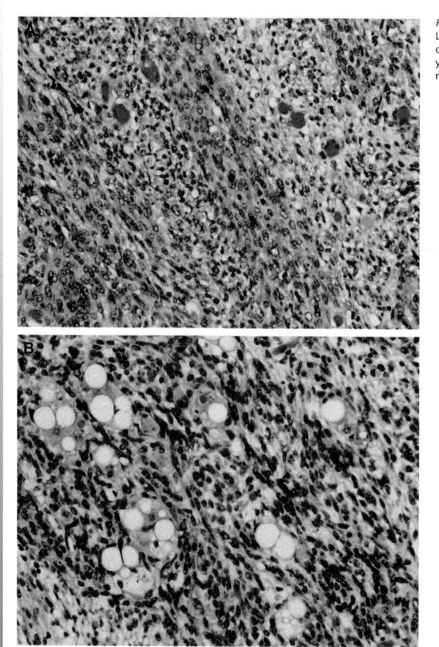

Fig. 25. (A, B) Sertoli-Leydig cell tumor, poorly differentiated (hematoxylin-eosin, original magnification ×200).

Fig. 26. Ovarian fibroma.

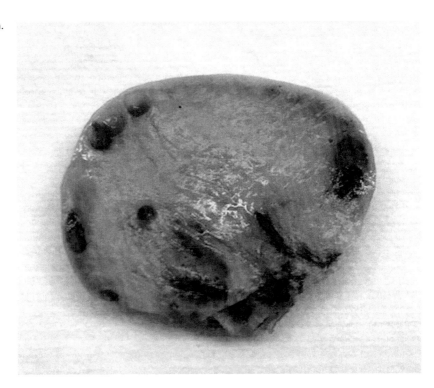

Fig. 27. Ovarian the-coma.

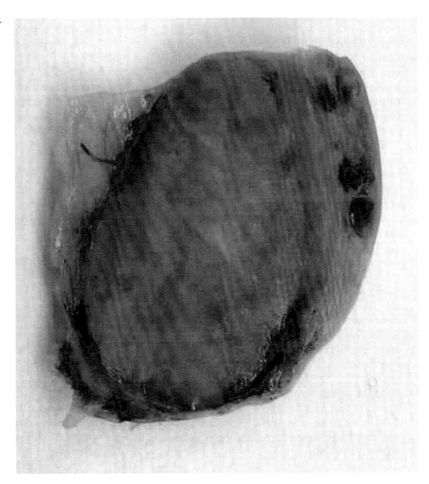

REFERENCES

1. Scully RE, Young RH, Clement PB. Tumors of the ovary. Maldeveloped gonads, fallopian tube and broad ligament. Washington, DC: Pathology AFlo; 1998.
2. Prat J, editor. Pathology of the ovary. Philadelphia: Saunders; 2004.
3. Mills SE, editor. Histology for pathologist. 2nd edition. Philadelphia: Lippincott Williams and Wilkins; 1997.
4. Burandt E, Young RH. Thecoma of the ovary: a report of 70 cases emphasizing aspects of its histopathology different from those often portrayed and its differential diagnosis. Am J Surg Pathol 2014; 38(8):1023–32.
5. Baiocchi G, Manci N, Angeletti G, et al. Pure Leydig cell tumour (hilus cell) of the ovary: a rare cause of virilization after menopause. Gynecol Obstet Invest 1997;44(2):141–4.
6. Yetkin DO, Demirsoy ET, Kadioglu P. Pure Leydig cell tumour of the ovary in a post-menopausal patient with severe hyperandrogenism and erythrocytosis. Gynecol Endocrinol 2011;27(4):237–40.
7. Kron B. Fibro-thecoma of the ovary with pleural effusion and ascites. Sem Hop 1973;49(18):1318–9, [in French].
8. Shen Y, Liang Y, Cheng X, et al. Ovarian fibroma/fibrothecoma with elevated serum CA125 level: a cohort of 66 cases. Medicine (Baltimore) 2018; 97(34):e11926.
9. Chan WY, Chang CY, Yuan CC, et al. Correlation of ovarian fibroma with elevated serum CA-125. Taiwan J Obstet Gynecol 2014;53(1):95–6.
10. Pirschner F, Bastos PM, Contarato GL, et al. Gorlin syndrome and bilateral ovarian fibroma. Int J Surg Case Rep 2012;3(9):477–80.
11. Khodaverdi S, Nazari L, Mehdizadeh-Kashi A, et al. Conservative management of ovarian fibroma in a case of Gorlin-Goltz syndrome comorbid with endometriosis. Int J Fertil Steril 2018; 12(1):88–90.
12. Zhang J, Young RH, Arseneau J, et al. Ovarian stromal tumors containing lutein or Leydig cells (luteinized thecomas and stromal Leydig cell tumors)—a clinicopathological analysis of fifty cases. Int J Gynecol Pathol 1982;1(3):270–85.
13. Garcia Jimenez A, Castellvi J, Perez Benavente A, et al. Ovarian fibrosarcoma: clinicopathologic considerations about the intraoperative and post-surgical procedures. Case Rep Med 2009;2009:802817.
14. Irving JA, Alkushi A, Young RH, et al. Cellular fibromas of the ovary: a study of 75 cases including 40 mitotically active tumors emphasizing their distinction from fibrosarcoma. Am J Surg Pathol 2006;30(8):929–38.

15. Zhao C, Barner R, Vinh TN, et al. SF-1 is a diagnostically useful immunohistochemical marker and comparable to other sex cord-stromal tumor markers for the differential diagnosis of ovarian Sertoli cell tumor. Int J Gynecol Pathol 2008;27(4):507–14.
16. Rabban JT, Zaloudek CJ. A practical approach to immunohistochemical diagnosis of ovarian germ cell tumours and sex cord-stromal tumours. Histopathology 2013;62(1):71–88.
17. Vang R, Bague S, Tavassoli FA, et al. Signet-ring stromal tumor of the ovary: clinicopathologic analysis and comparison with Krukenberg tumor. Int J Gynecol Pathol 2004;23(1):45–51.
18. Matsumoto M, Hayashi Y, Ohtsuki Y, et al. Signet-ring stromal tumor of the ovary: an immunohistochemical and ultrastructural study with a review of the literature. Med Mol Morphol 2008;41(3):165–70.
19. Clement PB, Young RH, Hanna W, et al. Sclerosing peritonitis associated with luteinized thecomas of the ovary. A clinicopathological analysis of six cases. Am J Surg Pathol 1994;18(1):1–13.
20. Irving JA, McCluggage WG. Ovarian spindle cell lesions: a review with emphasis on recent developments and differential diagnosis. Adv Anat Pathol 2007;14(5):305–19.
21. Damajanov I, Drobnjak P, Grizelj V, et al. Sclerosing stromal tumor of the ovary: a hormonal and ultrastructural analysis. Obstet Gynecol 1975;45(6): 675–9.
22. Kawauchi S, Tsuji T, Kaku T, et al. Sclerosing stromal tumor of the ovary: a clinicopathologic, immunohistochemical, ultrastructural, and cytogenetic analysis with special reference to its vasculature. Am J Surg Pathol 1998;22(1):83–92.
23. Bennett JA, Oliva E, Young RH. Sclerosing stromal tumors with prominent luteinization during pregnancy: a report of 8 cases emphasizing diagnostic problems. Int J Gynecol Pathol 2015;34(4):357–62.
24. Guo L, Liu T. Ovarian sclerosing stromal tumor with minor sex cord elements. Chin Med J (Engl) 1995; 108(12):935–7.
25. Roth LM, Sternberg WH. Ovarian stromal tumors containing Leydig cells. II. Pure Leydig cell tumor, non-hilar type. Cancer 1973;32(4):952–60.
26. Irving JA, Lee CH, Yip S, et al. Microcystic stromal tumor: a distinctive ovarian sex cord-stromal neoplasm characterized by FOXL2, SF-1, WT-1, cyclin D1, and beta-catenin nuclear expression and CTNNB1 mutations. Am J Surg Pathol 2015;39(10):1420–6.
27. Deshpande V, Oliva E, Young RH. Solid pseudopapillary neoplasm of the ovary: a report of 3 primary ovarian tumors resembling those of the pancreas. Am J Surg Pathol 2010;34(10):1514–20.
28. Kurman RJ, Carcangiu ML, Herrington CS, et al, editors. WHO Classification of tumors of the ovary. Lyon (France): IARC; 2014.

29. Sternberg WH, Roth LM. Ovarian stromal tumors containing Leydig cells. I. Stromal-Leydig cell tumor and non-neoplastic transformation of ovarian stroma to Leydig cells. Cancer 1973; 32(4):940–51.

30. Hayes MC, Scully RE. Ovarian steroid cell tumors (not otherwise specified). A clinicopathological analysis of 63 cases. Am J Surg Pathol 1987;11(11): 835–45.

31. Chetkowski RJ, Judd HL, Jagger PI, et al. Autonomous cortisol secretion by a lipoid cell tumor of the ovary. JAMA 1985;254(18):2628–31.

32. Young RH. Sex cord-stromal tumors of the ovary and testis: their similarities and differences with consideration of selected problems. Mod Pathol 2005; 18(Suppl 2):S81–98.

33. Young RH, Scully RE. Ovarian sex cord-stromal tumors with bizarre nuclei: a clinicopathologic analysis of 17 cases. Int J Gynecol Pathol 1983;1(4):325–35.

34. Shah SP, Kobel M, Senz J, et al. Mutation of FOXL2 in granulosa-cell tumors of the ovary. N Engl J Med 2009;360(26):2719–29.

35. Al-Agha OM, Huwait HF, Chow C, et al. FOXL2 is a sensitive and specific marker for sex cord-stromal tumors of the ovary. Am J Surg Pathol 2011;35(4): 484–94.

36. Wang Y, Karnezis AN, Magrill J, et al. DICER1 hotspot mutations in ovarian gynandroblastoma. Histopathology 2018;73(2):306–13.

37. Young RH, Dickersin GR, Scully RE. Juvenile granulosa cell tumor of the ovary. A clinicopathological analysis of 125 cases. Am J Surg Pathol 1984;8(8): 575–96.

38. Kalfa N, Ecochard A, Patte C, et al. Activating mutations of the stimulatory g protein in juvenile ovarian granulosa cell tumors: a new prognostic factor? J Clin Endocrinol Metab 2006;91(5):1842–7.

39. Auguste A, Bessiere L, Todeschini AL, et al. Molecular analyses of juvenile granulosa cell tumors bearing AKT1 mutations provide insights into tumor biology and therapeutic leads. Hum Mol Genet 2015;24(23):6687–98.

40. Bessiere L, Todeschini AL, Auguste A, et al. A hotspot of in-frame duplications activates the oncoprotein AKT1 in juvenile granulosa cell tumors. EBioMedicine 2015;2(5):421–31.

41. van Meurs HS, Schuit E, Horlings HM, et al. Development and internal validation of a prognostic model to predict recurrence free survival in patients with adult granulosa cell tumors of the ovary. Gynecol Oncol 2014;134(3):498–504.

42. Suri A, Carter EB, Horowitz N, et al. Factors associated with an increased risk of recurrence in women with ovarian granulosa cell tumors. Gynecol Oncol 2013;131(2):321–4.

43. Farkkila A, Andersson N, Butzow R, et al. HER2 and GATA4 are new prognostic factors for early-stage ovarian granulosa cell tumor-a long-term follow-up study. Cancer Med 2014;3(3):526–36.

44. Korzets A, Nouriel H, Steiner Z, et al. Resistant hypertension associated with a renin-producing ovarian Sertoli cell tumor. Am J Clin Pathol 1986; 85(2):242–7.

45. Oliva E, Alvarez T, Young RH. Sertoli cell tumors of the ovary: a clinicopathologic and immunohistochemical study of 54 cases. Am J Surg Pathol 2005;29(2):143–56.

46. Tavassoli FA, Norris HJ. Sertoli tumors of the ovary. A clinicopathologic study of 28 cases with ultrastructural observations. Cancer 1980;46(10):2281–97.

47. Yamamoto S, Sakai Y. Ovarian Sertoli-Leydig cell tumor with heterologous hepatocytes and a hepatocellular carcinomatous element. Int J Gynecol Pathol 2018, [Epub ahead of print].

48. Sahoo TK, Kar T, Kar A, et al. Poorly differentiated Sertoli-Leydig cell tumour of ovary with heterologous elements. J Clin Diagn Res 2017;11(5):XD01–2.

49. Mooney EE, Nogales FF, Bergeron C, et al. Retiform Sertoli-Leydig cell tumours: clinical, morphological and immunohistochemical findings. Histopathology 2002;41(2):110–7.

50. Heravi-Moussavi A, Anglesio MS, Cheng SW, et al. Recurrent somatic DICER1 mutations in nonepithelial ovarian cancers. N Engl J Med 2012;366(3):234–42.

51. Gui T, Cao D, Shen K, et al. A clinicopathological analysis of 40 cases of ovarian Sertoli-Leydig cell tumors. Gynecol Oncol 2012;127(2):384–9.

52. Young RH. Ovarian sex cord-stromal tumours and their mimics. Pathology 2018;50(1):5–15.

53. Prat J, Young RH, Scully RE. Ovarian Sertoli-Leydig cell tumors with heterologous elements. II. Cartilage and skeletal muscle: a clinicopathologic analysis of twelve cases. Cancer 1982;50(11):2465–75.

54. Young RH, Scully RE. Ovarian Sertoli-Leydig cell tumors with a retiform pattern: a problem in histopathologic diagnosis. A report of 25 cases. Am J Surg Pathol 1983;7(8):755–71.

55. Schultz KAP, Harris AK, Finch M, et al. DICER1-related Sertoli-Leydig cell tumor and gynandroblastoma: clinical and genetic findings from the International Ovarian and Testicular Stromal Tumor Registry. Gynecol Oncol 2017;147(3):521–7.

56. Zhang X, Shen D, Wang Y. Detection of the DICER1 hotspot mutation alongside immunohistochemical analysis may provide a better diagnostic measure for ovarian Sertoli-Leydig cell tumors. Pathol Res Pract 2018;214(9):1370–5.

57. Lim D, Oliva E. Ovarian sex cord-stromal tumours: an update in recent molecular advances. Pathology 2018;50(2):178–89.

58. Meurgey A, Descotes F, Mery-Lamarche E, et al. Lack of mutation of DICER1 and FOXL2 genes in microcystic stromal tumor of the ovary. Virchows Arch 2017;470(2):225–9.

59. Rose PG, Rubin RB, Nelson BE, et al. Accuracy of frozen-section (intraoperative consultation) diagnosis of ovarian tumors. Am J Obstet Gynecol 1994;171(3):823–6.

60. Cox HY, Cracchiolo B, Galan M, et al. Pitfalls of frozen section in gynecological pathology: a case of endometrial tumor with sex cord-like elements. Int J Surg Pathol 2018;26(4):327–9.

61. Burris A, Hixson C, Smith N. Frozen section diagnostic pitfalls of Sertoli-Leydig cell tumor with heterologous elements. Case Rep Pathol 2018;2018: 5151082.

Germ Cell Tumors of the Female Genital Tract

Elizabeth D. Euscher, MD

KEYWORDS

- Germ cell • Teratoma • Yolk sac • Dysgerminoma • Embryonal carcinoma • Ovary • Uterus • Vulva

Key points

- Ovarian germ cell tumors are a histologically diverse group of neoplasms with a common origin in the primitive germ cell. The vast majority are represented by mature cystic teratoma.

- Histologic overlap between patterns encountered in the various germ cell tumor subtypes as well as with somatic carcinomas can pose diagnostic challenges.

- Judicious use of immunohistochemistry can reliably distinguish between germ cell tumor subtypes.

- Extragonadal germ cell tumors primary in extragonadal locations within the gynecologic tract (ie, uterus, vagina, vulva) can mimic more commonly encountered somatic tumors at these sites. Awareness of extragonadal germ cell tumors and use of immunohistochemical stains facilitate correct diagnosis.

ABSTRACT

Ovarian germ cell tumors are a histologically diverse group of neoplasms with a common origin in the primitive germ cell. The vast majority are represented by mature cystic teratoma. In the minority are malignant germ cell tumors including immature teratoma, dysgerminoma, yolk sac tumor, embryonal cell carcinoma, and choriocarcinoma. This article reviews the histologic and immunohistochemical features of the most common ovarian germ cell tumors. The differential diagnoses for each are discussed.

OVERVIEW

Germ cell tumors of the ovary are the second most frequently encountered ovarian neoplasms following surface epithelial tumors. They are a histologically heterogeneous group with common origins in the primitive germ cell that can show features reminiscent of the primordial germ cell (ie, dysgerminoma) to differentiation into embryonic structure (ie, teratoma). In the ovary, most germ cell tumors are represented by mature teratoma; malignant ovarian germ cell tumors constitute only a fraction of germ cell tumors. Although germ cell tumors typically arise in the gonads, they may also arise at extragonadal sites typically in midline structures along the presumed migration path of germ cells during embryogenesis. This review describes the most commonly encountered germ cell tumors in the gynecologic tract both of gonadal and extragonadal origin.

TERATOMATOUS GERM CELL TUMORS OF THE OVARY

MATURE TERATOMA

Accounting for 90% of all ovarian tumors in premenarchal girls and 60% of all ovarian neoplasms in women younger than 20, mature cystic teratoma is the most common germ cell tumor arising in the ovary.[1] Most are diagnosed during the reproductive

---

Disclosure Statement: Nothing to disclose.
Department of Pathology, The University of Texas M.D. Anderson Cancer Center, 1515 Holcombe Boulevard Unit 85, Houston, TX 77030, USA
E-mail address: Edeusche@mdanderson.org

Surgical Pathology 12 (2019) 621–649
https://doi.org/10.1016/j.path.2019.01.005
1875-9181/19/© 2019 Elsevier Inc. All rights reserved.

years, but they also occur in children or post menopause.[2] Typically these tumors present with symptoms associated with a pelvic mass, but up to 60% may be asymptomatic.[2,3] Unusual presentations peculiar to mature teratoma include neuropsychiatric syndrome secondary to autoimmune encephalitis due to antibodies against the N-methyl-D-Aspartate receptor (anti-NMDAR),[4,5] opsoclonus-myoclonus syndrome, juvenile dermatomyositis-like syndrome, seronegative polyarthritis/tenosynovitis,[6] and memory deficits due to anti-Ri antibodies.[7] Although usually unilateral, mature teratoma can be bilateral in 13.2% of cases.[1] In addition, synchronous tumors involving the ovary plus another anatomic site such as the fallopian tube, omentum, pouch of Douglas, or mediastinum have been reported. Rare familial cases have been reported.[1]

Ovarian teratomas may become quite large with sizes exceeding 30 cm.[2] Typical tumors are cystic (unilocular or multilocular), although rarely may be predominantly solid.[8] The cysts are usually filled with yellow to tan-brown sebaceous material and hair; some tumors may have additional features such as teeth, seen in approximately one-third of cases, or a polypoid nodule emanating from an inner surface (Rokitansky protuberance) (**Fig. 1**). Rarely, components of mature teratoma form a mass resembling a poorly formed human fetus within a cystic space: fetiform teratoma.[9]

Microscopically, this neoplasm is usually composed of elements from all 3 germ cell layers:

ectoderm (ie, squamous epithelium, skin/adnexal structures, brain, peripheral nervous system tissue, cerebellum, and choroid plexus), mesoderm (ie, fat, bone, cartilage, teeth, blood vessels, smooth muscle, lymphoid tissue, skeletal muscle), and endoderm (ie, respiratory and gastrointestinal epithelium, thyroid, and salivary gland tissue), although often ectodermal derivatives predominate (**Fig. 2**).

MONODERMAL TERATOMA

Struma Ovarii

The most common monodermal teratoma, representing approximately 3% of all ovarian teratomas, is struma ovarii.[10] For a designation of struma ovarii, more than 50% of the teratoma is composed of thyroid tissue.[10] Up to one-third of patients have ascites (pseudo-Meigs syndrome), and approximately 5% of patients have hyperthyroidism.[10] Usually the thyroid is not enlarged with radioiodine uptake noted in the pelvis, but low or absent in the thyroid.[11]

Struma ovarii is composed of variably sized thyroid follicles embedded in a stroma that may be ovarian or teratomatous, edematous, or fibrous.[12,13] The thyroid tissue may undergo similar changes to those encountered in the thyroid, including adenomatous change,[13] papillary hyperplasia,[14] thyroid-type adenoma appearance, proliferative changes (ie, densely hypercellular thyroid tissue with follicular, trabecular, or solid

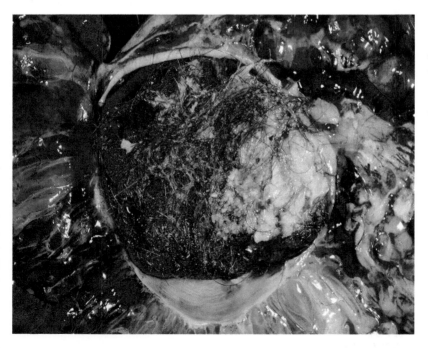

Fig. 1. Mature teratoma, cystic structure with hair and sebaceous material; this example has a component of mucinous borderline tumor, note mucoid areas at bottom and left of cyst.

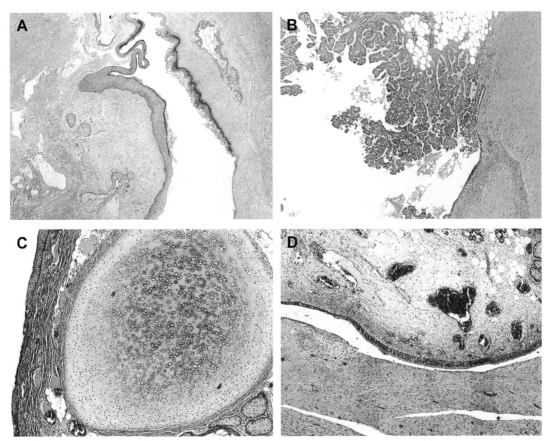

Fig. 2. Mature cystic teratoma. (*A*) Squamous epithelium and sebaceous glands. (*B*) Choroid plexus. (*C*) Cartilage. (*D*) Respiratory epithelium.

growth patterns),[15] prominent cystic changes,[13] changes of toxic goiter associated with clinical hyperactivity, Hashimoto thyroiditis, prominent microfollicles, or oxyphilic cytoplasmic changes[10] (Fig. 3).

Thyroid-type carcinomas, most commonly papillary carcinoma followed by follicular carcinoma, may arise in ovarian struma ovarii.[13,14,16] Papillary carcinoma is characterized by enlarged, overlapping nuclei with optically clear nuclei, nuclear pseudoinclusions, nuclear grooves, and an irregular nuclear membrane. Papillary architecture is at least focally (>1%) present in its classic form (Fig. 4). In the follicular variant of papillary thyroid carcinoma, the same nuclear features are present but follicular architecture predominates (at least in 99% of the tumor).[17] Highly differentiated follicular carcinoma of ovarian origin (HDFCO) describes the rare occurrence of normal-appearing ovarian thyroid tissue associated with extraovarian disease (see Fig. 4). The presence of any cytologic atypia and/or vascular invasion within the ovarian tumor is not in keeping with a diagnosis of HDFCO,

and these cases are best classified as follicular carcinoma. HDFCO replaces an older term: "peritoneal strumosis." HDFCO is usually seen at the time of presentation of the ovarian struma ovarii; however, rarely struma ovarii allegedly confined to the ovary has recurred intraperitoneally as well as distantly, including the lung, from months to many years after removal of the ovarian lesion.[13,17,18] Most of these cases have had either no peritoneal or omental sampling or secondary pathology review for diagnosis confirmation. Very rarely a thyroid-type tumor with solid growth, necrosis, and/or ≥5 mitoses per 10 high power fields can be seen in struma ovarii.[17]

Thyroid differentiation is highlighted by reaction to antibodies directed at thyroglobulin and thyroid transcription factor−1 (TTF-1).[13] Classic papillary thyroid carcinoma arising in struma ovarii may have a *BRAF* mutation. It is presumed that, as in primary thyroid carcinoma, this finding indicates more aggressive disease.[11] *BRAF* mutation has not been identified in the follicular variant of this neoplasm.[13]

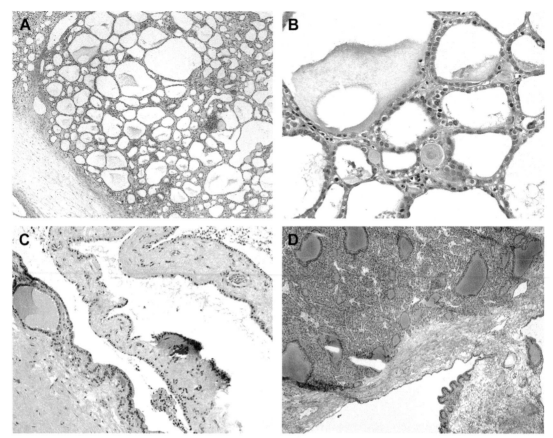

Fig. 3. Struma ovarii. (*A*) Thyroid follicles of varying size. (*B*) Higher power, follicles lined by bland, cuboidal epithelium. (*C*) Prominent cystic change. (*D*) Adenomatous change.

Differential diagnostic considerations include other tumors with papillary or follicular architectural features. Serous cystadenoma or borderline tumor can have architectural overlap with struma ovarii with cystic changes and/or papillary carcinoma. For those cases mimicking papillary carcinoma, nuclear features are usually absent. In addition, serous tumors are only rarely associated with mature cystic teratoma,[13] and usually at least a few normal thyroid follicles are seen at the periphery of a papillary carcinoma in struma ovarii. By immunohistochemistry, serous epithelium is positive for WT-1 but usually negative for TTF-1 with the reverse being true for strumal neoplasms. Notably, both tumor types are positive for PAX-8, so this stain will not aid in the differential diagnosis. Sex cord stromal tumors with a microfollicular or trabecular pattern can simulate the architectural features of a thyroid-type neoplasm in the ovary, and in the case of adult granulosa cell tumor will have overlapping cytologic features. Helpful immunohistochemical stains include inhibin, calretinin, or SF-1 to exclude sex cord lineage and

TTF-1 to confirm thyroid tissue. Endometrioid carcinoma may simulate a microfollicular pattern in some cases, and rarely can have expression of TTF-1.[19] Additional immunohistochemical markers, such as hormone receptors, attention to nuclear detail, and associated endometriosis, when present, may all be helpful in making this distinction. Metastatic thyroid carcinoma should be considered in a patient with a synchronous (or history of) primary thyroid carcinoma and in whom the ovarian tumor lacks associated benign thyroid tissue or teratomatous elements.[13]

Struma ovarii is usually benign; however, some cases lacking any suspicious feature can recur (ie, HDFCO). On the other hand, histologic evidence of malignancy does not always equate to aggressive behavior, particularly when the tumor is confined to the ovary. There are no formal guidelines with respect to the need for follow-up of patients with struma ovarii or thyroid-type malignancies arising within struma ovarii. Patients with the latter require long-term monitoring of serum thyroglobulin. Given the potential for a

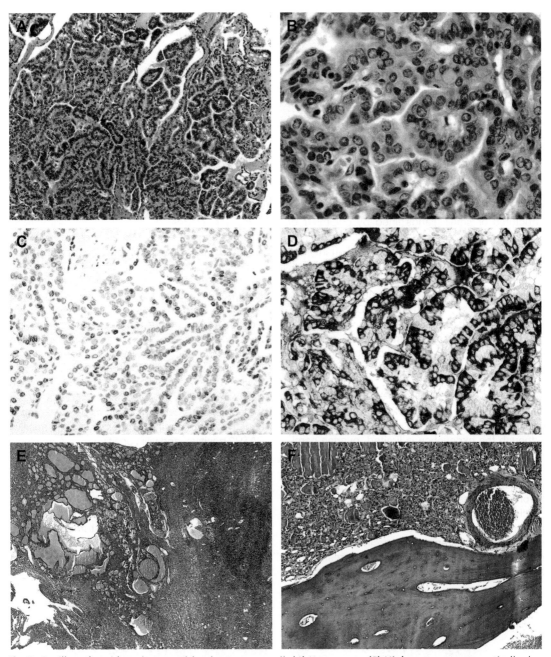

Fig. 4. Papillary thyroid carcinoma arising in struma ovarii. (*A*) Low power. (*B*) Higher power, note optically clear nuclei, nuclear grooves and nuclear overlap. (*C*) TTF-1 positive. (*D*) Thyroglobulin positive. (*E*) Bland thyroid tissue in ovary, HDFCO with (*F*) bone metastasis.

rare case of HDFCO, consideration to long-term follow-up in cases of apparently benign struma ovarii may be given.[11]

Carcinoid

Ovarian carcinoid tumor is rare, yet is the second most common type of monodermal teratoma. They occur over a wide age range but are most common in the peri-menopausal or early postmenopausal years.[20] Most patients will present with symptoms related to an abdominal mass, but classic carcinoid syndrome related to secretion of serotonin like substances (ie, facial flushing, bronchospasm, diarrhea, edema) has been reported more commonly with insular carcinoid over other architectural patterns.[21]

The most common pattern is insular carcinoid characterized by small acini and nests of polygonal cells with uniform round or oval nuclei with finely distributed chromatin (**Fig. 5**). The trabecular pattern is less common, with cells arranged in trabeculae or ribbons. Carcinoid tumor may be seen in pure form but more commonly is associated with other tumor types including mature cystic teratoma/struma ovarii, mucinous tumor, Brenner tumor, or Sertoli-Leydig cell tumor.[22,23] Strumal carcinoid is the presence of carcinoid, usually insular or trabecular, and thyroid tissue, which at least focally is admixed. The rare mucinous carcinoid is characterized by acinar structures or small glands lined by columnar or cuboidal cells intermixed with goblet cells. The mucinous component may be malignant and contain signet ring cells.[22] As with neuroendocrine tumors at other sites, ovarian carcinoid has expression of 1 or more neuroendocrine markers: chromogranin, synaptophysin, or CD56.[24] Expression of pankeratin and keratin 7 is variable. The carcinoid component is distinguished from any associated sex cord or thyroid component by absent staining for inhibin, calretinin, and SF1 or TTF-1, respectively. Both insular carcinoid tumors and mucinous carcinoids of the ovary express CDX2 limiting use of this marker to exclude a metastatic carcinoid from the gastrointestinal tract. Although the experience is limited, ovarian carcinoids appear to be PAX-8 negative.[24]

The primary diagnostic consideration is exclusion of metastatic carcinoid to the ovary. Features favoring a metastasis include a clinical history of carcinoid tumor at another anatomic site, bilaterality, multinodular growth pattern, extraovarian disease, and persistence of carcinoid syndrome following removal of the tumor. The presence of an associated teratoma, Brenner tumor or sex cord stromal tumor, as well as a unilateral tumor, supports an ovarian origin.[22]

Somatic-Type Tumors Arising in Teratomas

Malignant transformation is rare, occurring in 0.17% to 3.5% of mature cystic teratomas.[2,25] It has been reported over a wide age range but is more frequent in postmenopausal patients.[1,25] In approximately 80% to 90% of such cases, the somatic tumor will be squamous cell carcinoma (**Fig. 6**).[26] Prognosis depends on tumor stage, ranging from a 5-year survival of 75% for unruptured stage 1 tumors to 25%, 12%, and no survivors, for stages II, III, and IV, respectively. Adenocarcinomas (usually gastrointestinal type, respiratory less frequent) are seen in approximately 7% of cases.[27] In addition to intestinal-type adenocarcinoma, mature cystic teratomas can harbor the full spectrum of mucinous neoplasia, including cystadenoma, borderline tumor, and intraepithelial carcinoma.[28,29] All of these mucinous neoplasms can be associated with pseudomyxoma ovarii and/or peritonei[28,29] and have overlapping histologic and immunohistochemical features with a primary mucinous neoplasm from the appendix or lower gastrointestinal tract. Mucinous tumors arising in the context of a teratoma tend to be cytokeratin 7 negative, cytokeratin 20 positive, CDX2 positive, SATB2 positive, and villin positive.[28–30] A mucinous neoplasm overgrowing an ovarian teratoma should be a diagnostic consideration when a diagnosis of a secondary ovarian tumor from the appendix or lower gastrointestinal tract is contemplated. The distinction is made on clinical grounds.

A wide range of other somatic tumors have also been described but are rare. Among this list are melanocytic lesions, skin adnexal tumors, and tumors of the central nervous system.

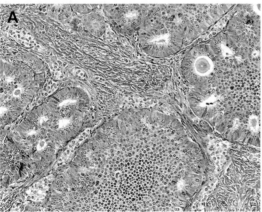
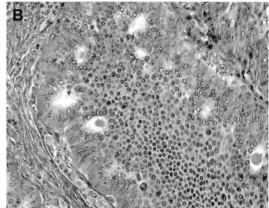

Fig. 5. Insular carcinoid. (*A*) Nests and acini. (*B*) Higher power showing finely distributed ("salt and pepper") chromatin.

Fig. 6. Squamous cell carcinoma arising in a mature cystic teratoma (inset, higher power).

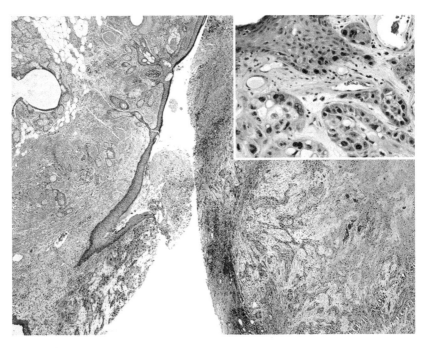

- Melanocytic lesions (compound and blue nevi) and melanoma[31]: Microscopically, melanoma is composed of epithelioid and/or spindle cells arranged in sheets and nests. Pigment deposition, a lentiginous pattern, macrofollicles, a pseudopapillary pattern, necrosis, rhabdoid cells, lipoblastlike cells, tumor giant cells, and signet-ring like cells can be seen. Melanoma arising in an ovarian teratoma has a similar immunoprofile to melanoma at other sites including expression of one or multiple melanocytic markers, such as S100, HMB-45, MelanA, and SOX10.[32] Melanoma arising in teratoma tends to exhibit aggressive behavior.[32]
- Skin adnexal lesions and tumors including sebaceous hyperplasia, sebaceous gland adenoma (one associated with Muir-Torre syndrome), sebaceous carcinoma, microcystic adnexal carcinoma, trichoadenoma, pilomatrixoma, and Paget disease have been described in ovarian teratomas.[33,34]
- Nervous system neoplasms: The full spectrum of nervous system tumors has been reported in association with ovarian teratoma, including astrocytic (glioblastoma, pilocytic astrocytoma) and oligodendroglial tumors,[35–39] central neurocytoma,[40] choroid plexus papilloma,[41] atypical choroid plexus papilloma,[41,42] and primitive tumors of the neuroectoderm (medulloblastoma, desmoplastic medulloblastoma, embryonal tumor with multilayered, neuroblastoma).[35,43–45] Some

investigators regard these neoplasms as monodermal teratomas[12,46]; however, these neuroectodermal neoplasms, with the exception of ependymoma, are almost always associated with mesodermal and endodermal elements suggesting that these neoplasms represent a tumor arising in one of the many components of a teratoma (glial or neural tissue) rather than a true monodermal teratomas. Even in the context of a teratoma, these tumors retain their prototypic histologic features. Tumors with astrocytic or oligodendrocytic differentiation express glial fibrillary acidic protein (GFAP),[35,45] whereas the primitive tumors may be positive for synaptophysin, neurofilament, and focally positive for GFAP.[35] The primitive neuroectodermal tumors described previously are of the central type and do not have the distinct membranous CD99 expression or t(11;22) (q24;q12) translocation characterizing peripheral primitive neuroectodermal tumor (PNET/Ewing sarcoma).[47] Choroid plexus papilloma has staining for synaptophysin, neuron specific enolase, transthyretin with focal staining for pankeratin and keratin 7.[42] Oligodendroglioma is distinguished from neurocytoma by expression of GFAP and absence of synaptophysin expression, whereas the reverse is true for the latter. Despite the histologic similarity, ovarian astrocytomas do not have the *IDH* mutation associated with most grade I and II central nervous system diffuse astrocytomas.[45] Because of their rarity, experience with nervous system tumors in teratomas is limited. Low-grade astrocytic/oligodendrocytic neoplasms confined to the ovary appear adequately treated by conservative surgery alone (ie, salpingo-oophorectomy). In contrast, the recommendation for high-stage, low-grade tumors and any high-grade tumor is chemotherapy.[35,45] Ultimately, prognosis depends on the tumor stage and grade of differentiation.[35]

IMMATURE TERATOMA

Immature teratoma is distinguished from its mature counterpart by the presence of immature neuroepithelium. Patients range from younger than 1 year to 58 years and most commonly present with an abdominal mass.[48,49] Some patients have mildly increased alpha-fetoprotein (AFP). These tumors are typically large (median size, 18 cm) and unilateral with areas of hemorrhage and necrosis (**Fig. 7**). Occasionally, a synchronous or metachronous mature cystic teratoma will be found in the contralateral ovary.[49]

Microscopically, immature neuroepithelium is arranged in sheets or rosettes and has conspicuous mitotic activity (**Fig. 8**). To determine the tumor grade, the slide with the greatest amount of immature neuroepithelium is reviewed under ×40 (×4 objective and ×10 eye piece) magnification. Foci from multiple slides may not be added. In addition, foci of ependymal tubules, retinal tissue, cerebellum, lymphoid tissue, or fetal-appearing mesenchymal tissue should not be mistaken for immature neuroepithelium. The initial grading scheme for immature teratoma was 3-tiered:

- Grade 1: amount of immature neuroepithelium occupies up to but does not exceed 1 low-power (×40) microscopic field.
- Grade 2: amount of immature neuroepithelium occupies more than 1 low-power (×40) microscopic field, but does not exceed 3 low-power fields.
- Grade 3: amount of immature neuroepithelium occupies more than 3 low-power (×40) microscopic fields.

Subsequently, a 2-tier grading system for immature teratoma was implemented:

- Low grade (amount of immature neuroepithelium on a single slide, <1 low-power field)
- High grade (amount of neuroepithelium on a single slide exceeds 1 low-power field)

The 2-tier system was found to reduce interobserver variability and thus is the one used for medical management.[48] It should be noted that not infrequently small foci of yolk sac tumor may be encountered adjacent to immature neuroepithelium. The presence of such foci (ie, up to 3 foci measuring up to 3 mm, each) in an otherwise low-grade (grade 1) immature teratoma does not affect prognosis.[48] When foci of immature neuroepithelium coalesce such that foci do not need to be added and instead form a distinct mass, the tumor is regarded as a central-type PNET rather than an immature teratoma.

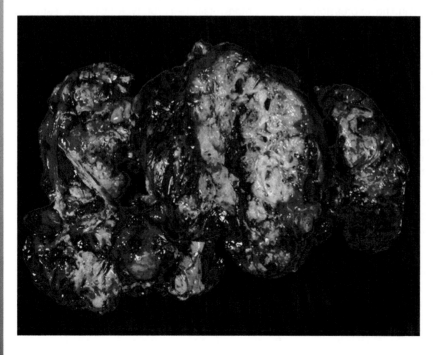

Fig. 7. Gross appearance, immature teratoma. Solid and cystic tumor with hemorrhage and necrosis.

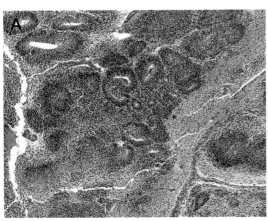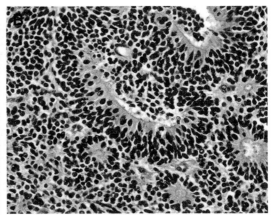

Fig. 8. Immature neuroepithelium in an immature teratoma. (*A*) Low power; (*B*) high power.

The treatment for immature teratoma is surgical and usually fertility sparing depending on the age of the patient. Use of adjuvant therapy also varies according to the patient's age.[50] The 5-year survival is almost 100% for early-stage disease and at least 75% in advanced-stage disease.[51] In the pediatric population, the 5-year overall survival is 99%.[44]

EXTRAOVARIAN LESIONS IN OVARIAN TERATOMAS

Both mature and immature teratoma may have extraovarian findings, which do not impact stage or prognosis and include the following:

- Granulomatous reaction in the peritoneum secondary to leakage of cyst contents.[52]
- Melanosis peritonei: grossly visible, focal or diffuse brown or black pigmentation in the peritoneum. The pigment is contained within macrophages and is usually melanin but may also be hemosiderin. The finding is often associated with rupture of a mature cystic teratoma. The differential diagnosis includes the rare case of metastatic melanoma to the omentum.[53] Use of SOX-10 immunohistochemistry will highlight melanoma and facilitate the correct diagnosis.
- Gliomatosis peritonei: multiple nodules of mature glial tissue are present on the peritoneal surface (**Fig. 9**) and occasionally within lymph nodes (nodal gliomatosis).[54,55] More commonly seen in association with immature teratoma, it may also be seen in mature cystic teratoma or mixed germ cell tumors. It is hypothesized that gliomatosis peritonei originates from pluripotent peritoneal cells stimulated by growth factors produced by the primary tumor that induce glial

differentiation.[56] Gliomatosis peritonei can be detected either initially or subsequent to diagnosis.[57] Rarely gliomas may arise in association with gliomatosis peritonei or foci of gliomatosis peritonei may be associated with growing teratoma syndrome.

GROWING TERATOMA SYNDROME

Although much more common in male than female patients, growing teratoma syndrome is the phenomenon of enlarging, extragonadal mature teratoma that appear during or after chemotherapy for malignant gonadal germ cell tumor, including immature teratoma, following normalization of serum AFP and/or human chorionic gonadotropin (HCG).[51,58,59] Typically, growing teratoma syndrome occurs within 5 years of the initial diagnosis of the gonadal tumor but intervals of more than 20 years have been reported. The retroperitoneum is the most common site of involvement. Up to 3% of cases may undergo malignant transformation. The treatment of this condition is surgical debulking.[51]

NONTERATOMATOUS GERM CELL TUMORS OF THE OVARY

DYSGERMINOMA

Second in incidence to teratoma with respect to all ovarian germ cell tumors, dysgerminoma is the most common malignant germ cell tumor of the ovary,[60,61] affecting mostly patients in the second to third decade.[60,62] Dysgerminoma may be associated with dysgenetic gonads and sexual maldevelopment including within the context of Turner syndrome, testicular feminization, and triple X syndrome.[63,64] In gonadal dysgenesis, dysgerminoma arises from a gonadoblastoma, most commonly

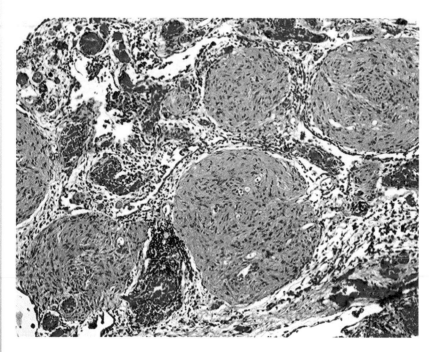

Fig. 9. Gliomatosis peritonei.

from a streak gonad, and occasionally from an intra-abdominal testis.[52] Dysgerminoma is almost always associated with an elevated serum lactic dehydrogenase, usually isoenzymes 1 and 2. Elevation of serum β-HCG and AFP has also been reported.[60,65–68]

Classically, dysgerminoma is a unilateral, solid, fleshy, cream-colored tumor (**Fig. 10**). The presence of calcification suggests an underlying gonadoblastoma.[52] Perhaps as a reflection of

associated gonadal dysgenesis, the contralateral ovary may be affected in up to 15% of cases.[60] Most of the time, the presence of contralateral ovarian involvement is seen grossly, but on occasion involvement may be limited to microscopic disease.[69]

The tumor is composed of polygonal cells, with clear or eosinophilic cytoplasm, visible cell membranes, large nuclei with vesicular chromatin, and an angulated or "squared off" nuclear membrane

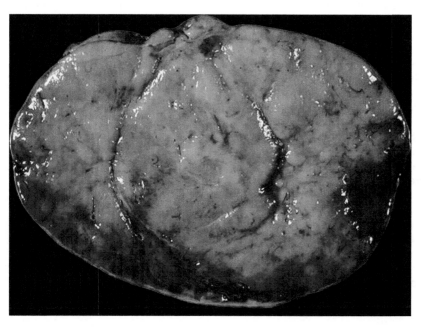

Fig. 10. Dysgerminoma, gross image; cream-colored, fleshy tumor.

and prominent nucleoli (**Fig. 11**).[61] Cells may be arranged in sheets, nests, cords, trabeculae, or single cells less commonly in follicle-like or pseudoglandular spaces that may contain eosinophilic material. Most cases have conspicuous mitotic activity.[60] Intervening stroma ranges from thin, collagenous strands to fibrous tissue bands of variable thickness containing lymphocytes and sometimes lymphoid follicles and plasma cells. Up to 20% of cases have a granulomatous reaction in the stroma that occasionally may be sarcoid-like. The presence of granulomatous inflammation in lymph nodes of a patient with dysgerminoma suggests the presence of metastatic dysgerminoma.[52] Some dysgerminomas have scattered syncytiotrophoblastic giant cells, which may be seen throughout the tumor or as clusters adjacent to fibrous bands.[70]

Dysgerminoma has the following characteristic immunohistochemical profile: SALLA-4 (diffuse, nuclear expression), OCT4 (nuclear expression), D2-40 (membranous and cytoplasmic expression), and CD117 (strong, membranous expression in approximately 80% of cases)[71–73] (**Fig. 12**).The expression of CD117 may correlate with the presence of a *KIT* mutation, identified in 27% to 53% of cases, most commonly in exon 17 rather than exon 11.[72–74] The therapeutic significance of such a finding remains to be determined. Other immunohistochemical markers that may be expressed in dysgerminoma include AFP (focal),[68] cytokeratin (focal dotlike to diffuse cytoplasmic staining in up to a third of cases).[24,71] Because epithelial membrane antigen (EMA) is not expressed in dysgerminoma, it may be used as an exclusionary marker for ovarian carcinoma.[24] HCG highlights the syncytiotrophoblastic giant cells observed in 3% of dysgerminomas,[70] which may correlate with the finding of an elevated serum β-HCG.[24] Recently described is focal nuclear immunoreactivity for NUT protein (<1% to 20% of the cells) in 93% of dysgerminomas.[75] **Table 1** outlines commonly used immunomarkers to diagnose dysgerminoma and other germ cell tumors.

The differential diagnosis includes an ovarian surface epithelial carcinoma, other germ cell

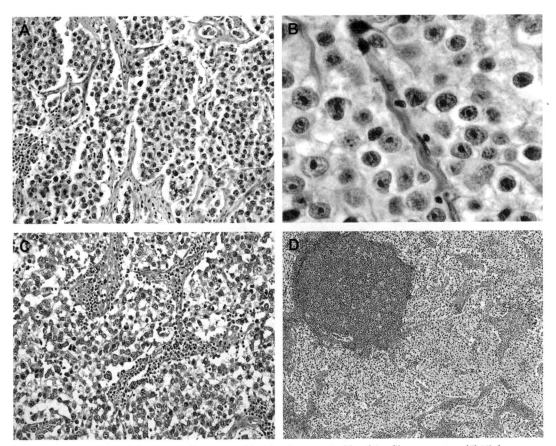

Fig. 11. Dysgerminoma. (*A*) Tumor cells arranged in islands separated by thin, fibrous septae. (*B*) Higher power image showing polygonal cells with distinct cell borders and eosinophilic to clear cytoplasm. (*C*) Lymphocytes present within fibrous septae. (*D*) May occasionally have prominent lymphoid follicles.

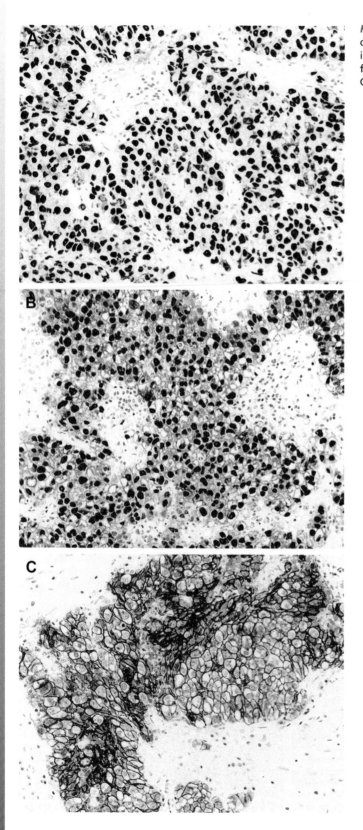

Fig. 12. Immunoperoxidase staining in dysgerminoma. (*A*) Strong, nuclear staining for SALL-4. (*B*) Strong nuclear staining for OCT4. (*C*) Membranous staining for CD117.

Table 1
Commonly used immunohistochemical markers in the diagnosis of ovarian germ cell tumors

Immunomarker	Description	Immature Teratoma (NEP)	Dysgerminoma	Embryonal Carcinoma	Yolk Sac Tumor	Choriocarcinoma
SALL4	Nuclear stain; broad marker of malignant GCTs; pluripotency marker, nonspecific	+ (variable intensity)	+	+	+	–
OCT4	Nuclear stain; transcription factor maintains embryonic stem cell pluripotency	–	+	+ (but may be lost after chemotherapy)	–	–
CD117	Membranous staining;	–	>85% +	–	+/– (some solid YST express)	–
D2-40	Membranous and cytoplasmic staining; marks podoplanin (expressed in germ cells)	–	+	+/–	–/+ (rare YST express)	–
CD30	Membranous staining	–	–	+ (but may be lost after chemotx)	–	–
SOX2	Nuclear staining; transcription involved in totipotency, responsible for neuronal differentiation	+	–	+	–	–

(continued on next page)

Table 1
(continued)

Immunomarker	Description	Immature Teratoma (NEP)	Dysgerminoma	Embryonal Carcinoma	Yolk Sac Tumor	Choriocarcinoma
AFP	Cytoplasmic staining (granular); may be focal to patchy; specific; expressed in primary yolk sac before specialized differentiation	–	–	–	+	–
Glypican-3	Cytoplasmic staining; secreted by secondary yolk sac; good specificity for YST vs other GCT but can be expressed in clear cell CA	–	–	–	+	+/–
HCG	Cytoplasmic staining	–	– (dysgerminoma cells); syncytiotrophoblast positive	–	–	+ (syncytiotrophoblast)

Abbreviations: AFP, α-fetoprotein; GCT, germ cell tumor; HCG, human chorionic gonadotropin; NEP, neuroepithelium.

tumors, small cell carcinoma of hypercalcemic type, and lymphoma.

- Clear cell carcinoma: Dysgerminoma may mimic the solid architectural pattern of clear cell carcinoma as well as the glandular pattern when pseudoglandular features are present. In addition, up to 20% of clear cell carcinomas may have a plasmacytic or lymphoplasmacytic stromal infiltrate.[76,77] This combination of features can cause diagnostic difficulty. By hematoxylin-eosin staining, a typical clear cell carcinoma will exhibit at least focally areas of papillary architecture as well as areas of stromal hyalinization, features that are not associated with dysgerminoma. In difficult cases, immunohistochemical studies facilitate the correct diagnosis (ie, dysgerminoma is positive for SALLA4, OCT4, CD117, and D2-40, whereas clear cell carcinoma is positive for EMA and PAX-8).[24]
- Yolk sac tumor or embryonal carcinoma: Either tumor may be considered in the differential diagnosis of dysgerminoma when it contains few inflammatory cells, has sheets of cells with dense, eosinophilic, or amphophilic cytoplasm, and/or has increased nuclear crowding. All of these tumors have expression of SALL-4, and embryonal carcinoma and dysgerminoma both express OCT4. Differentiating markers between embryonal carcinoma and dysgerminoma include CD30 and SOX10 in the former and CD117 and D240 in the latter. Yolk sac tumor has expression of glypican 3 and AFP lacking expression of the other markers.[24]
- Choriocarcinoma: Aggregates of syncytiotrophoblastic cells admixed with the fairly uniform, polygonal, mononuclear cells of dysgerminoma can raise the possibility of choriocarcinoma. However, the distinct biphasic pattern of choriocarcinoma is not present in dysgerminoma.
- Small cell carcinoma, hypercalcemic type: Dysgerminomas may have pseudoglandular spaces that can mimic the folliclelike spaces of small cell carcinoma of the ovary, hypercalcemic type (SCCOHT). Expression of germ cell immunohistochemical markers will exclude small cell carcinoma of hypercalcemic type from consideration. Conversely, lack of expression of SMARCA4 is a defining feature of SCCOHT but expression is retained in germ cell tumors including dysgerminoma.
- Lymphoma: This diagnosis is considered when the inflammatory infiltrate obscures the tumor cells. Use of SALL4 and OCT4 will highlight the dysgerminoma cells.

The overall 5-year survival following a diagnosis of ovarian dysgerminoma is more than 90%, with good outcomes reported even in patients presenting at advanced stage. Approximately 20% of stage 1A patients experience recurrence.[78]

YOLK SAC TUMOR

Yolk sac tumor is the second most common malignant ovarian germ cell tumor.[79] It occurs over a wide age range, although most patients are young (median age 19). In its pure form, this tumor is rare in women older than 50.[79–81] Almost all patients have an elevated serum AFP. This is a rapidly growing tumor; approximately one-third of patients have extraovarian spread at presentation.[82]

Yolk sac tumor most commonly affects only one ovary and is usually a soft, tan to yellow or gray tumor with areas of hemorrhage and necrosis (**Fig. 13**). Tumors with polyvesicular-vitelline pattern may have a honeycomb appearance grossly.[83] Microscopically, yolk sac tumor typically exhibits a combination of 2 or more of the following architectural patterns[82] (**Fig. 14**):

- Microcystic/reticular: In this pattern, a loose meshwork of small interconnecting spaces is lined by occasionally flattened, primitive tumor cells with a variable amount of clear or light eosinophilic cytoplasm. Tumor nuclei have irregularly distributed chromatin, prominent nucleoli, and conspicuous mitotic activity.[49] Reticular areas usually merge with variably sized cysts lined by flattened cells with a deceptively bland appearance.
- Papillary: This pattern may be associated with Schiller-Duval bodies in which rounded to elongated papillae with a connective tissue core and a single central vessel protrude into a cystic space lined by flattened to cuboidal epithelium. Schiller-Duval bodies (**Fig. 15**) are variably present, ranging from up to 75% of cases in some series to as low as 20% in others.[82,84,85]
- Solid: Cells are closely packed and may have clear or eosinophilic cytoplasm. Hyaline globules may be prominent. Awareness of this growth pattern is important to avoid confusion with other solid tumors with clear cytoplasm, such as dysgerminoma.
- Festoon: Undulating cords and columns of primitive germ cells with a drapelike pattern characterize this pattern.
- Polyvesicular-vitelline: This rare pattern is recognized by cysts and glandlike structures lined by flattened cells merging with columnar cells. The glandlike strictures may have

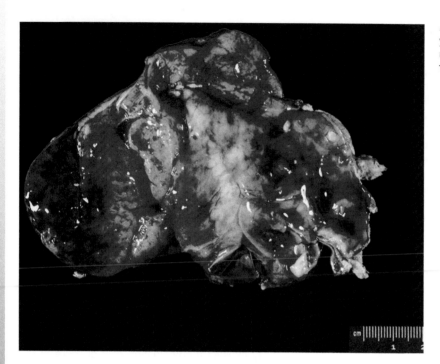

Fig. 13. Gross image, yolk sac tumor. Hemorrhagic cystic and solid tumor.

eccentric constriction. Cells may have cytoplasmic vacuoles or mucin. Often the surrounding stroma is abundant.

- Glandular pattern: This pattern reflects the capacity of yolk sac tumor to histologically reproduce endodermal somatic derivatives with glandular morphology (ie, endometrioid, intestinal/enteric, respiratory). Subnuclear and/or supranuclear cytoplasmic vacuoles are commonly identified.
- Hepatoid: Also a pattern reflecting an endodermal somatic derivative, hepatoid pattern is characterized by large polygonal cells with abundant eosinophilic cytoplasm arranged in aggregates separated by thin fibrous bands.

Other features include the presence of eosinophilic, periodic acid-Schiff (PAS)-positive, diastase-resistant intracellular and extracellular hyaline bodies and parietal differentiation characterized by abundant basement membrane–like material surrounding small groups and individual tumor cells.[61] Some patients have had a synchronous or metachronous mature cystic teratoma, ipsilateral or contralateral.[80] In addition, yolk sac tumor can coexist with dysgerminoma.[82]

When evaluating a potential yolk sac tumor by immunohistochemistry (**Fig. 16**), one should include a marker of primitive germ cell differentiation (ie, SALL-4 [nuclear staining]) and a marker considered specific to yolk sac tumor (ie, glypican-3 [variably distributed cytoplasmic staining] or AFP [cytoplasmic staining]) (see **Fig. 16**). Of note, glypican-3 is not entirely specific to yolk sac tumor and stains a subset of clear cell carcinoma. In contrast, AFP is considered highly specific to this diagnosis but the overall sensitivity may be as low as 60%.[24] A recently described marker, ZBTB16, has been considered as a sensitive and specific biomarker for yolk sac tumor.[86] Additional markers demonstrating evidence of differentiation, particularly enteric, also may be used, including CDX2 (nuclear staining seen in 40% of glandular yolk sac tumor),[87] villin (microcystic and glandular patterns), and HepPar-1 (glandular and hepatoid patterns[88]). Nuclear expression of GATA-3 is seen in the so-called primitive patterns of yolk sac tumor (reticular, papillary, and polyvesicular-vitelline), but not in the glandular variant.[89] Potential exclusionary markers include Keratin 7 and EMA, although yolk sac tumors with a glandular pattern may be focally positive for these markers.[88] PAX-8, Napsin A, and hormone receptors are typically not expressed in yolk sac tumor.[88,90]

The varied histologic appearance and resemblance to some somatic tumors can result in diagnostic difficulty. However, the proper clinical context of the ovarian tumor and presence of serum AFP will facilitate the correct diagnosis much of the time. In nonpediatric patients, clear cell and endometrioid carcinoma pose the greatest diagnostic challenge. Both carcinomas may have associated endometriosis. In the case of

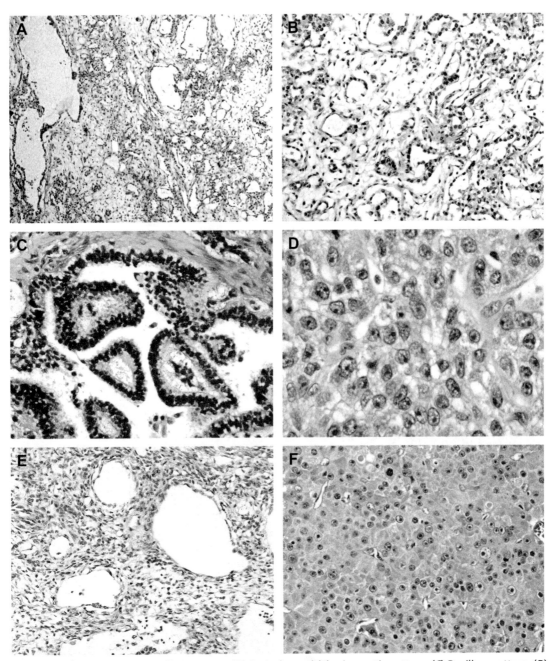

Fig. 14. Histologic patterns in yolk sac tumor. (*A*) Reticular and (*B*) microcystic pattern. (*C*) Papillary pattern. (*D*) Solid architecture. (*E*) Polyvesicular-vitelline pattern. (*F*) Hepatoid pattern.

clear cell carcinoma, the varied architectural patterns, lack of concordance between mitotic activity and cytologic atypia, and stromal hyalinization are useful histologic features to make this distinction. For endometrioid carcinoma, the presence of squamous metaplasia and the lack of primitive-appearing nuclei are useful histologic features.[82] Expression of PAX8 can distinguish endometrioid and clear cell carcinoma from yolk sac tumor. In

addition, clear cell carcinoma may have expression of NapsinA, and endometrioid carcinoma usually has expression of hormone receptors. Although there can be overlap with yolk sac tumor, expression of cytokeratin 7 and EMA is usually much stronger in carcinoma. Last, glypican 3 may be expressed in clear cell carcinoma so should not be used to distinguish this diagnosis from yolk sac tumor.[91] In cases of other germ

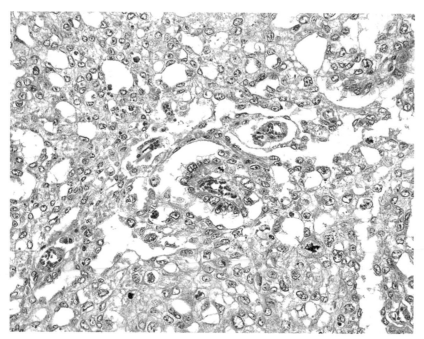

Fig.   15. Schiller-Duval body.

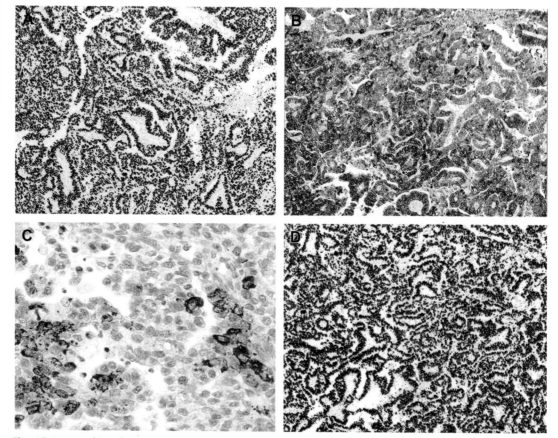

Fig. 16. Immunohistochemistry in yolk sac tumor. (*A*) SALL-4, nuclear expression. (*B*) Glypican-3, cytoplasmic expression. (*C*) Focal AFP expression. (*D*) Diffuse nuclear staining for CDX2.

cell tumors with overlapping histologic features, immunoperoxidase studies, as discussed in each respective section, facilitate diagnosis.

The 5-year survival rate for patients with yolk sac tumor decreases with increasing stage from 96% for stage I tumors to 25% for stage IV. Of note, the presence of a prominent polyvesicular-vitelline pattern may be associated with a more indolent behavior.[83] Apparent somatically derived yolk sac tumors seem to be less responsive to the standard chemotherapy used for malignant germ cell tumors.[92]

SOMATICALLY DERIVED TUMORS WITH GERM CELL TUMOR DIFFERENTIATION

Yolk sac tumor also may occur as a somatically derived tumor in the setting of an epithelial malignancy; that is, they originate from malignant stem cells present in somatic tumors of the ovary.[56] The histologic features are identical to yolk sac tumor of germ cell origin, although there is a propensity toward more frequent glandular pattern.[8] Such tumors typically arise in perimenopausal or postmenopausal women, and the presence of an associated somatic carcinoma provides support to the somatic derivation of this group of yolk sac tumor. Endometrioid carcinoma,[88,93–96] high-grade serous carcinoma,[90,96] clear cell carcinoma,[8,96] and carcinosarcoma[97] have all been reported. The term, "somatically derived yolk sac tumors" has been proposed for this group to distinguish them from true germ cell tumors.[96]

EMBRYONAL CARCINOMA

In its pure form, embryonal carcinoma of the ovary is exceedingly rare; most cases are seen in conjunction with one or more other germ cell tumor types.[61,84] Most patients are young (median 14 years). Serum levels of AFP and HCG may be elevated at presentation.[98]

Embryonal carcinoma is composed of predominantly sheets of large, pleomorphic cells with amphophilic, variably vacuolated cytoplasm with well-defined cell membranes. Within sheets of cells, papillary formations and glandlike structures may be observed. Nuclei have irregularly distributed chromatin, one or more prominent nucleoli, and exhibit crowding (**Fig. 17**).[61,84] Mitotic activity is high and atypical mitoses are frequent. Syncytiotrophoblast cells may be seen at the periphery of sheets of tumor cells or within surrounding stroma. The stroma can be loose or dense and fibrous. Intracellular and extracellular eosinophilic hyaline globules can be seen. Occasionally, glands with an intestinal appearance or foci of mature squamous epithelium and cartilage can be seen within the stroma.[84]

As with dysgerminoma and yolk sac tumor, embryonal carcinoma has nuclear expression of SALLA4. It also has expression of CD30 (membranous expression), OCT4 (diffuse, strong nuclear expression), and SOX2 (nuclear expression) (**Fig. 18**). The sensitivity of OCT4 is higher than CD30 for embryonal carcinoma. Of note, loss of OCT4 and CD30 expression has been observed following chemotherapy.[24] Associated syncytiotrophoblast cells are highlighted by HCG whereas AFP may be expressed in the embryonal carcinoma cells as well as in the hyaline globules.[84] Embryonal carcinoma usually exhibits membranous staining for AE1/AE3, whereas EMA is usually negative.[24]

Other diagnostic considerations include the following:

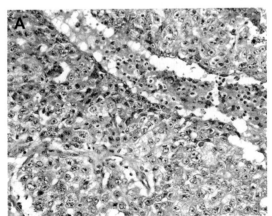 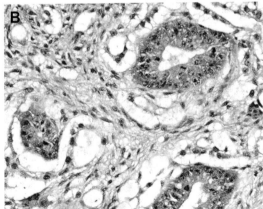

Fig. 17. Embryonal carcinoma. (*A*) Sheets of large primitive cells. (*B*) Embryonal carcinoma represented by atypical glandular elements admixed with yolk sac tumor.

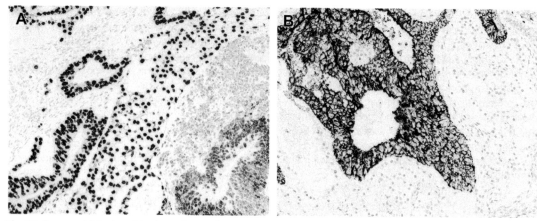

Fig. 18. Immunohistochemistry in embryonal carcinoma. (*A*) Nuclear expression of SALL-4. (*B*) Membranous staining for CD30.

- Yolk sac tumor usually has a variety of architectural patterns including those not associated with embryonal carcinoma (ie, reticular/microcystic, polyvesicular vitellin, and festoon).[84] Immunoperoxidase studies may facilitate diagnosis, as yolk sac tumor typically does not express OCT4 or SOX2. In addition, some investigators have found that the staining pattern of AE1/AE3 in yolk sac tumor is cytoplasmic rather than the membranous staining observed in embryonal carcinoma.[24]
- Dysgerminoma, compared with embryonal carcinoma, has smaller cells and fewer pleomorphic nuclei. In addition, dysgerminoma has characteristic fibrous stroma with lymphocytes. Dysgerminoma and embryonal carcinoma both express OCT4; however, expression of CD117 in dysgerminoma and CD30 in embryonal carcinoma will distinguish the two. Last, expression of keratin is less diffuse in dysgerminoma.[24]
- Choriocarcinoma is a diagnostic consideration, as embryonal carcinoma also may have syncytiotrophoblastic cells. However, choriocarcinoma has a characteristic biphasic admixture of syncytiotrophoblastic and cytotrophoblastic cells. Hemorrhage is also a frequent finding, which is not typical of embryonal carcinoma.[84] In difficult cases, inhibin highlights cytotrophoblastic cells.[24]
- Undifferentiated carcinoma enters into the differential diagnosis of metastatic tumor following chemotherapy due to loss of CD30 and OCT4 expression in embryonal carcinoma. However, expression of SALL4 is usually retained and can facilitate the correct diagnosis.[24,61]

Compared with other germ cell tumors, embryonal carcinoma has a worse outcome, and chemotherapy is standard of care regardless of the stage of disease.[99] The 5-year survival for stage I cases is 50%.[84]

CHORIOCARCINOMA

Pure, nongestational choriocarcinoma is rare; most nongestational cases are seen in the context of a mixed germ cell tumor.[100] Choriocarcinoma in the ovary associated with gestation (ie, associated with ovarian ectopic pregnancy or metastatic from a uterine or fallopian tube primary) is relatively more common. Most patients are diagnosed in their second or third decades of life,[101,102] presenting with abdominal pain, abdominal mass, or vaginal bleeding and an elevated HCG. Isosexual precocity has been reported in up to 50% of the premenarchal patients.[100]

Histologically, choriocarcinoma is characterized by a biphasic admixture of cytotrophoblast and syncytiotrophoblast (**Fig. 19**). Rare cases of nongestational choriocarcinoma of the ovary have arisen in association with an epithelial neoplasm of the ovary (serous carcinoma, mucinous cystadenoma, mixed high-grade carcinoma).[103]

Syncytiotrophoblast cells are positive for HCG, whereas inhibin is expressed in cytotrophoblast cells.[24] When the distinction between gestational and nongestational choriocarcinoma is unclear, molecular genotyping may assist in the distinction: nongestational tumor matches patient tissue and has allelic imbalances; gestational choriocarcinoma has biparental or androgenetic origin.[104]

The distinction between gestational and nongestational choriocarcinoma is important, as single-agent methotrexate may be the treatment of choice for the former but should not be used in the latter. It has been suggested that nongestational choriocarcinoma may be relatively resistant to chemotherapy; however, most patients respond

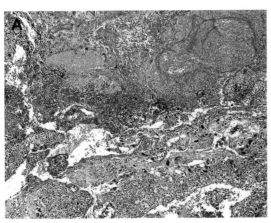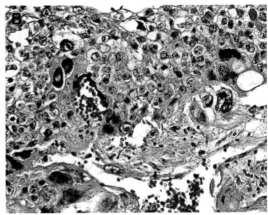

Fig. 19. Choriocarcinoma. (*A*) Low power, hemorrhagic tumor. (*B*) High power showing characteristic admixture of syncytiotrophoblast and mononuclear cytotrophoblast cells.

to combination chemotherapy.[101,105] Both gestational and nongestational choriocarcinoma tend to develop early hematogenous metastases to different organs (lungs, liver, brain, vagina).[100] The rare tumors arising in association with an ovarian surface epithelial neoplasm are biologically aggressive with most patients dying of disease within 24 months after diagnosis.[103]

EXTRAGONADAL GERM CELL TUMORS

Extragonadal germ cell tumors typically occur in midline structures and account for 2% to 5% of germ cell tumors in adults. Although they have identical histologic features to germ cell tumors in their gonadal counterparts, the rarity of these tumors, the unexpected location, and tendency to mimic somatic tumors combine to pose significant diagnostic challenge.[91,106] Yolk sac carcinoma, mature/immature teratoma, embryonal carcinoma and nongestational choriocarcinoma have all been reported in the vulva, vagina, and uterus, although mostly as case reports and small series.[91,107–123] Proposed mechanisms for the histogenesis of extragonadal yolk sac tumors include the following: (1) misplaced or arrested migration of germ cells during embryogenesis, (2) reverse migration of germ cells, (3) abnormal or retrodifferentiation of somatic tumor cells to more primitive ones, (4) specialized differentiation from a somatic carcinoma, (5) arising from residual fetal tissue following incomplete abortion, and (6) metastasis from an occult primary germ cell tumor of the gonad.[91,107] Each proposal has merit depending on the tumor location and to some extent type. For example, in the vulva, the leading hypothesis for germ cell tumor histogenesis is misplaced/aberrant germ cell migration along the gubernaculum.[107] In the uterus, residual fetal tissue may explain the development of some teratomas. However, the association of yolk sac tumor with somatic carcinomas in many of the reported cases supports the idea of a somatic origin for these tumors either through specialized or retrodifferentiation.[107] Special considerations with respect to the best characterized types of extragonadal gynecologic germ cell tumors (yolk sac tumor, teratoma) are outlined as follows.

YOLK SAC TUMOR

Yolk sac tumor is the most common germ cell tumor occurring in extragonadal sites within the female genital tract. In the vagina, yolk sac tumor is seen almost exclusively in young (≤2 years) girls. In contrast, endometrial yolk sac tumor is most commonly observed in postmenopausal women.[91,107] In the classic setting of vaginal yolk sac tumor in a young girl, the diagnosis is often fairly straightforward. The diagnosis of yolk sac tumor primary in the vulva or endometrium is much more difficult, as more commonly encountered somatic carcinomas, such as clear cell, endometrioid, mucinous carcinomas, or even a metastatic carcinoma are usually the first diagnostic consideration due to their increased frequency and overlapping morphologic and immunohistochemical features with yolk sac tumor. Like their gonadal counterparts, yolk sac tumor at extragonadal sites will frequently display a variety of architectural patterns (**Fig. 20**). Cells have primitive-appearing nuclei characterized by hyperchromaticity with homogeneous chromatin and peculiar supranuclear and subnuclear cytoplasmic vacuolization. Some cases have eosinophilic, PAS-positive, diastase-resistant intracellular and extracellular hyaline bodies. Schiller-Duval bodies are conspicuous in only a

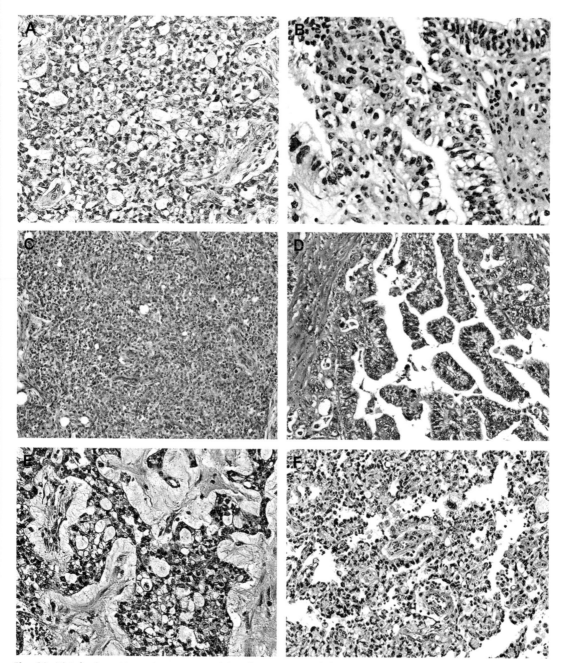

Fig. 20. Histologic patterns in extragonadal yolk sac tumor. (*A*) Microcystic/reticular pattern. (*B*) Glandular pattern, note supranuclear and subnuclear vacuoles. (*C*) Solid pattern. (*D*) Papillary pattern. (*E*) Areas of myxoid stroma that may be encountered in uterine extragonadal yolk sac tumor. (*F*) Schiller-Duval like bodies.

minority of cases.[91] Yolk sac tumor at extragonadal sites also may be seen in combination with other types of germ cell tumor (immature teratoma and embryonal carcinoma) or a somatic carcinoma. The key to avoiding the diagnostic pitfall of confusing yolk sac tumor with a somatic carcinoma begins with an awareness of the entity and an attention to the histologic features. A panel of immunoperoxidase studies often can confirm the diagnosis, but must include both inclusionary and exclusionary markers of germ cell/yolk sac differentiation (**Fig. 21**). SALL-4 is a pluripotential marker of germ cell differentiation but is not specific for yolk sac tumor. Due to its lack of specificity for yolk sac tumor as well as the tendency for weak, nuclear staining for SALL-4 in some somatic

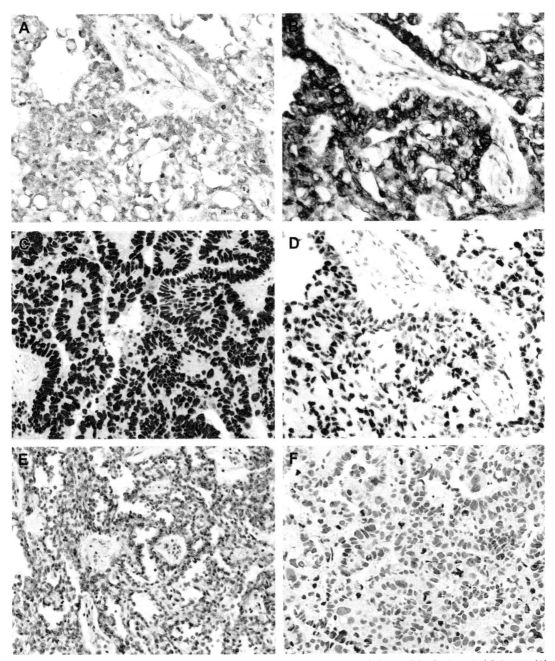

Fig. 21. Immunoperoxidase studies used in extragonadal yolk sac tumor. (*A*) AFP. (*B*) Glypican-3. (*C*) SALL4. (*D*) CDX2. (*E*) Cytokeratin 20. (*F*) Cytokeratin 7.

adenocarcinomas, this marker should be used in conjunction with a panel of immunoperoxidase stains. Only strong, diffuse nuclear staining for SALL-4 in the area of concern should be interpreted as a positive result. Yolk sac–specific markers such as AFP and glypican-3 should be included in the panel as well as markers of intestinal differentiation (cytokeratin 20, CDX2, villin), which have been reported in yolk sac tumors. AFP is very specific for a diagnosis of yolk sac tumor but is not very sensitive, and when staining is present, may be only focal. In contrast, glypican-3 is a sensitive marker staining 90% of yolk sac tumors but has overlapping expression with clear cell carcinoma. For this reason, exclusionary markers such as cytokeratin 7, estrogen receptor, and PAX8 also should be included. Markers used in the diagnosis of clear cell carcinoma (NapsinA and HNF1β) are not typically expressed in yolk sac tumor.[91] **Table 2** summarizes immunohistochemical stains used to distinguish yolk sac tumor from somatic carcinomas in the differential diagnosis.

As the diagnosis of yolk sac tumor is often not expected in patients with abnormal vaginal bleeding or a labial mass, particularly in patients beyond adolescence, a serum AFP is frequently not obtained before surgery. However, in the few reported cases with this information, AFP was typically elevated either preoperatively or at the time of recurrence, including some endometrial tumors thought to be somatically derived.[91] The behavior of vulvar yolk sac tumor is variable, although with a trend toward improved survival with modern chemotherapy.[91] It remains to be determined whether the presence of yolk sac tumor in an otherwise somatic carcinoma worsens the prognosis beyond that of the somatic carcinoma when the latter is already high grade or presents at an advanced stage.

TERATOMA

Teratoma outside of the ovary is rare. Few cases have been reported in the vagina, most of which contain ectodermal elements, such as squamous epithelium, sebaceous glands, hair follicles, and teeth. A rare case had cartilage. Lesions may be cystic or polypoid; none have exhibited malignant behavior.[113] An immature teratoma with inguinal lymph node metastasis was reported in the vulva.[108] Mature and immature teratomas have both been reported in the uterus (**Fig. 22**). Reports

of immature teratoma presenting with non-puerperal uterine inversion have been reported likely due the pedunculated nature of most of these tumors.[116,117]

Given the heterogeneity of endometrial tumors, the differential diagnosis of uterine teratoma includes endometrioid adenocarcinoma with heterologous elements, uterine carcinosarcoma, and uterine PNET. The rosettelike structures of immature neuroepithelium may simulate the glandular structures of endometrioid adenocarcinoma. The presence of a fibrillary background and associated glial cells highlighted by GFAP distinguishes the former. The presence of primitive-appearing mesenchyme separating rosettelike structures is an additional diagnostic feature that may be seen in immature teratoma. The presence of both glandular and mesenchymal components observed in uterine teratoma may lead to the consideration of carcinosarcoma. In contrast to carcinosarcoma, the epithelial component in a teratoma usually has a heterologous appearance (ie, thyroid tissue or respiratory/gastrointestinal differentiation). In a mature teratoma, both the epithelial and mesenchymal elements are histologically benign. Immature neuroepithelium is not characteristic of carcinosarcoma with the exception of a rare case of carcinosarcoma with a component of PNET. Distinguishing immature teratoma from PNET is challenging, as both entities may have immature neuroepithelial structures. In PNET, a proliferation of monotonous small round blue cells is the predominant histologic finding. In addition, PNETs typically lack associated, benign, mature elements

---

Table 2
Immunoperoxidase studies distinguishing extragonadal yolk sac tumor from more commonly encountered gynecologic epithelial tumors

	Yolk Sac Tumor	Clear Cell CA	Endometrioid CA	Mucinous CA (GYN Origin)
Cytokeratin 7	−/+	+++	++	+++
Cytokeratin 20	+/−	−	−/+	+
EMA	−/+	+++	+++	++
PAX-8	+/−	+++	+++	−/+
Estrogen receptor	−	−	+++	
Napsin	−	+++	−/+	−
mCEA	Unk	+/−	+/−	++
AFP	++	−/+	−	−
Glypican-3	+++	+/−	−/+	−
GATA-3	+++	−	−/+	Unk
Villin	++	−	−/+	+/−
CDX2	++	−	−/+	+

Abbreviations: AFP, α-fetoprotein; CA, carcinoma; EMA, epithelial membrane antigen; GYN, gynecologic; mCEA, monoclonal carcinoembryonic antigen; Unk, unknown.

Fig. 22. Immature teratoma in endometrium; inset, immature neuroepithelium at higher power.

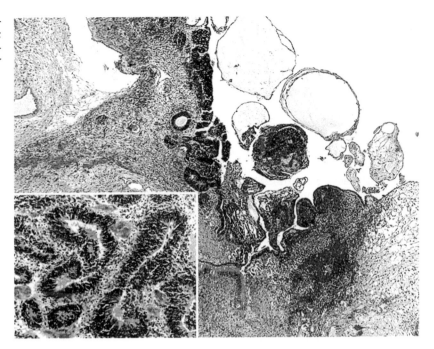

associated with teratoma. Mature teratomas have shown no metastatic potential, although there has been a single report of malignant transformation of glandular and thyroid components.[118] Immature teratomas have been associated with aggressive behavior.[106,116]

REFERENCES

1. Nezhat C, Kotikela S, Mann A, et al. Familial cystic teratomas: four case reports and review of the literature. J Minim Invasive Gynecol 2010;17(6):782–6.

2. Comerci JT Jr, Licciardi F, Bergh PA, et al. Mature cystic teratoma: a clinicopathologic evaluation of 517 cases and review of the literature. Obstet Gynecol 1994;84(1):22–8.

3. Benjapibal M, Boriboonhirunsarn D, Suphanit I, et al. Benign cystic teratoma of the ovary: a review of 608 patients. J Med Assoc Thai 2000;83(9): 1016–20.

4. Dalmau J, Gleichman AJ, Hughes EG, et al. Anti-NMDA-receptor encephalitis: case series and analysis of the effects 'of antibodies. Lancet Neurol 2008;7(12):1091–8.

5. Dulcey I, Cespedes MU, Ballesteros JL, et al. Necrotic mature ovarian teratoma associated with anti-N-methyl-D-aspartate receptor encephalitis. Pathol Res Pract 2012;208(8):497–500.

6. Ibarra M, Chou P, Pachman LM. Ovarian teratoma mimicking features of juvenile dermatomyositis in a child. Pediatrics 2011;128(5):e1293–6.

7. Fadare O, Hart HJ. Anti-Ri antibodies associated with short-term memory deficits and a mature cystic teratoma of the ovary. Int Semin Surg Oncol 2004;1(1):11.

8. Thurlbeck WM, Scully RE. Solid teratoma of the ovary. A clinicopathological analysis of 9 cases. Cancer. 1960;13:804-11.8 patients. J Med Assoc Thai 2000;83(9):1016–20.

9. Goldberg HR, Allen L, Kives S. Fetiform teratoma in the ovary of a 7-year-old girl: a case report. J Pediatr Adolesc Gynecol 2017;30(2):256–8.

10. Roth LM, Talerman A. The enigma of struma ovarii. Pathology 2007;39(1):139–46.

11. Ross DS, CD, Mulder JE. Struma ovarii. UpToDate; 2017.

12. Prat J, Carinelli SG, et al. In: Kurman RJ, Herrington CS, et al, editors. WHO monodermal teratomas and somatic-type tumours arising from a dermoid cyst. 4th edition. France: International Agency for Research on Cancer (IARC); 2014.

13. Wei S, Baloch ZW, LiVolsi VA. Pathology of struma ovarii: a report of 96 cases. Endocr Pathol 2015; 26(4):342–8.

14. Robboy SJ, Shaco-Levy R, Peng RY, et al. Malignant struma ovarii: an analysis of 88 cases, including 27 with extraovarian spread. Int J Gynecol Pathol 2009;28(5):405–22.

15. Shaco-Levy R, Peng RY, Snyder MJ, et al. Malignant struma ovarii: a blinded study of 86 cases assessing which histologic features correlate with aggressive clinical behavior. Arch Pathol Lab Med 2012;136(2):172–8.

16. Shaco-Levy R, Bean SM, Bentley RC, et al. Natural history of biologically malignant struma ovarii:

analysis of 27 cases with extraovarian spread. Int J Gynecol Pathol 2010;29(3):212–27.

17. Garg K, Soslow RA, Rivera M, et al. Histologically bland "extremely well differentiated" thyroid carcinomas arising in struma ovarii can recur and metastasize. Int J Gynecol Pathol 2009;28(3):222–30.

18. Roth LM, Karseladze AI. Highly differentiated follicular carcinoma arising from struma ovarii: a report of 3 cases, a review of the literature, and a reassessment of so-called peritoneal strumosis. Int J Gynecol Pathol 2008;27(2):213–22.

19. Kubba LA, McCluggage WG, Liu J, et al. Thyroid transcription factor-1 expression in ovarian epithelial neoplasms. Mod Pathol 2008;21:485–90.

20. Reed NS, Gomez-Garcia E, Gallardo-Rincon D, et al. Gynecologic Cancer InterGroup (GCIG) consensus review for carcinoid tumors of the ovary. Int J Gynecol Cancer 2014;24(9 Suppl 3):S35–41.

21. Soga J, Osaka M, Yakuwa Y. Carcinoids of the ovary: an analysis of 329 reported cases. J Exp Clin Cancer Res 2000;19(3):271–80.

22. Baker PM, Oliva E, Young RH, et al. Ovarian mucinous carcinoids including some with a carcinomatous component: a report of 17 cases. Am J Surg Pathol 2001;25(5):557–68.

23. Robboy SJ, Norris HJ, Scully RE. Insular carcinoid primary in the ovary. A clinicopathologic analysis of 48 cases. Cancer 1975;36(2):404–18.

24. Rabban JT, Zaloudek CJ. A practical approach to immunohistochemical diagnosis of ovarian germ cell tumours and sex cord-stromal tumours. Histopathology 2013;62(1):71–88.

25. Rathore R, Sharma S, Arora D. Clinicopathological evaluation of 223 cases of mature cystic teratoma, ovary: 25-year experience in a single tertiary care centre in India. J Clin Diagn Res 2017;11(4):EC11–4.

26. Rubio A, Schuldt M, Chamorro C, et al. Ovarian small cell carcinoma of pulmonary type arising in mature cystic teratomas with metastases to the contralateral ovary. Int J Surg Pathol 2015;23(5):388–92.

27. Wheeler L, Westhoff GL, O'Keefe MC, et al. Adenocarcinoma with breast/adnexal and upper gastrointestinal differentiation arising in an ovarian mature cystic teratoma: a case report and review of the literature. Int J Gynecol Pathol 2016;35(1):72–7.

28. Vang R, Gown AM, Zhao C, et al. Ovarian mucinous tumors associated with mature cystic teratomas: morphologic and immunohistochemical analysis identifies a subset of potential teratomatous origin that shares features of lower gastrointestinal tract mucinous tumors more commonly encountered as secondary tumors in the ovary. Am J Surg Pathol 2007;31(6):854–69.

29. McKenney JK, Soslow RA, Longacre TA. Ovarian mature teratomas with mucinous epithelial neoplasms: morphologic heterogeneity and association with pseudomyxoma peritonei. Am J Surg Pathol 2008;32(5):645–55.

30. Perez Montiel D, Arispe Angulo K, Cantu-de Leon D, et al. The value of SATB2 in the differential diagnosis of intestinal-type mucinous tumors of the ovary: primary vs metastatic. Ann Diagn Pathol 2015;19(4):249–52.

31. Kuroda N, Hirano K, Inui Y, et al. Compound melanocytic nevus arising in a mature cystic teratoma of the ovary. Pathol Int 2001;51(11):902–4.

32. Ueng SH, Pinto MM, Alvarado-Cabrero I, et al. Ovarian malignant melanoma: a clinicopathologic study of 5 cases. Int J Surg Pathol 2010;18(3):184–92.

33. Moulla AA, Magdy N, Francis N, et al. Rare skin adnexal and melanocytic tumors arising in ovarian mature cystic teratomas: a report of 3 cases and review of the literature. Int J Gynecol Pathol 2016;35(5):448–55.

34. Shintaku M, Nakagawa E, Tsubura A. Extramammary Paget's disease arising in a mature cystic teratoma of the ovary: immunohistochemical expression of androgen receptor. Pathol Int 2011;61(8):498–500.

35. Kleinman GM, Young RH, Scully RE. Primary neuroectodermal tumors of the ovary. A report of 25 cases. Am J Surg Pathol 1993;17(8):764–78.

36. den Boon J, van Dijk CM, Helfferich M, et al. Glioblastoma multiforme in a dermoid cyst of the ovary. A case report. Eur J Gynaecol Oncol 1999;20(3):187–8.

37. Skopelitou A, Mitselou A, Michail M, et al. Pilocytic astrocytoma arising in a dermoid cyst of the ovary: a case presentation. Virchows Arch 2002;440(1):105–6.

38. Ud Din N, Memon A, Aftab K, et al. Oligodendroglioma arising in the glial component of ovarian teratomas: a series of six cases and review of literature. J Clin Pathol 2012;65(7):631–4.

39. Liang L, Olar A, Niu N, et al. Primary glial and neuronal tumors of the ovary or peritoneum: a clinicopathologic study of 11 cases. Am J Surg Pathol 2016;40(6):847–56.

40. Hirschowitz L, Ansari A, Cahill DJ, et al. Central neurocytoma arising within a mature cystic teratoma of the ovary. Int J Gynecol Pathol 1997;16(2):176–9.

41. Kihara A, Iihara K, Murata K, et al. Choroid plexus papilloma arising in a mature cystic teratoma of the ovary: a short case report and literature review. Pathol Int 2015;65(10):563–5.

42. Quadri AM, Ganesan R, Hock YL, et al. Malignant transformation in mature cystic teratoma of the ovary: three cases mimicking primary ovarian

epithelial tumors. Int J Surg Pathol 2011;19(6): 718–23.

43. Reid HA, van der Walt JD, Fox H. Neuroblastoma arising in a mature cystic teratoma of the ovary. J Clin Pathol 1983;36(1):68–73.

44. Wey SL, Chen CK, Chen TC, et al. Desmoplastic medulloblastoma arising from an ovarian teratoma: a case report and review of the literature. Int J Surg Pathol 2013;21(4):427–31.

45. Liang JJ, Malpica A, Broaddus RR. Florid cystic endosalpingiosis presenting as an obstructive colon mass mimicking malignancy: case report and literature review. J Gastrointest Cancer 2007;38(2–4): 83–6.

46. Morovic A, Damjanov I. Neuroectodermal ovarian tumors: a brief overview. Histol Histopathol 2008; 23(6):765–71.

47. Kawauchi S, Fukuda T, Miyamoto S, et al. Peripheral primitive neuroectodermal tumor of the ovary confirmed by CD99 immunostaining, karyotypic analysis, and RT-PCR for EWS/FLI-1 chimeric mRNA. Am J Surg Pathol 1998;22(11): 1417–22.

48. O'Connor DM, Norris HJ. The influence of grade on the outcome of stage I ovarian immature (malignant) teratomas and the reproducibility of grading. Int J Gynecol Pathol 1994;13(4):283–9.

49. Norris HJ, Zirkin HJ, Benson WL. Immature (malignant) teratoma of the ovary: a clinical and pathologic study of 58 cases. Cancer 1976;37(5): 2359–72.

50. Gershenson DM, Frazier AL. Conundrums in the management of malignant ovarian germ cell tumors: toward lessening acute morbidity and late effects of treatment. Gynecol Oncol 2016;143(2): 428–32.

51. Merard R, Ganesan R, Hirschowitz L. Growing teratoma syndrome: a report of 2 cases and review of the literature. Int J Gynecol Pathol 2015;34(5): 465–72.

52. RH CPaY. In: CPaY RH, editor. Germ cell tumors of the ovary. Philadelphia: Saunders Elsevier; 2008. p. 118, [Chapter 15].

53. Lim CS, Thompson JF, McKenzie PR, et al. Peritoneal melanosis associated with metastatic melanoma involving the omentum. Pathology 2012; 44(3):255–7.

54. Nogales FF, Preda O, Dulcey I. Gliomatosis peritonei as a natural experiment in tissue differentiation. Int J Dev Biol 2012;56(10–12):969–74.

55. Kim NR, Lim S, Jeong J, et al. Peritoneal and nodal gliomatosis with endometriosis, accompanied with ovarian immature teratoma: a case study and literature review. Korean J Pathol 2013;47(6):587–91.

56. Nogales FF, Dulcey I, Preda O. Germ cell tumors of the ovary. An update. Arch Pathol Lab Med 2014; 138:351–62.

57. Liang L, Zhang Y, Malpica A, et al. Gliomatosis peritonei: a clinicopathologic and immunohistochemical study of 21 cases. Mod Pathol 2015; 28(12):1613–20.

58. Kato N, Uchigasaki S, Fukase M. How does secondary neoplasm arise from mature teratomas in growing teratoma syndrome of the ovary? A report of two cases. Pathol Int 2013;63(12):607–10.

59. Djordjevic B, Euscher ED, Malpica A. Growing teratoma syndrome of the ovary: review of literature and first report of a carcinoid tumor arising in a growing teratoma of the ovary. Am J Surg Pathol 2007;31(12):1913–8.

60. Bjorkholm E, Lundell M, Gyftodimos A, et al. Dysgerminoma. The Radiumhemmet series 1927-1984. Cancer 1990;65(1):38–44.

61. Ulbright TM. Germ cell tumors of the gonads: a selective review emphasizing problems in differential diagnosis, newly appreciated, and controversial issues. Mod Pathol 2005;18(Suppl 2):S61–79.

62. Gordon A, Lipton D, Woodruff JD. Dysgerminoma: a review of 158 cases from the Emil Novak Ovarian Tumor Registry. Obstet Gynecol 1981;58(4): 497–504.

63. Schwartz IS, Cohen CJ, Deligdisch L. Dysgerminoma of the ovary associated with true hermaphroditism. Obstet Gynecol 1980;56(1):102–6.

64. Kemp B, Hauptmann S, Schroder W, et al. Dysgerminoma of the ovary in a patient with triple-X syndrome. Int J Gynaecol Obstet 1995;50(1):51–3.

65. Kapp DS, Kohorn EI, Merino MJ, et al. Pure dysgerminoma of the ovary with elevated serum human chorionic gonadotropin: diagnostic and therapeutic considerations. Gynecol Oncol 1985;20(2): 234–44.

66. Brettell JR, Miles PA, Herrera G, et al. Dysgerminoma with syncytiotrophoblastic giant cells presenting as a hydatidiform mole. Gynecol Oncol 1984;18(3):393–401.

67. Cormio G, Seckl MJ, Loizzi V, et al. Increased human chorionic gonadotropin levels five years before diagnosis of an ovarian dysgerminoma. Eur J Obstet Gynecol Reprod Biol 2018;220:138–9.

68. Sekiya S, Inaba N, Takamizawa H, et al. Human chorionic gonadotropin and alpha-fetoprotein in sera and tumor cells of a patient with pure dysgerminoma of the ovary. A case report with radioimmunoassay and immunoperoxidase. Acta Obstet Gynecol Scand 1987;66(1):75–8.

69. Kurman RJ, Norris HJ. Malignant germ cell tumors of the ovary. Hum Pathol 1977;8(5):551–64.

70. Zaloudek CJ, Tavassoli FA, Norris HJ. Dysgerminoma with syncytiotrophoblastic giant cells. A histologically and clinically distinctive subtype of dysgerminoma. Am J Surg Pathol 1981;5(4):361–7.

71. Nogales FF, Quinonez E, Lopez-Marin L, et al. A diagnostic immunohistochemical panel for yolk

sac (primitive endodermal) tumours based on an immunohistochemical comparison with the human yolk sac. Histopathology 2014;65(1):51–9.

72. Hoei-Hansen CE, Kraggerud SM, Abeler VM, et al. Ovarian dysgerminomas are characterised by frequent KIT mutations and abundant expression of pluripotency markers. Mol Cancer 2007;6:12.

73. Cheng L, Roth LM, Zhang S, et al. KIT gene mutation and amplification in dysgerminoma of the ovary. Cancer 2011;117(10):2096–103.

74. Hersmus R, Stoop H, van de Geijn GJ, et al. Prevalence of c-KIT mutations in gonadoblastoma and dysgerminomas of patients with disorders of sex development (DSD) and ovarian dysgerminomas. PLoS One 2012;7(8):e43952.

75. Iacobelli JF, Charles AK, Crook M, et al. NUT protein immunoreactivity in ovarian germ cell tumours. Pathology 2015;47(2):118–22.

76. Kato H, Hatano Y, Makino H, et al. Clear cell carcinoma of the ovary: comparison of MR findings of histological subtypes. Abdom Radiol (NY) 2016; 41(12):2476–83.

77. Shintaku M, Dohi M, Yamamoto Y, et al. Ovarian clear cell carcinoma with plasma cell-rich inflammatory stroma: cytological findings of a case. Diagn Cytopathol 2017;45(2):128–32.

78. Vicus D, Beiner ME, Klachook S, et al. Pure dysgerminoma of the ovary 35 years on: a single institutional experience. Gynecol Oncol 2010;117(1): 23–6.

79. Lange S, Livasy C, Tait DL. Endodermal sinus tumor of the ovary in an 86 year old woman. Gynecol Oncol Case Rep 2012;2(2):65–6.

80. Kurman RJ, Norris HJ. Endodermal sinus tumor of the ovary: a clinical and pathologic analysis of 71 cases. Cancer 1976;38(6):2404–19.

81. Rittiluechai K, Wilcox R, Lisle J, et al. Prognosis of hepatoid yolk sac tumor in women: what's up, Doc? Eur J Obstet Gynecol Reprod Biol 2014; 175:25–9.

82. Young RH. The yolk sac tumor: reflections on a remarkable neoplasm and two of the many intrigued by it-Gunnar Teilum and Aleksander Talerman-and the bond it formed between them. Int J Surg Pathol 2014;22(8):677–87.

83. Young RH, Ulbright TM, Policarpio-Nicolas ML. Yolk sac tumor with a prominent polyvesicular vitelline pattern: a report of three cases. Am J Surg Pathol 2013;37(3):393–8.

84. Kurman RJ, Norris HJ. Embryonal carcinoma of the ovary: a clinicopathologic entity distinct from endodermal sinus tumor resembling embryonal carcinoma of the adult testis. Cancer 1976;38(6): 2420–33.

85. Nogales FF, Prat J, Schuldt M, et al. Germ cell tumour growth patterns originating from clear cell carcinomas of the ovary and endometrium: a comparative immunohistochemical study favouring their origin from somatic stem cells. Histopathology 2018;72:534–47.

86. Xiao GQ, Li F, Unger PD, et al. ZBTB16: a novel sensitive and specific biomarker for yolk sac tumor. Mod Pathol 2016;29(6):591–8.

87. Nogales FF, Preda O, Nicolae A. Yolk sac tumours revisited. A review of their many faces and names. Histopathology 2012;60(7):1023–33.

88. Nogales FF, Bergeron C, Carvia RE, et al. Ovarian endometrioid tumors with yolk sac tumor component, an unusual form of ovarian neoplasm. Analysis of six cases. Am J Surg Pathol 1996;20(9): 1056–66.

89. Schuldt M, Rubio A, Preda O, et al. GATA binding protein 3 expression is present in primitive patterns of yolk sac tumours but is not expressed by differentiated variants. Histopathology 2016;68(4): 613–5.

90. Varia M, McCluggage WG, Oommen R. High grade serous carcinoma of the ovary with a yolk sac tumour component in a postmenopausal woman: report of an extremely rare phenomenon. J Clin Pathol 2012;65(9):853–4.

91. Ravishankar S, Malpia A, Ramalingam P, et al. Yolk sac tumor in extragonadal pelvic sites: still a diagnostic challenge. Am J Surg Pathol 2017; 41:1–11.

92. Kabukcuoglu S, Arik D. Ovarian endometrioid adenocarcinoma with a yolk sac tumor component in a postmenopausal woman. Eur J Gynaecol Oncol 2016;37(6):867–9.

93. Lopez JM, Malpica A, Deavers MT, et al. Ovarian yolk sac tumor associated with endometrioid carcinoma and mucinous cystadenoma of the ovary. Ann Diagn Pathol 2003;7(5):300–5.

94. McBee WC Jr, Brainard J, Sawady J, et al. Yolk sac tumor of the ovary associated with endometrioid carcinoma with metastasis to the vagina: a case report. Gynecol Oncol 2007;105(1): 244–7.

95. Abe A, Furumoto H, Yoshida K, et al. A case of ovarian endometrioid adenocarcinoma with a yolk sac tumor component. Int J Gynecol Cancer 2008;18(1):168–72.

96. McNamee T, Damato S, McCluggage WG. Yolk sac tumours of the female genital tract in older adults derive commonly from somatic epithelial neoplasms: somatically derived yolk sac tumours. Histopathology 2016;69(5):739–51.

97. Garcia-Galvis OF, Cabrera-Ozoria C, Fernandez JA, et al. Malignant Mullerian mixed tumor of the ovary associated with yolk sac tumor, neuroepithelial and trophoblastic differentiation (teratoid carcinosarcoma). Int J Gynecol Pathol 2008;27(4):515–20.

98. Nakakuma K, Tashiro S, Uemura K, et al. Alpha-fetoprotein and human chorionic gonadotropin in

embryonal carcinoma of the ovary. An 8-year survival case. Cancer 1983;52(8):1470–2.

99. NCCN. Ovarian cancer including fallopian tube cancer and primary peritoneal cancer. NCCN National Comprehensive Cancer Network; 2017.

100. Heo EJ, Choi CH, Park JM, et al. Primary ovarian choriocarcinoma mimicking ectopic pregnancy. Obstet Gynecol Sci 2014;57(4):330–3.

101. Goswami D, Sharma K, Zutshi V, et al. Nongestational pure ovarian choriocarcinoma with contralateral teratoma. Gynecol Oncol 2001;80(2):262–6.

102. Park SH, Park A, Kim JY, et al. A case of nongestational choriocarcinoma arising in the ovary of a postmenopausal woman. J Gynecol Oncol 2009;20(3):192–4.

103. Hafezi-Bakhtiari S, Morava-Protzner I, Burnell MJ, et al. Choriocarcinoma arising in a serous carcinoma of ovary: an example of histopathology driving treatment. J Obstet Gynaecol Can 2010;32(7):698–702.

104. Savage J, Adams E, Veras E, et al. Choriocarcinoma in women: analysis of a case series with genotyping. Am J Surg Pathol 2017;41(12):1593–606.

105. Choi YJ, Chun KY, Kim YW, et al. Pure nongestational choriocarcinoma of the ovary: a case report. World J Surg Oncol 2013;11:7.

106. Saffar H, Nili F, Malek M, et al. Primary immature teratoma of the uterus with peritoneal and lymph node involvement, case report. J Obstet Gynaecol 2017;37:1096–8.

107. Euscher ED. Unusual presentations of gynecologic tumors. Arch Pathol Lab Med 2017;141:293–7.

108. Mamoon N, Mushtaq S, Akhter N, et al. Immature teratoma of the vulva with an inguinal lymph node metastasis: report of a case and review of literature. Int J Gynecol Pathol 2010;29(2):197–200.

109. Abudaia J, Habib Z, Ahmed S. Dermoid cyst: a rare cause of clitorimegaly. Pediatr Surg Int 1999; 15(7):521–2.

110. Bhatt M, Braga LH, Stein N, et al. Vaginal yolk sac tumor in an infant; a case report and literature review of the last 30 years. J Pediatr Hematol Oncol 2015;37:e336–40.

111. Gibson AA. Embryonal carcinoma of vagina in infancy. Arch Dis Child 1973;48:163.

112. Fernandez-Pineda I, Spunt SL, Parida L, et al. Vaginal tumors in childhood: the experience of St. Jude Children's Research Hospital. J Pediatr Surg 2011;46:2071–5.

113. Vural F, Vural B, Paksoy N. Vaginal teratoma: a case report and review of the literature. J Obstet Gynaecol 2015;35:757–78.

114. Wong T, Fung E, Yung AWT. Primary gestational choriocarcinoma of the vagina: magnetic resonance findings. Hong Kong Med J 2016;22: 181–3.

115. Berry E, Hagopian GS, Lurain JR. Vaginal metastases in gestational trophoblastic neoplasia. J Reprod Med 2008;53:487–92.

116. El Youbi MBA, Mohtaram A, Kharmoum J, et al. Primary immature teratoma of the uterus relapsing as malignant neuroepithelioma: case report and review of the literature. Case Rep Oncol Med 2013; 2013:971803.

117. Gomez-Lobo V, Burch W, Khanna PC. Nonpuerperal uterine inversion associated with an immature teratoma of the uterus in an adolescent. Obstet Gynecol 2007;110:491–3.

118. Newsom-David T, Poulter D, Gray R, et al. Case report: malignant teratoma of the uterine corpus. BMC Cancer 2009;9:195.

119. Iwanaga S, Shimada A, Hasuo Y, et al. Immature teratoma of the uterine fundus. Kurume Med J 1993;40:153–8.

120. Ansah-Boateng Y, Wells M, Poole DR. Coexistent immature teratoma of the uterus and endometrial adenocarcinoma complicated by gliomatosis peritonei. Gynecol Oncol 1985;21:106–10.

121. Kamgobe E, Massinde A, Matovelo D, et al. Uterine myometrial mature teratoma presenting as a uterine mass: a review of the literature. BMC Clin Pathol 2016;16:5–8.

122. Cappello F, Barabato F, Tomasino RM. Mature teratoma of the uterine corpus with thyroid differentiation. Pathol Int 2000;50:546–8.

123. Spatz A, Bouron D, Pautier P, et al. Primary yolk sac tumor of the endometrium: a case report and review of the literature. Gynecol Oncol 1998;70: 285–8.

Moving?

Make sure your subscription moves with you!

To notify us of your new address, find your **Clinics Account Number** (located on your mailing label above your name), and contact customer service at:

Email: journalscustomerservice-usa@elsevier.com

800-654-2452 (subscribers in the U.S. & Canada)
314-447-8871 (subscribers outside of the U.S. & Canada)

Fax number: 314-447-8029

Elsevier Health Sciences Division
Subscription Customer Service
3251 Riverport Lane
Maryland Heights, MO 63043

*To ensure uninterrupted delivery of your subscription, please notify us at least 4 weeks in advance of move.

Printed and bound by CPI Group (UK) Ltd, Croydon, CR0 4YY

03/10/2024

01040306-0006